Classic Cases
in Medical Ethics

*Accounts of Cases that Have Shaped Medical Ethics,
with Philosophical, Legal, and Historical Backgrounds*

Classic Cases in Medical Ethics

Accounts of Cases that Have Shaped Medical Ethics, with Philosophical, Legal, and Historical Backgrounds

FOURTH EDITION

Gregory E. Pence
Professor of Philosophy
School of Medicine
University of Alabama at Birmingham

Boston Burr Ridge, IL Dubuque, IA Madison, WI New York
San Francisco St. Louis Bangkok Bogotá Caracas Kuala Lumpur
Lisbon London Madrid Mexico City Milan Montreal New Delhi
Santiago Seoul Singapore Sydney Taipei Toronto

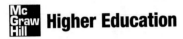

Higher Education

CLASSIC CASES IN MEDICAL ETHICS: ACCOUNTS OF CASES THAT HAVE SHAPED MEDICAL
ETHICS, WITH PHILOSOPHICAL, LEGAL, AND HISTORICAL BACKGROUNDS

This book is printed on acid-free paper.

2 3 4 5 6 7 8 9 0 FGR / FGR 0 9 8 7 6 5 4 3

ISBN 0-07-282935-4

Publisher: *Christopher Freitag*
Sponsoring editor: *Jon-David Hague*
Marketing manager: *Lisa Berry*
Project manager: *Jill Moline*
Production supervisor: *Janean Utley*
Designer: *Sharon C. Spurlock*
Supplement associate: *Kate Boylan*
Photo research coordinator: *Alexandra Ambrose*
Cover design: *Linda Robertson*
Interior design: *Linda Robertson*
Typeface: *10/12 Palatino*
Compositor: *G&S Typesetters*
Printer: *Quebecor World Fairfield Inc.*

Library of Congress Cataloging-in-Publication Data

Pence, Gregory E.
    Classic cases in medical ethics : Accounts of cases that have shaped medical ethics, with
philosophical, legal, and historical backgrounds/Gregory E. Pence.
        p. cm.
    Includes index.
    ISBN 0-07-282935-4 (softcover : alk. paper)
    1. Medical ethics—Case studies.   I. Title
R724.P36 2004
174' 2—dc21   2003044513

http://www.mhhe.com

About the Author

GREGORY E. PENCE is a Professor of Philosophy in the School of Medicine and Department of Philosophy at the University of Alabama at Birmingham, where he has taught since 1976. He has written *Who's Afraid of Human Cloning?* (1998), *Designer Food: Mutant Harvest or Breadbasket of the World?* (2002), *Re-Creating Medicine: Ethical Issues at the Frontiers of Medicine* (2000), and *Brave New Bioethics* (2003) and edited *Flesh of My Flesh: The Ethics of Cloning Humans—A Reader* (1998) and *The Ethics of Food* (2002) (all published by Rowman & Littlefield). He has cowritten *Seven Dilemmas in World Religions* with G. Lynn Stephens (Paragon, 1995). He has published articles in *Bioethics, American Philosophical Quarterly, Canadian Journal of Philosophy, The New York Times, Wall Street Journal, Newsweek,* and *Journal of the American Medical Association.* He has also edited *Classic Works in Medical Ethics: Core Philosophical Readings,* a companion anthology to this work (McGraw-Hill, 1995). He also directs the BS/MD program at UAB.

Contents

Part Two
CLASSIC CASES ABOUT THE BEGINNING OF LIFE

Part Three
CLASSIC CASES ABOUT RESEARCH AND
EXPERIMENTAL TREATMENTS

Part Four
CLASSIC CASES ABOUT INDIVIDUAL RIGHTS
AND THE PUBLIC GOOD

Preface

This new, fourth edition reflects several big changes. First, and like no other issue in decades, since the birth of the lamb Dolly was announced in early 1997, cloning has dominated bioethics. For that reason, and because this author has some unique national expertise on this topic, the new edition contains two new chapters on the ethics of cloning: the first on cloned embryos and stem cells, the second on reproductive cloning.

So much has happened since the last edition with assisted reproduction (AR) that a new rewrite of this chapter would have been necessary even if Dolly had not been cloned. The new chapter on AR includes material previously in a separate chapter on surrogacy as well as new material about the ethics of paying for sperm, eggs of young women, adopted babies, surrogacy, and other reproductive services.

The old chapter on ethics and AIDS previously focused on mandatory testing and the case of Kimberly Bergalis, but the new chapter concentrates on stopping the spread of this lethal disease across the planet. How to stop this spread is perhaps our paradigmatic case in the ethics of international medicine and world public health. This chapter surveys conflicting theories about how to stop HIV's spread and, more pessimistically, whether it will be possible to do so.

I rearranged the four chapters that focus on the beginning of human life to reflect the order in which these topics burst into American life. So I began with abortion in the early 1970s, moved to assisted reproduction in the 1980s and 1990s, and ended with the two chapters on cloning. The section on surrogate motherhood in previous editions now lies within the chapter on assisted reproduction. Continuing controversies about abortion that originated in the early 1970s explain why embryonic cloning now symbolizes the power of faith-based constituencies to shape national medical policy.

To make room for the additions, and to eliminate redundancy, the two chapters on the first heart transplant and artificial heart have been combined into one—on the ethics of adult heart replacement. The three core chapters on death and dying have had their cases updated and include new sections on palliative care, disability groups, and the problem of depression in physician-assisted dying. These chapters and all others have been edited to improve their flow.

All in all, this edition has four completely new chapters.

As with previous new editions, and so far as possible without violating privacy or the wishes of the people involved, each chapter's central case has been updated. A gratifying trend has been the participation of many key people in these chapters in verifying details and correcting any mistakes. In particular, I have communicated with Dax Cowart, Elizabeth Bouvia (through her lawyer), Jack Kevorkian's lawyers, Kenneth Edelin, and Nancy Wexler. Others have also communicated to me who were indirectly involved in these cases, such as Russ Fine (Larry McAfee), Nancy Cummings (God Committee), and Norman Fost (Johns Hopkins cases). I am grateful for the cooperation of all these people, who continue to make this a much better text than it would have been without them.

An important new section focuses on the Jesse Gelsinger case (in the chapter on ethics and genetics), which could have itself been a whole chapter. My student Satya Shreenivas, now in our medical school, wrote an excellent paper for me on this case in a 2001 seminar (later published in the *Monash Bioethics Review*). Other new sections focus on Edward Taub's breakthrough in constraint-induced therapy for stroke victims, scandals in research ethics (deaths of Ellen Roche and the lead-paint study on black children, both at Johns Hopkins), hand transplants, new Abicor artificial heart recipients, UNOS and the rule of rescue, separating conjoined twins at birth (the case in England), Kendra's law in New York (for violent homeless patients), the Carr case in Georgia (mother kills adult sons with Huntington's disease), and states with successful CHIP programs to get medical coverage to poor kids.

Throughout several editions of this book, several users have provided great feedback, including Lance Stell (Davidson University), Mark Yarborough, (University of Colorado), and Louis Pojman (United States Military Academy). Stuart Rachels (at my sister institution, the University of Alabama-Tuscaloosa) provided superogatory commentary on two thirds of the chapters and especially on the first chapter on ethical theory.

McGraw-Hill picked an extraordinary group of professors to review the last edition, many of whom have been using *Classic Cases* for a decade. In particular, I want to thank and acknowledge Paul T. Durbin at the University of Delaware, Lynn Lindholm at the University of North Dakota, David Karnos at Montana State University-Billings, Daniel Holbrook at Washington State University, Albert Flores at California State University-Fullerton, and Marlene Spencer at Valencia Community College. Disability advocate Karen Sadler has also helped me through the years.

Several gifted students in the BS/MD program at UAB helped me with this new edition. During the summer of 2002, my full-time research assistant for this book, Pooja Agarwal, was a spectacular summer research assistant. For someone just out of high school, her ability to write, research, and edit material was amazing. Jason Lott also contributed to this edition before he went off to Oxford, and to a much greater extent, my later part-time, temporary research assistant, Matt Malone, who contributed heartily, especially on the sections in genetics and finance. I thank all these extraordinary students for helping me in this research-journey.

At McGraw-Hill, I thank Jon-David Hague, Ken King, Allison Rona, and Jill Moline for helping me push out the fourth edition.

As always, I am eager to hear from students and professors using this book, so please email me at the address below with any and all comments.

Gregory E. Pence
pence@uab.edu

CHAPTER 1

Moral Reasoning and Ethical Theories in Medical Ethics

PART ONE: MORAL REASONING

A. Common Mistakes in Moral Reasoning

There are well-known pitfalls into which students often fall in discussing issues in contemporary ethics, and one that is peculiar to medical ethics. In the following brief section, these mistakes are covered.

Begging the Question is to assume to be true what should be proved to be true. It is obviously easier to just assume a contentious point under debate than to do the hard work of proving it. Even if we can't prove a point, we must attempt to give reasons for it. To simply state that our given position is *obvious* is to avoid giving such reasons and not intellectually respectable.

Begging the question occurs frequently in debates about who is and who is not a person in those cases at the margins that involve comatose humans, human embryos and fetuses, and non-human animals. For example, someone may say, in referring to a nine-day-old human embryo, "No mere bit of cells the size of a dot could be a person." This debater has assumed that the size of a being, not its genes, DNA, or potential, determines its personhood, but that assumption needs both to be made explicit and defended. Similarly, someone might assert that "Anyone who calls a Crisis Center and says he is planning to commit suicide should be committed because he is not in control of his mind." This also begs the question because we have assumed that all suicides are irrational without even inquiring about the reasons a caller has for wanting to die (there may be cases of rational suicide, e.g., where a person is in the last stages of cancer and still mentally competent).

In general, question-begging statements are designed to mask the need for reasons or an argument. Unmasking such statements sometimes involves identifying and justifying key premises—both factual and evaluative—in our arguments.

Approaching the Arguments: Premises, Conclusions, and the Fact-Value Gap   In moral reasoning, a conclusion about a moral issue is supposed to follow logically from certain premises. If the premises logically support the conclusion, the argument is said to be *valid*. In practical reasoning, validity should not be confused with truth: *Validity* refers to the form of an argument, whereas *truth* refers to the content of its premises. A *sound* argument is one that has both valid form and true premises.

In any moral argument, the conclusion will of course be evaluative. Such a conclusion can be based entirely on evaluative premises, or it can be based on some combination of evaluative and factual (nonevaluative) premises. But a moral argument can *never* be valid if the evaluative conclusion is derived from solely factual premises. Moral conclusions commonly state that something "ought" or "should" be the case; factual premises, on the other hand, state that something "is" the case. A point made famous by the eighteenth-century philosopher David Hume is that an "ought" conclusion cannot be validly derived from only "is" premises. A valid moral argument, therefore, must have at least one evaluative premise, so that the evaluative element in the conclusion is not pulled out of the air from factual premises but "flows through" the argument from the evaluative premise or premises to the evaluative conclusion.

In addition, if a moral argument includes a factual premise, in order to be valid it must somehow connect the factual and evaluative elements. The connection can take the form of a separate *connecting fact-value premise,* or it can be part of a larger premise.

Drawing an evaluative conclusion from solely factual premises—or omitting the fact-value connection if any premise is factual—is an error, sometimes called the *is-ought problem* or the *naturalistic fallacy;* more simply, it is called *jumping the fact-value gap.*

For example, suppose that someone says, "First, a fetus has a brain wave after 25 weeks of gestation," and "Second, a conscious adult has a brain wave," and then draws the conclusion, "Killing a fetus after 25 weeks gestation is as wrong as killing a conscious adult." The crucial point with regard to ethical reasoning is that, while either the first or the second statement is entirely permissible as a *premise,* the two statements together do not lead to the conclusion: They are both factual, whereas the conclusion is evaluative. In other words, this is not a valid moral *argument,* because it has jumped the fact-value gap; something important is missing.

By contrast, here is a valid argument:

Premise 1 (factual). A human fetus has a brain wave after 25 weeks of gestation.

Premise 2 (connecting fact-value premise). A human with a brain wave is a person.

Premise 3 (evaluative premise). Killing a person is morally wrong.

Conclusion (evaluative). Therefore, killing a fetus with a brain wave is morally wrong.

As noted above, it would be permissible to combine premises 1 and 2 as "A human with a brain wave is a person (connecting fact-value premise)," if the fact about fetal brain waves is understood. The traditional format for such an argument is:

1. A human with a brain wave is a person.
2. Killing a person is morally wrong.
3. Therefore, killing a human with a brain wave is morally wrong.

When a moral argument is valid—that is, when its premises are made explicit and lead properly to the conclusion—we can see it clearly, and we can also see exactly where we agree or disagree with it. In this example, for instance, it becomes clear that either the evaluative premise or the connecting fact-value premise could apply not only to abortion but also to euthanasia; this gives us a perspective from which we may or may not accept these premises.

It is helpful to understand that in a valid argument, each key term must be defined in the same way throughout. To define a key term in more than one way is to commit the fallacy of *ambiguity.* Obviously, then, defining a key term factually in a premise but evaluatively in the conclusion commits two fallacies: ambiguity and jumping the fact-value gap.

Jumping the fact-value gap is in essence a special version of begging the question because the evaluative nature of the conclusion (the question) is "begged" by being assumed in the factual premises. This naturalistic fallacy is sometimes inadvertent, but it often appears when people do not want to make the real premises of their argument explicit. When hidden premises (assumptions) are revealed, these premises must be justified, and that can be a difficult job.

Reductio Ad Absurdum is an argumentative strategy used so often in moral debates that it deserves early notice. Literally meaning *reduce to the absurd,* this strategy takes a premise of an argument and tries to show that it has ridiculous or absurd implications. For example, to the person who believes that nine-day-old embryos are persons, a *reductio* reply might be, "So you would baptize all the embryos that fail to survive to become fetuses? And you think Heaven has millions of embryos?"

If the advocate of the premises accepts that the implication is absurd or ridiculous, then he must either give up the premise that is the basis for the implication (perhaps by changing the premise) or deny that the absurd implication really follows from the premise. In some situations, a proponent may reject the "absurdness" of the implication. For example, in arguing about whether nonhuman animal pain should count in our moral calculus, someone who disagrees might try a reductio by saying, "If you believe that, you can't eat hamburgers and hot dogs!" But the proponent of animal rights might accept this implication and not think it "absurd" at all but merely a consistent implication for living of his general position.

Ad Hominem   When discussion in ethics works best, people give objective reasons for their views. Sometimes people get frustrated with this difficult task and try to short-cut the process by making attacks on another person. Often such attacks impugn the personal behavior of opponents and suggest negative things about them. *Ad hominem* literally means "to the human" and suggests a personal attack on an opponent.

Suppose two people are arguing about a single-payer system of medical finance. The first, a physician, opposes such a system, while the second, a lawyer, favors it. Suppose that after an initial attempt at refuting the physician's reasons, the lawyer says, "You physicians just fear a single-payer system because you're afraid that your high incomes will change under a new system." The lawyer here has made a personal attack on the physician by implying that the physician's reasons against a single-payer system are badly motivated, in this case, by greed. (Of course, if the physician replied, "And you lawyers just want a complicated system so everyone will have to go to court all the time and make you rich," then he or she too would have committed an *ad hominem* fallacy.)

Avoiding the Evaluative Premise   When it comes to discussing moral issues in medicine, one common fallacy among medical students and physicians is to persevere in acquiring and discussing facts while never mentioning the underlying moral premise. Perhaps because such people shy away from open moral disagreement (in order to get along) or because their training has emphasized the acquisition of facts, there is a mistake that often occurs where people argue more and more about the facts surrounding a moral issue and never explicitly discuss the ethics of the moral issue. This is a mistake because, for real discussion and any hope of progress, the real moral issue must be identified and discussed.

For example, and as we shall discuss at the end of Chapter 7 where abortion is discussed, a new movement has started to teach young women that possible pregnancies can be prevented after unprotected sex by immediately using common birth control pills in doubled dosages. This method works by preventing a very early human embryo from implanting on the uterine wall, after conception has occurred and the embryo has traveled down the fallopian tubes.

This method is called *emergency contraception* by its proponents, but conceptionist critics (this is, people who believe moral personhood begins at human conception) argue that this method is an abortion. Medical students and physicians often retort that no abortion occurs because there is no "pregnancy." And why is there no pregnancy? Because many medical dictionaries define pregnancy as starting when the human embryo successfully implants on the uterine wall (mainly because many embryos do not successfully so implant).

But why should we let a dictionary define our moral views? After all, dictionaries were not written to provide moral guidance. The medical dictionary also is defining pregnancy partly in terms of likelihood of successful continuation of embryonic development and not making a statement about the moral status of the being before implantation.

A similar approach is to claim that, just as birth control pills act by preventing pregnancy, so their use after conception is also merely "contraception" because they are similarly (and only) "preventing" pregnancy, not creating abortions. (And so it also follows that physicians prescribing birth control pills for such purposes are not in the business of doing abortions.)

The point is that no recourse to semantics or fact gathering will advance think-ing in this example if the real moral issue (premise) is avoided. In fact, just the opposite occurs because the real moral issue—the possible personhood of a very early embryo—is avoided or begged by semantic obfuscation about contraception. Ultimately, someone has to have the guts or clarity to state, "I don't believe that early human embryos have moral status" or to state the opposite. Only then will we see the evaluative premise at stake and then we can begin to give reasons for or against that premise. But it won't help to endlessly deal just in facts or definitions.

B. Other Aspects of Moral Reasoning

Moral Disagreement   As we shall see in Chapter 2, the Quinlan and Cruzan cases directly involved *moral disagreement:* that is, conflicting standards of morality and conflicting judgments about particular issues. In the case of Karen Quinlan, the nuns who were administrators at the hospital believed that morality is founded on unchanging standards given by God, whereas Karen's parents and their parish priest believed that moral rules must change in order to be compassionate. In the case of Nancy Cruzan, the attorney general of Missouri believed far more than Nancy's parents did that the state should protect vulnerable incompetent patients. Indirectly, these cases also involved general philosophical questions about moral-ity: Where does morality come from? Is there such a thing as moral truth? If dif-ferent standards exist by which to judge an issue, how are we able to live together?

When reasonable people need to discuss moral conflicts and general questions about morality, philosophical reflection can sometimes help. For instance, we can ask (as Socrates asks in the dialogue *Euthyphro*) whether morality depends on a god or gods, or whether it can exist independently. If we believe that morality de-pends on a deity, we must then go on to ask—to specify—how we know that any particular moral rule is that deity's will. If we turn to a source such as the Bible, we need to ask which of various interpretations we will choose, and how we will jus-tify that choice. To engage in such *moral reasoning,* it is useful to consider several concepts.

Moral Pluralism   Almost everyone realizes that people espouse different views about religion, morality, and the good life. This *sociological thesis* that people have different values is not controversial but fact. What is controversial is the thesis of *moral pluralism,* the claim that many nonequivalent values exist that are all correct.

Moral pluralism is seen in the statement, "That may be true for you but it's not for me." Moral pluralism adopts a skeptical stance on the ability of moral discus-sion and education to lead us to the same values.

While sociological pluralism is compatible with the existence of absolute moral values, moral pluralism is not. As for the former, absolute moral values could exist but most people could be ignorant of them. Moral pluralism denies that they even exist.

How moral values might be true or false is a deep and difficult topic in ethical theory. How, even if those values were true, two different individuals might both come to understand them as true is a similar topic (the first topic is metaphysical, the second, epistemological).

Fortunately, to do bioethics we need not decide about the truth or falsity of moral pluralism. From the above discussion, we can draw two conclusions: first, we can acknowledge both sociological pluralism and the difficulty of answering the moral pluralist's claim that there are no universal, absolute values and even if there were, there is no way for most of us to know them and agree about them. Second, this acknowledgment should make us humble about how passionately we champion our own absolute views or how passionately we champion any particular ethical or religious theory. We could, after all, be incorrect.

Moral Truth   Pluralism raises the question whether there is or is not such a thing as truth in ethics. It is worth noting that this question goes back at least as far as the fifth century before the Christian, or Common, era (B.C.E.), when Socrates debated it with the Sophists; and it has also been a primary focus of ethical theory throughout the second half of the twentieth century. In part, this question has to do with the limitations of reasoning in ethics. Although moral truth is a rather difficult concept and is not the subject of this book, saying something about it at this point will be helpful.

Moral philosophers differ greatly about whether there is any truth at all in ethics. *Moral skeptics* believe that no objective ethical truth is possible. Against this is the position that a moral idea or statement can be true; ethical theories which hold that moral statements can be true (or false) in some objective way include *cognitivism, realism,* and *naturalism*. In theories like these, however, moral truth is not necessarily characterized by universal agreement. To put this second position another way, the premise, "If a statement is morally true, everyone will agree about it" does not necessarily hold. (This idea is not really startling: Consider that in science there are also truths which are known only to a small, highly educated elite.) The ancient Greeks, for instance, developed a naturalistic ethical theory called *perfectionism*, which assumed that people will not always agree about moral truths because some people are wiser than others.

Worldviews and Moral Issues   A *worldview* is a comprehensive concept of life: Worldviews include overall philosophies of life such as religions, political theories such as Marxism or feminism, psychological theories such as Freudianism or behaviorism, and specific ethical theories such as utilitarianism. It is sometimes thought that a worldview will provide answers or solutions to all moral issues, but this is not necessarily true.

To begin with, some people believe that no one worldview or ethical theory could be good enough to capture the complicated reality of contemporary moral life. As a practical matter, we may be able to find small bits of truth even without discovering a true worldview or developing a completely satisfactory ethical theory. If we refused to act without the moral certainty of a worldview, we would be paralyzed. In actuality, throughout our lives we do formulate moral judgments as best we can when we make decisions and face crises: when we marry, give birth, raise children, and bury our dead. We may not be certain about what we should do, but most of us get by.

Keep in mind that most of us do not arrive at adulthood with a pure worldview. Most of us have inherited bits and pieces of different worldviews from different cultures, views which may have been reshaped or discarded by larger, pluralistic societies. Though there are some total communities (such as the Amish, Orthodox Jews, Jehovah's Witnesses, conservative Catholics, and the Primitive Baptist Church), even those of us who are raised in them may question our world-views when confronted with very different moral ideas—as we typically are when we enter college.

Nor is it necessarily a bad thing that we don't have one all-encompassing worldview, because most such worldviews are simplistic and rigid. In bioethics, good judgments require knowledge of complex concepts, general facts, and specifics of each case, and the ability and willingness to balance different values. To impose a single, absolute worldview on an issue in bioethics would violate the rights of those involved and would therefore lead to many undesirable outcomes.

Similarly, it is not necessarily a bad thing that we can't figure out one monistic answer to a question such as "What makes an act right?" People and people's lives may be more complex than monistic answers to such questions would allow. Absorbing different aspects of several worldviews gives us more flexibility to adapt to changing situations in the modern world. Accepting parts of many ethical theories gives us different insights into moral issues without binding us to one rigid view.

Intuition and Moral Reflection   Suppose that we think in terms of moral pluralism, understand that moral truth may not presuppose universal agreement, and recognize that for most people a worldview may not solve moral issues. How, then, is reasoning possible in ordinary morality?

The answer, as suggested above, is pragmatic, or practical. Not all of us have to agree on everything in order to agree on one particular thing. We can take specific cases one at a time; within each case, we can take specific arguments one at a time; and within each argument, we can sometimes even take specific premises one at a time.

In ethics, basic core beliefs are called *intuitions*. We all carry intuitions around inside us, and these come from many sources, including our own feelings. Ethical reasoning must always start somewhere, and intuitions are often our basis for accepting or rejecting premises in moral arguments; sometimes our intuitions themselves can serve as premises in such arguments. Some of our intuitions go together—in which case they are said to be *consistent*—but some contradict each other. We always need to see what our intuitions imply, how they may contradict other intuitions, how they compare with known facts, and how they compare with the views of people we respect.

In essence, seeing these aspects of our intuitions is *moral reflection*. Moral reflection is what allows us to accept or reject each premise of an argument; it is what allows us to find a good answer in a specific case. We should not be surprised if the premises we accept or reject, and the decisions we make in specific cases, vary as we gain more knowledge and experience in life; and we should not be surprised if some of our decisions change as a result of the process of moral reflection itself.

Moral reflection is a slow process, and it will not please those zealots who are impatient for moral progress and who want to uplift humanity rapidly by achieving moral consensus. But given the limitations on our powers of reasoning in ethics, we may have no other choice than to adopt this slow process. Even if we accept moral pluralism, even if we cannot discover moral truth, and even if we cannot develop a perfect ethical theory, we still need rules by which to live. We still need to live with people who have different ideas, without thinking of those people as evil or terrible—and without resorting to force to solve our disagreements.

Delimiting Moral Issues

Mill's Principle of Harm　The nineteenth-century political philosopher John Stuart Mill wrote *On Liberty* in 1859. This classic work contains an admirable distinction between private life and public morality—a distinction based on the concept of harm.

Mill believed that a civilized society must promote certain ideas and discourage certain vices. He also believed that a society can do this while granting individuals a sphere of private belief and action immune from interference by government. Mill saw that the power of the nation-state can be dangerous when used against the individual, and he held that governments and their agents—such as the police—should be forbidden to meddle in private life. Equally, he held, the majority should be prevented from becoming tyrannical: It should be forbidden to impose its social or religious beliefs on a dissenting minority.

Where is the line to be drawn between private life and public morality? Mill's rough rule of thumb is called his *harm principle.* According to this principle, private life encompasses those actions of an adult that are purely personal and that do not put other people at risk of harm.

In private life, as defined by this principle of harm, there should be no interference by government—even for a person's own good. For example, consider a certain form of sexual activity between two consenting adults: Even if other people consider this activity immoral, for Mill it will not be a moral question if no one else is affected.

Personal Life, Morality, Public Policy, and Legality　Building on Mill's work, this book will make a distinction among four areas: (1) personal life, (2) morality, (3) public policy, (4) legality.

Issues of *personal life* are purely private and affect no one else.

When someone else is affected, issues move from the personal area to the second area, the realm of *morality.*

When society attempts to promote certain values while at the same time tolerating individuals' personal disagreement with those values, issues move into the third area, *public policy.* Actions in the area of public policy—like those in the area of morality—do affect other people's interests. However, negative actions in this area are not necessarily considered immoral; similarly, if some positive action is encouraged by public policy, omitting to perform that action would not be considered immoral. For example, consider alcohol. Though society tends to discourage drinking (as by taxation) and regulate it (alcohol cannot be sold to minors), people may in general drink without being seen as immoral. For another example, consider adoption. Society would like adults to adopt needy children (and may offer tax incentives to encourage adoption), but no one thinks it immoral for a childless couple not to adopt a baby.

When society decides to promote certain actions and discourage certain other actions without tolerating individual disagreement, issues move into the fourth area, *legality*. In this area, some actions (such as paying taxes) are compulsory and others (theft, murder) are forbidden. Omitting a legally compulsory action or committing a legally forbidden action is punishable by the force of the state. In general, the more harmful an action is considered, the more likely it is to fall into the area of legality.

The effect of these distinctions is to limit the range of morality from two ends: first, by carving out a zone of private, personal life; and second, by allowing society to encourage and discourage behaviors without explicit moral judgment. In summary, then:

- *Personal Life:* Concerns actions that are purely private and affect no other person (or persons).
- *Morality:* Concerns interpersonal actions—situations where one person's actions affect other people.
- *Public Policy:* On the one hand, concerns actions which affect other people negatively, but which society tolerates, though it attempts to discourage such actions (as by education). On the other hand, concerns actions which affect other people positively and which society attempts to encourage (as through incentives).
- *Legality and Illegality:* Concerns positive actions which are, by law, compulsory; and negative actions which are, by law, forbidden. Penalties (such as fines and incarceration) are imposed for omitting compulsory actions or performing forbidden actions.

Here are some further examples: Smoking is a personal issue; smoking in your child's room is a moral issue; taxing tobacco products heavily is a public policy issue; prohibiting the sale of cigarettes to minors is a legal issue. To repeat: According to these distinctions, *not every issue is moral.* An issue such as masturbation, or littering in one's own car, or individual and family religious beliefs, is not a moral issue at all.

It should be understood that although these distinctions will be used in this text, they would not be recognized—as Mill's more general distinction might not be recognized—in some evaluative frameworks or worldviews. For example, a fanatical teetotaler might see no reason to tolerate drinking by anyone, even in private; and Roman Catholicism forbids the use of contraceptive devices by married couples (a stand reaffirmed by the Pope in 1993). There are various reasons for such disagreement. In some worldviews, everything in life may be seen as a moral issue: That is, the "personal" area is always the "moral" area. Other frameworks may make a distinction between personal and moral issues but may come to different conclusions about what actually falls into each area; for example, such a framework might consider not only harm to others but also self-harm as a matter of morality. Another framework might assume that there is simply no such thing as self-harm distinct from harm to others, that when we harm ourselves we also in some sense harm others.

As we shall see, the Quinlan case may have arisen in part because the hospital and the Catholic hierarchy on the one hand and Karen Quinlan's family on the other did not agree on a distinction between personal and moral issues. It is worth pointing out, in this regard, that other religiously affiliated hospitals may reject distinctions assumed by a patient or a patient's family and mandate their own values within their own walls. Patients and families need to be aware of this, since they may not agree with the policies of a hospital to which they have been referred.

PART TWO: ETHICAL THEORIES AND MEDICAL ETHICS: A HISTORICAL OVERVIEW

The Greeks and the Virtues

The teaching of the major ancient Greek philosophers—Socrates, Plato, and Aristotle—as well as the general culture of fifth-century (B.C.E.) Athens—advocated virtue ethics, the ethical theory that emphasizes acquiring good traits of character. Virtue theory applied to medicine emphasizes creating physicians with such traits.

Our English word *ethics* derives from the Greek *ethos,* meaning "disposition" or "character." *Ethos* was an inseparable part of the Greek phrase *ethike aretai* (literally "skills of character"). The Greek word *arete* means at once "excellence," "good," and "skill." Our modern "ethics" builds on, but differs from, *ethike aretai* because two millennia of later theories of ethics built other meanings onto the original concept.

From at least as early as the time of Homer (sometime from eighth- to sixth-century B.C.E.), presocratic Greek ethics emphasized *ethike arete* in performing a role well. That is to say, the scope of ethical inquiry was limited to the roles one fulfilled. If one wanted to know about ethics, one asked about the traits of a good soldier, physician, mother, or ruler. For example, one would ask, "What is the goal of being a soldier?" Answer: "To defend one's country." Then one asks, "What excellences are needed to defend one's country?" Answer: "Physical strength, courage, skill in using weapons, organization in fighting in groups, temperance, and cunning."

Such ethics were teleological. In other words, they assumed that things developed towards a natural goal. In Greek medicine, if we want to know what makes a good physician, we need to know the purpose of medicine. That purpose is to heal the sick. What virtues are needed to do so? Answer: compassion, knowledge of healing, and skill in human relations.

Role-defined ethics remain powerful today and are the basis on which more universal principles build. For example, medical students first try to live by virtues of that role.

Socrates, Plato, and Aristotle, in a combined move of ethical genius, attempted to transcend role-defined ethics and to argue that there were distinctive *ethika aretai* of a good person. What are they? In their view, they were the cardinal (primary) virtues of courage, temperance, wisdom, and justice (in dealing with people). These are the distinctive excellences necessary to function best in human society.

The implication of this view for medical ethics is that moral inquiry must not only ask, "What virtues should a good physician possess?" but also, "What virtues should a good person possess who happens to be a physician?" The narrow questions is, "What should a good physician do?" The broader question is, "What should a *good person* do?"

Not all physicians in ancient times agreed about the role of a good physician, and here looms one of the great divides in medical ethics. Hippocrates and his brethren adopted not only a patient-centered ethics but also a sanctity-of-all-life worldview, holding that physicians should neither perform abortions nor assist in euthanasia of any kind. But most ancient Greek physicians took a *naturalistic* approach that was a precursor to the scientific worldview. In other words, they advocated forming conclusions based on what one could see and feel. These physicians did not practice medicine based on assumptions about gods and goddesses or about an afterlife, so they were more oriented to helping patients in the here-and-now. Accordingly, they often helped terminally ill patients to die. Most such Greek physicians adopted a quality-of-life view, believing that it was futile to maintain a life of pain and suffering that had little chance of amelioration. It is unclear whether their aid was role-defined, or whether it stemmed from compassion. In either case, the majority of naturalistic physicians used their factual knowledge and technical skills for very different evaluative ends than their Hippocratic counterparts.

Christian Ethics, Christian Virtues

By the fourth century C.E., Christianity had added its theological virtues of faith, hope, and charity to the list of human virtues. The paradigmatic virtue of compassion (charity) that many today associate with a good physician comes in part from Christianity's emphasis on helping others. The etymological root of "compassion" means to "to suffer with," as Jesus of Nazareth is held by Christians to have suffered with, and for, humans on the cross.

Here we have two differences of emphasis that later came to be fused. Where naturalistic physicians emphasized technical competence in curing disease, religious physicians emphasized compassion in *being with* patients. When the limits of technical competence had been reached—as they were often reached very soon during these centuries—compassion became the supreme virtue. Both traditions contributed to today's definition of good physicians: Every patient wants a physician who is both knowledgeable and merciful.

Virtue ethics in medicine also underlies the apprentice system of medical education, in which young medical students gradually assume more responsibility by assisting older physicians in treating patients. The attending physician teaches the resident, who teaches the intern, who teaches the third-year student. What is taught, theoretically, is not only how to perform a procedure but also how to be compassionate, wise, courageous, and patient-centered.

What would virtue ethics say about a particular issue in medical ethics? The general answer is that with every new case, the physician-in-training should imitate the reasoning and empathy of good physicians. Thus confronted with a 14-year-old patient who refuses to eat after being partially paralyzed after an auto accident, most experienced physicians are likely to say, "Let's work with him until he's of legal age, then he can decide for himself. By that time, he'll probably find a reason to live."

It should be emphasized that Socratic virtues also celebrated an elitist, anti-democratic ethics that scorned the ordinary person and his worth. The Greeks believed themselves superior to all the peoples they had conquered. Aristotle's student, Alexander the Great, attempted to instill Greek values, culture, and language in everyone, and he had no tolerance for the cultures of other, "inferior" peoples. The Greek ethics that Alexander inherited was perfectionistic, aristocratic, and meritocratic. In this sense, the quality-of-life attitude of ancient Greek physicians was elitist and perfectionistic, whereas the sanctity-of-life ethic of Hippocratic physicians was much less so.

In contrast to Greek elitism, the three great religions of the West emphasize duties to the poor and sick: The rabbinic ethics of Bar Hillel stress acts that help one's fellow man; Jesus says that as you treat the poor, so you treat Him; and Mohammed made the *zakat*, the tax on property for the poor, one of the pillars of Islam. So for a Jew, Christian, or Moslem, a good physician is first a Jew, Christian, or Moslem, and second a physician.

As such, a good Christian physician must care for the poor as part of his duties as a physician. To put this point in more religious terms, the physician's license, knowledge, and wisdom is not a proprietary right to make money but an instrument of a higher calling from God. In the movie, *Chariots of Fire*, the Presbyterian Olympic runner says, "I run not for me but to glorify the Lord" and for this reason refuses to compete on the sabbath. Similarly, to use a medical degree only to make money is to abase a degree given in trust for a higher cause.

One area in which the contrast between religious and nonreligious ethics in medicine becomes salient is in thinking about genetics. Greek ethics advocated eugenics ("good birth"). Plato advocated mystery-shrouded mating festivals where those men judged to be "most perfect" would impregnate similar females. For Plato, breeding would be arranged to perfect humanity, not by choice or for love. Just as the Greeks improved the stock of their animals by selective breeding, so Plato wanted to improve humans. Just as the young Greek gentleman should try to perfect his body and life as a work of art, so human society should try to perfect itself by creating better children.

In contrast, the three western religious traditions have preached for centuries that the goal of human life has been either to create a God-based society on earth or to save the most souls for the afterlife. Accordingly, western religions have resisted attempts to tamper with the genes of humans, asserting that humans were created in the image of God and denying that humans should try to perfect themselves through genetics. (In modern times, however, some liberal believers have argued that eliminating genetic disease is not sinful.)

Applying virtue ethics to medical ethics has several limitations. One is that it has little to say about how to make particular, ethical decisions, aside from the injunction to imitate good physicians. Another limitation is that as ethics becomes more role-defined, the less it meets universal standards. Finally, both religious and nonreligious theories of the virtues tend to emphasize the status quo over fundamental, social change. One outcome is that physicians adopting a traditional role tend to be paternalistic, treating patients as children and overruling their decisions.

Natural Law Theory

It has become a truism that when the Romans conquered Greece (in the second century B.C.E.), they themselves were conquered by many aspects of Greek culture. The Stoic philosophers of Roman times elevated one aspect of the Greek world-view to a higher level. Rules for human beings, the Stoics argued, were so embedded in the texture of the world that they were "law" for humans. These came to be known as "natural laws." They were apprehended by unaided reason, in other words, without Scripture or divine revelation.

Behind the notion of a natural law, of course, is that of a hidden law-giver. In the thirteenth century, Thomas Aquinas synthesized many aspects of Aristotelianism with what had become orthodox teachings of the Christian church. Aquinas made explicit the connection between God and the natural laws of the world: A rational god made the world work rationally and gave humans reason to discover his rational, natural laws. Studying ethical theory was a rational process of discovery about the world that revealed rules about how humans should act. Correct *descriptions* of the world would yield correct *prescriptions* about how to act. To act rationally was to act morally, which in turn was to act in accordance with natural law.

One thing that these rules commanded was to go against one's natural feelings. St. Augustine taught in the fourth century C.E. that human nature was contaminated by sin and, as such, human feelings were mired in lust, sloth, avarice, and the other deadly sins. In stunning contrast to modern times, Aquinas held that thinking about ethics was emphatically *not* about examining one's feelings. Instead, it was a matter of following rules laid down by God and his agents, the clergy and theologians of the Church.

An example of natural law theory in medical ethics concerns homosexuality. Aquinas believed that God made two sexes for procreation and that it was natural and rational for a man and woman to mate to have children. On the other hand, for two people of the same gender to have sex (or form a lifelong union) was contrary to natural law, and hence, immoral.

One problem with natural law theory is seen in the above example in that what is considered "against natural law" may vary over the centuries. Many rational people today do not consider homosexuality to be unnatural, especially because it has been practiced since the beginning of human history and because some great cultures, such as the ancient Greeks, celebrated it as ideal.

As another example of problems of natural law theory, consider sex in marriage. Augustine held that the *only* permissible justification for sexual relations between a man and a wife was to produce children. Modern Catholic teaching is very different, and regards loving sexual relations between man and wife as natural and good, even when there is no desire to have children. Indeed, the Catholic Church today holds *in vitro* fertilization to be immoral precisely *because* no act of loving sex is involved between man and woman.

Natural law theory bequeathed to medical ethics the famous *doctrine of double effect*. This doctrine held that if an action had two effects, one good and the other evil, the action was morally permitted: (1) if the action was good in itself or not evil, (2) if the good followed as immediately from the cause as did the evil effect, (3) if only the good effect was intended, and (4) if there was as important a reason for performing the action as for allowing the evil effect. For example, exceptions could be made to the rule banning abortions in cases of an ectopic pregnancy (an embryo growing in a fallopian tube) and a cancerous uterus (where uterus and fetus had to be removed together). In both cases, this doctrine would allow abortions if the direct intention was to save the life of the mother. Similarly, the doctrine of double effect would not allow physicians to assist in executions, since it would not allow a direct intention to assist in the taking of a life, although it might allow a physician to be present to ease the suffering of a prisoner in the event of a botched execution.

Also derived from the natural law tradition is the *principle of totality,* which covers what kinds of changes may be made to the human body: Changes are permitted only to ensure the proper functioning of the total body. The underlying idea is that one's body is not something that one owns, but that one holds in trust for God: "The body is the temple of the Lord." So a gangrenous leg may be amputated or a cancerous breast removed, because the fundamental health of the body is at risk from these threats. According to this principle, we are given our bodies as they are for a reason and we should not change our bodies for frivolous reasons. Thus the principle of totality rules out all forms of sterilization to prevent pregnancy — vasectomy, tubal ligation, and hysterectomy — because producing pregnancy is a natural function of the bodies of men and women. The principle also forbids cosmetic surgery solely to change one's appearance, such as breast reduction, breast augmentation, rhinoplasty, and liposuction.

This principle is more deeply embedded in our thinking than we may at first think. When a news photograph in 1996 showed a mouse whose genetic system had been altered to grow a human ear on its back, many people felt disgust at seeing this mouse-with-human-ear. This disgust arose from a sense that the creation of this being had violated the bodily integrity of both humans and mice.

Social Contract Theories

Social contract theory, or contractarianism, is essentially secular, independent of belief in God. Contractarians assume that people are fundamentally self-interested and that moral rules have evolved for humans to get along with one another. It is rational for humans to agree to such rules because otherwise, everyone will pick up the sword and be worse off.

Social contract theory does not separate ethics from politics. Indeed, hypothetical political bargaining is viewed as the foundation of the kind of behavior that is allowed as ethical. (*Hypothetical* because contractarians do not believe people ever came together to make the basic social contract.) Plato described one early kind of hypothetical social contract in the *The Republic,* but the philosopher who really gave this theory weight was the Englishman, Thomas Hobbes (1588–1679).

Hobbes believed that the most detestable condition for humans was the state of nature, a premoral agglomeration of self-interested individuals for whom life was (he said, famously) "solitary, poor, nasty, brutish, and short." By the use of their reason, people realize that each is better off in a society of moral and legal rules backed by the force of opinion and law. They therefore form a social contract to create "society" to better themselves.

Contractarianism can support both minimal and maximal government. To oversimplify, let us contrast two extreme champions of contractarianism: Libertarians and Rawlsians.

Libertarians favor government for defense and for very limited public works, perhaps not even including national parks or a public interstate road system (we could have private, toll roads). They disfavor government programs such as Medicare, Medicaid, disability insurance, food stamps, and welfare. Libertarians oppose forced taxation by the government, especially when it redistributes property and income from rich to poor. They champion the property rights of the status quo, but tend to be silent about how those enjoying the status quo acquired their property. Libertarian philosophers such as Harvard's Robert Nozick see forced taxation as equivalent to forced labor, that is, to slavery.

Accordingly, Libertarians oppose mandatory F.I.C.A. taxes on all workers' pay for Medicare and for the Hospital Insurance Trust Fund. Even though federal programs such as Medicare have made American physicians rich, libertarian physicians would rather have no government control over their business. Presumably, in a libertarian society, physicians would be reimbursed only in cash.

Critics say that in such a system, fewer hospitals would be built, elderly patients would frequently forgo procedures for lack of money (as never happens under Medicare), and physicians would earn far less money. It is also true that in such a system physicians would be controlled by no federal regulations.

Rawlsians are named for John Rawls, a Harvard colleague of Nozick. Rawls believes that the social contract should have moral restraints imposed on it. The most important restraint is what Rawls called the "veil of ignorance," meaning that in the hypothetical social contract, no one would know his or her age, gender, race, health, number of children, income, wealth, or other arbitrary personal information. Rawls' theory is contractarian in that it assumes that people are self-interested and are forced to form a social contract to choose the basic institutions of their society; on the other hand, it is Kantian (as we shall see in the next section) in that it imposes impartiality on the choosers.

Rawls argues, controversially, that the only rational way to choose under the veil of ignorance is as if one might be the least well-off person in society (because a person doesn't know anything personal under the veil, he doesn't know what place in society he occupies). This justifies the choice of his famous *difference principle:* Choosers should opt for institutions creating equality unless a difference favors the least well-off group. Everyone should be trained in medicine unless training only a few is better for the least well-off. The choice of the difference principle, as the archprinciple of this theory of justice, can be seen as the imposition of the golden rule on the choice of the structure of society.

Rawlsian justice entails that every citizen should have equal access to medical care unless unequal access favored the poor (an unlikely prospect!). Rawlsian justice attempts to reduce the natural inequalities of fate; hence, it is especially important that children and those with genetic disease have good medical care. Let us consider these two classes combined: children with genetic disease. Their care takes up a large share of resources in children's hospitals, and costs for their care may be deliberately excluded in for-profit insurance plans. Nevertheless, for Rawls, such children deserve good medical care as a matter of justice.

Indeed, as genetics reveals new insights every year, we stand now under a real, not hypothetical, genetic veil of ignorance about our future illnesses and those of our children and grandchildren. The coming decade will identify much more precisely who is susceptible to genetic disease and who is not. In the future, it may be much more difficult for those with familial lines of genetic disease to purchase private medical insurance. Some of the people now attacking national medical plans may find themselves at risk.

Libertarians favor private medical insurance plans in which the healthy do not subsidize the unhealthy. Rawlsians see "healthy" and "unhealthy" as arbitrary distinctions, due more to genetics and fate than individual merit. Libertarians would allow for-profit companies to practice experience rating, whereby citizens with preexisting illness may be excluded (and genetic disease is increasingly being defined in this way). Rawlsians favor community rating, whereby risk and premium rates are spread over all members of a large community, such as a state or nation (for example, a federal, single-payer system).

Kantian Ethics

John Rawls is a modern Kantian using a social contract methodology. Immanuel Kant (1724–1804) published during the Enlightenment (that is, about the time of the American Revolution), and believed in the power of humans to use reason to solve their problems.

Kant was raised by conservative Protestant parents and was strongly oriented to conservative religious ethics until he studied science at his university, whereupon he became skeptical of his former beliefs. He continued to believe that many of the basic values and attitudes of Christian ethics were correct, but then he had a problem of how to justify those values. His solution was to base those values on abstract reason rather than on metaphysical beliefs about God or an afterlife.

The distinctive elements of Kantian ethics are these:

a. Ethics Is Not a Matter of Consequences but of Duty.   Why an act is done is more important that its good or bad results. Specifically, an act must be done from the right motive, and the right motive is the desire to do one's moral duty. In its emphasis on motives and not consequences, Kant's ethics are Christian.

Kant's ethics are an ethics of duty (also called *deontological,* from *deontos,* duty) because they emphasize not having the right desires or feelings, but acting correctly according to obligation. Only acts done from duty, and not, say, from compassion, are praiseworthy. For Kant, the correct motive for treating a patient well is not because a physician feels like doing so, but because it is the right thing to do. When we act morally, Kant says, reason tells feelings what to do. Contrary to popular culture, we should not consult our feelings about what to do but reflect upon what is our duty.

Kant says the only thing valuable in the world is a good will, the trait of character indicating a willingness to choose the right act simply because it's right. But how do we know what is right? What is our duty? Kant gives two formulations.

b. A Right Act Has a Maxim that Is Universalizable.   An act is right if one can will its "maxim" or rule to be acted on by all others. "Lie to get out of keeping a promise" cannot be so willed because if everyone acted this way, promise-keeping would mean nothing.

c. A Right Act Always Treats Other Humans as Ends-in-themselves, Never as a Mere Means.   To treat another person as an "end in himself" is to treat him as having absolute, infinite moral worth, not relative worth. His welfare cannot be sacrificed to the good of others or to my own desires. So patients cannot unwittingly be used as guinea pigs in dangerous medical experiments to advance knowledge.

Consider the case of a pulmonary resident who discovers that he missed a small lesion three months previously on the x-ray of a 48-year-old patient. The patient now has level four untreatable cancer. The patient says, "I guess that cancer just grew out of nowhere because it wasn't there three months ago." Should the resident tell the patient the truth? A consequentialist might argue that he should not because it could do no good for the patient.

But for Kant, the answer is clear: The patient must be told the truth. Why? The only universalizable rule is "Always tell patients the truth." Such a rule is the basis of trust and of treating patients as "ends in themselves." If the physician was a patient, he would want to know the truth. The resident may *feel* that he shouldn't reveal the truth but his reason will tell him what his duty is.

d. People Are Only Free When They Act Rationally.   Kant would agree that much of how we act is governed by our emotions and other, nonrational parts of upbringing. But controversially, Kant denies that we are truly acting morally when we do the right thing because we are accustomed to it, because it feels right, or because our society favors the act. The only time a person can act morally is when she exercises her rational, free will to understand why certain rules are right and then chooses to bind her actions to those rules. Kant calls the capacity to act this way, *autonomy.* For him, it gives humans higher worth than animals.

It follows for Kant that very few people act morally. Kant accepts that fact. It was also true that in early Christianity, very few people were thought to be capable of salvation. The purity of Kant's view entails a moral elitism for the few who can successfully follow Kantian ethics.

e. Problems in Kantian Ethics.   Kantian ethics has several problems. First, Kant is regarded as the supreme rationalist in ethics because he claimed that anyone who disagreed with his view was guilty of a logical contradiction. But the utilitarian lifeboat commander, when he will not let everyone board to save those in the boat, does not contradict himself (he can will the maxim, *All those in control of lifeboats should maximize survivors, even if it means denying access to some in the water.*)

Kant is generally regarded as failing in his Enlightenment project. His critic and contemporary, the Scottish skeptic, David Hume, came close to arguing that ethics is really *emotivism*. Charles Darwin and the father of psychiatry, Sigmund Freud, later agreed with Hume that reason is the tip of the moral iceberg because much of ethical life is emotional and not changeable by reason. Emotivism and Kant's rationalism are the two extreme views on the issue of the place of reason in ethics.

Other problems of Kantian ethics remain. For one thing, it fails to tell us how to resolve conflicts between competing, universalizable maxims. Its best answer is to try to universalize whatever ad-hoc solution to the conflict seems appropriate. But then our sense of what is appropriate, not our ability to universalize without contradiction, is the test of an act's morality. For another thing, it seems ridiculous to imply that consequences never count morally. Many critics believe that Kantians indirectly appeal to consequences in thinking about what to universalize. Finally, the ideal of treating each person as if he had infinite value is not always practical: It does not tell us how to deliberate about trade-offs when, by definition, some humans will die in triage situations and cannot be treated as "ends in themselves."

f. Kantians Reply.   Nevertheless, Kant provides useful insights to medical ethics. He would favor using a lottery to distribute a lifesaving but expensive new drug that most patients will be unable to obtain. He would argue that the captain of the lifeboat should draw straws to decide who gets to stay in the boat. His emphasis on people as "ends in themselves" explains the outrage that people have felt when learning of scandals involving medical experimentation, such as research done by Nazi physicians. Finally, perhaps Kant's most important legacy to modern medical ethics is his emphasis on the "autonomous will" of the free, rational individual as the seat of moral value. Autonomy explains why informed consent is necessary to legitimate participation in an experiment. When combined with the emphasis on personal liberty in our democracies, Kant's emphasis on autonomy sets the stage for modern medical ethics.

Utilitarianism

Utilitarianism originated in the late 18th and early 19th century England as a secular replacement for Christian ethics. Jeremy Bentham (1748–1832) and John Stuart Mill (1806–1873) were its two chief theorists. The essential idea of utilitarianism is that right acts should produce the greatest amount of good for the greatest number of people, which is called "utility."

The Puritans in England and America wanted to organize society so that everyone had to obey their rules, but utilitarians saw morality as a human construct that should minimize harms of humans to each other and maximize group welfare. For Christians, Jews, or Muslims, morality is inconceivable without God's existence, but not so for utilitarians.

Likened to the counterculture movement of students in the 1960s and 1970s, utilitarianism was a reform movement intended to humanize outmoded institutions. Developed by social reformers Jeremy Bentham and James Mill (the father of John Stuart Mill), it focused on large, practical changes that could benefit the vast majority of people who were not aristocrats.

Utilitarianism did not urge people to turn the other cheek and hope for justice in another life, nor did it exalt those virtues so cherished by England's aristocracy: stylish dress and manners, personal honor, literacy, scientific and artistic accomplishment, and patriotism. The foundation for reform came in 1832 in eliminating pocket boroughs under the control of one great landlord and in extending the vote to the 20 percent of the adult male population who had some property (property-less males and women still had no vote). Utilitarian reformers also campaigned against slavery in the British empire and the intolerable factory conditions made famous by Charles Dickens in novels such as *Hard Times*. (Their Factory Act forbade employment of children under age nine in cotton mills and declared that 13-year-olds could work no more than 12 hours a day.) Similar bills were passed to make mining and industrial machinery less lethal to workers.

They also attacked the penal system, passed the Corn Laws, ended debtor's prison, opposed capital punishment for petty thefts, and advocated the vote for women. They urged public hospitals for the poor, proper sewage disposal, the penny post so that everyone could send and get mail, and created a central board of health, so that municipalities could create facilities for clean water, waste disposal, and sewers.

Utilitarianism's essence can be summed up in four basic tenets:

1. *Consequentialism:* Consequences count, not motives or intentions.
2. *The maximization principle:* The number of people affected by consequences matters; the more people, the more important the effect.
3. *A theory of value* (or of "good"): Good consequences are defined by pleasure *(hedonic utilitarianism)* or what people prefer *(preference utilitarianism)*.
4. *A scope-of-morality premise:* Each being's happiness is to count as one and no more.

For utilitarians, right acts produce the (2) greatest amount of (3) good (1) consequences for the (2) greatest number of (4) beings.

Each of these tenets can be controversial. Bentham emphasized that the meaning of the fourth tenet was whether a being could suffer, not whether it was human or animal. As such, utilitarianism includes animals in its calculations of the *greatest number.*

To the modern utilitarian Peter Singer (and author of the famous *Animal Liberation*), utilitarianism was in advance of its time in not differentiating between the sufferings of humans and those of animals. Utilitarianism also seems to imply that every being's happiness on the planet matters, not just beings of my society. Singer also says that morality doesn't stop at the borders of his country.

Virtue ethicists and Kantians regard a person's motives as a sign of his character. John Stuart Mill says that the drowning man doesn't care why the lifeguard is swimming out to sea to rescue him, just that the lifeguard is coming. Utilitarians think motives only count insofar as they tend to produce the greatest good.

In medicine, it makes a difference whether a physician listens because she really cares about patients or because she's found that having satisfied patients is an effective way to maximize income. A utilitarian might argue that if the physician's techniques are good enough, whether she really cares about her patients matters very little; in either case, the behavior produces good consequences to real people.

Utilitarianism is also a theory of value (that is, a theory about what is a harmful consequence and about what is a good one). The simplest theory of value is *hedonic utilitarianism,* which equates a good consequence with pleasure, and harm with pain. *Negative utilitarianism* focuses on relieving the greatest misery for the greatest number, as in famine relief. *Positive utilitarianism* focuses on benefiting humanity. Utilitarian theorists debate whether some things are intrinsically valuable, such as pride and honor, or whether they are good only because they create good feelings in people over the longrun. Another view is called *preference utilitarianism,* and its adherents believe that utility is maximized by furthering the actual preferences that people have. Finally, *pluralistic utilitarians* hold that many different things or states are valuable.

The maximization tenet can get utilitarians into trouble. Wouldn't utilitarianism be willing to violate the traditional sanctity-of-life principle to save many people? Here, Utilitarians bite the bullet. They think that the Nazi generals who tried to kill Hitler in 1944 at Wolf's Lair were justified. They think that on the expedition to the South Pole, commander Robert Scott should have allowed his crew member with the gangrenous leg to die, rather than slowing down the whole party by carrying the injured man, which resulted in the death of all. They think that if an FBI sniper saw a terrorist about to detonate a bomb in a skyscraper full of innocent people, the sniper should shoot the terrorist.

These are the easy cases. The hard ones come in population policy. If more happiness is better than less, why shouldn't we create the maximal number of people on the planet? So long as each new life has more happiness than misery, and so long as everyone else's life has at least the same, shouldn't we produce more? This "total view" of utilitarianism is universally seen as what philosopher Derek Parfit calls "The Repugnant Conclusion," because we think the average happiness is more important. But it is difficult to see why utilitarianism entails maximizing average happiness and not the total good, so it may be stuck with this counterintuitive implication.

More specifically to medical ethics, wouldn't utilitarianism permit the sacrifice of an innocent, healthy person to transfer his organs to four patients who needed them to live? Aren't four people alive better than one? If consequences and number of lives define morality, what's morally wrong with doing so? Yet it certainly seems morally wrong to chop up an innocent patient this way.

One traditional reply among utilitarians is to distinguish between *act* and *rule* utilitarianism. Rule utilitarians believe that normal moral rules, such as "First, do no harm" in medicine, maximize utility over the decades. Act utilitarians advocate judging each act's utility. Some act utilitarians think rule utilitarianism has a dilemma: If there are exceptions, then you ultimately have act utilitarianism (since you never know in advance whether a particular situation needs to be judged as an exception); if there are no exceptions, then you are close to a Kantian and only a nominal utilitarian. If "First, do no harm" has no exceptions in medical ethics, it may explain why it is wrong to chop up an innocent person to transplant his organs to four others.

In medicine, the two areas where utilitarianism applies most powerfully are public health and triage situations. It is likely that improvements in public health have helped more people live longer (created more "utility") than all the drugs and surgeries ever invented. The English physician John Snow might have agreed: In 1849 he advocated clean water to prevent cholera epidemics, which were spread by contaminated water. (It took 40 years and many more cholera epidemics for Snow's ideas to prevail.) It doesn't matter why Snow improved the water supply, only that he did and that many millions of people now live decades longer.

Triage involves the apportionment of scarce resources during emergencies when circumstances preordain that not all victims will live. Because consequences count, utilitarianism says a physician should not treat each patient equally, but should focus only on those whom he can actually benefit. Rigorous application of this principle gives utilitarianism its famous hard edge: A physician should abandon those who will *die* even if he helps and, just as ruthlessly, abandon those who will *live* without his help. He should help only those who waver between life and death and for whom he can make the difference. The goal is to save the maximal number of lives.

This point illustrates an ambiguity in sanctity-of-life ethics. Traditionally, sanctity-of-life ethics such as Kant's emphasize the absolute value of each individual, implying that the physician should at least comfort those who are beyond his help. But utilitarian-triage ethics maximizes the value of life in saving the maximal number of people who will eventually live.

Principles and Medical Ethics

One modern method of analysis is to analyze a dilemma or case of medical ethics in terms of four powerful principles. According to advocates of this method, deciding what is the right thing to do in a particular case involves applying and balancing all four principles. These principles are clearly chosen as a distillation of the ethical theories described above.

What do each of the principles mean? *Autonomy* refers to the right to make decisions about one's own life and body without coercion by others. This principle celebrates the value that democracies place on allowing individuals to make their own decisions about whom to marry, whether to have children, how many children to have, what kind of career to pursue, and what kind of life they want to live. Insofar as is possible in a democracy, and to the extent that their decisions do not harm others, individuals should be left alone to make fundamental medical decisions that affect their own bodies and lives.

John Stuart Mill was a political theorist as well as an ethical theorist. In his most famous work of politics, *On Liberty* (1859), he defends "one very simple principle," his so-called *harm principle:* that "the only purpose for which power can rightfully be exercised over any member of civilized community, against his will, is to prevent harm to others. His own good, either physical or moral, is not a sufficient warrant . . . . Over himself, over his own body and mind, the individual is sovereign."

Such political individualism corresponds to personal autonomy in ethics. Since the beginnings of modern medical ethics in the early 1960s, autonomy has meant the patient's right to make her own decisions about her body, including dying and reproduction.

The ethics of autonomy evolved as a rejection of paternalistic ethics. During the patient rights movement in the early 1960s in America, paternalistic physicians were scorned as sexist octogenarians who would impose their rigid traditions on a more enlightened, freethinking, younger generation. Both secular and religious versions of virtue ethics tend to be paternalistic, especially when they emphasize the physician's greater wisdom and when they teach young physicians to follow the lead of older physicians in ignoring wishes of patients. These traditional, somewhat rigid, secular and religious roles of good physicians contrast starkly with the dominant value of more universal, modern theories of ethics, including the principle of individual autonomy.

In the first two decades of bioethics (1962–1982), autonomy was considered by many bioethicists to be the supreme value above all others, grounding the right of competent adults to end their lives when they choose and to decline to participate in dangerous experiments. Since then, bioethicists have realized that other values are also important, which must be weighed with autonomy in dictating answers in particular cases.

Beneficence, "doing good to others," is clearly tied to the Judaeo-Christian-Muslim virtue of compassion and helping others. The application of the principle of beneficence comes to the fore in efforts to distinguish therapeutic from nontherapeutic experiments on patients. If a physician means to help diabetic patients, an experiment on diabetic patients (with their consent) is justified by this principle. If the experiment is nontherapeutic, some other justification is required.

Beneficence can be seen both as a principle and a virtue for physicians. Physicians receive special powers, income, and prestige from society. In return they are asked to dedicate their careers to helping others. Medical training requires this trait as demands on a student increase between premedical years and residency. Self-sacrifice is part of medicine. Ideally, physicians should want to help others, but if the internal desire is lacking, they should still help others from a sense of duty. The principle of beneficence spells out this duty.

Beneficence may sometimes come into conflict with autonomy (as, indeed, any of these principles may conflict with each of the others in a particular case). Consider the involuntary psychiatric commitment of schizophrenic, homeless people. Is it better to let such people wander the cold streets of a big city, or to incarcerate and medicate them against their will? Should we let them "die with their rights on" or inject them with sedatives and antipsychotic drugs "for their own good"? Maybe we should do nothing at all and not risk making them worse off. After all, who are we to say that it is "beneficent" to do so? Maybe homeless schizophrenics want to stay as they are. How beneficence and autonomy are balanced in particular cases is not easy to understand. (Indeed, since John Stuart Mill advocated both utilitarianism and the value of autonomy, critics have wondered whether his views were actually consistent.)

Nonmaleficence, "not harming others," echoes an ancient maxim of professional medical ethics, "First, do not harm." Above all, this maxim implies that if a physician is not technically competent to do something, he shouldn't do it. So medical students should not harm a patient by practicing on them (unless the patient

ing the 1980s, feminist philosophers began to question whether many ways
ing were *the* ways or merely *male* ways. Contractarianism, Kantianism, and
ınism all looked like male theories, too abstract, too intellectual, and
false to the ordinary experience of many women. What was missing was
is on values such as cooperation, nurturing, and bonding.

vard education professor Carol Gilligan showed that many women ana-
hical dilemmas differently from men. Subsequently, feminist theorists ar-
d theories of ethics whose central notions were not rights or universaliza-
t caring, trust, and relationships. This so-called "ethics of care" may be
red a branch of virtue ethics that promotes the "female" virtues of caring,
ıg, trust, intimate friendship, and love. Even among feminist theorists, this
nt is controversial because some theorists believe that such virtues are not
t in women by nature but exist only because they are encouraged in most
by traditional, sexist gender roles.

e might view the ethics of care as a corrective to the previous emphasis in
:heory on abstract, semilegalistic concepts. Alternately, one might consider
cs of care as reflecting a modern turning inward to the family and to those
one, fighting battles close at hand and letting far-off concerns such as world
take care of themselves. Finally, one might view this approach as taking a
ıodest, minimalist approach to morality—a kind of "within-my-circle-of-
ıships" approach—in which moral concerns usually arise among those one

haps the ethics of care is best seen as an antidote to moral views that are cast
terms of rights, utility, and duty. It is not yet a complete ethical theory, for
not tell us how to treat people we do not know or care about. This is an im-
: criticism in medical ethics because much of medicine is about treating
•rs, at least when patients first meet a physician. It may be retorted that good
.ans should care for all their patients, but the meaning of "care" gets too di-
·/hen someone claims they care about everyone they meet. Nor does this
yet tell us how to resolve conflicts among those we care about, such as when
le physician is torn between checking on a patient and being with her
·er at the birth of her first grandchild. This theory, however, is still very
.and in coming decades, may have more to offer.

Based Reasoning

physicians and medical ethicists do not find any of the theories described
very useful to their practice of medicine. To force the complexities of many
ıl cases into a preconceived, abstract framework is often to be guilty of over-
fication, and when that happens, the truth is rarely discovered.

the past decade a new approach has been articulated that bases moral rea-
, on paradigms or model cases. These paradigmatic cases serve as a basis
vhich a person can generalize to other, similar cases; for example, both Karen
ın and Nancy Cruzan were young women who went into lifelong comas
"persistent vegetative states" after, respectively, a drug overdose in 1975
ı automobile accident in 1983. In both cases, parents decided after many
.s that their daughter's biography was over and wanted to end the mere life

consents): Patients are there to be helped, not to help students
least, patients should not leave an encounter with a physician v
were before. This crucial principle of medical ethics prohibits c
petence, and dangerous, nontherapeutic experiments.

The principle of nonmaleficence also accords with Mill's h
contractarianism: Both of these are minimalist moralities impl
and society should not attempt to shape all citizens' lives fo
worldview. In a fundamental sense, the first obligation we have
other alone, especially those who do not want our help, advice
That means, above all else, not harming others by unsolicited ir

The last principle, *justice*, has both a social and political
cially, it means treating similar kinds of people similarly (this is
mal element" of the larger principle). A just physician treats eac
regardless of his insurance coverage.

Politically, the principle amounts to distributive justice, an
to the allocation of scarce medical resources. Because there ar
justice, this principle is not self-evident. For example, Rawls's t
mands that medicine serve the worse off people. But another v
with simple egalitarianism: Medicine is just if it treats each
course, that goal would not be easy to achieve either, and doing
way towards realizing Rawls's ideal. At the very least, it would
of equal access to medical care for every citizen, such that
would not be a factor (as it is now) in selection of which patier
transplant. Finally, justice can be interpreted in a libertarian se
one with the ability to pay the same. In this sense, it means not 1
cannot pay.

It is obvious that interpretation of the principle of justice is
when an interpretation of this principle must be used with tl
ciples in a particular case. However, in the most normal sense, j
sicians to treat patients impartially, without bias on account o
ality, or wealth. Even in such a minimal sense, justice requires
behavior among physicians.

Feminist Ethics: The Ethics of Care

In the early 1970s a modern version of feminism shook Amer
foundations and buttressed its sister movement, the patient
Both movements attempted to take patients' decisions about th
away from physicians—especially male physicians—and g
tients control.

The landmark book was *Our Bodies, Ourselves,* by a g
women patients in Boston who had access to one of the grai
say, most self-satisfied—medical centers in the world, Ha
couldn't get the information they wanted in down-to-earth,
guage, they published a "how-to" manual covering everythir
to abortions. Successive editions sold millions upon million
rise to the areas of publishing now called "alternative medici

of the remaining body. Karen Quinlan's case focused on removal of a respirator; Nancy Cruzan's on removal of a feeding tube. Both cases resulted in landmark legal decisions in, respectively, 1976 and 1990.

Advocates of case-based reasoning believe that study of these two famous cases can teach us a lot about how ethics in medicine has actually worked over the last two decades. Paradigms are bedrock cases from which we generalize in ever-expanding circles of similarity. By understanding and analyzing arguments on both sides—about killing and letting die, ordinary versus extraordinary treatment, forgoing versus withdrawing treatment, standards of brain death, and models of proxy consent for making decisions about incompetent patients—we can hope to increase our understanding of related issues in medical ethics.

Because thousands of patients may end up in comas like those of Karen Quinlan and Nancy Cruzan, studying how decisions were handled in their famous cases can teach us how to handle future cases better. Case-based reasoning is very similar to the method of case-analysis of some famous business schools and the traditional teaching on rounds in medical schools. It is much the same as an ancient method of theological reasoning called "casuistry," and some bioethicists with theological training today use this word to describe this orientation.

Case-based reasoning does not deny that ethical theories and moral reasoning play roles in moral life. When these are relevant to a case, they must be discussed. It is just that when they are relevant, we need not study ethical theory to see their relevance. If a patient has been abused in a nontherapeutic, psychiatric experiment, we do not need to understand much about the principle of justice to understand that the patient has been abused. In short, how all the different ingredients of the ethical recipe go together to bake a good result can be judged only in terms of the complex details of each case, not in terms of preset formulas.

Case-based reasoning does deny that any overarching ethical principle of morality can guide us in making day-to-day ethical decisions in medicine. Each situation or case will present a unique array of people, interests, conflicting principles, incompatible role-duties, strong passions, and concerns about the larger good, about resources, about institutional policies, and about political consequences. Each set of circumstances will require what the Greeks called *phronesis*, or practical judgment, to find the optimal solution for all parties.

PART ONE

Classic Cases about Death and Dying

CHAPTER 2

Comas

Karen Quinlan and Nancy Cruzan

With the hindsight of a quarter-century, we know now that the cases of Karen Quinlan and Nancy Cruzan galvanized America's interest in medical ethics and, indirectly, the world's. Why is that so? The answer is that the cases made public many questions that had previously only vexed physicians inside medicine: Does a person die when only machines keep her body alive? What are the rights of families to decide when medical intervention ceases to become treatment and starts to become torture? Does actively killing a patient differ morally from omitting intervention necessary to continue life? What is the role of the courts, physicians, and families in making such decisions?

So this chapter introduces concepts central to this book: standards of brain death; definitions of personhood; problems of safeguarding incompetent patients from overzealous families; problems physicians have getting families to come to grips with medical realities; and the ethics of killing versus letting die.

The Quinlan case started in 1975 and some of its real issues remained misunderstood for a long time. Fifteen years later, the Cruzan case resulted in the first landmark decision by the U.S. Supreme Court on the rights of dying patients. This chapter describes these cases in some detail, their ethical and legal issues, and how these issues have evolved over the last 25 years.

THE QUINLAN CASE

The Medical Situation: Karen Quinlan's Coma

In April of 1975, Karen Quinlan had just turned 21. A perky, independent young woman, she had recently left her adoptive parents' home in New Jersey against their wishes and moved in with two male roommates a few miles away. Her friends described her as a wild, free spirit who lived recklessly. They also alleged that Karen experimented with heroin, cocaine, and methadone, although Karen's parents denied this.[1] Once Karen lost control of her car going around a curve, went over a cliff, slid down a ravine, and walked away unhurt; she told her parents it was no big deal.

On April 15, a few nights after moving out of the family home, Karen cele-brated a friend's birthday at a local bar. After a few gin and tonics, she suddenly seemed faint and was taken home. Her friends put her to bed, where she immedi-ately slept. When they checked on her 15 minutes later, she wasn't breathing. (Her friends never said why they had felt a need to check her condition.) While one of her roommates called an ambulance, the other started mouth-to-mouth resuscita-tion. Though Karen did not respond, a policeman did later get her breathing, and her color returned, but not her consciousness.

The Role of Drugs   When Karen was admitted after midnight to the intensive care unit (ICU) at Newton Memorial Hospital in New Jersey, a bottle of Valium was found in her purse; some pills were missing from it, suggesting that Karen had consumed both Valium and alcohol that evening. Karen had also been dieting for several days and, at admission, weighed only 115 pounds.

Valium is a benzodiazapine (so are Lithium, Ativan, and Xanax). As a class of antianxiety drugs, benzodiazapines act on specific nerve receptors in the brain and are considered safer than barbiturates, which have been around since 1912 when physicians first used phenobarbitol.

Both benzodiazapines and barbiturates are *synergistic* with alcohol, meaning the effects of both drugs intensify in combination. Alcohol *potentiates* these drugs, making their effects much stronger, and in some cases, more deadly. Radical hippie Abbie Hoffman intentionally killed himself in 1989 by taking 150 phenobarbitol pills and then drinking a fifth of hard liquor. The actor River Phoenix unintention-ally killed himself in 1993 by mixing barbiturates, alcohol, and benzodiazapines. Synergistic effects increase on an empty stomach.

The later court transcript contradicts itself about the exact drugs Karen con-sumed. Attending physician Robert Morse testified that, "She had some barbitu-rates, which was normal, 0.6 milligrams; toxic is 2 milligrams, and the fatal dose about 5 milligrams percent"[sic].[2] Consulting neurologist Julius Korein, whom the Quinlans hired, testified that Karen's drug screen "was positive for quinine, nega-tive for morphine, barbiturates and other substances. A subsequent test for Valium and Librium was positive."[3] (No one else mentioned Librium.) Court prosecutor George Daggett testified that Karen had taken tranquilizers with alcohol shortly before becoming unconscious.[4] The Quinlans denied that the drug screen showed barbiturates: "The early urine and blood samples, taken on the day Karen was brought to the hospital, revealed only a "normal therapeutic" level of aspirin and the tranquilizer Valium in her system."[5]

Although the parents never wanted their adopted daughter's death to be seen as drug-related, the death most likely resulted from a synergistic reaction of bar-biturates, benzodiazapines, and alcohol on an empty stomach. Their cumulative effects suppressed her breath, caused loss of oxygen to the brain, and thus, after 30 minutes or so, destroyed large parts of her brain.

Respirators   Nine days after admission to Newton Memorial, Karen's medical status had not changed and she was transferred to the much larger St. Clare's Hos-pital, a Catholic institution in Denville, New Jersey. Unlike Newton, St. Clare's had pulmonologists and neurologists on its staff.

A small respirator, also called a *ventilator*, kept Karen breathing during her first days of hospitalization. It also prevented aspiration of vomit into her lungs, which could cause pneumonia.

Respirators began to be used in medicine during the 1960s and by 1975 had become common in cases of emergency and trauma. The respirator's use in the Quinlan case showed that the *criteria of death* needed clarification. Because the brain must have a fresh supply of oxygenated blood to live, lack of such oxygenated blood (*anoxia*) quickly damages the brain and, over enough time, destroys it. The traditional definition of death—where the body stops breathing and the person is declared dead—indirectly *assumed* brain death as inevitable, but now a respirator prevented this.

The small respirator that forced air into her lungs hardly made Karen appear as a Sleeping Beauty. Karen's sister, Mary Lou, knew that Karen was comatose but wasn't prepared for what she saw when she visited the hospital:

> Whenever I thought of a person in a coma, I thought they would just lie there very quietly, almost as though they were sleeping. Karen's head was moving around, as if she was trying to pull away from that tube in her throat, and she made little noises, like moans. I don't know if she was in pain, but it seemed as though she was. And I thought—if Karen could ever see herself like this, it would be the worst thing in the world for her.[6]

Sometimes she would choke, sit bolt upright with her arms flung out and her eyes wide open, appearing to be in intense pain. Eventually her breathing stabilized, but even then she didn't breath deeply enough to sigh. Without breathing to a sigh, the lower sacs of her lungs risked infection. Hence she was put on a larger respirator that gave her "sigh volume." This larger respirator required a tracheotomy (a hole cut surgically in the throat or trachea) to which her mother, Julia Quinlan, reluctantly agreed.

This more powerful respirator altered her appearance. At a later hearing, her lawyer testified about Karen in September 1975 that:

> Her eyes are open and move in a circular manner as she breathes; her eyes blink approximately three or four times per minute; her forehead evidences very noticeable perspiration; her mouth is open while the respirator expands to ingest oxygen, and while her mouth is open, her tongue appears to be moving in a rather random manner; her mouth closes as the oxygen is ingested into her body through the tracheotomy and she appears to be slightly convulsing or gasping as the oxygen enters her windpipe; her hands are visible in an emaciated form, facing in a praying position away from her body. Her present weight would seem to be in the vicinity of 70–80 pounds.[7]

Comas   Karen Quinlan, of course, was in a coma, but what does that mean? The word *coma* is vague, with many meanings across a continuum. On one end of this continuum, a coma is like extended sleep. While we don't say a person goes into a coma when he goes to sleep, if he failed to awaken for two days, we would. Comas disrupt the body's natural sleep/wake cycle.

Many people awake from comas. Minor head injuries, allergic reactions, and surgery may create long disruptions of consciousness. The brain may be healing while comatose.

On the other hand, some comas are irreversible and tantamount to brain death. Some physicians use "coma" to represent the last and lowest level of function of the brain prior to death. Nevertheless, comas should never be confused with brain death. Despite popular belief at the time, under New Jersey law in 1975 Karen was not brain-dead.

One serious form of coma is called *persistent vegetative state* (PVS). PVS is a generic term covering a type of deep unconsciousness that is almost always irreversible if it persists for a few months. In this case, although Karen was unconscious, her eyes sometimes opened and she would suddenly seem to laugh or cry. Furthermore, her eyes were *disconjugate,* i.e., they moved in different, random directions at the same time. Despite eye movements, she was thought to be *decorticate:* Karen's brain could not receive input from her eyes. She had slow-wave—*not* isoelectric, or "flat"—electroencephalograms (EEGs).

At one time, a patient in such a condition would simply starve to death; but in the late 1960s, crude intravenous and nasogastric feeding tubes began to be used. Initially, an intravenous tube fed Karen, but as her condition persisted, the rigidity of her muscles made it difficult to insert and reinsert such a tube into her veins. Five months after her admission, in September 1975, she required a nasogastric feeding tube.

Julia Quinlan disliked this feeding tube:

> They were feeding her a high caloric diet—which seemed completely unreasonable, especially since her body didn't always accept the food. Often she would vomit. . . . And she was more agitated than she'd ever been. I wouldn't have thought it possible that Karen's head could writhe so much. It was as though her body was in a vise, and her head was caught in a whirlpool.[8]

This invasive (possibly painful?) feeding tube, along with the respirator, for many people symbolized an oppressive medical technology that unnaturally prolonged dying. Although unknown during her lifetime, Karen Quinlan posthumously became a world-famous symbol of the wrong way to die.

A hired security force vigilantly kept Karen from being photographed, thus never allowing her condition to penetrate public consciousness. During the wait for the later court verdict, a national tabloid offered the Quinlans $10,000 for just one picture. They refused because they wanted their daughter to be remembered as she had lived rather than as a coma patient. Ignorant artists even portrayed her in newspapers and magazines as a normal girl resting peacefully so that most people never understood the horrible nature of her deterioration.

Given her real condition, Karen had little chance of ever regaining consciousness. Nevertheless, St. Clare's felt that they owed a "1 in a million" chance of recovery to a helpless, incompetent patient. However, their parish priest assured them that Catholics need not endure *extraordinary means* in dying (such as the big respirator)—so Pope Pius XII had declared in 1957.

After awhile, it became clear that, as her heart was strong, she no longer needed the ICU's cardiac monitor. Against her parents' wishes Karen was moved out of the ICU and placed in a corner of the emergency room (ER), where the staff could respond if she vomited. The ER was a logical, if somewhat cold, solution, which upset her father, Joseph Quinlan, who wanted her back in the ICU.

Karen's family took many months to accept the judgment that Karen would never regain consciousness. Finally, they understood that her mind was gone, and that she was much the same as being dead. They also agreed that she would never have wanted her body to continue in such a condition. The Quinlans averred that Karen had twice said that if anything terrible happened to her, she did not want to be kept alive as a vegetable on machines.

So the Quinlans decided to remove the respirator and to let Karen's body die. They had no idea that their long struggle to reach this decision would be the easy part.

We mentioned above that the use of respirators in the Quinlan case revealed new ethical problems about brain death. Besides using them in combination with a feeding tube, now other problems surfaced: how active could ethical physicians be in *withdrawing* respirators and feeding tubes? To some physicians, such withdrawals felt like killing vulnerable patients. Were such feelings justified? Isn't it a physician's job to look out for vulnerable patients? What if the patient's family feels differently than the physician? How should such a conflict be resolved and where?

The Legal Battle

The Legal Background   The legal environment at the time of the Quinlan case needs to be explained, especially the effect of the Kenneth Edelin case in Massachusetts (discussed in detail in Chapter 7). Back in 1975, no ethics committees existed, so no other recourse existed but to go to court.

Abortion had been legalized in 1973, when the Supreme Court decided in *Roe* v. *Wade* that states could pass laws banning abortion only *after* viability of the fetus. The Court did not directly state that a fetus is a person at viability, but its decision did stipulate where states could draw the line between legal and illegal abortions.

At the time a senior resident in obstetrics at Boston City Hospital, Kenneth Edelin, performed a very late second-trimester abortion by hysterotomy at the request of a pregnant teenage girl. In 1975, in a sensationalistic trial, a jury convicted Edelin not of homicide but of manslaughter: The jury understood *Roe* v. *Wade* to mean that a viable fetus is a person, believed that Edelin had not done everything possible to save a viable fetus, and thus found that he had acted illegally.

Sentenced to a year of probation, Dr. Edelin also risked losing his license if his appeal failed. This verdict traumatized Edelin: his medical career could be over before it started and he could be hard to employ anywhere as a convicted felon.

Edelin had been convicted just a few weeks before Karen Quinlan's admission to St. Clare's. As the Quinlan case developed during 1975, Edelin's appeal was pending, and things looked bad for him.

An overview of possible stages of a court case will also help us understand the Quinlan legal battle. In a state case, the first stage takes place in a court of limited jurisdiction: a probate, district, or municipal court. After judgment is delivered there, an appeal can be directed to a circuit court. Next, state appellate courts hear cases (e.g., in Alabama the Court of Civil Appeals and the Court of Criminal Appeals). At the state level, the court of last resort is usually called the *state supreme court.*

A separate court system hears federal cases. The federal system has two independent, intermediate steps: district courts and courts of appeals. A court of appeals usually has three judges, but a district court often has just one judge. Nationally, the court of last resort is the Supreme Court of the United States.

State or federal cases can be tried either as violations of *civil law* (such as malpractice) or as violations of *criminal law* (such as assault and battery). Each state's criminal code defines homicide and manslaughter, and such definitions differ from state to state. Clauses in state statutes about self-defense, brain death, and legalized withdrawal of medical treatment describe *exceptions* to homicide.

The First Hearing   The lawyers for the physicians in the Quinlan case must have seen parallels between their case and Edelin's case. In Edelin's case, a patient wanted a fledgling physician to kill another being (a late-term human fetus) who might legally be considered a person. In the Quinlan case, parents were asking fledgling physicians to bring about the death of a being (comatose patient) who was legally still a person. The lawyers also may have thought that Edelin's conviction set a precedent.

Everyone wondered in both cases why senior medical staff had ducked these cases and let such young physicians take the heat. The doctors in Karen Quinlan's case, Robert Morse and his colleague Arshad Javed, had just begun their medical careers. Morse had completed his residency in neurology only 10 months earlier; Javed had graduated from a medical school in Pakistan and had completed an American fellowship in pulmonary medicine 2 years before being assigned to Karen's case.

It is not hard to understand why, in the context of Edelin's conviction, Morse and Javed became nervous about possibly crossing the line between legality and illegality. First, in 1975 the American Medical Association (AMA) equated withdrawing a respirator in order to allow death to occur with *euthanasia* (mercy killing), and then equated that with murder. Remember that in early 1976, no federal or state court had decided anything about death and dying that clarified the rights of patients or their families.

Second, Dr. Morse also feared a malpractice suit if the Quinlans later changed their minds. One common definition of malpractice in the United States is "departure from normal standards of medical practice in a community," and in 1975—when almost all physicians felt it their duty to continue treatment until the very last moment of life—actively assisting in the death of a comatose patient would have been such a departure.

This definition of malpractice raises the interesting philosophical issue of whether a physician can change standards of treatment without committing malpractice; it would seem that, unless the entire medical community changes at one fell swoop, any such changes by a progressive physician would leave him or her open to such charges.

To get Karen's respirator disconnected, Joseph Quinlan sought counsel at a Legal Aid office, which represented clients who could not afford a lawyer. (Because she was no longer a minor and was indigent, Karen qualified for Legal Aid). A young, idealistic attorney named Paul Armstrong took the case. Judge Robert Muir of New Jersey probate court first heard the case; later, the New Jersey Supreme Court heard the case without intermediate appeals. (State supreme courts sometimes do so when the case may set a precedent.)

Armstrong needed to find some legal basis for letting Karen die. Neurologists testified that Karen's condition was irreversible and that her chances of returning to normal were minuscule. So Armstrong first argued, incorrectly, that Karen was legally brain-dead. Judge Muir scolded him and made it clear that since Karen's brain stem was still functioning, she did not meet New Jersey's "total brain" standard of brain death.

Armstrong also argued unsuccessfully on the basis of an alleged right to die in the Constitution of the United States, but in 1975, no Supreme Court decision had ever interpreted the Constitution to imply such a right, even for *competent* patients, much less for *incompetent* patients such as Karen Quinlan (15 years later, the high court would change this in its *Cruzan* decision—see below).

The simplest and easiest legal route for the Quinlans would have been to obtain guardianship of Karen and then have her moved to another hospital, where the respirator could have been disconnected. As one legal commentator declared, Armstrong may have botched the case by not pursuing this quiet strategy; instead, he immediately raised the dramatic issue of letting Karen die:

> In the hands of a conscientious but regrettably inexperienced 30-year-old lawyer, Paul Armstrong, the Quinlan family got very dubious legal advice. For the question of *guardianship* could have been pursued prior to and separate from the question of *treatment refusal.*[9]

By immediately announcing to Judge Muir that Joseph Quinlan wanted to disconnect Karen's respirator, Armstrong tied Muir's hands. A guardian must protect the interests of his or her ward; in this case, the ward was a vulnerable patient, and the question whether that patient was still a person had by no means been settled. Given Armstrong's announcement, Muir could not have appointed Joseph Quinlan Karen's guardian without prejudging whether Karen was now not a person.

In logical terms, lawyer Paul Armstrong begged several questions. *Begging the question* in logic is the fallacy of assuming the truth of what should be proven. It often occurs when controversial topics are at issue and people get too excited to lay out their evidence for a position. It is also a cheap trick in debate. First, Armstrong had begged the question by assuming that PVS should be equated with brain death, but the law had never interpreted brain death that way and to do so would have been a big leap, so this position should have been argued, not assumed. Second, what course of action really was in Karen's best interests? Armstrong begged the question by assuming it was to be dead, but again, would she really not have wanted to stay alive with some chance of regaining consciousness? Third, he also begged the question of who best represented Karen's interests: her parents or some appointed advocate? Armstrong erred in just assuming that Karen's father should play this role, especially when the result was life or death for Karen. Consequently, Judge Muir appointed another lawyer, Daniel Coburn, as Karen's guardian *ad litem* ("for this suit or action").

The Courtroom Drama   Daniel Coburn, Karen's guardian, opened the case in Judge Muir's court with a verbal salvo:

> I have one simple role in this case . . . and that is, to do every single thing that I can do as a skilled professional to keep Karen Quinlan alive. . . .
>
> We talk about facts. Karen Quinlan is not brain dead. She's nowhere near being "brain dead," if that's the accepted standard. . . .
>
> There's another facet. . . . There are thousands of Karen Quinlans out there. I've received thousands of phone calls from all over the world about people . . . where there was no hope, and they recovered. They have been brain damaged, and they are educable, although they may have some retardation. But they are still alive. These people don't want Karen Quinlan dead. I don't want Karen Quinlan dead. . . .
>
> As to the theory that she's not really leaving this earth—that she's just getting to the next world a little bit sooner—in all frankness to the court, and I'm not trying to be flippant, my attitude is that if the Quinlans want an express, I'm going to take the local. . . .
>
> As far as the legal basis for this, I've heard "death with dignity," "self-determination," "religious freedom"—and I consider that to be a complete shell game that's being played here. This is euthanasia. Nobody seems to want to use the word. I'm going to use the word, whether it's euthanasia or a variation of it. . . .
>
> One human being, by conduct, or lack of conduct, is going to cause the death of another human being.[10]

Ralph Porzio, the flamboyant attorney for Karen's doctor Robert Morse, implored Judge Muir "not to impose an execution—a death sentence" on Karen. He asked, "Once you admit that a person is alive, legally and medically, and once you make a determination that a life must come to an end, then where do you draw the line?"[11] Porzio held that Karen should not be killed on the basis of someone else's assessment of her quality of life: "Fresh in our minds are the Nazi atrocities. Fresh in our minds are the human experimentations. Fresh in our minds are [sic] the Nuremberg Code." Porzio cited the sanctity of life as "the cornerstone of Western culture . . . and our Western religions," and asserted that turning off Karen's respirator would be "like turning on the gas chamber." He didn't "care where the idea [of mercy killing] comes from, whether it comes from Rome or from Mecca or from Salt Lake City, the end result is still the same." He compared Morse's refusal to disconnect the respirator to the civil disobedience of Socrates and Thomas More, reminding the Court that "we are not gods." In closing, he held nothing back:

> So let us then, in this hour of trial as we begin, so conduct ourselves that when the eyes grow dim and when our own lives shall fade, and when men and women in some distant day shall gather to warm their hands over the fires of memory, they may look back—they may look back and say of us: They searched for truth, they nurtured justice, they knew compassion; but above all, above all, they walked with honor and wore the garments of understanding.

Privately, the two young physicians must have winced while their lawyer used such rhetoric because they had always sympathized with the plight of the Quinlans and had always agreed that Karen's chances of regaining consciousness were miniscule. Nevertheless, once they plunged into the adversarial legal system, lawyers on both sides swept them into their courtroom theatrics. The physicians had no choice but to go along with these unsettling tactics of the courtroom.

Morse himself testified that no medical precedent allowed him to disconnect Karen's respirator. The neurologist Julius Korein testified that he had seen about 50 patients in PVS and that all of them were better off than Karen; he described Karen as having no mental age at all and as being like "an anencephalic monster."[12] Famous neurologist Fred Plum, author of the then-definitive textbook, *Stupor and Coma*, confirmed Korein's diagnosis; Plum described Karen as "lying in bed, emaciated, curled up in what is known as flexion contracture. Every joint was bent in a flexion position and making one tight sort of fetal position. It's too grotesque, really, to describe in human terms like fetal."[13]

In November 1975, almost 7 months after Karen's original admission, Judge Muir decided that Coburn should continue as Karen's guardian and that the respirator should not be disconnected. Muir said that Karen's own wishes were unknown because they had never been written down, and that her parents' testimony about her wishes could not be taken as final if it entailed her death. He also ruled that no constitutional right to die existed.

The New Jersey Supreme Court Decision   Armstrong ultimately argued successfully before the New Jersey Supreme Court by appealing to the Constitution's implied right to privacy. The phrase *right to privacy* is misleading because it seems to refer to private actions; in fact, it refers to the liberty of an American to decide purely personal issues without interference from government. The U. S. Supreme Court in 1965 first recognized a right to privacy in *Griswold* v. *Connecticut,* when it found unconstitutional state laws banning physicians from giving contraceptives to married couples. The *Griswold* court said for a state government to say women and couples couldn't use contraception to avoid having children violated the fundamental liberty of personal life that was assumed throughout the Constitution and that made the lives of Americans the envy of many people around the world.

Several weeks later, the New Jersey State Supreme Court heard the case and testimony about the role of physicians in deciding matters of life and death. The justices then expressed surprise at the importance placed by physicians on the distinction between disconnecting a respirator and not starting it. At the time, the official position of AMA was that it was permissible not to put a patient on a respirator; but once a patient was on a respirator, it was not permissible to take that patient off if the intention was to allow death to occur. The justices found this line of reasoning "rather flimsy."

Additionally, lawyers for the physicians argued that once a physician accepted a patient, an absolute duty to pursue the patient's welfare became "attached" to the physician, such that the physician could never, ever pursue death. However, Julius Korein (the neurologist who had testified for the Quinlans in the lower court) now testified that physicians privately used "judicious neglect" in letting terminal patients die and that this was an "unwritten standard" in medicine.

Korein's testimony opened this issue to legal and public scrutiny. In doing so, he ignited controversies that would rebound around America for the next two decades, for not everyone agreed with everything that the *Quinlan* justices would decide.

The justices pressed the hospital's lawyers about the physician–patient relationship. Why couldn't Morse and Javed allow Karen to be transferred to another hospital, where other physicians could disconnect her? The lawyers for the hospital hemmed and hawed, but finally just said that St. Clare's thought it would be immoral to do so.

In January 1976, after 2 months of deliberation, the New Jersey Supreme Court ruled unanimously in favor of the Quinlans. The Constitution's implied right to privacy (liberty) allowed the family of a dying incompetent patient to decide to let that patient die by disconnecting life support. Because the Supreme Court of the United States had not yet made a comparable decision, New Jersey was thus the first to apply the right to privacy in a case of "letting die." The New Jersey court also allowed Joseph Quinlan to become Karen's guardian, gave legal immunity to Morse and Javed for disconnecting Karen's life support, and suggested (though it did not require) an advisory role for ethics committees in hospitals composed mostly of laypeople to help in future cases.

This last suggestion is interesting because the ensuing decades have seen a proliferation of hospital ethics committees (HECs). But the court may have been guilty of a fantasy here in thinking that such committees could keep such cases out of the legal system. For consider: how many laypeople would have understood the real issues of the Quinlan case in 1975 without all the publicity? Indeed, some of the real issues only emerged after the legal battle. So could such a committee really help physicians decide such cases, especially if a primary fear of physicians was legal liability? Finally, as we will see below, some of the issues in the case were more subtle than it first appeared.

The Aftermath   At both the lower-court and the higher-court level, the Quinlan case generated immense publicity; and it involved many different county, state, and hospital officials as well as private lawyers. The AMA and many physicians understandably hated not only the publicity, but the presence of lawyers; most physicians felt that tragic cases like Karen's should be kept out of the courts.

Given the traditional definition of malpractice, they also wanted (somewhat inconsistently) immunity from prosecution before they would break new ground in cases involving dying patients. Over the next 15 years, several big legal cases in state courts about death and dying were instigated precisely by physicians sympathetic to families who wanted prior, blanket legal protection from suit. It is easy to see why physicians both sought and scorned the courts in such cases.

Pulling the Plug or Weaning from a Respirator?   In April 1976, 4 months after the higher-court decision, machines still helped Karen Quinlan's body breathe. By then, decubitus ulcers had eaten through her flesh, exposing her hip bones. Why

Karen was still alive at this point is one of the least understood and most interesting aspects of this case.

According to the Quinlans, Morse resisted implementing the decision of the New Jersey Supreme Court, because "this is something I will have to live with for the rest of my life."[14] A nun who worked in an administrative position was more blunt: "You have to understand our position, Mrs. Quinlan. In this hospital we don't kill people."[15] To this, Julia Quinlan replied, "Why didn't you tell me 10 months ago? I would have taken Karen out of this hospital immediately."

The administrators at St. Clare's were not by any means alone in their position. Catholic hospitals saw the Quinlan decision as another step down a slippery slope that had started 3 years earlier with the American legalization of abortion in 1973. During the trial, the Vatican theologian Gino Concetti criticized the Quinlans: "A right to death does not exist. Love for life, even a life reduced to ruin, drives one to protect life with every possible care."[16] A pulmonary specialist at Catholic University in Rome said that removal of the respirator "would be an extremely dangerous move by her doctors, and represents an indirect form of euthanasia."[17]

Instead of simply disconnecting Karen's respirator, Morse and Javed decided to try to wean her from it. *Weaning* means to gradually train the patient off the machine by building up different muscles or teaching a patient new techniques. The tired, confused Quinlans and their inexperienced lawyer did not understand what this meant, and the real implications would become painfully clear over the next 10 years.

A more experienced lawyer would have obtained a *writ of habeus corpus* ("you should have the body"), which is designed to protect Americans from false imprisonment. A writ of habeus corpus can be issued by a local judge, and it works very quickly; if they had gotten such a writ, the Quinlans could have transferred Karen to a hospital where she would have been allowed to die.

Eventually, Javed had Karen off the respirator for 4 hours; then, after intensive work over many weeks, for 12 hours. By late May of 1976, Karen was off the respirator altogether. This weaning created some confusion in the general public: Some people took it to mean that Karen had gotten better; others took it to mean that Karen's physicians had "pulled the plug" and that a miracle must have occurred because she hadn't died. Both impressions were false.

How the Case Ended   St. Clare's hospital now wanted to transfer Karen immediately to any other facility, and a desperate search ensued for a nursing home. The New Jersey Medicaid office forced one nursing home to accept Karen on June 9, 1976. At this point, Karen had been unconscious for 14 months.

Not until June 13, 1986, after more than 10 years in the nursing home, was Karen Quinlan's body declared dead. For several months before that, Karen had had pneumonia; and the Quinlans had declined antibiotics to reverse it. Julia Quinlan maintained a vigil at her daughter's bedside and saw the last moment of Karen's biological life.

Paul Armstrong became famous and later tried other right-to-die cases before the New Jersey Supreme Court. Robert Morse died in a small plane crash in 1987.

THE CRUZAN CASE

Nancy Cruzan's case led to a landmark decision by the United States Supreme Court in June 1990.[18] Before this decision, 20 states had recognized the right of competent patients to refuse medical life support, and all these states (with the exception of New York and Missouri) had recognized the right of surrogates to make decisions for incompetent patients.[19] The *Cruzan* decision by the United States Supreme Court was the first to explicitly recognize the rights of dying patients.

The Patient: Nancy Cruzan's Coma

Nancy Cruzan, at the age 24, lost control of her car around midnight on a lonely, icy country road in Missouri on January 11, 1983.[20] She was thrown 35 feet from the car and landed face-down in a water-filled ditch. Paramedics arriving on the scene found that her heart had stopped. They injected a stimulant into the heart and then shocked it into restarting; but because her brain had been anoxic for perhaps 15 minutes, Nancy Cruzan was in PVS.[21]

For 7 years, Nancy remained in this state. Over time, her body became rigid, her hands curled tightly, and her fingernails became like claws. In a state much like Karen Quinlan, Nancy could take nothing by mouth and somebody turned her every two hours to prevent ulcers. According to her family, much of the time she drooled, causing her hair, pillow, and sheets to be wet. Her care cost the state of Missouri $130,000 a year.

Where the Quinlan case focused on withdrawal of a respirator, the Cruzan case focused on withdrawal of a feeding tube. Because she could not swallow, Nancy could not be fed by mouth. Loss of ability to swallow signals a key decision in the care of incapacitated patients, especially those with dementia or neurological diseases. Before feeding tubes began to be used in the 1960s, the natural course for such patients was starvation and then death. With a feeding tube, this natural deterioration of the body can be put on hold for years, even decades.

Legally or morally, is a PVS patient owed food and water? Karen Quinlan's parents evidently thought so; they never withdrew the nutrition that kept Karen's body alive. Nancy's parents, Joe and Joyce Cruzan, thought otherwise: they sought permission in court to disconnect their daughter's feeding tube.

The Case

Legal Background to the Cruzan Decision   In discussing the Cruzan case, it is necessary to understand three standards of legal evidence. The minimum standard is *preponderance of evidence;* a more rigorous standard is *clear and convincing evidence;* the most rigorous standard—the standard used for serious felonies—is *beyond a reasonable doubt.*

Preponderance of evidence simply means that there is more evidence one way than the other; in some cases, this simply means there is some evidence one way or the other. Clear and convincing denotes more rigorous evidence, and, in cases of dying, it means a declaration such as an advanced directive (living will) or durable power of attorney. Finally, beyond a reasonable doubt requires the most evidence and, of course, is used in trials of homicide to establish guilt and where the accused is presumed innocent.

Early Decisions   The Cruzans won their case in probate court; but upon direct review, the Missouri Supreme Court reversed the decision, and this reversal had to do with the standard of clear and convincing evidence. Simply put, because Nancy Cruzan's parents could not produce an advanced directive (living will) and because only the two parents and a sister testified, the Cruzans did not produce enough evidence to be "clear and convincing" about Nancy's true wishes. In particular, Joe Cruzan emphasized that Nancy was a fighter and strong-willed, and as such, it was hard to see Nancy might not want to fight to return to life.

The Missouri Supreme Court concluded that the state had an interest in preserving life—regardless of "quality of life—and that before medical support could be withdrawn from an incompetent patient, its standard of clear and convincing evidence had to be met, no matter how strongly the family felt otherwise.

The U.S. Supreme Court Decision   In reviewing this Missouri decision, the United States Supreme Court did much more than adjudicate this practical case. Indeed, it made three very important declarations.

First, and most generally, it recognized a right of a *competent* patient to decline medical treatment, even if such refusal led directly to the patient's death. *Cruzan* was the first time the Supreme Court decided that the Constitution gave Americans a liberty interest to be free of unwanted medical support. The reporter covering the Supreme Court for *The New York Times* wrote:

> The framers of the Constitution, who prohibited the Government from depriving a person of "life" or "liberty" without due process of law, had little reason to envision a day when the very act of sustaining a life might itself be a deprivation of liberty.[22]

And yet, she went on to say, modern medical technology had done precisely that.

Second, the Supreme Court also found that withdrawing a feeding tube did not differ from withdrawing any other kind of life-sustaining medical support. Hence some state laws permitted forgoing or withdrawing respirators but not artificial nutrition.

Third, with regard to *incompetent* patients, the Supreme Court held in *Cruzan* that a state *could, but need not,* pass a statute requiring the clear and convincing standard of evidence about what a formerly competent patient would have wanted done if he or she became incompetent for a long time. Because Missouri had such a standard, its law was constitutional. Because the Cruzan family had not met that standard, Nancy's feeding tube could *not* be removed.

How did the Supreme Court see its first decision on death and dying? Justice Sandra Day O'Connor concurred, "Today we decide only that one state's practice does not violate the Constitution. The more challenging task of crafting appropriate procedures for safeguarding incompetents' liberty interests is entrusted to the 'laboratory' of the states."[23] She thus suggested that state legislatures and state courts should *balance* the rights of families to make such decisions for incompetent relatives with protection of the interests of such vulnerable patients.

The *Cruzan* decision said nothing about another category where a state might make a law about withdrawing medical treatment from never-competent patients, such as people with profound mental retardation. Because of past abuses, it is reasonable to expect that in these cases only state laws with the most rigorous standards of proof will pass the Supreme Court's review. The Supreme Court might well choose to require for such cases the same standard used in criminal law of beyond a reasonable doubt.[24]

To summarize the three standards of evidence:

(1) Preponderance of evidence (most permissive)
(2) Clear and convincing evidence (permitted by *Cruzan*)
(3) Beyond a reasonable doubt (least permissive; perhaps necessary with incompetents)

Reactions to *Cruzan*   Reactions to the Supreme Court *Cruzan* decision ran along two lines: legal commentators welcomed it; medical commentators hated it.

Most legal scholars supported the new conservative position of this Rehnquist Court on its role with regard to the Constitution. The proper function of the Supreme Court, according to the law professor Charles Baron, was not as a super legislature over the states or even "to promulgate uniform rules of state law. Instead, the U.S. Supreme Court should only have the minimal power to strike down state laws that conflict with either federal law or the U.S. Constitution."[25] In other words, not every bad or undesirable state law is necessarily unconstitutional.

Texas law professor John Robertson went so far as to say that Nancy Cruzan could not be harmed and hence had no interests in the case. He argued that the real claim in *Cruzan* had nothing to do with Nancy Cruzan's right to die or her right to privacy (her liberty interests); instead, the case was about the Cruzan family's right to be free of the emotional burden of maintaining her body in a state institution.[26]

Both Baron and Robertson agreed that the previous legal standard of *substituted judgment* (the standard applied by the New Jersey Supreme Court in Quinlan) was a mockery in such cases "[leading] us to pretend that we are merely complying (however reluctantly) with the wishes of the patient. The result in most states is mere lip service to substituted judgment. Almost any evidence is deemed sufficient to establish a preference for death over PVS. Or families are empowered to express patient preferences for death—with few questions asked."[27]

In contrast, the usual standard used in such cases was that of *best interests of the patient*. So in the *Cruzan* case, would the best interests of Nancy be to live on in such a state and subject her family to such a burden? Most people would say no, although this judgment is not open-and-shut since the State of Missouri argued that Nancy's best interests entailed continued feeding.

A different kind of reaction came from physicians who worked with families of vegetative and hospice patients. They emphasized the misery that families in New York and Missouri have to suffer if they could not meet the clear-

and-convincing standard. Neurologist and ethicist Ronald Cranford of Minnesota said:

> We should realize what the law is in Missouri . . . that once medical treatment is started (at least for artificial nutrition and hydration), it can't be stopped. [And to allow such a state to use the "clear and convincing standard" is] "unworkable, unfair, and cruel to so many families who will experience the utter helplessness of the Cruzans. It will place an enormous burden on society, which will spend hundreds of millions of dollars each year for a condition that no one in their right mind would ever want to be in."[28]

Hospice physician Joanne Lynn emphasized in Missouri and New York, "the suffering of the patient and family, the costs, the kind of life that can be gained, are all to count for nothing. If life can be prolonged, then it will have to be."[29]

How the Case Ended   Five months after the Supreme Court's decision in *Cruzan*, on December 14, 1990, physicians legally removed Nancy Cruzan's feeding tube, and she died.

As it turned out, Nancy had been divorced just before her accident, and she had some old friends who knew her only by her married name, Nancy Davis. When her case first became widely known, her friends had not realized that "Nancy Davis" was the "Nancy Cruzan" of the headlines.[30] Later, as nationwide publicity grew, they learned her real identity and came forward. But by then, they were too late to testify about Nancy's wishes because the appeals process was under way and the judges were discussing larger issues. However, after the major decision, the case was reheard in a lower court and Nancy's friends were offering new testimony. In that hearing, the lower court decided that the state's clear-and-convincing standard for evidence had now been met.[31]

Joe Cruzan, Nancy's father, had suffered from depression for years. Six years after Nancy's death, he committed suicide by hanging himself.

ETHICAL ISSUES: FROM BRAIN DEATH TO MEDICAL FUTILITY

Communication and Control

The Quinlan and Cruzan cases involved not only moral conflicts but also conflicts about control of medical treatment.

In the Quinlan case, one such issue had to do with Karen's transfer from a small community hospital—Newton Memorial—to St. Clare's. When approached about transferring Karen, the Quinlans didn't understand the consequences of a transfer. So what are they?

At a local hospital, patients and families deal with physicians they know, trust, and have chosen themselves. Once transferred to a large, impersonal, tertiary care hospital, patients and families deal with medical personnel who are strangers, who are assigned to their cases by the luck of the draw, and whose sense of professionalism within a specialty may conflict with the family's wishes (i.e., "they may do things that way at a little community hospital but we don't do it that way *here!*")

Another issue that often arises when a patient is transferred has to do with hospital policies, since different hospitals and many specialties have their own internal rules. Ideally, hospitals would post their policies, including those about care of the dying, and inform patients and their families in advance about such policies. In reality, however, patients and families rarely know about hospital policies before an admission or transfer takes place. For example, when the Quinlans were asked to give their informed consent and sign papers allowing Karen to have the tracheotomy required for the larger respirator, they did not know about St. Clare's policy that once a patient was on such a respirator, the respirator could not be removed. Such ignorance of hospital policy raises an interesting question about informed consent, which is legally required before a physician or hospital can give a patient drugs or perform surgery. How could a hospital obtain informed consent from a family facing a crucial decision without giving the family information about its policy of not withdrawing respirators or feeding tubes? Similarly, when the Cruzans signed papers allowing Nancy to be transferred to a state-run hospital, they did not realize that such facilities in Missouri would not remove a feeding tube from a PVS patient.

Standards of Brain Death

People have always feared that they might be declared dead prematurely and buried alive. In the eighteenth century, gruesome stories circulated about exhumations that found frantic scratches on the inside lids of coffins. In the nineteenth century, some legislatures required a delay before burial, and in 1882 an undertaker named Kirchbaum attached periscopes to coffins so that a person who woke up after being buried might signal for help.[32] Many people were buried with cowbells which they could ring if they awakened underground.

As previously mentioned, for thousands of years, the definition of death included cessation (almost simultaneously) of breathing and heartbeat. When breathing stopped, cardiac *anoxia* (lack of oxygen) would begin; this would be followed by cessation of the heart and then by *ischemia* (lack of blood flow to an area). Ischemia of the brain destroys brain tissue very rapidly. This is the traditional *whole-body standard* of death.

This whole-body standard became inappropriate when ventilators allowed respiration of brain-damaged patients. Before them, heart-lung machines could maintain immobilized patients. As early as 1967, when surgeon Christiaan Barnard transplanted Denise Darvall's heart into a dying patient named Louis Washkansky (discussed in Chapter 11), the question arose whether Denise Darvall had really been dead before her heart was removed. She obviously hadn't been declared dead by the whole-body standard since her healthy heart was exactly what was wanted for transplantation. Medicine needed a new standard of death, specifically of *brain death*, to determine when organs could be removed from a still-living body.

Although first described in the medical literature in 1959, brain death did not really become operational until Barnard transplanted a heart in late 1967.[33]

Shortly after that event, an ad hoc committee at Harvard Medical School developed the Harvard criteria of brain death.[34] The Harvard criteria operationally defined brain death as behavior that indicated unawareness of external stimuli, lack of bodily movements, no spontaneous breathing, lack of reflexes, and two isoelectric (nearly flat) electroencephalogram (EEG) readings 24 hours apart. These criteria required a loss of virtually all brain activity (including the brain stem, and hence breathing). The Harvard criteria personified caution: indeed, no one declared dead by these criteria has ever regained consciousness. (One could truly say, "If you're Harvard dead, you're really dead.") The extreme conservatism of the Harvard standard certainly disappoints people waiting for organ transplants from donors who must be declared brain dead: Relatively few potential donors (dying patients with healthy organs) have met the Harvard standard during the last 25 years.

Another standard of brain death is the *cognitive criterion.* This criterion identifies a philosophical core of properties of persons and assumes that without such a core, a human body is no longer a person; the core properties commonly include reason, memory, agency, and self-awareness. For example, neurological disorders such as Alzheimer's or Lewy body disease destroy brain cells at a high rate so that over a decade not much of the higher person remains. The cognitive criterion has the greatest potential to generate organs for transplantation. So far, however, this criterion has been considered too controversial and too vague to be adopted by any state, although countless families in fact act on it when they use it to agree to reduce treatment to speed a patient's death.[35]

A third standard of brain death, the *irreversibility standard,* falls between the Harvard and cognitive criteria. According to this standard, death occurs simply when unconsciousness is irreversible. Operationally, this judgment would be made by a neurologist and another physician. The irreversibility standard would allow PVS patients to be declared dead after several years (perhaps, in some cases, after several months). At the time of the first heart transplant in 1968, this standard was thought to be too broad.

The *Uniform Brain Death Act (UBDA)* attempted to provide a consistent definition of brain death that all states could use so that, for instance, a patient could not be dead in New Jersey, be taken across the George Washington Bridge, and be declared resurrected and alive in New York.[36] According to the UBDA standard, death occurs when there is irreversible loss of *all* brain function.

The UBDA may not have gone far enough. If it had been in effect in New Jersey during the Quinlan case or in Missouri during the Cruzan case, it would not have changed the outcome. Both Karen Quinlan and Nancy Cruzan had a functioning brain stem, and so neither of them would have met the UBDA standard.

To sum up standards of brain death:

- *Harvard Criteria.* Operational definition based on loss of nearly all brain functioning, with two nearly flat EEGs. Most conservative and least conducive to generate transplantable organs.
- *Cognitive Criterion.* Definition based on loss of core mental properties without which a body is no longer to be considered a person. Most liberal; most conducive to generate organs for transplant.
- *Irreversibility Standard.* Defines death as occurring when unconsciousness is irreversible (operationally, when PVS has lasted over 1 year). Less conservative than the Harvard criteria but not so liberal as the cognitive criterion; moderately conducive to obtaining organs for transplant.

One remarkable fact slowly becoming known during the Quinlan case, and again revealed years later when videotapes of patients like Nancy Cruzan were televised, is that a *person can be dead whose heart is beating and whose eyes are open and moving.*

In popular culture, some people believe that a uniform, metaphysical event with physical manifestations, marks death and perhaps as the counterpart of a similar event at the beginning of life. Some people would have described these metaphysical events as the entrance and departure of a soul. The occurrence of such metaphysical events of course cannot be proven, and even if they do occur, they seem to have no physical manifestations.

In medical reality, the definition of death is not so much a matter of discovery as a kind of decision that families and their physicians make. It is hence not so much an event as a process.

As it turns out, the phrase *brain death* misleads us in many ways. Newspapers commonly refer to someone as being "brain-dead" for months until "life support" is removed, after which the patient is said to "expire." Reformers such as North Carolina medical ethicist Lance Stell believe that such terms incorrectly imply that a patient could be dead in two different ways and that there are degrees of being dead. Such equivocation creates confusion about the epistemological criteria for declaring death, and implies that someone might die more than once. Stell thinks a more accurate phrase would be "death by neurological criteria." A being that meets these criteria, he says, "is not a patient but a cadaver." [37]

Proposals to redefine brain death today express conflicting needs of doing everything possible for an incompetent patient, allowing families to experience closure and control of a loved one, obtaining organs for transplantation, and preventing exorbitant medical costs. These opposed needs create controversies.

On the one hand, practical reformers want to end public uncertainty over brain death, expand the number of organs available for transplantation by having a universally accepted, practical definition of brain death, save the medical system money by not maintaining comatose patients, and help families move on after the death of a relative. On the other side, patient advocates want to give patients every chance of recovery.

Chances of Awakening from PVS

It is very important here to pay attention to the fact that several studies have documented that patients can recover after being comatose for over a year. In a study published in 1994 by the Multi-Society Task Force on PVS, of 434 adults with traumatic head injuries, seven made good recoveries and regained consciousness after being in PVS for more than 12 months.[38] None have ever done so after being comatose for 30 months (Karen and Nancy were in PVS longer than that). The above Task Force, after an extensive study of many cases of PVS patients, concluded that "recovery of consciousness from a post-traumatic persistent vegetative state is unlikely after 12 months in adults and children." It thus implied that medical maintenance of these patients after 12 months was futile because unconsciousness was irreversible.

Nevertheless, the seven recoveries warn against any quick judgment that a patient's condition is "irreversible." Indeed, some people would want to be given this

7 in 434 chance of recovery if they became a PVS patient. To date, however, no state has accepted the irreversibility standard.

In a more recent study of 19 patients with severe head injuries and persisting post-traumatic unawareness, 58 percent (11 patients) recovered within the first year and 5 percent (1 patient) within the second.[39] In another study of 34 patients with anoxic coma, 2 patients with "malignant EEG's" (the worst classification, where patients were expected to die based on lack of brain wave activity) eventually made a "good recovery."[40]

During the last decade, several people have awakened from PVS or PVS-like comas. On February 11, 1996, ex-policeman Gary Dockery of Chattanooga, Tennessee, garnered national attention when he emerged out of his coma of 8 years to talk for a few hours to his sons and family (after which he lapsed back into coma and died a year later in April).[41] On July 8, 1999, after lapsing into a coma during her pregnancy with twins, Maria Hernandez of Los Angeles awoke a month later and gave birth. (Compare this case to that of Nancy Klein [end of Chapter 7], where aborting her fetus brought her out of coma.) Sixteen years earlier, Patricia White Bull became comatose while delivering her fourth child and could not speak, swallow, or move much, but suddenly awakened to full consciousness on Christmas Eve 1999.

Whether anoxia or trauma causes the coma seems to make a difference in prognosis. More patients seem to emerge, especially in the first few months, after coma caused by trauma than by anoxia.

Whether any chance at all exists of coming out of PVS after a year, especially coma caused by anoxia, remains controversial within medicine. Probably such cases do occur but are extremely rare. That anyone at all comes out of long-term comas matters morally because it changes the prognosis from an absolute certainty to a probability. Families prefer to hear physicians say that the patient has "no" chance of recovery rather than a "miniscule" one because the later allows some hope to families.

PVS patients may eventually help us learn more about the anatomical basis of human consciousness. Neurologists now believe that consciousness has two components: wakefulness (or arousal) and awareness. On this analysis, PVS patients can be described as wakeful but not aware.

Mercy

In cases like Karen Quinlan's or Nancy Cruzan's, the Golden Rule might imply that, "If I ended up in a condition like Karen's or Nancy's, I would want to die, and I hope that those around me would be merciful enough to let me die. If I could somehow possibly be 'conscious' in such a state, I wouldn't want to go on. I wouldn't want to be imprisoned in such a body for months or years, which would be worse than being buried alive. Mercy requires us to make dying humane, not an endless torture."

Such a thought illustrates how the Golden Rule is ambiguous because some people might want a chance to recover, even if it is very slight. Doing whatever someone else wants must take into account that people differ in their personalities and wants.

The Quinlans and the Cruzans did argue that allowing Karen and Nancy to die would be merciful. The issue of mercy is relevant in these and similar cases because we can't know for certain that such patients do not feel—we cannot be certain that they do not experience sensations such as pain and discomfort; we may not even be certain that they do not experience distress, fear, frustration, loss, or other tormenting emotions.

In one 1996 survey of 250 medical directors of nursing homes and 250 neurologists, 30 percent of these physicians believed that PVS patients experienced pain.[42]

For example, Karen Quinlan's limbs were at first tied down, but her head moved violently, as if she were trying to dislodge the nasogastric feeding and ventilator tubes. That's why some of Karen's family—and their lawyer—said that Karen looked as if she were in pain. Julia Quinlan said, "[It] seems as if she's in pain by her facial expressions"; and, "They say she doesn't feel pain, but I wondered if they really knew."[43]

The question whether these phenomena were intentional behavior or merely reflexes raises philosophical as well as medical issues. *Intentional behavior* indicates an organism seeking some goal, such as freedom from pain, and might indicate awareness. As the seventeenth-century philosopher René Descartes noted, consciousness (awareness) in others is always an *inference* from outward behavior; it cannot be directly observed. Unconsciousness, or lack of consciousness, is also an inference. If we claim—as some people do—that flies aren't conscious, this is an inference from flies' behavior and from the comparative anatomy of flies and humans. As far as flies are concerned, we can make such inferences easily. In the case of a human being, however, a lot is at stake if we are wrong.

Consider *locked-in syndrome*, where patients are so extensively paralyzed that they can control nothing except blinking their eyes. Nevertheless, and perhaps unfortunately, these patients are perfectly conscious. This syndrome may have led to some live burials in the past. Could anything be more terrible to imagine than that? Perhaps: suppose that Karen Quinlan's mind was alive for 10 years inside her apparently comatose body.

Although a minority of neurologists believe that PVS patients experience pain, most do not. In the similar case of Paul Brophy in 1986, the American Academy of Neurology wrote:

> No conscious experience of pain and suffering is possible without the integrated functioning of the brain stem and cerebral cortex. Pain and suffering are attributes of consciousness, and PVS patients like Brophy do not experience them. Noxious stimuli may activate peripherally located nerves, but only a brain with the capacity for consciousness can transfer that neural activity into an experience.[44]

According to the Multi-Society Task Force on PVS, scanning devices show that brain activity of PVS patients falls far below that of patients with locked-in syndrome, and extensive neurological examinations of PVS patients during autopsies reveals deep lesions incompatible with awareness.[45]

Although these neurological findings may be reassuring, they do not resolve the issue of mercy. Even if there is only a small chance of awareness of pain, such a chance raises the issue of relief of misery for a vulnerable, incompetent patient.

Eventually, the cases of Karen Quinlan and Nancy Cruzan came to symbolize mercy as an issue for both patients and families. These cases seemed to represent an inversion of values in medicine: instead of doing what families wanted, medicine did what bureaucracies required; instead of a dignified death, breathing machines and feeding tubes maintained existence; instead of a quick death, there was slow withering over a decade of an emaciated body. On top of all that, the chance that a shell of a person might still exist in pain was too much for most people. For many people, the long dyings of these two patients were merciless.

PVS Patients: Costs of Care

The Multi-Task Force Study in 1994 estimated that in the United States between 10,000 and 25,000 adults and between 4,000 and 10,000 children were in PVS.[46] It is unclear how the neurologists arrived at this estimate, but it is likely incorrect partly (as this Task Force noted) because of lack of accepted, uniform diagnostic criteria for PVS. Even so, in France in 1973 the prevalence of PVS in the general population was 2.5/100,000 and a similar incidence was found in Japan of 2.0/100,000. The above figure from the Multi-Task Force Study puts the ratio at 4–10/100,000, but if the ratio from France and Japan holds for America, only about 5,000 adults would be in PVS in America and perhaps 2,000 children.

Costs per patient per year ranged then between $24,000 and $120,000.[47] The longest case of PVS so far has been that of Rita Greene, who became comatose in 1952, at age 24, after open-heart surgery in D.C. General Hospital in the District of Columbia and whose body still lives in a nursing home in West Virginia.[48]

PVS patients initially require round-the-clock monitoring by hospital personnel. Karen Quinlan and Nancy Cruzan required 24-hour nursing (in case an airway became clogged, leading to suffocation), expectorants and anticonvulsive drugs, changes of urinary catheters and tubes removing fecal waste, flexing of their muscles to prevent contractions, washing the body, brushing the teeth, treating dental cavities to prevent lethal mouth infections, and treating other infections with antibiotics.

When a hospital is left with a PVS patient after having done all it can, these facts create moral dilemmas for the hospital and the family. What is to be done with the patient? Few nursing homes will admit PVS patients, since the care these patients require is far beyond what most such homes can provide, especially if patients cannot swallow and are maintained by feeding tubes. In any case there is virtually no medical insurance that would cover long-term care of a PVS patient in a nursing home. Hardly any family can afford this care, which might easily cost $150,000 a year.

Kinds of Medical Support

Extraordinary versus Ordinary Treatment   In the years between the Quinlan case and the Cruzan case, physicians and philosophers debated whether certain levels of medical support had moral significance. The first concerned whether patients could be harmed by not receiving extraordinary, as opposed to ordinary, treatment. In 1957, a group of anesthesiologists asked Pope Pius XII what they owed dying patients. The pope said that they need not take heroic steps to keep such patients alive: patients were owed merely ordinary, but not extraordinary, treatments.

Unfortunately, the word *extraordinary* is equivocal as end points of a continuum that shifts with medical progress. In 1967, when Christiaan Barnard first transplanted a human heart, his heart-lung bypass machine was extraordinary. That machine was the forerunner of the large, bulky ventilator that kept Karen Quinlan breathing. Today, miniaturized ventilators—some small enough to be used with premature babies—are used everywhere in medicine. Yesterday's extraordinary treatment has become today's ordinary treatment, rendering the distinction much more fluid and unhelpful than it might at first seem.

Artificial Nutrition and Hydration   During the 1960s, artificial feeding of comatose patients was considered a temporary treatment. Patients unable to swallow were nourished by means of flexible plastic tubing which conveyed artificial, carefully balanced liquid nutrients to the gastrointestinal (GI) tract. Eventually, however, this treatment became an accepted way of indefinitely sustaining the bodies of dying and chronically ill patients.

In the 1980s, some people believed that whatever might be said about extraordinary and ordinary care in the future, providing food and water would always be considered ordinary and humane. They felt that such basic care was morally owed to PVS patients.

Arguments abounded in the 1980s for and against withdrawing nutrition and hydration. Some states allowed removal of respirators but not of feeding tubes, and champions of a sanctity-of-life worldview saw removal of feeding and hydration tubes as the immediate cause of death and hence as mercy killing. One such philosopher argued in 1983 that providing food and water to PVS patients is the ordinary care "that all human beings owe each other"; another argued at about the same time that such feeding involves "the most fundamental of all human relationships," and that "to tamper with, or adulterate, so enduring and central a moral emotion" is "a most dangerous business."[49]

On the other side are those who see artificial feeding either as prolonging the inevitable—dying—or as sustaining the body of a patient who is in fact already dead. People who argued this way gave little weight to the symbolic value of feeding and thought that equating withdrawal of nutrition with murder was conceptually confused. According to this view, the moral question here is simple: Does artificial feeding and hydration *benefit* or *burden* the patient?

It should be noted that, despite common beliefs to the contrary, neither dehydration nor starvation distresses semiconscious, dying patients. Patients near death not on nutritional support seem more comfortable than patients on whom such support is forced. One important national commission noted in 1983 that loss of appetite is "almost the norm in the latter stages of terminal illness" and concluded, "Only rarely should a dying patient be fed by tube or intravenously."[50] Indeed, such feeding may actually make the patient suffer and thus harm him or her.

The reality of feeding a chronically vegetative patient is not like spooning chicken soup into the mouth of a patient who is simply weak. Most vegetative patients have no swallowing reflexes, so they cannot be fed by mouth. Therefore, an artificial liquid diet must be mechanically introduced into their bodies. Artificial feeding is done in three basic ways: (1) by a temporary nasogastric tube run up the nostrils and down into the gastrointestinal tract; (2) by a permanent intravenous feeding line, surgically attached to one of the major veins of the chest; (3) by a surgically implanted gastrostomy tube. With many kinds of feeding tubes, patients must be tied down to avoid dislodging the line. All feeding tubes carry the risk of infection; with many, such a large volume of fluid is needed to supply the nutrients that other problems are caused. The chicken-soup image can distort people's impression of a PVS case. Karen Quinlan's sister, for example, thought that her comatose sister would look like Sleeping Beauty and was shocked by the emaciated figure she saw. By the time of Nancy Cruzan's case in 1990, improvements in artificial feeding would create the opposite effect: PVS patients now had rotund "Porky Pig" faces because of retention of fluids.

Furthermore, artificial feeding also requires medical support. Many physicians involved in caring for PVS patients during the late 1970s decided that artificial nutrition was by no means natural feeding, and that the artificial procedures were not simply "care" but highly sophisticated medical treatment. By the 1990s, most physicians had come to feel that artificial IV feeding lines for PVS patients were comparable to ventilators: both were advanced medical technology. The *Cruzan* decision in 1990 agreed with this view.

Not everyone agreed with the emerging idea that artificial nutrition and hydration is just another form of medical treatment, which can ethically be withdrawn for PVS patients. Several physicians and members of the clergy in conservative religions opposed such withdrawal.[51] However, most state courts now allow withdrawal of artificial nutrition and hydration. By 2000, sanctity-of-life champions for the most part had abandoned or changed their views about end-of-life treatment and shifted their attention to embryos, abortion, and stem cell research.

Withdrawing Treatment and Forgoing Treatment   During the last two decades, a central moral debate has concerned the degree to which a physician may be involved in hastening the death of a dying patient. One cause of this debate was a declaration by AMA in 1973 (two years before *Quinlan*):

> The intentional termination of the life of one human being by another—mercy killing—is contrary to that for which the medical profession stands and is contrary to the policy of the American Medical Association.
>   . . . The cessation of the employment of extraordinary means to prolong the life of the body when there is irrefutable evidence that biological death is imminent is the decision of the patient and/or immediate family.[52]

In this statement, the word *extraordinary* is ambiguous, and AMA policy did not clarify it. Are all patients on ventilators receiving extraordinary care? Is a physician who withdraws a dying patient's ventilator without the family's consent with the intent of termination of life guilty of mercy killing? What if the physician withdraws a feeding tube?

Concern about the possibility of being considered guilty of mercy killing led some physicians to *forgo* the use of ventilators and artificial feeding. Since withdrawal of such care might be seen as intentional termination of life (mercy killing), it was far easier to forgo medical support than to withdraw it. This reasoning created an odd situation, in which physicians would *forgo* the same treatment that they would not *withdraw*.

To others, it seemed that patients could be harmed both by the AMA's policy and by the interpretation that an extraordinary treatment could be forgone but not withdrawn. They believed that because the outcome is never certain, a patient is morally owed extraordinary treatment—both a ventilator and artificial feeding, for example—in order to see if recovery is possible. Also, some people argued that, regardless of whether a ventilator or a catheter was ordinary or extraordinary medical support, nobody really thought that a physician who withdrew such a device "killed" a terminally ill patient. In such a situation, we would say—if the patient had cancer—that cancer killed the patient, not the physician.

Kinds of Cases

When we engage in moral reasoning about people who are dying, it is helpful to distinguish among different kinds of cases. Consider how a society might ideally make decisions about death and dying. First, the courts would deliberate about *competent adult* patients with terminal diseases, defining these patients' right to refuse treatment. Second, the courts might rule on whether competent adults have a right to refuse medical treatment who are *not* terminally ill but desire to die because accidents or disease give them miserable quality of life (e.g., patients such as Elizabeth Bouvia and Larry McAfee, discussed in Chapter 3). Third, the courts might move to a very different kind of case, in which a surrogate or proxy is making decisions for a patient who once was but is no longer competent—an *incompetent but formerly competent* patient. A fourth kind of situation would include decision making by a surrogate for infant and child patients: in general, the category of *presently incompetent but later to be competent* patients. Finally, the courts would rule on whether or not special standards are needed for *never competent* patients (such as severely retarded babies and adults). Some of these cases raise difficult ethical questions with regard to evaluating quality of life, since what a competent person may see as an inferior quality of life may be perceived differently by an incompetent patient.

In summary, here are kinds of cases from easiest to judge to hardest:

(1) Competent patients who are terminally ill.
(2) Nonterminal competent patients with miserable quality of life.
(3) Formerly competent patients who are permanently incompetent.
(4) Patients who have never been competent and who never will be.

One would expect the reasons justifying a decision to die would need to be stronger as one moves down from (1) to (4).

In the *Quinlan* case, the decision of the New Jersey Supreme Court ran two different kinds of cases together, and looking back, we can see some confusion in this decision.[53] As we noted, the New Jersey Supreme Court based its decision partly on the right to privacy (liberty) as established by the United States Supreme Court in *Griswold* v. *Connecticut* in 1965, a right that, in a medical context, would presumably apply only to *competent* patients. But the standard of substituted judgment also grounded the decision that Karen's respirator could be disconnected, according to which relatives or friends can *substitute their judgment* for that of an *incompetent* patient.

Consequently, this decision had at least two major problems. First, how did the family's right to exercise substituted judgment derive from *Griswold*? Critics felt that the New Jersey court had jumped too quickly from married people's right to control their own reproduction (the situation in *Griswold*) to the parents' right to let an adult, comatose child die—since there had then been no intervening decisions about whether competent adults (terminally ill or not) had a right to hasten their own death by refusing medical treatment.

Given that quick, big jump, critics justifiably wondered what was next? Giving parents the right to make life-or-death decisions for never competent patients? Retarded babies?

Another problem had to do with the standard of substituted judgment itself, which is notoriously loose and subjective.[54] This standard (later used by several other state supreme courts) presumes that decisions made by a patient's family or friends will reflect what the patient himself or herself would have wanted done. In the *Quinlan* case, however, it was unclear whether Karen Quinlan had ever expressed a wish not to have her life prolonged if she became comatose, or even a wish that her parents should act for her in such a situation.

In any case, the implied liberty interest in the Constitution connoted by the right to privacy most obviously applies to competent patients and their rights to determine their own medical destinies. Ideally, our courts would have first laid out that right and then later tackled incompetent patients. But life is messy and things didn't happen that way, as the *Quinlan* decision showed. It took 15 years to get things somewhat straightened out by the *Cruzan* decision.

UPDATE

Advance Directives

One of the most controversial ethical and legal aspects of the Quinlan case was whether to withdraw medical support when the patient's wishes were not known. The fact that Karen Quinlan's wishes were unproven led some critics to condemn her family's decisions. Legal critics also said that *parens patria*, the ancient duty of courts to protect incompetents (a principle that had been accepted in English/ American law for centuries), had been abandoned by this court.

The *Quinlan* case caused written *advance directives* to become popular. Such advance directives can take several forms. A *living will* informs physicians about conditions under which a person would or would not want medical support continued. A *values inventory* specifies what a person values in life and may be useful to a patient's family and physicians if they must make decisions for that person. A *durable power of attorney* assigns to someone else the right to make financial and life-and-death medical decisions if the person becomes incompetent. In those states that allow it to be applied to medical decisions, durable power of attorney is the most powerful device for protecting the rights of dying people; however, not all states have statutes creating powers of attorney for proxy medical decisions. By 1990, 43 states had statutes recognizing some version of advance directives.[55] The decision in the *Cruzan* case emphasized that such a document would be crucial in meeting the "clear and convincing" standard required by New York and Missouri.

In December 1991, the Health Care Financing Administration (HCFA) required all American hospitals to ask incoming patients if they had, or wanted to sign, an advance directive. This requirement increased the use of advance directives and has forced hospitals to specify their policies about honoring such directives.

A major problem of advance directives is that most people do not accurately predict how they will feel later when they are actually near death. According to an important 1995 study, most competent people change their minds when actually faced with a decision to decline treatment and die, despite having predicted the opposite about themselves many years before.[56]

If this is true for competent patients, what can we infer about the wishes of incompetent patients? Neither the best interests standard nor the substituted judgment standard are decisive: If a patient has a small chance of coming out of a yearlong coma, aren't his best interests in being kept alive? If he had known these odds, would he have wanted to be given the chance? Whose judgment substitutes for his, especially if his choice was made in semi-ignorance?

Advance directives often do not cover nonterminal, though permanently comatose, patients. Only a few advanced directives are thorough enough and specify whether food and water is included under unwanted medical treatment or name a specific person to be a proxy for the incompetent patient. Because such directives are only requested of patients upon admission to hospitals, most people under 30 do not have one.

Hospital Ethics Committees

Although Hospital Ethics Committees (HECs) have become popular in the last decades, they have only a limited role in resolving these decisions because of inherent problems about their powers, role, and membership. Almost all such committees are advisory, meaning that the physician of record on the case can ignore them. Because volunteers largely comprise such committees, the commitment of time of members is often very limited. Even with such caveats, such committees do wield some power, such that some physicians resist bringing cases to them. ("Wouldn't it hurt me," one said, "if I was being sued and it was on record that I went against the HEC recommendation?") Finally, consider that the composition of HECs can easily predict the outcome: One hospital can have a rubber-stamp committee by appointing weak people, or another, a strong, powerful committee by appointing strong personalities and giving them real power. The latter possibility worries most physicians: They ask whether we really want to practice medicine by committee? To take away power from the physician at the bedside?

HECs perhaps work best in institutions such as religious hospitals or the Veterans Administration hospitals where nurses, physicians, clergy, and ethicists work together to make policies consistent, educate staff, and, on occasion, consult on cases. These committees are largely internal to the hospital, not ones with many volunteers or laypeople.

Ethics of Withdrawing Support

In 1975, Karen Quinlan's physicians—Morse and Javed—were upholding the official position of AMA: that withdrawing medical support from a patient was the same as "active euthanasia." In 1986, the AMA changed its policy to reflect a new understanding of chronically comatose patients supported by ventilators and artificial nutrition. Now it was ethically possible for a physician, after consulting with the family, to withdraw a ventilator and feeding tubes from an irreversibly comatose patient. This new AMA policy did not say that being irreversibly comatose was equivalent to being brain dead. Criteria for ethical removal of medical support differ from a state's legal standard of brain death. Physicians, under AMA policy, can remove support from patients who are not legally dead under a state's laws.

The *Cruzan* case, unlike the *Quinlan* case, focused on removal of a feeding tube. As noted earlier, the *Cruzan* Supreme Court (1990) saw no difference between withdrawing artificial nutrition and withdrawing other kinds of medical support.

Medical Futility

In December 1991, Helga Wanglie, age 87, had been in PVS for eight months, sustained by a ventilator and a feeding tube, at Hennepin County Hospital in Minneapolis, Minnesota.[57] At the hospital the physicians' decision to withdraw treatment opposed the wishes of the patient's husband, Oliver Wanglie, who refused his permission for discontinuation of her respirator and feeding tube.

The *Wanglie* case was unusual for two reasons. First, since Helga Wanglie's medical insurance covered her hospitalization, the hospital would actually lose money by withdrawing artificial life support. Second, the case involved an ethical and philosophical dispute about whether a medical team could be forced by a family member to continue care it regarded as futile. When Helga Wanglie died, the legal case ended, and the Hennepin County physicians did not continue to seek a precedent in the courts; however, about half a dozen other cases of medical futility were heard by courts and hospital ethics committees.[58]

In Massachusetts in a nasty court suit, physicians were sued in the 1989 *Gilgunn* case for removing medical support they unanimously believed to be futile. Even though the jury agreed that Caroline Gilgunn would have wanted to remain on life support, the physicians won in 1995 because the court agreed that patients could not force physicians to render futile treatment.

During the 1990s, *medical futility* was widely discussed. The concept is semi-evaluative, but this aspect can be obscured by the desire of clinical physicians for an objective standard for ending care.[59] It is noteworthy that those who brought the *Wanglie* case were mainly *physician bioethicists:* When bioethics first developed, few physicians entered the field, but this has changed over the last two decades.

Medical futility held out the promise in 1990 that a descriptive concept could help physicians and families easily make decisions about treatments of minimal benefit at the end of life, but a decade later, most physicians and bioethicists had realized that the promise masked too many ethical and emotional issues. Today, the "medical futility movement" has largely waned.

Pressure from families for presumably futile care is rare. Most American patients and their families now decline treatment when their physicians advise them that there is no realistic chance of recovery. A study in 1994 that followed over 4,000 patients whose condition was diagnosed as life-threatening or terminal found that only 14 percent of them were resuscitated after being near death. This figure was far less than most physicians predicted and far less than it would have been a decade earlier, when most of those patients would have been resuscitated.[60]

In the same year as this 1994 study, Richard Nixon died of a stroke and Jacqueline Kennedy Onassis of cancer. Both deaths symbolized a new attitude toward declining medical interventions in terminal situations. Richard Nixon had left instructions that he was not to be connected to a respirator or resuscitated; and Jacqueline Onassis, when she was told that no further medical treatment would help her, simply went home to die.

Hugh Finn

Controversy erupted in 1998 when the Republican Governor of Virginia disputed a wife's right to remove the feeding tube of her husband, Hugh Finn, who had been in PVS for 3 years.[61] Hugh Finn, a former television anchorman in Louisville, Kentucky, had prepared a document stating that he would not want to live in a persistent vegetative state sustained by a feeding tube. Unfortunately, before he could sign it, a terrible automobile accident severed his aorta and left his brain anoxic for many minutes. His resulting coma left him unable to eat, care for himself, or communicate.

Or so it seemed, until a nurse claimed that he had said "Hi" to her when she smoothed his hair. This prompted Hugh's brother John to challenge a request by Hugh's wife, Michelle, to remove his feeding tube so Finn's story could end. John was joined in this suit by Hugh's parents. John lost in court, but Governor James S. Gilmore III asked the Virginia Supreme Court to overrule a lower court order permitting removal of the feeding tube. Gilmore ordered that such a removal would be "mercy killing or euthanasia." The high Court agreed with the lower court judge that removal would merely "permit the natural process of dying" and not be mercy killing or euthanasia.

In the similar case in Alabama in the 1990s of Correan Salter, opponents fought against the next-of-kin's wishes in part because it is so difficult to believe that a person is not present in a body with open, moving eyes. Mrs. Salter had signed an advanced directive, but lent it to a friend, who lost it. Mrs. Salter's coma lasted 7 years, but because no advanced directive could be produced, Judge Pamela Baschab ruled that the "clear and convincing standard" of *Cruzan* had not been met (which had never previously been taken to be the legal standard in Alabama), and hence, the feeding tube could not be removed.

In these two cases, two points are noteworthy. First, opponents may make it almost impossible for a patient in PVS to die if no advanced directive is present. Even though no one has ever emerged from PVS of 3 years' duration, opponents hope that, miraculously, someone might still be alive "in there." Second, in this hope the logic is curious, because there is a dilemma here, acceptance of either horn of which argues for removal of the feeding tube. If someone is not "in there," then the arguments are moot. On the other hand, if someone is "in there," then arguments for mercy perhaps should win, for who would want to exist as a flicker of consciousness inside a paralyzed body, unable to speak or move, for 3, 7, or 20 years?

FURTHER READING

Margaret Battin, *The Least Worst Death: Essays in Bioethics at the End of Life*, Oxford University Press, New York, 1993.

Joanne Lynn, ed., *By No Extraordinary Means: The Choice to Forgo Life-Sustaining Food and Water*, expanded ed., 1989, Indiana University Press, Bloomington, 1989.

Pat Milmoe McCarrick, "Scope Note 7: Withholding or Withdrawing Nutrition or Hydration," National Reference Center for Bioethics Literature at the Kennedy Institute of Ethics, Georgetown University, Washington, D.C., updated, November 1986.

Sherman Nuland, M.D. *How We Die: Reflections on Life's Final Chapter* (Vintage books, 1995).

Web Links/Medi

Coma Recovery Association, Inc. — ww.comarecovery.org/

Karen Ann Quinlan Hospice, Inc. — www.karenannquinlanhospice.org/

CHAPTER 3

Requests to Die

Elizabeth Bouvia and Larry McAfee

*T*his chapter discusses the cases of Elizabeth Bouvia and Larry McAfee, two people with nonterminal physical disabilities who decided that they no longer wanted to live.

BACKGROUND: PERSPECTIVES ON SUICIDE

Greece and Rome

Ancient Greek aristocrats strove not simply to live, but to live with nobility, honor, excellence, and beauty. They believed that "the unexamined life is not worth living," and that "the really important thing is not to live but to live well." They thought that philosophy would give them the wisdom to approach death in the same way as life (the word *philosophy* means "love of wisdom"). Plato records Socrates as saying, "True philosophers make dying their profession, and . . . to them of all men, death is least alarming. . . . So if you see one distressed at the prospect of dying, it will be proof that he is a lover not of wisdom but of the body."[1]

Socrates' own death is one of the most famous in history: Sentenced to die for his beliefs, Socrates could have fled his beloved Athens but instead chose to drink the poison hemlock. At his death scene, he talked about the nature of death with his friend Cebes. In this discussion, Cebes says that it is easy not to fear death if one is convinced of life after death, but he himself believes that the soul "may be dispersed and destroyed on the very day that the man himself dies [and] may be dissipated like breath or smoke, and vanish away, so that nothing is left of it anywhere. . . . No one but a fool is entitled to face death with confidence, unless he can prove that the soul is absolutely immortal and indestructible." Socrates replies that the soul may indeed be immortal, but if it is not, then death is like a sleep from which one never awakes. If death is sleep, there is nothing to fear in death, because no one will exist who can feel pain or miss life.

Hemlock is a poison that acts (like nicotine) by decreasing circulation at the extremities, creating the sensation of distal numbness, and eventually stopping the heart. During Socrates' and Cebes' abstract discussion, the hemlock has been taking effect on Socrates, working up from his toes to his legs. As the discussion ends, the state poisoner finds that since Socrates' thighs are numb, he will die in minutes, when the poison reaches his heart. As his friends begin to cry, Socrates says, "Calm yourselves and try to be brave!" He dies moments later and his admiring follower, Plato and the author of this account, writes, "Such . . . was the end of our comrade, who was, we may fairly say, of all those whom we knew in our time, the bravest and also the wisest and most upright man."

Centuries later, in ancient Rome, the emperor Marcus Aurelius (portrayed in the 2000 movie *Gladiator*) and the slave-philosopher Epictetus celebrated suicide as more courageous than an undignified life of pain. The Roman Stoics defended the *argument for the open door:* "If the room is smoky, if only moderately, I will stay; if there is too much smoke, I will go. Remember this, keep a firm hand on it, the door is always open."[2] Seneca wrote about old age: "If it begins to shake my mind, if it destroys my faculties one by one, if it leaves me not life but breath, I will depart the putrid or the tottering edifice."[3] (The argument for the open door would be revived in the twentieth century by the existentialist philosopher Jean-Paul Sartre, who emphasized that choice—even the choice of staying alive each day— is inescapable.[4])

Jesus and Augustine

According to the New Testament, Jesus prohibited killing and advocated pacifism; but the primary focus of his message as presented in the gospels—contrary to widespread belief—was not to impart a morality to live by but rather to establish a new spiritual relationship with God. His dominant message is: repent of sin, ask forgiveness of God, be born again, and be ready for the dawning kingdom of God, which will come very soon. In Matthew, he says to his disciples, "There be some standing here, which shall not die, till they see the Son of Man coming in his kingdom."[5] As Alasdair MacIntyre writes in his *Short History of Ethics:*

> The paradox of Christian ethics is precisely that it has always tried to devise a code for society as a whole from pronouncements which were addressed to individuals or small communities to separate themselves off from the rest of society. This is true both of the ethics of Jesus and of the ethics of St. Paul. Both Jesus and St. Paul preached an ethics devised for a short interim period before God finally inaugurated the Messianic kingdom and history was brought to its conclusion. We cannot, therefore, expect to find in what they say a basis for life in a continuing society.
>
> . . . St. Paul's dislike of marriage as other than expedient ("It is better to marry than burn") is not so inhumane as unhistorically minded secularists have made it out to be, if it is understood in terms of the pointlessness of satisfying desires and creating relationships which will hinder one from obtaining the rewards of eternal glory in the very near future. . . . [But] the crucial fact is that the Messianic kingdom did not come, and that therefore the Christian church ever since has been preaching an ethics which could not find application in a world where history had not come to an end.[6]

To begin with, Jesus' original views are open to different interpretations. Also, whatever his original views were, they must differ significantly from modern

Christian doctrines, which are complex and vary widely. Furthermore, in its nearly 2,000 years, Christianity itself has become fragmented into different churches, denominations, and sects; and its doctrines have been profoundly interpreted and reinterpreted. Although many Christian theologians and church leaders have made confident assertions, they have often disagreed with each other, and there seems to be no way for us to know which of them is *the* Christian truth.

Certain key ideas of the organized religion now called Christianity were actually formed not by Jesus but by later thinkers. Some of these ideas were developed in the fourth century of the Christian or Common era (C.E.), by Augustine, who condemned suicide as "detestable and damnable wickedness."

The Bible contains no explicit prohibition of suicide (in fact, it seems to condone the suicides of Saul and Judas), and Augustine based his condemnation on the sixth commandment (Exodus 20:13), best known today as translated in the King James version: "Thou shalt not kill." However, a more accurate translation of either the Hebrew or the Greek words would be: "Thou shalt not commit wrongful killing"—and in this translation the commandment offers much less guidance, because there is a question which killings are wrongful and which are not. (Only a few pages after the ten commandments, at Exodus 23:23, God commands Moses to lead the Israelites in attacking neighboring tribes such as the Hittites and does not distinguish between killing enemy soldiers and killing civilians.)

Augustine distinguishes between *private killing* and killing that is carried out at the orders of a divine or divinely constituted authority. Private killing, or killing undertaken "on one's own authority," is never right[7], but according to Augustine, not all killing is private. God may command a killing, and when this is the case, full obedience is required. Such a command may take two forms: It may come directly from God (as when God commands Abraham to sacrifice Isaac) or it may be required by a just law. With either form, the individual who does the killing does not do it on his or her own authority but is simply an "instrument," a sword in God's hand, and thus is not morally accountable.

This reasoning underlies the permissibility of capital punishment and killing in war: Both are performed by people who are acting in accordance with law. The worldly Ambrose had already said that Christians could kill in war, and Augustine went even further by condoning war against heretics. Frederick Russell in *The Just War in the Middle Ages* says that through Augustine, "the New Testament doctrines of love and purity were accommodated to the savagery of the Old Testament and pacifism was defeated."[8]

Augustine apparently did not condone killing in self-defense, although present-day Catholic moral theology does allow it for persons who are not capable of attaining the "higher way" of self-sacrifice.[9]

One problem with Augustine's view is that he gives no explanation of how he knows that certain forms of killing are ordered by God and other forms are forbidden. How do we know that he is not begging the question when he assumes that the sixth commandment forbids suicide? In Protestant Christianity (which of course developed much later than Augustine), this problem becomes even more serious, since the interpretation of God's will is a more individual process.

It may seem natural to ask whether it really matters that Jesus did not talk about suicide, or that Augustine's argument presents difficulties. Does all that have anything to do with modern Christianity? Isn't it enough to know the general intent of Jesus's teachings and the present Christian view about suicide? The answer is, perhaps not.

With regard to applied ethics, such problems increase. Quakers, Mennonites, and the Amish, for example, have always rejected Augustine's position and followed the original pacifism of the early church. How do they know that Augustine was mistaken? Today, some devout Christians support capital punishment but reject suicide. How do they know that suicide is sinful but killing a criminal is not?

Some people, of course, simply believe that God's will is whatever they have been taught; and some also believe that questioning God's will is blasphemy, an insult to God. This approach holds danger in medical ethics. As Paul Badham writes:

> As Church Historian, I am very conscious of how Christians of previous ages have vehemently denounced medical practices which today no Christian would dream of questioning. For centuries Christians forbade giving of medicine, the practice of surgery, the study of anatomy, or the dissection of corpses for medical research. Later the practice first of inoculation and then of vaccination faced fierce theological condemnation, as did the initial use of quinine against malaria. The introduction of anesthesia, and above all the use of chloroform in childbirth, were seen as directly challenging the divine edict that "in pain you shall bring forth children" (Genesis 3:16), and hence were violently denounced from pulpits throughout Britain and the U.S.A.[10]

Bioethics today faces problems which could never have been imagined by the people who wrote the Bible: patenting genes, defining brain death, withdrawing advanced medical technology, financing medical care, experimenting on animals. However, if everything has a purpose, then our ability to think critically exists for a purpose. If we believe in God, is it blasphemy to believe that we were given minds to reflect on these questions? The philosophical approach to bioethics assumes that for those who seek God's will, reasoning and knowledge of history are compatible with their quest.

Western Philosophers

Aquinas   The thirteenth-century philosopher and theologian Thomas Aquinas held that suicide is sinful for several reasons; in fact, he considered it the most dangerous of sins because it left no time for repentance. Aquinas felt that suicide is wrong because life is a gift from God and only God can take life back (ever since, Thomists have argued vigorously for this view). He also argued that suicide hurts the community by depriving it of talented people, and that it is sinful because it deprives children of their parents. Finally, Aquinas said, suicide is unnatural, going against the instinct of self-preservation.

Montaigne, Spinoza, and Donne   The French essayist Michel de Montaigne in the sixteenth century, the Dutch philosopher Baruch Spinoza, and the English poet John Donne in the seventeenth condoned suicide. Montaigne concluded his essay "To Philosophize Is to Learn How to Die" by saying, "If we have learned how to live properly and calmly, we will know how to die in the same manner."[11] Spinoza wrote, "A free man, that is to say, a man who lives according to the dictates of reason alone, is not led by the fear of death."[12] Donne wrote, "When the [terminal] disease would not reduce us, [God] sent a second and worse affliction, ignorant and torturing physicians."[13]

Kant   The German philosopher Immanuel Kant strongly opposed suicide. He based this conclusion on several arguments.

First, for Kant an act is right if it represents or is based on a maxim (rule) that can be *universalized,* that is, a rule we would want everyone to act on. Kant argued that suicide cannot be universalized, because its motive is self-interest (for instance, escaping pain); for Kant, self-interest can never justify an action. Since we cannot universalize the maxim that people may commit suicide, suicide is immoral.

Second, Kant argued that suicide is immoral because people should always be treated as *ends in themselves,* never as *mere means.* He reasoned that treating oneself as an "end" entails recognizing one's own free will as an absolute (rather than a relative) value, but destroying oneself by committing suicide means destroying that freedom of will. "Man's freedom cannot subsist except on a condition which is immutable. This condition is that man not use his freedom against himself to his own destruction."[14]

Third, Kant argued that a person "who does not respect his life even in principle cannot be restrained from the most dreadful vices." In other words, if I do not respect my own life, I cannot really respect anything at all; to respect the general principle that life is sacred, I must respect the sacredness of my own life.

Finally, like Aquinas, Kant held that we have a moral duty to live because our lives are not really our own possession: "Human beings are sentinels on earth and may not leave their posts until relieved by another beneficent hand. God is our owner; we are His property."

Hume   In the eighteenth century, Scottish philosopher David Hume—Kant's contemporary—argued that suicide "is no transgression of our duty to God" and made the somewhat humbling observation, "The life of a man is of no greater importance to the universe than that of an oyster."[15] In his famous "Essay on Suicide," he disagreed with Augustine and Aquinas, who had both held that suicide violates the will of God. Especially for dying patients, Hume believed, voluntary death is not a sin: "A house which falls by its own weight, is not brought to ruin by [God's] providence."[16] Hume believed that if God had made the world through the laws of causality—the laws of physics, medicine, etc.—then disease merely expressed the natural working of such laws.

Hume also attacked the idea that suicide is blasphemous. To Kant's view that we have a station in life which is assigned by God and which we must not give up, Hume replied, "It is a kind of blasphemy to imagine that any created being can [by taking his own life] disturb the order of the world. Any suicide is insignificant to the workings of the universe and it is blasphemy to think otherwise." To Hume, it was self-indulgent to think that the world's smooth functioning required one's own continued existence.

Against Aquinas's argument that suicide harms the community, Hume argued:

> A man who retires from life does no harm to society; he only ceases to do good; which, if it is an injury, is of the lowest kind. All our obligations to do good to society seem to imply something reciprocal. I receive benefits of society, and therefore ought to promote its interests; but when I withdraw myself altogether from society, can I be bound any longer? But [even] allowing that our obligations to do good were perpetual, they have certainly some bounds; I am not obliged to do a small good to society at the expense of a great harm to myself: when then should I prolong a miserable existence, because of some frivolous advantage which the public may perhaps receive from me?

Mill   John Stuart Mill presented his *principle of harm* in *On Liberty* (1859), in one of the most famous passages in western political philosophy:

> [There is] one very simple principle, [that is] entitled to govern absolutely the dealings of society with the individual in the way of compulsion and control, whether the means used is physical force in the form of legal penalties, or the moral coercion of public opinion. That principle is, that the sole end for which mankind are warranted, individually or collectively, in interfering with the liberty of action of any of their number, is self-protection. That the only purpose for which power can be rightfully exercised over any member of a civilized community, against his will, is to prevent harm to others. His own good, either physical or moral, is not a sufficient warrant. . . . The only part of the conduct of any one, for which he is amenable to society, is that which concerns others. In the part which merely concerns himself, his independence is, of right, absolute. Over himself, over his own body and mind, the individual is sovereign.[17]

According to Mill's principle, with regard to our own lives and bodies, we can do whatever we want, so long as others are not harmed. Mill distinguished between *self-regarding* and *other-regarding* acts and argued that only other-regarding acts are subject to moral criticism.

Interestingly, Mill's analysis can be used both for and against suicide. On one hand, it can be can argued that taking one's own life is clearly self-regarding; in fact, suicide is often described as the ultimate private issue. On the other hand, it can also be argued that one should not commit suicide because suicide is an other-regarding act.

It does seem that most acts of suicide are other-regarding in some way: When someone commits suicide, parents, children, friends, colleagues, physicians, students, and others are deeply affected. In fact, since motives for suicide include spite and malevolence, a suicide may be deliberately other-regarding—it may be intended to hurt other people by making them feel guilty, sorry, or incompetent. On the basis of Mill's principle of harm, such a motivated suicide would not be excusable.

What about a suicide that inadvertently harmed others? There is a general problem with Mill's principle. Very few of our actions are completely self-regarding, and it is arguable that anyone who contemplates suicide should be aware of that.

As John Donne wrote, "No man is an island, entire of itself; every man is a piece of the continent, a part of the main."

When the American feminist Charlotte Perkins Gilman killed herself in 1935, she left a note saying that she preferred "chloroform to cancer." In an essay published posthumously, she wrote: "The record of a previously noble life is precisely what makes it sheer insult to allow death in pitiful degradation. We may not wish to 'die with our boots on,' but we may well prefer to 'die with our brains on.'"[18]

We do not know whether Gilman's husband, children, and friends agreed with her decision to kill herself, but we certainly know they did not view her act as purely self-regarding.

Hume might reply that a man who "withdraws" from society does little harm, and if he thereby prevents great harm to himself from continued life, the risk-benefit ratio is justified. Yet Hume's view of suicide seems most to apply to lifelong bachelors such as he was, not to a 36-year-old mother with three small kids, husband, and her own parents—all of whom would miss her terribly if she took her own life.

The Modern Era

A century ago, only the poor and people without families went to a hospital to die; today, more than 80 percent of Americans die in hospitals. Before the Harrison Act of 1914, Americans could legally purchase heroin and other opiates to lessen the pain of terminal illnesses such as cancer; today, this is not possible. Before World War II, most people died of sudden-onset, acute diseases such as pneumonia and cholera. Today, most people live longer and die more slowly from emphysema, diabetes, cardiomyopathy, cancer, and coronary artery disease. Because of changes like these, choosing to end one's life has become a prominent issue.

In the late nineteenth century and the twentieth century, suicide has come to be seen as a medical, psychological, or social problem rather than as a moral issue. Some nineteenth-century physicians had imputed suicide to heredity, imbalances in body chemistry, or even the shape of the head; around the turn of the century, Émile Durkheim analyzed it in terms of sociology rather than pathology. Today, suicide is associated with emotional disorders such as clinical depression.

THE BOUVIA CASE

The Patient: A Woman with Cerebral Palsy

In September 1983, Elizabeth Bouvia's father drove her from Oregon to Riverside General Hospital in California, where she was diagnosed as suicidal and admitted to the psychiatric ward as a voluntary patient. She stated that she wanted "just to be left alone and not bothered by friends or family or anyone else and to ultimately starve to death." "Death is letting go of all burdens," she said. "It is being able to be free of my physical disability and mental struggle to live."[19] She claimed that at least once she had already attempted suicide.

Twenty-five years old and almost totally paralyzed from cerebral palsy, Elizabeth Bouvia had never had the use of her legs. She had some control over her right hand (enough to operate a battery-powered wheelchair and to smoke cigarettes) and enough control of her facial muscles to chew, swallow, and speak.

Her life had never been easy. After her parents divorced when she was 5 years old, she lived with her mother until age 10, when her mother placed her in a children's home. The following account comes from two physicians:

> For their 18th birthday, some children receive cars and gifts. When [Elizabeth Bouvia] turned 18, her father, a postal inspector, told her that he would no longer be able to care for her because of her disabilities. The chief of psychiatry at Riverside says that what she did next showed great drive and promise. She gathered her requisite amount of state aid and lived on her own in an apartment with a live-in nurse. Although she earlier had dropped out of high school, she completed her general equivalency degree and went on to graduate from San Diego State University with a bachelor's degree in 1981. She even entered a master's program at the university's School of Social Work, but left in 1982 over a disagreement about her field work placement.
>
> . . . For eight months, she worked as a volunteer in the San Diego placement program, but she has never been employed for salary or wages.
>
> . . . During the last year, Ms. Bouvia faced a series of devastating events. In August, 1982, she married an ex-convict, Richard Bouvia, with whom she had been corresponding by mail. Together they conceived a child, but a few months later she suffered a miscarriage.
>
> . . . Her husband's part-time job did not provide enough income for the two to live decently, so they called her father to ask for help. He declined to aid them, Richard Bouvia said. They next went to Richard Bouvia's sister in Iowa to ask for help. That did not work out for long, and soon they ended up back in Oregon, where Richard Bouvia still could not find work. At that point, he abandoned her, stating—according to pleadings in the case—that he "could not accept her disabilities, a miscarriage, and rejection by her parents."
>
> . . . A few days later, Elizabeth Bouvia got a ride to Riverside General and wheeled herself into the emergency room, complaining that she wanted to commit suicide.[20]

In addition to her problems with her husband and father, she had severe degenerative arthritis, which caused great pain even though she was paralyzed. As a resident of California (she had lived in Riverside as well as in Oregon), she was eligible for Medi-Cal, a substantial supplement to Medicaid for the indigent.

The Legal Battle: Refusing Sustenance

Elizabeth Bouvia's first attending physician, for the 4 months from September to late December, was Donald Fisher, chief of psychiatry at Riverside Hospital. Since Fisher was unwilling to let her starve herself to death as she intended, she contacted the American Civil Liberties Union (ACLU) and also telephoned a reporter. Richard Scott of Beverly Hills, who was both a physician and a lawyer, took her on as a *pro bono* (charity) case.

In the first hearing—before a California probate judge, John Hews—Fisher testified that he believed his patient would eventually change her mind, that he would not let her starve, and that he would force-feed her if necessary: "The court cannot order me to be a murderer nor to conspire with my staff and employees to murder Elizabeth."[21] Elizabeth Bouvia asked Judge Hews to enjoin the hospital from feeding her.

At this point, the Bouvia case "escalated into a public debate":

> Disabled individuals held vigils at the hospital to convince her to change her mind. Bouvia's estranged husband hitchhiked to Riverside from Iowa, retained lawyers, and asked to be named her legal guardian. He charged the ACLU with using his wife as a "guinea pig." She filed for divorce. Columnist Jack Anderson's offer to raise funds for Bouvia's treatment was rebuffed. Richard Nixon sent a letter to Bouvia to "keep fighting." A meeting with President Reagan was discussed. Two neurosurgeons offered free surgery to help her gain the use of her arms. A convicted felon volunteered to shoot her.[22]

In December 1983, the day after the closing arguments had been completed, Judge Hews decided to allow the force-feeding. Hews acknowledged that the patient was rational, sincere, and fully competent; his decision was based on the probable effects *on others* of allowing her to starve: the "profound effect on the medical staff, nurses, and administration of the hospital," as well as the "devastating effect on other . . . physically handicapped persons."[23] Hews indicated that his decision was influenced by Advocates for the Developmentally Disabled, which had held candlelight vigils outside Riverside Hospital, fearing that if Elizabeth Bouvia died, other disabled people would choose to do the same. This attitude was also expressed by a lawyer at the Law Institute for the Disabled, who asserted that Elizabeth Bouvia symbolized a "social problem" of disabled people (they are told by society that they cannot be productive) and said, "She needs to learn to live with dignity."[24] Elizabeth Bouvia's lawyer described Hews as having accepted "the Chicken Little defense that the sky would fall if Ms. Bouvia wasn't force-fed."[25]

Habeeb Bacchus, associate chief of medicine at Riverside Hospital, became Elizabeth Bouvia's second physician (indigent patients and those in university hospitals have different physicians each month, as the attending physician changes). Bacchus worried that letting her die would depress other disabled people: "Being allowed to die when there's no need for her to die—this is a dangerous precedent. Patients might wonder, 'Am I next slated to be allowed to die?'"[26] Judge Hews allowed the force-feeding to continue under Bacchus, holding that since the patient was not terminally ill and could live for decades, "there is no other reasonable option."

Columnist Arthur Hoppe felt otherwise:

> I had the feeling that the judge, the doctor, and the hospital had found Elizabeth Bouvia guilty—guilty of not playing the game. It was as though the Easter Seal Child had looked into the camera and said being crippled was a lousy deal and certainly nothing to smile about.[27]

The law professor George Annas also disagreed bitterly with Hews:

> The judge's decision begs the question: Is there a reasonable option? In the adversary proceeding played out in California, no one seemed to search for reasonable options. The county, in fact, consistently took the most extreme position. It continually threatened to eject Ms. Bouvia from the hospital by force, and leave her out on the front sidewalk, hoping someone would pick her up and take her away. Almost from the beginning, the county and hospital made it clear that they did not care whether she lived or died but, because of their own fear of potential legal liability, would not let her die at Riverside Hospital.[28]

While Elizabeth Bouvia appealed, physicians in California argued about her. Laurens White, who later became president of the California Medical Association, said, "The most troublesome thing about this [case is that] Mrs. Bouvia's First Amendment rights may hit somebody else's medical ethics right between the eyes. . . . Refusal to take water and food is not suicide. Providing care while a patient is doing this is a tough thing, but I think she should have the right to do it. Forcing her to eat is battery."[29] With regard to Fisher's original force-feeding, White said, "He's full of it. . . . He's just completely off the wall about this." Bacchus retorted: "It is very simple. Physicians, if they err, should err on the side of saving life. When it comes to criminal charges, wrongful death is more of a crime than battery, so there you have it."[30]

Force-feeding Elizabeth, a plastic tubing was inserted in her mouth, but she bit through it. Thereafter, four attendants held her down and inserted a plastic tube through her nose into her stomach and a liquid diet was pumped in. Annas commented on this gruesome scene:

> I do not believe competent adults should ever be force-fed; but efforts at persuading the individual to change his or her mind, and offering oral nutrition should continue. If a court determines, however, that invasive force-feeding is required, . . . then to [prevent] hospitals from becoming the most hideous torture chambers, some reasonable limit must be placed on this "treatment."[31]

Elizabeth Bouvia lost her first appeal to have the lower-court decision reversed, and she left Riverside Hospital on April 7, 1984. What happened at that point has been interpreted differently by different commentators. So how did these commentators interpret these events?

On September 22, 1985, Elizabeth Bouvia entered Los Angeles County-USC Medical Center (the hospital with the largest number of beds in the United States), where physicians installed a morphine pump to control the pain caused by her worsening arthritis. At this public hospital, staff accepted her declaration that she would eat and live; she was not force-fed; and she was not required to socialize with other patients.

After 2 months, she was transferred to nearby High Desert Hospital, another public hospital. Although apparently she ate voluntarily at High Desert, her physicians there decided that she wasn't eating enough and began force-feeding her. Their rationale was that "since she is occupying our space, she must accede to the same care which we afford every other patient admitted here, care designed to improve and not detract from chances of recovery and rehabilitation."[32] Several critics thought it odd to say that a patient who "occupies" hospital "space" must do what the hospital dictates. (That would make an interesting slogan for a hospital's advertising.)

The question whether or not the patient was eating enough is of some importance, because she soon petitioned the courts again to have the forced feeding stopped. At this time, she weighed only 70 pounds. A consultant on nutrition had noted on her chart that a weight of 75 or 85 pounds "might be desirable," and her physicians wanted to achieve an ideal weight of 104 to 114 pounds. Keep in mind that because of her paralysis, her muscle mass was slight, and so her ideal body weight would be much lower than normal for a person of her height (5 feet).

At the new hearing, a new judge—Judge Warren Deering— interpreted her weight as evidence of starvation and as "not motivated by a bona fide right to privacy but by a desire to terminate her life."[33] Deering held that the right to privacy (defined as the "right to be left alone") did not apply to suicide by starvation, and that any treatment necessary to preserve life could be forced on her. "Saving her life is paramount," he said.

Elizabeth Bouvia appealed again, and the California Court of Appeal found in her favor. The justices said that she could refuse life-sustaining medical treatment: "A desire to terminate one's life is probably the ultimate exercise of one's right to privacy."[34] Moreover, they found "no substantive evidence to support the [lower] court's decision." Judge Deering (like Judge Hews) had taken into account the fact that this patient could live for decades more, but the appeals court completely dismissed this factor: "This trial court mistakenly attached undue importance to the amount of time possibly available to [Elizabeth Bouvia], and failed to give equal weight and consideration for the quality of that life; an equal, if not more significant, consideration." The appeals court concluded:

> This matter [Deering's decision against Bouvia] constitutes a perfect paradigm of the axiom: "Justice delayed is justice denied." Her mental and emotional feelings are equally entitled to respect. She has been subjected to the forced intrusion of an artificial mechanism into her body against her will. She has a right to refuse the increased dehumanizing aspect of her condition. . . . The right to refuse medical treatment is basic and fundamental. It is recognized as part of the right of privacy protected by both the state and federal constitutions. Its exercise requires no one's approval. It is not merely one vote subject to being overridden by medical opinion.
>
> . . . [A precedent has been established that when] a doctor performs treatment in the absence of informed consent, there is an actionable battery. The obvious corollary to this principle is that a competent adult patient has the legal right to refuse medical treatment. [Moreover,] if the right of the patient to self-determination as to his own medical treatment is to have any meaning at all, it must be paramount to the interests of the patient's hospital and doctors. . . . The right of a competent adult patient to refuse medical treatment is a constitutionally guaranteed right which must not be abridged.
>
> . . . In Elizabeth Bouvia's view, the quality of her life has been diminished to the point of hopelessness, uselessness, unenjoyability, and frustration. She, as the patient, lying helplessly in bed, unable to care for herself, may consider her existence meaningless. She is not to be faulted for so concluding. . . . As in all matters,

lines must be drawn at some point, somewhere, but that decision must ultimately belong to the one whose life is the issue.

Note especially the statement that *the right of a competent adult patient to refuse medical treatment is a constitutionally guaranteed right which must not be abridged.* With regard to force-feeding, the wording of the decision was very strong:

> We do not believe it is the policy of this State that all and every life must be preserved against the will of the sufferer. It is incongruous, if not monstrous, for medical practitioners to assert their right to preserve a life that someone else must live, or more accurately, endure, for "15 or 20 years." We cannot conceive it to be the policy of this State to inflict such an ordeal upon anyone.

Moreover, the appeals court added that "no criminal or civil liability attaches to honoring a competent, informed patient's refusal for medical service."

If nothing else, Elizabeth Bouvia—frail, small, alone, and barely able to move—had won a remarkable victory for other patients. She had wrested from the appeals court the first clear statement (it preceded the *Cruzan* decision by 5 years) that competent, adult patients have a constitutional right to refuse medical treatment in order to die.

Commentators on the Case

Commentaries on the *Bouvia* case show how passion imbues so-called "objective" accounts.

Two physicians writing in the *Archives of Internal Medicine* gave the following description:

> The standoff continued until April 7, when Ms. Bouvia unexpectedly checked herself out of the hospital. The hospital bill for the 217 days, excluding physicians' fees, was more than $56,000, paid by Riverside County and by the State of California. Ms. Bouvia went to the Hospital del Mar at Playease de Tijuana, Mexico, known for amygdalin (Laetrile) treatments for cancer. She believed the staff would help her die. Her new physicians, however, became convinced that she wanted to live. Two weeks later, Ms. Bouvia left the hospital, hired nurses, and moved to a motel. Three days later, with friends, a reporter, and an intern from Hospital del Mar at her side, she gave up her plan to starve herself to death and took solid food. Ms. Bouvia said that she wanted treatment, including surgery to reduce muscle spasms. As of August 1985, Ms. Bouvia's location and plans were not known. Her case was complicated further by the revelation that the newspaper reporter who covered the case most closely had a contract with Ms. Bouvia for a book, television, and movie rights to her story.[35]

This account emphasizes Elizabeth Bouvia's unexpected departure from the hospital, the size of her hospital bill, the public expense of her bill, the agreement of her Mexican physicians with her American physicians in refusing to honor her wish to die, her seemingly arbitrary decision to give up her plan of starving herself, and her contract with a reporter for book and film rights to her story. (There was never a movie or book.)

In contrast, here is law professor George Annas's account of the same events:

Two years ago this column dealt with Elizabeth Bouvia's unequal and doomed struggle.... After losing both in the hospital and in the courtroom, Ms. Bouvia fled to Mexico on April 7, 1984, to seek her death. She was soon persuaded that Mexican physicians and nurses would be no more sympathetic to her plan than those at Riverside, and so returned to California. Because of the brutal force feeding she had endured at Riverside, she was afraid to return there. Since no other facility would admit her unless she agreed to eat, she resigned herself to eating and entered a "private care" location. There she remained, without incident, for more than a year.[36]

Differences can also be found in accounts of the earlier events in the Bouvia case. For instance, this is how Derek Humphrey of the Hemlock Society described the start of the case:

Her troubles multiplied. The graduate school where she had been studying refused to readmit her, and her brother was drowned in a boating accident. Not long after, Elizabeth had a miscarriage, and she learned her mother was dying of cancer.

... Determined once again to be in charge of her fate, she asked her father to take her to the county hospital in Riverside, near Los Angeles (an area where she had friends), for an examination. She checked herself into the psychiatric ward and told physicians she wanted to die by starvation. Elizabeth specifically asked that, until she died, she be looked after normally and given painkillers when her arthritis was troublesome.[37]

The disability advocate Paul Longmore, who argues that the Bouvia case reflects rank prejudice against the disabled, describes the early phases as follows:

The very agencies supposedly designed to enable severely physically handicapped adults like her to achieve independence . . . become yet another massive hurdle they must surmount, an enemy they must repeatedly battle but can never finally defeat.

. . . [When she tried to go on internship,] the SDSU [San Diego State University] School of Social Work refused to back her up. They wanted to place her at a center where she would only work with disabled people. She refused. Reportedly, one of her employers told her she was unemployable, and that, if they had known just how disabled she was, they would never have admitted her to the program. . . .

The attorneys brought in three psychiatric professionals to provide an independent evaluation. None of them had any experience or expertise in dealing with persons with disabilities. In fact, Elizabeth Bouvia had never been examined by any psychiatric or medical professional qualified to understand her life experience. . . . Her examiners prejudicially concluded that because of her *physical* condition she would never be able to achieve her life goals, that her [physical] disability was the reason she wanted to die, and that her decision for death was reasonable. . . . [Judge Hews] too declared that Ms. Bouvia's physical disability was the sole reason she wished to die.[38]

These accounts all appeared in scholarly journals, presumably objective. However, the two physicians portray Elizabeth Bouvia as irresponsible; Annas and

Humphrey portray her as a helpless heroine fighting a cold bureaucracy; and Longmore sees her as a victim of a prejudiced system and of misguided, do-gooder lawyers. Note also that the physicians refer to her as "Bouvia," Humphrey calls her "Elizabeth," and Longmore uses "Elizabeth Bouvia" or "Ms. Bouvia." The physicians say that "she got a ride" to Riverside, as if she had hitchhiked to some arbitrary location; Humphrey, by contrast, says that her father took her to a place "where she had friends." Longmore emphasizes her desire to be independent; Humphrey emphasizes her physical pain and social trauma. Longmore suggests that society is prejudiced against disabled people and that Elizabeth Bouvia's disability is not so much her problem as society's problem. Humphrey writes from a point of view "inside" Elizabeth Bouvia; the physicians write from the viewpoint of hospital staff members who must accept patients presenting "management problems."

The Aftermath

After her victory in court, Elizabeth Bouvia did not kill herself. Some caring people had come forward and offered to help her die. These new friends seem to have showed her that life could be worth living, and gradually she came to change her mind.

THE McAFEE CASE

The Patient: A Quadriplegic Man

At 29 years old Larry McAfee became almost completely paralyzed (a C-2 quadriplegic) in a motorcycle accident on May 5, 1985. While he was riding on a dirt road at less than 10 miles per hour he hit a curve, fell over his motorcycle, snapped his head, and crushed his two top vertebrae on the bottom of his helmet.

He had been an adult student at Georgia State University in Atlanta, studying mechanical engineering, and an avid outdoorsman; on weekends, he had often motorcycled with other students in the mountains northwest of Atlanta.

Left with the use of only his eyes, mouth, and head, he could not clear his throat and sometimes had a sensation of choking. He could not breathe on his own (the muscles that control breathing were also paralyzed) and therefore needed a ventilator. He had no control over his bladder or bowels. He could feel no physical pleasure from any sexual activity, although he still experienced sexual desire. He had never married; according to statistics, single people who suffer spinal-cord injuries like his seldom marry (and those who are married at the time of their injury are almost always divorced later).[39]

The Case: Quality of Care and the Right to Die

The mass media presented the case of Larry McAfee only as a right-to-die issue involving his own perception of his quality of life, but inside medicine, the case also involved rationing care and medical finance.

McAfee had a $1 million health insurance policy, but he remained for over 1 year at the expensive Shepherd Spinal Center in Atlanta, where the average stay for C-1 to C-4 patients was 19 weeks; and later, at his apartment in Atlanta, he insisted on nurses who were three times more expensive than home health aides. After 16 months at home, he had used up his insurance benefits.[40] Some members of his family offered to take care of him, but he said that he did not want to burden them.

At this point, he was eligible for Medicaid (*not* Medi*care*), the fund in each state that pays for medical care for the indigent. According to Aaron Johnson, commissioner of Georgia's Medicaid office, McAfee wanted Georgia to pay for care for him in his apartment and refused to go to a much-less-expensive, state-controlled nursing home.[41] In other words, he wanted to be cared for at pubic expense but according to his own wishes.

Apparently, Larry McAfee was then dumped in the Aristocrat Berea nursing home outside Cleveland, Ohio—a facility that provided care for ventilator-dependent C-1 patients—with the state of Georgia paying. Officials at Aristocrat Berea said that they had acted in good faith, accepting him on a temporary, short-term basis because they had understood that no bed was available for him in Georgia. After 2 years, when it became clear to them that this had been a dump, they hustled him onto a plane bound for Georgia, whisked him to the emergency department (ED) at Grady Memorial Hospital in Atlanta (by federal law, patients cannot be denied admission to an ED), and went back to Ohio.

According to the administrator of Aristocrat Berea, Larry McAfee wouldn't make appointments for vocational rehabilitation and vented over conditions that no other patients complained about: "Larry was very demanding, wanted things precisely the way he wanted them. . . . I had nurses toward the end who just couldn't work with him anymore because they were just extremely, extremely frustrated."[42] He also noted that McAfee's family and friends were all in Georgia.

McAfee, however, claimed that he had been housed with demented, senile, and brain-damaged patients who, because of tight funds, were being "warehoused"—with only 1 or 2 staff members assigned to supervise as many as 30 to 40 patients. The easiest way to warehouse such patients is to keep them heavily sedated. McAfee said that he experienced intense loneliness and received inadequate personal care. "You're just a sack of potatoes," he said.[43]

After being returned to Atlanta in January 1989, Larry McAfee spent several miserable months in the intensive care unit (ICU) of Grady Memorial Hospital. Though he hated Grady Memorial, no other facility in Georgia would take him. During the summer of 1989, however, officials at Grady Memorial found that the patient—who was then 33 years old—could be accepted by Briarcliff Nursing Home in a suburb of Birmingham, Alabama, and he was voluntarily transferred to Birmingham. (Briarcliff was one of the few nursing homes in the country that accepted ventilator-dependent patients.)

Russ Fine, a disability advocate and director of the Injury Control Research Center at the University of Alabama at Birmingham (UAB), became aware of McAfee through an article that appeared in a Birmingham newspaper describing his petition for the right to end his life. Upon learning of McAfee's plight, Fine contacted the Briarcliff Nursing Home and asked to speak with McAfee. His request was denied by Briarcliff personnel who informed Fine that all inquiries were to be directed to McAfee's attorney, Randy Johnson, in Atlanta. Subsequently, Fine explained his interest in the case to Johnson and requested an opportunity to meet with McAfee. Three days following their conversation, Fine received a call from Johnson informing him that McAfee had agreed to meet with him later that same day. After a marathon, four-hour session McAfee finally agreed to allow Fine to "pursue some option on his behalf." Fine openly admitted to McAfee that he had no idea how he would proceed and said, later, that he thinks McAfee agreed to go along with his advocacy simply because "I wore him down . . . I outlasted him." In fact, at the end of their initial encounter, McAfee referred to Fine as "the most tenacious son-of-a-bitch he'd ever met."

Subsequently, Fine interviewed McAfee on a nightly radio talk show that he and his wife Dee co-hosted. According to Fine, Larry McAfee's treatment on Medicaid in Ohio, Georgia, and Alabama represents "everything that's wrong about the system that serves [severely] disabled people."[44] When he first met Larry McAfee, Fine was appalled to find him lying in bed staring at the ceiling. The patient had no voice-activated telephone and no television. All he could do was stare "at whatever happened to be in front of his face. From a quality of life standpoint, it was a devastating commentary on a society with a very advanced health-care system."[45] A reporter once arrived to find that McAfee's urinary catheter was not connected to a container and urine was spilling over the floor. Fine says, "These facilities were not equipped to take care of a patient such as Larry, with labor-intensive health-care requirements."[46]

The previous summer—5 years after a federal appellate court had found in favor of Elizabeth Bouvia—Larry McAfee decided to file suit in court for the right to die. He did not want to die by having his ventilator disconnected, since it had once been dislodged accidentally and he had experienced a terrifying sensation of suffocation (in fact, he also had a sense of suffocating at some other times).

On September 7, 1989, after a heart-wrenching 45-minute hearing in Fulton County Superior Court, Judge Edward Johnson found in Larry McAfee's favor. Johnson ruled that Larry could modify the "Puff-Sip" system (which ventilator-dependent patients use to control the movements of their motorized wheelchair) with circuitry that would allow Larry to disconnect the ventilator. It is interesting to note that, given McAfee's previous terror at the sensations of suffocation, this method of dying would seem to be very unappealing to him. Notably, Johnson also wrote that McAfee had "a right to be free from pain at the time the ventilator is disconnected."[47] During the hearing, all the parties had assumed that a decision for McAfee would result in his death within a few days; however, the state of Georgia appealed. On direct appeal, the Georgia Supreme Court affirmed Johnson's decision.

The Aftermath

Larry McAfee did not use his switch device to kill himself. Russ Fine, through his intervention and discussions with McAfee, convinced McAfee that life could be worth living. However, although McAfee decided to live, his problems of securing funding continued.

During the summer of 1989, while his assisted-suicide suit was pending in court, Larry McAfee had qualified for additional benefits under a special disability extension of Medicare, but these payments were to end in April 1990. Anticipating that, Fine persuaded officials of Birmingham's United Cerebral Palsy (UCP) to allow him to live temporarily in a nine-person group home run by UCP for the severely disabled; this home had a supported-employment program. Larry McAFee's stay in the UCP home began in April 1990 but was interrupted during May and June, when he was in a private hospital recuperating from surgery to remove a kidney stone. By July 1990, he had returned to the UCP home; but UCP officials had not received the funding they had hoped for and therefore announced that he would have to leave their facility soon. Officials at Grady Memorial Hospital in Atlanta, where he had run up a bill of $175,000, had no intention of taking him back. Under intense pressure from the media, officials in Georgia arranged for him to be transferred—in early July of 1990—to the Medical College of Georgia at Augusta, where he was promised most of what he wanted. The Medical College created an independent-living facility for Larry McAfee and five other disabled patients.

ETHICAL ISSUES: FROM AUTONOMY
TO SOCIAL PREJUDICE

The Concept of Assisted Suicide

Definitions   One question raised by the cases of Elizabeth Bouvia and Larry McAfee is what to call the intended action: suicide, rational suicide, assisted suicide, euthanasia, voluntary death, self-deliverance, or something else. To help sort out this semantic welter, two points can be made.

First, *euthanasia* usually means the killing of one person by another (or others) for allegedly merciful reasons. The two cases in this chapter cannot be said to involve euthanasia, then, since in each case the death would be initiated by the person herself or himself. Opponents of suicide sometimes lump it together with euthanasia, but that is a semantic sleight-of-hand designed to win an argument when more rational means have failed.

Second, it is inaccurate to say that a *terminally ill* patient who forgoes medical treatment thereby "commits suicide." It is true that the definition of *suicide* is now often broadened to include indirect ways of bringing about one's own death.[48] Nevertheless, it is still important to maintain the distinction between: (1) cases where an underlying disease is incrementally leading to death, and by choosing not to do everything possible, the patient accepts death at an earlier date; and (2) cases where a competent adult without a terminal illness causes his or her own death. Case 2 is appropriately called *suicide*. One reason to maintain the distinction between forgoing treatment in terminal illness and committing suicide is that if a death is classified as a suicide, many life insurance companies refuse to pay benefits. Another reason is that in all states, with the exception of Oregon, it is illegal to assist in a suicide. In three important cases—*Saikewicz, Conroy,* and *Colyer*—state supreme courts have decided that withdrawal of treatment in terminal illness is not suicide.[49]

Actually, the issue in the Bouvia and McAfee cases is probably best described as *assisted suicide*. Neither Elizabeth Bouvia nor Larry McAfee had a terminal disease (each could have lived another 20 or 30 years): hence the term *suicide*. They could not easily kill themselves, and so they needed help from others, especially medical staff members: hence the term *assisted*.

Arguments For and Against Assisted Suicide Opponents of assisted suicide have stressed that neither Elizabeth Bouvia nor Larry McAfee had a terminal illness (thus neither of them would meet one crucial condition of Hume's argument, a "house falling under its own weight") and that both of them were young. This meant that they might place some hope in medical progress, if they changed their minds and decided to live. It was also argued that neither of them really needed to die in a medical institution—that the duty of physicians and hospitals to comfort the sick and dying does not extend to disabled people who are neither sick nor dying, and that such disabled people cannot claim a right to have physicians and nurses help them kill themselves. These critics also point to the role of medicine as a bulwark against death, not a catalyst for dying.

In these two cases, also, opponents of assisted suicide argued that Elizabeth Bouvia and Larry McAfee may not really have wanted to die. Since they did not simply commit suicide quietly but instead made dramatic demands on public institutions, it was suggested, they may have been acting out and pleading for attention. In such a situation, medicine cannot just accede to the expressed wish of the patient, because it may not represent the patient's real wishes. It would not seem sensible, much less compassionate, to assist in the suicide of every distraught or depressed patient who comes to an ER and announces a desire to die.

Of course there are also religious arguments against assisted suicide. The Roman Catholic church opposes rational suicide; in 1990, the Catholic theologian Kevin O'Rourke argued that it is based on an illusion—the idea that human beings are totally in control of their lives and destinies.[50] O'Rourke believes that God has a plan for each person, and that this plan never includes suicide.

Advocates for *communitarian ethics* also oppose assisted suicide: They argue that severely disabled people should not simply be allowed to die; rather, society must provide humane institutions where these people can be loved. With regard to the community, opponents of assisted suicide can also argue that how society treats disabled people—whether its attitude is prejudiced or unbiased, what resources it is willing to expend, how it intends to cover the costs, and so on—is not an issue that medicine can solve or should be expected to solve.

On the other side, supporters of assisted suicide in cases like those of Elizabeth Bouvia and Larry McAfee argue that providing such assistance may, appropriately, be the final part of a continuum of good medical care. Normally, leaving a patient untreated—*patient abandonment*—is considered unethical and may even be a crime; and cutting short the continuum of care may be seen as a form of abandonment. The fact that a patient does not have a terminal disease is irrelevant, according to this argument. The real issue is whether or not the patient has an acceptable quality of life, and that is an evaluative judgment which can be made only by patients themselves. If physicians or others in effect make this evaluation by refusing to assist in suicide, that may be the worst kind of medical paternalism.

A Note on Unassisted Suicide   It is sometimes asked why patients such as Elizabeth Bouvia and Larry McAfee don't simply go off somewhere and kill themselves. One answer is that it's not easy to commit suicide when you want to die painlessly and aesthetically, and when you need to be sure that you accomplish what you intend. When you are already sick or disabled, suicide becomes even more difficult.

Most people don't know how to easily and cleanly kill themselves. Consider the attempted suicide of Robert McFarlane, a national security advisor during the administration of Ronald Reagan, at the time of the Iran-Contra hearings. McFarlane took somewhere between thirty and forty 5- to 10-milligram (mg) tablets of Valium, but he didn't die, and some people inferred that therefore he didn't really want to kill himself. An equally plausible explanation is that he didn't really know how to kill himself. In 1985, a physician, Robert Rosier, didn't even know how much morphine to give his terminally ill wife to bring about her death—and if a physician doesn't know, how could the rest of us expect to know what to do?[51]

Although suicide attempts by teenagers increased 300 percent between 1967 and 1982, only 1 in 50 attempts succeeded.[52] Elderly people are apparently more knowledgeable, though even they succeed only one in three times; Miami Beach, a popular retirement city, leads the United States in successful suicides. Women attempt suicide more than men but are less often successful; this may be because men tend to use violent means such as guns whereas women tend to use drugs.

It is a common mistake to infer ambivalent motives whenever a suicide is botched. Emergency room physicians can confirm that most people don't know how to kill themselves. Emergency medicine is full of stories of bizarre survivals (often related with gallows humor).[53] The hand holding the gun wobbles a fraction of an inch and leaves the would-be suicide a drooling zombie. "Jumpers" survive the fall from the Golden Gate Bridge because the drugs they have taken to give themselves courage also relax their muscles and thus soften the impact. One jumper—a woman—hits a parked car and not only does not die but does not even lose consciousness. The skirt of an elderly woman jumper catches on a balcony halfway down a skyscraper; she tries to fight off the fireman who reaches her on a ladder; he gets a medal and she gets a straitjacket.

Available methods for committing suicide present a grim picture. To begin with, Valium and other benzodiazapines—which figure prominently in many attempted suicides—rarely cause death when used alone because they are usually taken in insufficient quantities. Instead, the would-be suicide awakes with half his or her IQ.

People who try some other popular methods are just as likely to end up in the ER as dead. Carbon monoxide (CO) poisoning may not work because the car can stall or run out of gas; or the CO may not be concentrated enough to produce death, so that the person ends up in a coma. Slitting the wrists in a warm tub is not easy: the cuts are painful and must be made very deep and in the right place. Nor is this method certain: In the time between unconsciousness and death, the arm may move out of the water and the blood may coagulate. One ER physician observes, "Most slashers just get a trophy: a claw hand."

Some people are discovered in the act of committing suicide, especially those who choose a method that takes several hours. They may then wake up in an ER with a nasogastric tube down the throat, into which syrup of ipecac is pumped to induce vomiting; this is followed by injections of saline solution; next comes gastric lavage—alternate flooding and suctioning out of the stomach—and then granulated charcoal is pumped in to absorb the remaining toxins. These procedures are painful, messy, and unpleasant for patients who return to consciousness while they are in progress.

People may be reluctant to use certain methods if they want to spare the feelings of others, or if they want to be found in a reasonably dignified state after death. For instance, a drug overdose not only decreases respiration but also relaxes bowel and bladder control. Even messier is jumping off a building or shooting oneself in the head. Hanging is not foolproof: It is difficult to do correctly because the neck may not break and the victim, kicking in agony as he or she partially asphyxiates, may not die. If it succeeds, it also relaxes bowel and bladder control; and a man who dies by hanging himself will be found with an erect penis.

Rationality and Competence

One ethical issue in these cases was made famous by a play called *Whose Life Is It, Anyway?* which was later made into a movie (Elizabeth Bouvia had evidently seen the film version). Its hero, Ken Harrison, like Larry McAfee, is a quadriplegic who wants to die. Harrison offers rational arguments for suicide, but a psychiatrist reasons that those arguments are undercut by Harrison's "obvious intelligence." In other words, because Harrison is intelligent and sane enough to formulate a convincing case for suicide, he is too intelligent and sane to really want to die. Or, to put it another way, only if he were irrational would Harrison really decide to die; he could convince the psychiatrist of his rationality only by deciding to live.

In Elizabeth Bouvia's case the psychiatrist Nancy Mullen testified along similar lines: Mullen held that since the patient was seeking suicide, she must be incompetent to make medical decisions about her life and prospects; Mullen said that she herself could conceive of no situation where a person could make a "competent" decision to take his or her own life.[54] Carol Gill, a clinical assistant professor of occupational therapy (who herself used a wheelchair), argued similarly: She criticized ACLU for accepting the decision of "a handful of medical experts" that Elizabeth Bouvia was competent when she decided to starve herself.[55] It should be noted that Gill had not examined Elizabeth Bouvia before concluding that the patient was incompetent.

Mullen, Gill, and the psychiatrist in *Whose Life Is It, Anyway?* were all making the logical error called *begging the question.* A question is "begged" when the answer is assumed to be true rather than proved. In these cases, the "question" or point is whether a decision to die rather than lead an unsatisfactory life is irrational: that is, whether such a decision indicates mental illness, misinformation, faulty reasoning, or the like. Simply assuming that a decision to die is *necessarily* or *always* irrational—and hence incompetent—begs that question.

This is not to say, of course, that a decision to die is necessarily or always rational. Elizabeth Bouvia, for example, might in fact have been suffering from clinical depression, and psychological tests might have shown this. But Mullen and Gill did not base their arguments on this kind of consideration. They were not Elizabeth's Bouvia's therapists and were not among the professionals who were treating her. Mullen and Gill reacted to the content of the decision itself rather than to any psychological factors which they knew of firsthand and which might have influenced that decision. Actually, three psychiatric professionals who tested Elizabeth Bouvia did find her competent.[56]

With regard to the legal aspects of competence, in the United States a patient must be considered mentally competent until proven otherwise in a legal hearing, and no patient can be held in a hospital against his or her will without having been proven legally incompetent. (Chapter 15 discusses criteria for involuntary psychiatric commitment.) Typically, in a large urban hospital a lower-court judge will spend one day every one or two weeks ruling in competency hearings. In such hearings, two attending psychiatrists or residents usually testify for commitment; indigent patients have court-appointed lawyers.

In practice, hospitals sometimes break the law regarding competence. One well-known case was that of Donald ("Dax") Cowart in Texas in 1973. Cowart, a young bachelor, was burned over 67 percent of his body in a propane-gas explosion. As a former pilot, Dax understood burns and requested a gun to shoot himself when emergency medical technicians arrived at the scene of the explosion. His request was denied, and for 232 days he underwent excruciatingly painful treatments, against his will, in Parkland Memorial Hospital in Dallas. Although he was never declared incompetent, his physicians ignored his refusal to be treated; instead, they honored the wishes of his very religious mother and forced treatment on him. He was left blind, horribly disfigured, and with only partial use of his fingers.[57]

Autonomy

As we have seen, John Stuart Mill (in *On Liberty*) applied his principle of harm to define or delimit private or "self-regarding" actions. Mill held that so far as such actions are concerned, the individual should be *autonomous;* that the source of values is individual experiences and choices (in other words, values are not imposed by the state); and that the state should have no power to force an individual to act for the public good or even in his or her own best interest. In essence, Mill saw individual rights as conditions limiting what government may do to citizens.

During the early development of bioethics, this concept of individual autonomy became very important in the *patient rights movement.* According to the principle of autonomy, as applied to the right to die, a person who has not been proved incompetent has the right to make decisions about when to end his or her own life. Clearly, applying the principle of autonomy might lead to bad results in some specific cases; its general application, however, may lead to the "greatest good for the greatest number" of patients who want to die. If the principle is not extended to such patients, they can be forced to live inside a hospital; and it can be argued that there is little difference between this result and involuntary commitment of competent people to psychiatric wards—a practice for which psychiatrists in the former Soviet Union were widely condemned by their counterparts in the free world.

Applying the principle of autonomy in Elizabeth Bouvia's case, would suggest that the key question was not whether she was demonstrably competent or incompetent. Instead, the question would be simply whether there was any room for doubt about her incompetence; if there was room for doubt, she would have a right to autonomy and thus she herself rather than anyone else could control the decision to die.

Not everyone would agree that the principle of autonomy resolves a case like Elizabeth Bouvia's. For one thing, some observers considered her unstable—even if there was room for doubt that she was actually incompetent—and felt that assisted suicide in her case would therefore set a dangerous precedent. These critics saw something odd in her case: She seemed to want to kill herself only inside a hospital and did not take the opportunity to die outside, in private; and this seemed to indicate that after all there might be some psychiatric problem.

Another criticism related to the concept of autonomy is whether or not it can be genuinely applicable to severely disabled people in American society. We turn next to this issue.

One might also note contrarily that almost all the right-to-die authors cited in the historical survey were rich or aristocrats: Plato, Hume, Montesquieu, and Marcus Aurelius. What about powerless people lacking resources?

Modern bioethics has been accused of worshipping autonomy at the expense of other values such as community and family solidarity. Nowhere does this seem truer than in its glorification of assisted suicide by young individuals who are not terminally ill. Critics emphasize the lack of family relationships in all three cases of Elizabeth Bouvia, Larry McAfee, and Dax Cowart, citing how atypical are such cases of atomistic individuals without family ties.

Treating Symptoms and Depression

Despite emphasis in the bioethics literature to the contrary, some decisions to die really do stem from clinical depression. Although it is fallacious to say that every decision to die is irrational because it is a decision to die, it is also true that humane medicine will not let people needlessly die because of chemical imbalances in their brain.

This is even truer for young, nonterminal people such as Elizabeth Bouvia or Dax Cowart. Although wanting to die after being horribly burned or after losing most of one's physical abilities is understandable, people who are in the throes of depression frequently do not understand how they can come to feel much better. Modern psychiatry has some remarkable antidepressants that really do lift mood and change outlook on life. (Despite this fact, some people with severe limitations still persist in their decisions to die). Nevertheless, at the very least, antidepressants should be tried on all nonterminal patients who wish to die (this is actually a requirement of the Oregon law for terminally ill patients who wish to die—see next chapter).

A more subtle issue concerns depression stemming from inadequate resources for the disabled. Do we want to encourage society to be stingy by being generous in allowing disabled people to kill themselves? Do we want to give some families an easy way out? It seems that ethics requires some safeguards against too-quick assisted suicide, as shown by all the cases in this chapter where the patients decided to live when they obtained control of their case and better resources.

A different clinical issue concerns relief of symptoms. In this regard, psychiatrist and palliative care physician John Shuster says it is always important to ask patients who want to die, "What is the chief symptom that makes you want to die?"[58] He first argues that often that symptom is not what outsiders would predict. For example, a terminal patient once suffered from air hunger but his chief complaint, when asked, was not suffocation but how he missed going to a public park in his trailer (such visits were easily arranged with hospital volunteers). Second, Shuster argues that, with well-financed coverage, almost any symptom can be controlled, including pain, air hunger, itchiness, fatigue, and even boredom.

Raising the issue of inadequate resources puts physicians in an awkward place. On the one hand, they do not want to be instruments of torture to disable people who want to die. On the other hand, they do not want to acquiesce to unnecessary deaths of the disabled because a prejudiced, cheap society has the wrong attitude towards people with disabilities. In this regard, it is important to recognize that most institutions are still not anywhere near in compliance with the Americans with Disabilities Act (ADA), despite its being passed in 1991.

The catch, of course, is that to provide such great care, the patient must either be rich or have good insurance, or society must be generous. In conclusion, someone once remarked that the true measure of a society's civilization and humanity is how it treats its least well-off members. In that case, how many resources society commits to helping the disabled may be paradigmatic of that measure.

Social Prejudice and Physical Disabilities

Are there nonmedical conditions that make patients such as Bouvia and McAfee to want to die? Are such conditions, such as lack of resources, inevitable or preventable?

The disability advocate Paul Longmore, quoted earlier as a commentator on Elizabeth Bouvia's case and who is himself a ventilator-dependent quadriplegic, opposes voluntary death among the severely disabled. Longmore believes that the Bouvia case shows how a prejudiced system destroys the independence of disabled people, leaving them in a position where their so-called autonomous decisions to die are actually bogus.

By creating intolerable conditions for disabled people, Longmore holds, American society paints them into a corner. Such patients have only one decision left that can be consistent with their former autonomous selves: They can decide to die. Every other decision is made for them by others who keep them passive and dependent. In Longmore's words:

> Given the lumping together of people with disabilities with those who are terminally ill, the blurring of voluntary assisted suicide and forced "mercy" killing, and the oppressive conditions of social devaluation and isolation, blocked opportunities, economic deprivation, and enforced social powerlessness, talk of their "rational" or "voluntary" suicide is simply Orwellian newspeak. The advocates of assisted suicide assume a nonexistent autonomy. They offer an illusory self-determination.[59]

Longmore argues that in a different kind of society or in a different kind of hospital system—where people were given independence and their autonomy was maximized—disabled people would be less likely to choose to die. People could be given more choices about what and when to eat, when to be weighed, whom to see, and so on.

Some critics of autonomy see Elizabeth Bouvia's case as a failure on the part of society: a lack of caring, a situation in which a patient "slipped through the cracks" of an impersonal system. These critics see Elizabeth Bouvia as a tragic figure not primarily because of her physical situation but rather because of her social situation: Even as a hospitalized patient, she remained alone, and it was her aloneness that underlay her fierce assertion of her right to tear herself away from life.

On this analysis, to see Elizabeth Bouvia as simply a right-to-die case is to miss the heart of a much bigger issue. What made Elizabeth Bouvia want to die was the cumulative effect of centuries of prejudice against people who are physically disabled—prejudice that is virulently expressed in modern American society, which idealizes youth, beauty, sex, athleticism, fitness, and wealth. These are not the only values that make life worthwhile, but our culture lacks any strong expression of many other values, such as caring for others, erudition, creativity, and community.

Longmore argues in this way, and he also attacks several films that seem to covertly encourage severely disabled people to kill themselves as a highly rational response to their low quality of life. He cites *Annie Hall, Elephant Man,* and especially *Whose Life Is It, Anyway?* and claims that *Whose Life Is It, Anyway?* depressed Elizabeth Bouvia.

Specifically, Longmore maintains that Elizabeth Bouvia's problems resulted in part because she did not receive the maximum payments she was entitled to; he says that her county is notorious for its stinginess in benefits to disabled people. Furthermore, he says, the hospital where she was supposed to do her internship refused to comply with laws designed to ensure disability rights. He also believes that Elizabeth Bouvia was strongly discouraged from seeking work or marrying because benefits are reduced when a disabled person takes a job or marries. California's In-Home Supportive Services program allowed Elizabeth Bouvia to manage her own life at home while she was single; when she married, however, she became ineligible for the program: Her husband was now expected to care for her. Given these circumstances, Longmore thinks it is no wonder that Bouvia was later divorced or that she became discouraged about completing her training—for even in the unlikely event that she was able to overcome discrimination and find a job, she would then lose the benefits that allowed her to live on her own at home. Longmore concludes:

> This is a woman who aimed at something more significant than mere self-sufficiency. She struggled to attain self-determination, but she was repeatedly thwarted in her efforts by discriminatory actions on the part of the government, her teachers, her employers, her parents, and her society. Contrary to the highly prejudiced view of the appeals court, what makes life with a major physical disability ignominious, embarrassing, humiliating, and dehumanizing is not the need for extensive physical assistance, but the dehumanizing social contempt toward those who require such aid.

The case of Larry McAfee also raises the issue of social prejudice, although in his case that issue may have been somewhat clouded by his own personality. Was he a demanding, spoiled patient as some people described him, or was he a heroic figure who would rather die than live in the institutional squalor of publicly funded nursing homes?

Russ Fine, the disability advocate who intervened in the McAfee case, clearly believes that Larry McAfee's desire to die was mainly a result of severely inadequate physical and psychological care. McAfee said that if he couldn't get his own apartment he would rather die. According to Fine, McAfee "was very vocal about inferior nursing care, which was the rule, not the exception, in these marginal health-care facilities that had accepted these contracts."[60] Once, Fine had brought McAfee a Thanksgiving dinner and the two were watching a televised football game while waiting for McAfee's family to arrive. Fine was drowsing in an armchair when he suddenly realized that McAfee had stopped breathing. By the time the family arrived, nurses and aides were swarming over McAfee, trying to get him breathing. When he finally revived, Fine saw tears streaming out of his eyes. "He didn't really want to die," Fine concluded. "He was just terrified."[61]

It should be noted that Larry McAfee, like Elizabeth Bouvia, wanted to work, but this would have made him ineligible for most publicly funded assistance in housing or medical care.

Cases such as Bouvia's and McAfee's suggest that society often does give severely disabled people only three limited, grim choices: to become a burden on their families or friends, to live miserably in a large public institution, or to kill themselves. However, these three are not by any means the only possible options, and it can certainly be argued that society should explore and offer more and better choices.

Inadequate Independent-Living Facilities

For instance, small independent-living facilities known as *group homes* can be established; in such a facility (which is probably one of the best formats), a few home health aides can help disabled residents lead productive lives. Both Elizabeth Bouvia and Larry McAfee evidently would have accepted such an arrangement all along, and although bureaucrats didn't seem to know this, caring for Larry in a group home would have been cheaper than in a nursing home.

Not many group homes exist, however, and one of the main reasons is a reaction called NIMBY—"not in my back yard"—that is, neighborhood resistance to such homes. In the case of group homes for the disabled, such resistance seems to be based significantly on prejudice. Neighborhoods sometimes argue that group homes will create dangerous situations and lower property values, but this does not seem very convincing with regard to homes for people like Elizabeth Bouvia and Larry McAfee. Prejudice should surely not be allowed to prevent communities from giving their severely disabled members better choices than imprisonment in hospitals or death.

As we will discuss later, lobbying for adequate housing has become a major issue for advocates for the disabled and a defining issue of the "disability culture."

Allocating Scarce Medical Resources and the Rule of Rescue

The McAfee case involved the issue of funding, and therefore allocation, of medical resources. In this regard, the case illustrated several quirks in our medical system.

As we have seen, Larry McAfee's own private insurance benefits ran out quite soon; thereafter, his care was financed in various ways, principally by Medicaid. States determine levels of Medicaid support, and the level in any state can be too low to cover expenses of nursing-home care. In fact, only a very small number of nursing homes in the United States will admit ventilator-dependent patients like Larry McAfee, and virtually none will take ventilator-dependent Medicaid patients, since reimbursement for these Medicaid patients is so limited. It should also be noted that, according to federal regulations, Medicaid cannot be used for group homes or independent apartments; moreover, with regard to support for communal living for the disabled, Georgia is seen by many disability advocates as one of the least generous states. Medicaid regulations disallowing group and independent living arrangements have drawn considerable opposition: critics such as Paul Longmore have charged that Medicaid works to warehouse disabled people rather than to let them live independently and possibly work.

Social security was another, though modest, source of funding for Larry McAfee's care. Social security (which comprises more than one program) includes federally financed medical care for Americans over 65 (Medicare), and a welfare program for poor retirees and disabled young people—Supplemental Security Income (SSI). In 1992, SSI payments averaged $362 a month and were paid to 5.4 million elderly, disabled, or blind Americans.[62] Larry McAfee's SSI benefits increased his total reimbursement.

Still another source of payments, for a time, was a special extension of the Medicare disability program. This, however, had been repealed by Congress in November 1989 (in order to save money) and expired on April 10, 1990. Before their expiration, these benefits had been used for agency nurses (costing $3,000 a week) while Larry McAfee was in the Briarcliff Nursing Home.

United Cerebral Palsy (UCP) also provided some funding. As has been described above, UCP in Birmingham was persuaded by the disability advocate Russ Fine to admit Larry McAfee to a UCP group home there on a temporary basis. When he entered this group home, UCP initially paid for his agency nurses, but this was with the expectation that federal funding would soon be provided instead.

In Larry McAfee's case, disability advocates argued that he could live more cheaply as well as far more satisfactorily and with far better care in an independent-living facility; and he himself argued that Medicaid should at least help defray the cost of an independent-living facility by contributing the same amount that the Georgia Medicaid program would pay him for a nursing home. Accordingly, officials at UCP and some rehabilitation centers orchestrated an intense national campaign to make an exception for Larry McAfee. Such an exception would take the form of a presidential waiver for McAfee: That is, his care would be federally funded rather than paid for by the state Medicaid program. When Larry McAfee entered the nine-person UCP home on April 11, 1990, it was hoped that the president—then George Bush—would issue such a waiver for him; it was also hoped that the waiver would apply to care he would subsequently receive in Georgia if he returned there.

In mid-May, with the matter of the waiver still unsettled, Larry McAfee entered a hospital in Birmingham for removal of a large kidney stone. Since Medicaid pays for hospital care of acute conditions, this postponed for a while the problem of long-term funding, and he remained in the hospital for a month (an unusually long stay, clearly based on financial rather than medical considerations).

From June 15 to about July 10, Larry McAfee was back in the UCP home; but it had become clear to UCP officials in Birmingham that there would be no presidential waiver, and they had announced to the newspapers that he would have to leave their facility soon. Meanwhile, Russell Fine tried to get the president or the Georgia legislature to accept some kind of group arrangement for him.

About July 10, the Georgia legislature relented, and Larry McAfee was transferred to the Medical College of Georgia; the independent-living facility that was created there for him and the five other patients was an exception to Georgia's disability law and to its state Medicaid plan.

There are obviously a number of issues involved in this financial saga, but let us focus on only one, a phenomenon that bioethicists call the *rule of rescue*. The campaign to obtain a presidential waiver for Larry McAfee provoked considerable criticism and was seen as demonstrating that decisions about who should be helped are too often arbitrary. Two citizens, for instance, were disturbed when McAfee said that he would not return to a nursing home to "vegetate" and wanted Georgia to pay for his private apartment.[63] They complained:

> But why should McAfee be the only one singled out and given special attention, not to be in a nursing home, or that Medicaid should "open up" for? . . . McAfee "understands" that life is preferable, but it must be life with some dignity; in this case, *his* way or no way. McAfee says that if someone else won't pay for him to live *where and how* he chooses, he'd rather be dead. What about all the other people in the same situation?[64]

Critics like these hold that American society will rescue only someone like McAfee who manages to get into the national spotlight; it ignores all the others whose needs are just as great. (In McAfee's case, there were some 75,000 to 85,000 others.)

Larry McAfee and Elizabeth Bouvia both illustrate the rule of rescue. When one person's plight is made prominent by the news media, society tends to feel compelled to rescue that person, even if the rescue entails spending enormous amounts of scarce medical resources. In contrast, obscure people quietly go unrescued and live in abysmal conditions until they die. The rule of rescue in effect turns some crucial decisions over to the media: The editors of local newspapers and television news departments become gatekeepers, determining who will and will not be rescued. This is hardly the most rational way to distribute scarce medical resources.

UPDATE

In 1990, as noted in Chapter 2, the United States Supreme Court decided in *Cruzan* that no state may pass a law limiting the right of competent patients to decline medical treatment, even if declining treatment would hasten death. *Cruzan* built on previous appellate court decisions, including *Bouvia* and *McAfee,* and was a re-sounding victory for advocates of the right of competent adults to control their own death and dying.

In 1991, the Americans with Disabilities Act (ADA) went into effect. This legislation represents one of the most sweeping changes in the history of American law. Although at present it is still widely unenforced, its long-term effects will eventually integrate many Americans with disabilities—including those with cerebral palsy and spinal-cord injuries—into regular life.

A decade after Elizabeth Bouvia's victory in court, her body was described as "gnarled and useless."[65] She was living in California as a Medicaid patient, in a private hospital room with 24-hour care; the cost was $300 a day. A continuous dose of morphine was controlling her pain, and her weight was up to 100 pounds. Her life, she has said, is "a lot of needles and bags," and she spends most of her time watching television. On her own description, she would seem to be resigned to her fate: "I wouldn't say I'm happy, but I'm physically comfortable, more comfortable than before. There is nothing really to do. I just kind of lay here."

Ironically, Richard Scott, the physician and lawyer who represented Elizabeth Bouvia, committed suicide in August 1992. His wife said that he had battled depression for most of his life. When he died, Elizabeth Bouvia said, "Jesus, I wish he could have come in and taken me with him."

In 1993, Larry McAfee's story became the subject of *The Switch,* a CBS television movie. Gary Cole of the television series *Midnight Caller* starred as Larry McAfee; Russ Fine was portrayed only as a radio talk show host, not as an expert on rehabilitation. The producers had paid Russ and Dee Fine for rights to their story, but the Fines gave the money to Larry McAfee.[66] In January of 1993, according to Russ Fine, Larry McAfee was "real happy" about the movie and its national premiere. However, to keep the disability payments that funded his home, McAfee himself could not accept any of the profits. A few months later, authorities in Georgia didn't include McAfee's independent-living center in the state budget. At that time McAfee's center in Augusta housed five other patients and cost $116,000 per year; the overall budget from which it had been omitted was $8.9 million. When the Fines contacted the media, pointing out that the cost per person in the independent-living center was only $52 a day, the Georgia legislature found funds to continue the center for another year.

Tragically, in November 1993, Larry McAfee suffered two devastating strokes. The probable cause was a nursing error: a kink in his urinary catheter that caused urine to back up. Because of his paralysis, he could not feel what was happening; and the backup caused toxicity and high blood pressure.[67] McAfee survived but was left with only a little short-term memory. He had been planning to leave the independent-living facility for his own apartment but instead had to leave it for a long-term nursing home in Augusta. This nursing home was just the kind of place and fate that Larry McAfee had wanted to avoid when he won the right to use his "switch" and before he lost the ability to choose to use it. Larry McAfee died on October 6, 1995, not by his own hand or a "switch," but after becoming comatose for many months.

Elizabeth Bouvia was still alive in 1998 and appeared on *60 Minutes* on the tenth anniversary of her one and only other public appearance, another *60 Minutes* story on her case in March of 1988. She had been living in Riverside County hospital for 10 years, but in 1997, her new pro bono attorney Griffith Thomas, M.D., succeeded in getting all her disability payments put into a trust fund that in turn allowed her to live on her own with 24-hour in-home assistants.

In the interview, Elizabeth said that she still was in pain each day and needed to remain connected to the morphine drip, which was shown. She said she wished to be left alone and that she did not intend to be alive for another 10-year anniversary story by *60 Minutes* in 2008. She did not express gratitude for being forced to live and, 10 years later, still had great ambivalence about her life and being alive.

Eighteen years after the court granted Elizabeth Bouvia her plea to starve herself, she shared her current views on death and dying in an interview coordinated through her lawyer, Griffith Thomas. Bouvia still asserts that depression did not drive her attempts to starve herself. But instead, the decision was more rationally driven by her paralysis as well as her dependency on others for physical and financial care. It is not easy to starve oneself, and after repeated attempts, Elizabeth accepted that this method of dying was too difficult. She states in the interview:

> Refusing food and hydration WAS NOT a temporary impulse caused by life events, as has been implied. Contrary to what was said about me, I fully understood the consequences of my actions. But did the legal system or society consider the consequences of their actions? No sane person (terminal or otherwise) wishes to die. But during the process of death, one must accept the inevitable and let go.[68]

Elizabeth continues to wish that one day soon she will peacefully slip away. However, considering her physical limitations, if she does decide to end her suffering, starvation could be Elizabeth's only option.

Elizabeth claims that during the 3 years when she legally fought to die, doctors controlled her life. Some even threatened to coerce her into changing her mind. Furthermore, the media invaded the privacy of her family.

Today in an independent living facility, she has finally attained long-sought privacy and dignity. Elizabeth says that she simply makes the best of what she has; for her, dwelling on her disability or indigence only makes life more difficult.

Dax Cowart, the burn patient who had been treated against his will in Texas, became a millionaire from an out-of-court settlement with the gas company, graduated from law school in 1986, married a nurse he had known in high school, and became interested in two hobbies: ham radio and raising golden retrievers. He also became a frequent speaker for the Society for the Right to Die, arguing that even though he was glad to be alive today with his present blessings, his physicians had been morally wrong to treat him against his wishes. As he once said to this author, "If I should be so unlucky as to be burned that way again, and if I knew what was waiting at the end, I wouldn't go through that pain to get there."[69] He is now active as a trial lawyer. He frequently tells the story in public of his forced medical treatment in 1973 and 1974 in Texas, emphasizing the lack of empathy by his physicians in coercing him to endure 14 months of suffering and terrible pain.

It is, indeed, interesting to note that in the three most famous cases of nonterminal adults who wanted to die in medical facilities, all three patients changed their minds when they had a genuine opportunity to do so.

Paul Longmore continued to argue that too many people such as McAfee, were dying, and too many were going to see Dr. Kevorkian, because of inadequancies in the American health system. In a column in 1997, Longmore revealed that, as a result of childhood polio, his arms were paralyzed, his spine is curved, and he uses a ventilator as much as 18 hours a day.[70] He is an associate professor of history at San Francisco State University. He writes that his success would not have been possible without the ability to live independently on his own, which required many home health care aides. Fortunately, California's generous Medicaid program paid for his domestic aides (costing $15,000 a year) and he managed to avoid being disqualified from Medicare disability, which paid for his ventilator (costing $12,000 a year). Longmore's point is that he, too, might have wanted to die, had he lived in Georgia or Michigan, where he would not have been able to obtain a self-determined independent living facility and "probably would have found my life unendurable."

Disability Culture

Disabled people have reinvented themselves over the last decade, increasingly adapting a new militancy towards a society they see as prejudiced and selfish. Banding together in groups and houses, they assert their right to 24-hour attendants, access to public transportation, and good housing.[71]

They argue they have a condition, not an illness. Going further, some advocates say they have a new identity, a new culture. In the same way that some gay people use "Queer Nation" as an honorific phrase, so some people with disabilities use "Disability Culture" with pride as their new calling.

They argue that the disabled community is the only minority that anyone may join at any time. They point out that in 1962, when James Meredith sued to become the first black person to gain admission to the University of Mississippi, Edward V. Roberts had to sue as a quadriplegic to be admitted as a student to the University of California. But they believe that society over the past 40 years has far more successfully achieved integration of races than it has of the disabled.

So people with disabilities abound who see their life as a call-to-action to help their less assertive, disabled friends. They despise Mattel's "Share-a-Smile Becky" in a wheelchair (sold in some hospitals' gift shops) and demonstrate outside of classes of Princeton bioethicist Peter Singer, whose views on quality of life, they fear, will allow society to easily kill the disabled or deny them adequate resources.

Disability groups also hectored the Hemlock Society, which it accused of being sympathetic to the assisted death of nonterminal patients. It cites psychologist Faye Girsh, this Society's Executive Director, who testified on behalf of Bouvia in the original case, as well as this Society's support of Jack Kevorkian's killing of many nonterminal, female conditions beset by economic hardship; George DeLury, who in Manhattan in 1996 killed his wife in the late stages of multiple sclerosis; and Canadian Robert Latimer, who killed his 12-year old daughter with cerebral palsy in 1993. In particular, disability groups accuse the Hemlock society of being rich, well-insured, and more interested in maximizing autonomy of its members than in securing better conditions for the disabled.

For example, in the case of Robert Wendland before the California Supreme Court, a disability organization that calls itself "Not Dead Yet" filed an *amicus* brief against removing the feeding tube of this cognitive-disabled man who is neither terminal nor unconscious.

Robert Wendland, an auto-parts salesman from Stockton, CA, was left minimally conscious after awaking from a 17-month coma when his pickup truck rolled over in 1993. Fed through a tube, Robert could vaguely recognize people, follow basic instructions, and perform simple tasks such as writing his initials (which led some to question why he couldn't communicate his desires to others).[72] His wife, Rose, wanted to remove his feeding tube in 1995, claiming that Robert never would have wanted to exist in a vegetative state. However, his mother, Florence, opposed Rose and wanted to continue artificial feeding; moreover, Wendland's cognitive state was better than a vegetative state, making his alleged, prior statements about existing in a vegetative state less decisive.

The California medical community and 43 bioethicists supported Wendland's wife in her pursuit of her husband's "right to die." On July 18, 2001, Robert Wendland died from pneumonia. His mother and sister were present, but perhaps not his wife.

Three weeks later, the California Supreme Court ruled in the case to establish case law, holding that food and water can only be withheld from a semiconscious patient if a clear-and-convincing standard has been met. However, this *only* applies to conscious patients who are "not terminally ill, comatose, or in a persistent vegetative state." If Wendland had signed an advanced directive or assigned a proxy to his wife, Robert's treatment would have ended according to her wishes because the "clear-and-convincing" standard would have been met.

FURTHER READING AND RESOURCES

David Hume, "On Suicide" (1755), in Eugene Miller, ed., *Collected Essays of David Hume*, Liberty Classics, Indianapolis, Ind., 1986.
"Elizabeth Bouvia: 10 years later," *60 Minutes* Special, www.cbs.com.
"A Man of Endurance" *20/20* television show on March 22, 1999 on Donald Cowart's case. Call 1-800-CALL-ABC to order tape (around $30).
Pat Milmoe McCarrick, "Scope Note 18: Active Euthanasia and Assisted Suicide," *Kennedy Institute of Ethics Journal*, vol. 2, no. 1, March 1992.

CHAPTER 4

Physician-Assisted Dying

Oregon's Legalization

*I*n March of 1998, the first legal, physician-assisted death occurred in modern America when a terminally ill Oregon woman took her own life with lethal drugs prescribed by her physician. Citizens of Oregon had voted and fought over a decade to make this happen. Twenty-seven years before in 1971, a physician in Holland killed her terminally ill mother, igniting a course of events there which led to gradual legalization of physician-assisted dying until its complete legalization came in 2001.

Meanwhile in America, Dr. Jack Kevorkian became a lightning rod for physician-assisted dying. In the 1990s, he assisted over 100 patients to die before being finally jailed in 1999 for flouting the law. Critics saw his efforts, as well as developments in Oregon and Holland, as a descent into barbarism and as a return to the "euthanasia" of Nazi medicine.

This chapter reviews thirty years of these developments and the arguments about physician-assisted death. This debate has intensified after Attorney General John Ashcroft attempted to suspend licenses of physicians in Oregon who helped patients die.

BACKGROUND: ANCIENT GREECE AND THE HIPPOCRATIC OATH

The Hippocratic Oath, considered the origin of medical ethics, forbids physicians to kill patients. It began in ancient Greece at the time of Socrates in fifth century B.C.E. But did Hippocratic physicians represent most ancient Greek physicians? Almost certainly not.

In 1931, medical historian Ludwig Edelstein described Hippocrates as a disciple of the mathematician Pythagoras,[1] developer of the famous theorem, who worshipped numbers as divine and who held that all life was sacred. As his follower, Hippocrates did not represent most ancient Greek physicians.

Indeed, the Hippocratic *corpus*, or body of writings, does not represent the work of one man named Hippocrates, but was drawn from a number of his followers.

The practitioners of the Hippocratic school "possessed no legally recognized professional qualifications" and competed with gymnastic instructors, drug-sellers, herbalists, midwives, and exorcists.[2]

Many people today misunderstand the context of the original Hippocratic Oath or what it actually requires of physicians who swear by it. Few medical schools today use the original version (especially the pagan curse at its end!). Nor does the version given at medical graduation ceremonies necessarily reflect the values taught at that school. Let us see what the original oath actually makes physicians promise. Here is the complete text of Edelstein's translation:

> I swear by Apollo Physician and Asclepius and Hygeia and Panaceia and all the gods and goddesses, making them my witnesses, that I will fulfill according to my ability and judgment this oath and this covenant:
>
> To hold him who has taught me this art as equal to my parents and to live my life in partnership with him, and if he is in need of money, to give him a share of mine, and to regard his offspring as equal to my brothers in male lineage, and to teach his art—if they desire to learn it—without fee and covenant; to give a share of precepts and oral instruction and all the other learning to my sons and to the sons of him who has instructed me and the pupils who have signed the covenant and have taken this oath according to the medical law, but to no one else.
>
> I will apply dietetic measures for the benefit of the sick according to my ability and judgment; I will keep them from harm and injustice.
>
> I will neither give a deadly drug to anybody if asked for it, nor will I make a suggestion to this effect. Similarly I will not give to a woman an abortive remedy. In purity and holiness I will guard my life and my art. I will not use the knife, not even on sufferers of stone, but will withdraw in favor of such men as are engaged in this work.
>
> Whatever houses I visit, I will come for the benefit of the sick, remaining free of all intentional injustice, of all mischief and in particular of sexual relations with both female and male persons, be they free or slaves.
>
> What I may see or hear in the course of the treatment or even outside of the treatment in regard to the life of men, which on no account one must spread abroad, I will keep to myself holding such things shameful to be spoken about.
>
> If I fulfill this oath and do not violate it, may it be granted to me to enjoy life and art, being honored with fame among all men for all time to come; if I transgress it and swear falsely, may the opposite of all this be my lot.

This version does include swearing never to help dying patients who request death—and never to perform abortions—but that should be understood in context. Such vows were included because the Hippocratic school wanted to solidify its membership against competing healers; thus the oath also includes swearing not to perform surgery and (medical school instructors take notice!) not to charge students for teaching them medicine.

The prohibition against euthanasia by the Hippocratic school therefore set its members apart from most other physicians in ancient Greece, who were not opposed to letting patients die. Indeed, many Greek physicians excelled in helping patients die painlessly.

Two roots grounded the Greek attitude that patients could be helped to die. First the Greeks thought that life had certain natural limitations, beyond which it was folly to try to extend living. The concept of a *meson* or natural limit infused Greek culture, particularly architecture and theater. To attempt to go beyond *meson* was *hubris* [arrogance]—and invited the gods to strike one down.

The second root was practical: Physicians at that time simply did not know very much; also, they worried about being shown up by competitors. Consequently, they would often let terminal patients die in peace rather than attempt to heal them.

Despite all these problems, the Hippocratic oath does mean something because it symbolizes an ancient tradition of self-sacrifice and respect for human life. It also symbolizes commitment to the patient's welfare over the physician's convenience. Today, when too many physicians seem driven by money, have affairs with their patients, and divulge their patients' confidences, it seems wise to retain this symbolic commitment.

The Nazis and "Euthanasia"

Debates about physician-assisted dying often invoke Nazi Germany. German physicians during the Nazi era killed 90,000 patients in the name of "euthanasia" because of presumed mental or physical inferiority such as retardation. A related program, the so-called "final solution" to the problem of cleansing Germany of racially inferior non-Aryan stock, was kept more secret at the time: Under this program, the Nazis killed approximately 6 million Jews, 600,000 Poles, thousands of Gypsies, and thousands of homosexuals.

Leo Alexander, a New York psychiatrist who observed the Nuremberg trials, argued in 1949 in a famous article in the *New England Journal of Medicine* that the Nazis' "euthanasia" of people with disabilities and the later Nazi genocide—the mass murder of Jews and others—can both be traced to the same beginning: acceptance by German physicians of the idea that some people, because their quality of life is poor, are better off dead than alive.[3] Once one kind of person was killed because of unacceptable quality of life, Alexander argued, soon another kind of person was also killed.

In 1986, another New York psychiatrist, Robert Jay Lifton, argued similarly, although his "first step" differs from Lifton's:

> The Nazis justified direct medical killing by use of the . . . concept of "life unworthy of life," *lebensunwertes Leben*. While this concept predated the Nazis, it was carried to its ultimate racial and "therapeutic" extreme by them.
>
> . . . Of the five identifiable steps by which the Nazis carried out the destruction of "life unworthy of life," coercive sterilization was the first. There followed the killing of "impaired" children in hospitals, and then the killing of "impaired" adults—mostly collected from mental hospitals—in centers especially equipped with carbon monoxide. The same killing centers were then used for the murders of "impaired" inmates of concentration camps. The final step was mass killing, mostly of Jews, in the extermination camps themselves.[4]

People opposed to physician-assisted dying often cite Alexander and Lifton. They emphasize that physicians in Nazi Germany, especially professors in elite medical schools, took the first step.

J. C. Wilke argues that a few cases of merciful deaths for severely handicapped infants and children were the infamous first steps down the slope to the Holocaust.[5] In particular, the first case was the killing of a mentally ill child by his father in 1937, where the father was let off very lightly. This case was followed by another pivotal case in 1939 of an infant named Knauer, born blind and missing an arm and leg, investigated by Dr. Karl Brandt for Hitler, who issued clearance for Dr. Brandt to kill Knauer and all similar infants. Wilke claims these two test cases led to the first phase of deaths in Germany where many disabled children were killed (estimated by Wilke to be 6,000).

Many history professors reject these arguments, pointing out that German medicine had been blatantly racist for many decades before the Nazis and that anti-semitism had been in Germany for a thousand years. So the eventual mass murders did not result from a subtle, initially imperceptible shift in attitudes but from a widespread overt racism in the general population. Moreover, whatever steps led to the Nazi "euthanasia" program, the Nazi program had nothing in common with *voluntary* physician-assisted dying by *competent* patients in Holland or Oregon. Finally, in Nazi Germany, the term *euthanasia* camouflaged atrocities that were not good deaths but despicable murders.

So what, exactly, does the Nazi *euthanasia argument* involve in medical ethics? Answers to this question do not come easily because this argument actually contains many different claims, among them:

(1) Involuntary killings of people for *medical reasons* led to the Holocaust.

(2) Involuntary killings of people *by physicians* led to the Holocaust.

(3) Justifying medical killings of patients *for reasons of quality of life* led to the Holocaust.

(4) *Coercive, involuntary sterilization* of retarded, psychotic, and demented people led to the Holocaust.

(5) The *killing of impaired children* led to the Holocaust.

(6) Ideological desires to create better people (aka "A Master Race"), in other words, *eugenics,* led to the Holocaust.

(7) Deep *cultural racism and anti-Semitism* coupled with a Nietzschean elitist mentality, led to the Holocaust.

(8) Acceptance by physicians of a *new role of killers,* rather than healers, led to the Holocaust.

This chapter discusses most of these arguments after it describes the experiences of Oregon, Holland, and the case of Jack Kevorkian. (Sterilization and infanticide are discussed in the chapters about genetics and impaired babies.)

Because all its victims died involuntarily, and because no terminal patients died voluntarily by Nazi physicians, the relevance of the Nazi analogy to modern debates about dying is controversial. It would only be truthful to add, however, that people whose forebears experienced great evils—such as Jewish people, gays and lesbians, African Americans, native American Indians—are more likely to give weight to this analogy than those whose forebears did not.

Voluntary Euthanasia in the Netherlands

The Netherlands (Holland) began to decriminalize physician-assisted suicide in 1971 when the mother of physician Geertruida Postma suffered a cerebral hemorrhage, leaving the elderly woman partially paralyzed, deaf, and with gross speech deficits. As a people, the Dutch have always prized autonomy and mercy: "When I watched my mother, a human wreck, hanging in that chair, I couldn't stand it anymore," Postma testified at her trial.[6] So she then injected (in what has become the standard method) morphine to induce unconsciousness, and injected her mother with curare, killing her. After informing authorities, Postma was tried and found guilty of murder, but given only a suspended sentence.

Two years later in 1973, the Dutch Medical Association reached an agreement with Dutch prosecutors that physicians would not be prosecuted for murder if they abided by the following four guidelines (these were formalized further in 1984): (1) Only competent patients can request death. (2) The patient's request must be repeated, unambivalent, unpressured, and documented. (3) The physician must consult another physician for a second opinion. (4) The patient must be in unbearable pain or suffering, without likelihood of improvement.[7]

Notice that these guidelines do not allow killing of incompetent patients such as Karen Quinlan; nor do they allow killing of patients who are severely retarded. Note also that the patient's condition does not have to be terminal. In 1994, the Dutch Supreme Court held that unbearable *mental* suffering could also justify euthanasia. The Dutch do not, as Americans do, distinguish between assisted suicide and mercy killing.

By 1990, Holland had become an experimental ethics laboratory for the world to see if mercy killing by physicians would become (as one critic held) a "descent into barbarity." Its Remmelink Commission famously studied nearly two decades of data in this experiment and reported in 1990 that about 2 percent (2,300) of Holland's 130,000 deaths in 1990 were from euthanasia. Critics seized on the further report that another 1,000 deaths occurred in incompetent patients, and hence, violated the above guidelines.

The Commission's findings were a Rorschach test for both advocates and critics of physician-assisted death. Critics saw the extra thousand deaths as evidence of a slippery slope, claiming physicians had wrongly crossed a bright ethical line and kept going. Advocates took heart from two other facts found in this report: first, virtually 100 percent of the patients killed were terminally ill (most had been given between a week and a month to live), and second, physicians turned down two-thirds of requests for death from competent patients. After passage of a new law requiring physicians to notify authorities of any assisted deaths, a follow-up study in 1995 found much the same results.[8] Moreover, most of the thousand incompetent patients killed had cancer or AIDS, had previously expressed a wish to die should they become incompetent but became permanently incompetent suddenly without being able to die a planned death.

Several aspects of the Dutch experience caution against easy generalizations to North America. First, everyone in Holland has free medical care, including long-term nursing-home care, and thus no patient, physician, or family must decide on death for financial reasons. Second, Dutch patients have a physician who makes house calls, who has known them for years, whom they trust, and who will be the one they ask to help them die. To an extent that American physicians would envy, typical Dutch patients trust their physicians.

Some cases have pushed the limits, such as a physician who killed a woman in her twenties who had a decade of severe, uncontrollable anorexia. In another in May 1993, a physician assisted in the death of a severely depressed woman who had been traumatized by the death of her two children and the failure of her marriage.

Nevertheless, and after more than 30 years, the Dutch accept this new role for their physicians. The Dutch people resent the view of some American critics that to save money they dispatch their elderly relatives and the terminally ill. The Dutch tax themselves very heavily to pay for their national system of health care and pride themselves on a system that values autonomy and compassion for patients.

In April of 2001, after 30 years of agreements and semilegalization, Queen Beatrix signed a law passed by both legislative branches making physician-assisted death legal in Holland. After three decades, nearly 90 percent of Dutch citizens supported the new law.

The law lacked a controversial proposal allowing terminal 12- to 15-year olds the same right. It did include a right of patients in the early stages of dementia, amyotrophic lateral sclerosis (ALS), or other progressive diseases, to sign advanced directives allowing them to be killed at a later date.

During the 1990s, Dutch physicians rebuffed about 66 percent of patients who requested death. Patients who had assisted deaths generally had terminal cancer or end-stage ALS.

The Vatican and 10 percent of Dutch citizens and physicians condemned the legalization. In 2002, Belgium legalized the same, Switzerland legalized some kinds of physician-assisted dying and intensely debated complete legalization, and a commission in France recommended the practice for some extreme cases.

The Hemlock Society

In 1980 Derek Humphrey, a former British journalist, founded the Hemlock Society in the United States to help people with terminal illness die painlessly and with dignity. The society advocates limits on assisted suicide; it believes that laws should be liberalized only to assist dying for people who are both competent and terminally ill—not for chronic invalids, mental patients, or comatose patients.

The Hemlock Society is perhaps best known through its books, which are usually written by Derek Humphrey and give detailed instructions on how to kill oneself quickly and painlessly. No state has tried to ban the sale of these books, which are protected under the First Amendment. In 1991, Humphrey's *Final Exit* was a surprise best-seller and sold millions of copies.

The Hemlock Society and its publications have become popular because many Americans fear that their physicians will violate their wishes, forcing them to live their final days, months, or even years in pain, tethered to machines. As the writer and journalist Shana Alexander said about dying in a hospital, "When it comes to following my wishes, I trust my lawyer more than my physician."[9]

The Hospice Movement and Palliative Care

In the 1960s, two physicians—one working in the United States and the other in England—began a movement to change medicine so that it could accommodate the special needs of dying patients and their families. These two physicians were Elisabeth Kübler-Ross (who was born in Switzerland) and Cicely Saunders (born in Britain); their program was called the hospice movement. Many physicians in hospice argue that requests for physician-assisted dying arise only when patients do not know how modern hospice care works.

Kübler-Ross and Saunders developed special institutions that did not try to fight death but merely tried to make the dying patient as comfortable as possible. A hospice tries to give dying patients dignity and maximal control over the final months of their lives. Originally, hospices were special separate facilities, but the concept soon evolved to emphasize care in which most treatment is delivered by visiting nurses and physicians, allowing dying patients to stay at home.

As the result of the work of Kübler-Ross and Saunders, physicians are much more attuned today than they were 20 years ago to relief of pain and to the psychological needs of dying patients. In-home medical care, which includes hospice care, is now one of the fastest-growing fields of medicine, accounting for a large percentage of new jobs for nurses and aides. In the United States, Medicare (the program for people over 65) pays for hospice care for dying patients.

Within the last decade, a new movement inside medicine has developed called *palliative care*, the goal of which is to reduce the painful and undignified symptoms of the dying patient. Palliative therapy aims for maximal quality of life during the remaining weeks or months of life, and as such, may rule out full-dose radiation or chemotherapy in cancer patients (but may allow a short course of radiation to reduce a tumor to increase a patient's comfort).

DR. JACK KEVORKIAN AND DR. TIMOTHY QUILL

In June of 1990, Janet Adkins asked Jack Kevorkian, a retired pathologist, to help her die.

Janet Adkins, who lived in Oregon, was 54 years old. She loved music, sports and the outdoors, played tennis, and had hiked in the Himalayas—but now suffered the initial stages of Alzheimer's disease. For some time, she had been growing frustrated by her increasing inability to remember things, and she had found that she could no longer read the sheet music for her piano.

On average, people with Alzheimer's disease live 10 years after the onset of symptoms; in the final phase, which can last many years, such patients become vegetative. Alzheimer's disease is the fourth largest killer of Americans. Characterized by devastating loss of memory, resulting from irreversible degeneration of neural cells, it is incurable.

According to her husband, Ron Adkins, the diagnosis of Alzheimer's disease hit Janet Adkins "like a bombshell. . . . Her mind was her life." At the urging of her family, she tried THA (Tacrine), an experimental drug. According to her son Neil, "The drug didn't work. From then on, her mind was set. Quality of life was everything with her. She wanted to die with dignity intact." Janet Adkins had been a member of the Hemlock Society and strongly believed in its tenets.

Because assisted suicide was not illegal in Michigan then, where Kevorkian lived, Janet Adkins flew there with her husband and her three sons. Ambivalent about her intention to die, her family hoped that she might change her mind and had bought a round-trip ticket for her. In the end, however, the entire Adkins family supported her decision.

Jack Kevorkian, who was then 63, had grown up in Pontiac, Michigan, the son of Armenian immigrants, and had graduated from medical school in 1953. After finishing his residency, he worked from 1969 to 1978 in Detroit at Sarasota Hospital as director of laboratories. Later, he was employed at other hospitals, the last in southern California in 1982. When he retired from hospital work, he began to live on his social security benefits—$550 a month—and on his savings; his home was a tiny, two-room apartment above a florist's shop in Royal Oak, a suburban town near Detroit. For some years before Janet Adkins contacted him in 1990, Jack Kevorkian had actively publicized his views on physician-assisted death.

When Janet Adkins arrived in Michigan, Kevorkian and his two sisters interviewed her and her family for two hours; this was on June 3, 1990, a Saturday afternoon. None of the interviewers thought that Janet Adkins was irrational, depressed, or ambivalent about her decision to die; nor did any of them think that she could be helped by medicine. Janet Adkins and her family signed documents and made videotapes to prove that they were competent and understood what they were doing. Then the two families had a meal together to get to know each other better; after that, Janet Adkins and her family spent the night thinking things over.

The next day—Sunday afternoon, June 4, 1990,—Janet Adkins met Kevorkian alone and the two drove in his rusty 1968 Volkswagen van to a public park in north Oakland County, Michigan. Kevorkian had not been able to find any better place where he could help his patient kill herself. He had forthrightly told several clinics, churches, and funeral homes what he intended to do, and none of them would let him use their facilities. In desperation, he had decided on the park and had put a cot and his suicide device in the van.

The simple device in the van that would allow Janet Adkins to kill herself painlessly consisted of three intravenous (IV) bottles hung from an aluminum frame; Kevorkian called it a Mercitron. At the park, he connected an IV line to Janet Adkins and started a saline solution for fluid volume. Then she took over and pushed a switch that stopped the saline and released thiopental, a powerful sedative. The switch also started a six-second-timer which soon activated a drip of potassium chloride. The thiopental rendered Janet Adkins unconscious, and the potassium chloride killed her about one minute later. In effect, Kevorkian said, Janet Adkins had "a painless heart attack while in deep sleep." The whole process took less than 6 minutes.

Neither the Adkins family nor Kevorkian had anticipated the landslide of publicity that followed. The local district attorney prosecuted Kevorkian for murder. A local judge dismissed the case because there was no law against assisted suicide in Michigan, but he also ordered Kevorkian not to use the Mercitron again. (Since assisting suicide was not against the law, the judge's basis for issuing such an order was unclear.)

As an intern, Jack Kevorkian had begun to form his views on euthana-sia, when he cared for a middle-age woman with terminal cancer. He then be-came interested in death, and also in obtaining transplantable organs from pris-oners and dying patients—long before it was technically feasible to transplant organs.

During his residency at the hospital at the University of Michigan, he decried the waste of the bodies of condemned criminals and proposed that physicians ren-der such prisoners permanently unconscious and then use their bodies for risky medical experiments. He was forced to leave when university officials heard of his proposal. In his career as a pathologist, however, he never had any complaints filed against him.

While working as a hospital pathologist, he proposed that blood be trans-ferred directly from bodies of dead soldiers on a battlefield to wounded sol-diers lying nearby. In the decade before he became famous, he crusaded to let prisoners on death row become organ donors: "Each condemned prisoner could save five, six, seven lives. They're young, they're in good shape. What a waste."[10]

In 1986, he heard about the decriminalization of physician-assisted dying in the Netherlands. Instead of simply advocating the use of similar guidelines in the United States, he expanded "his death row proposal to include experimentation on willing patients who opt for euthanasia" and—under the mistaken impression that euthanasia had actually been legalized in the Netherlands—he went there to implement his proposal. (He found, of course, that euthanasia was not completely legal then in the Netherlands, and the Dutch rejected his ideas about allowing dy-ing patients to be used as subjects of medical experiments.)

Although Kevorkian has always sought ways to increase the availability of subjects for medical research and organs for transplantation, he never did medical research or surgical operations; nor has he ever been directly responsible for pa-tients in hospital beds. Thus his proposals about research subjects and organ trans-plants are more abstract than those of physicians in medical research who watch their patients die because of their inability to help.

Kevorkian's interest in assisting patients to die did not originally stem from compassion but from a desire to secure more organs for transplantation. He writes that when he was first contacted in 1989 by a patient with end-stage lung cancer, he felt "it only decent and fair to explain my ultimate aim": not to help patients achieve painless, dignified death, but to get terminal people to volunteer for "in-valuable experiments."[11] This aim would have constituted a new medical specialty, which he called "obitiary" or "medicide."

Jack Kevorkian has always been a loner and extremely independent. Except for a brief membership in one society of pathologists, he has scorned membership in medical societies: "Instinctively, as a student, I thought they were corrupt," he says. "I've been independent all my life."

After 1990, when he assisted at the death of Janet Adkins, Kevorkian received hundreds of letters a year from people whose suffering was of biblical proportions. Afraid to fly and hating to drive very far, he requires that his patients come to Royal Oak, the suburban town near Detroit where he lives. Thus he does not help anyone who is too ill to travel, which was a source of frustration for those who cannot find a way to get to Michigan. He accepts no money himself for helping patients; any donations go toward building a suicide center, the "Obitorium."

In the fall of 1991, Kevorkian assisted in the double suicide of two women patients, Sherry Miller and Marjorie Wanz: one with multiple sclerosis and another with chronic vaginal-pelvic pain. To comply technically with the order of the judge in the Adkins case, he used not the original Mercitron but a more sophisticated version of it. He was again indicted for murder, but again the charges were dismissed, since he still had not violated any Michigan law. However, his medical license in Michigan was suspended in November 1991.

With his license suspended, he could no longer obtain sodium pentothal and potassium chloride, and so he began using carbon monoxide (CO) with his next patients. In May of 1992, he helped another victim of multiple sclerosis to kill herself; this time the patient put on a mask in order to breath in the CO. Kevorkian came to believe that CO was a good way to commit suicide: The gas "has no color, taste, or smell; and it's toxic enough to cause rapid unconsciousness in relatively low concentration. Furthermore, in light complexioned people it often produces a rosy color that makes the victim look better as a corpse." After some trial and error, he began to teach patients to attach one end of a plastic tube to a canister of CO and the other to the kind of small plastic mask used in hospitals for oxygen therapy. When the gas is turned on and the patient breathes normally, death occurs within 5 minutes.

Many laypeople regard Jack Kevorkian as a folk hero, but most physicians and many medical ethicists denounced him. Asked about criticisms of his actions, he responds, "Why should I care what brainwashed ethicists and nonthinking physicians say?"[12] Nor has he worried about violating the Hippocratic oath; he calls physicians who follow these ancient ideas "hypocritic oafs."

In 3 years after the Adkins case, publicity about his other cases and his own eagerness to speak his mind made him a familiar figure in the American and Canadian media. After Janet Adkins's death, he appeared on television talk shows and news programs to publicize his invention, his ideas, and his services. He regards himself as a Socratic gadfly to the sluggish medical profession and compares himself proudly to the crusader Margaret Sanger, who was attacked by the medical profession for her work in birth control. He sees his struggle in heroic terms, comparing himself to Mahatma Gandhi, Martin Luther King, Jr., and Albert Einstein; he has even compared his early efforts at assisted dying to the birth of Christianity.

"Moreover, in sharp contrast to the timorous, secretive, and even deceitful intentions and actions of other medical euthanists on whom our so-called bioethicists now shower praise, I acted openly, ethically, legally, with complete and uncompromising honesty, and—even more important—I remained in personal attendance during the second most meaningful medical event in a patient's earthly existence."[13]

Kevorkian has sometimes been called a Dr. Frankenstein, but he does not consider himself a dangerous man and actually welcomes that comparison: "Frankenstein was benevolent, a dedicated researcher and doctor. He created this monster because he was interested in life and death. The monster was very loving."[14]

In the ensuing years, Kevorkian continued to advocate his cause through the mass media and to assist patients in committing suicide. In June 1995, he opened a "suicide clinic" in Michigan, but was soon evicted by the building's owner. In April 1996, he wore a colonial costume while being tried in court for the 1991 deaths of Sherry Miller and Marjorie Wanz to protest his prosecution under centuries-old common law. By 1998, he reached the milestone of having assisted 100 patients in committing suicide and had been acquitted in three trials involving five deaths.

In late 1998, *60 Minutes* aired a videotape that Dr. Kevorkian made of the assisted death of Thomas Youk, a 52-year old man suffering from Lou Gehrig's disease (ALS) who consented to both the death and the airing of his death on television. The appropriateness of showing Youk's death on national television became an issue in media ethics.

Kevorkian was charged with first-degree murder of Youk and convicted of second-degree murder. In April 13, 1999, Michigan judge Jessica Cooper sentenced Dr. Kevorkian. "Consider yourself stopped," she told him. For the death of Thomas Youk then 70 year-old Kevorkian was sentenced to 10–25 years in a Michigan state prison. That day, Kevorkian exchanged his street clothes for jail coveralls and was driven in a van (much like the one in which he helped Janet Adkins to die) to the State Prison of Southern Michigan at Jackson.

At his trial, he said he had helped over 130 patients to die since the case of Janet Adkins. Geoffrey Fieger, his previous attorney (whose brother, Dirk, sings for The Knack—"My Sharona"), did not represent Kevorkian in his the trial because "Kevorkian has turned self-destructive."

In November of 2001, the Michigan Court of Appeals affirmed Kevorkian's murder conviction. In April 2002, the Michigan Supreme Court refused in a 6–1 decision to hear Kevorkian's request for a new trial.

Kevorkian's new lawyer, Mayer Morganroth, planned to appeal to the federal courts and ultimately to the U. S. Supreme Court (although he did not say on what grounds). Kevorkian will be eligible for parole in May 2007. He has had no public interviews since entering prison.

•

In 1990, "Diane", a patient of Timothy Quill, an internist in Rochester, N.Y., asked him to help her die and he agreed to do so. This case differed significantly from the typical case of Jack Kevorkian.

As a young woman, Diane had survived vaginal cancer and had overcome alcoholism.[15] In 1990 At age 45, she suffering from leukemia, and had been a patient of Quill's for over 3 years, then suddenly developed acute myelomonocytic leukemia—one of the very worst kinds.

Quill explained to Diane that she had a 25 percent chance of long-term survival if she endured treatment. The treatment would consist of three weeks of induction chemotherapy (75 percent of patients respond to this and 25 percent die); then consolidation chemotherapy (another 25 percent die after this, so that the net survival rate becomes 50 percent); and finally bone marrow transplantation (requiring whole-body radiation and two months of hospitalization—another 25 percent die of graft-versus-host-disease, so that the net survival rate drops to 25 percent). For the last treatment to work well, a well-matched bone marrow donor would be needed. All these treatments would cause infections, loss of hair, and nausea. With no treatment, death would occur in days, weeks, or at most several months.

As is customary, the oncologists—who believe that any delay is dangerous in cases like this—began making plans "that afternoon" to insert a Hickman catheter into Diane to start chemotherapy. However Diane resisted being rushed in this way (a typical reaction among independent patients). On reflection, she decided that a 25 percent chance of long-term survival was not worth so toxic a course of therapy, especially because the hospital had no closely matched bone marrow donor. Disturbed by Diane's rejection of treatment, Quill apparently felt more positively about the 25 percent chance of survival. He had known her for 3 years, considered her mentally acute, and knew that her family supported her decision.

A few days after she had decided to forgo treatment, Diane began to worry intensely about a lingering death and concluded that when the time came she wanted barbiturates so that she could kill herself. Quill worried that her "preoccupation with her fear of lingering death would interfere with Diane's getting the most out of the time she had left." Having ruled out irrational depression, he wrote a prescription for barbiturates and told her how to use them for both sleep and suicide.

Diane then experienced three tumultuous months. Her son stayed home from college, and her husband worked at home. Several times she became weak or developed infections but bounced back. Near the end, Diane had two weeks of relative calm, followed by rapid decline.

Because Diane now faced what she feared most, increasing discomfort, dependence, and hard choices, Quill knew that her end had come:

> When we met, it was clear that she knew what she was doing, that she was sad and frightened to be leaving, but that she would be even more terrified to stay and suffer. In our tearful goodbye, she promised a reunion in the future at her favorite spot on the edge of Lake Geneva, with dragons swimming in the sunset.[16]

Quill published an account of Diane's death in a respected medical journal, was prosecuted for murder after his article appeared, but a grand jury refused to indict him.

His case contrasts in several ways with those of Jack Kevorkian: Timothy Quill had known Diane well and had been treating her for a long time; he first offered her a course of treatment that might allow her to survive; he helped her die privately and at the time, without publicity; he preserved her anonymity; he presented his account in an established medical forum; and he was not a specialist in assisted dying. Many physicians who strongly oppose Jack Kevorkian have lauded Timothy Quill.

RECENT LEGAL DECISIONS

In 1993, a bill was signed making assisted suicide illegal in Michigan, but Michigan's Court of Appeals threw it out in 1994. Meanwhile in the American West, states repeatedly tried to legalize physician-assisted dying. After intense, public opposition by the Catholic church, bills to legalize physician-assisted dying were narrowly defeated in California in 1992 and in Washington state in 1991. In May of

1994, federal Judge Barbara Rothstein struck down a law in Washington state banning assisted suicide, holding that the Fourteenth Amendment (guaranteeing equal protection of liberty) was broad enough to cover not only a woman's right to end a pregnancy but also a terminal patient's right to physician-assisted dying.[17]

In Canada, Sue Rodriquez, a 43-year-old victim of Lou Gehrig's disease, led a campaign to legalize physician-assisted suicide. Her case went to Canada's highest court, which in 1994 held 5 to 4 that sanctity of life outweighed personal autonomy and freedom from suffering. One poll said that 77 percent of Canadians agreed with Rodriquez, who despite the court's ruling killed herself with a physician's surreptitious help.[18]

In 1996, the Ninth and Second Circuit Court of Appeals in federal law held unconstitutional laws banning physician-assisted suicide in Washington and New York. In New York, Timothy Quill and other physicians successfully argued (*Quill v. Vacco*) that it was discrimination against dying patients that some could decide to die by having a ventilator or feeding tube removed, but others, who were terminal but neither ventilator- nor feeding tube-dependent, could not. In other words, Dr. Quill and others argued that it was irrational to allow physicians to kill by withdrawing treatment but not to kill by more active means.

In the Washington case, a district attorney appealed Judge Rothstein's 1994 decision to the Court of Appeals for the Ninth Circuit. The Supreme Court's *Cruzan* decision in 1990 had held that a fundamental liberty interest of citizens forbids states from making laws that restrict the rights of competent patients to refuse medical treatment, even if such refusal means their death. Building on this decision, judges of the Ninth Circuit on March 7, 1996 ruled that a fundamental liberty interest in the Constitution was broad enough to allow a state to decriminalize physician-assisted dying.

In June 1997, the U.S. Supreme Court rejected both lines of argument. In *Quill v. Vacco*, it decided that "the distinction between assisting suicide and withdrawing life-sustaining treatment, a distinction widely recognized and endorsed in the medical profession and in our legal traditions, is both important and logical; it is certainly rational. . . ."[19] The court specifically rejected the argument that it is inconsistent to allow refusal of life-sustaining treatment but disallow assisted suicide, saying the distinction was neither arbitrary nor irrational. (It did not really justify this assertion).

In *Washington* v. *Glucksberg*, the Court held that the traditional interpretation of liberty, protected in the due process clause of the Fourteenth Amendment, should only be expanded if the rights and interests in question are "deeply rooted in this nation's history and tradition." Not surprisingly, a right to assisted suicide was not found by the Court to be so. The Court also recognized the AMA's claim that legalization of physician-assisted dying would threaten the integrity of the medical profession, hurt the disabled and poor, and possibly start a slippery slope.

These decisions only said that a fundamental right to die did not exist in the Constitution, such that state laws banning assisted suicide would violate such a right. The decisions left open the door for a state to legalize physician-assisted suicide. In this way, these decisions mirrored what *Cruzan* said about laws about incompetent patients, i.e., states could, but need not, pass a certain kind of law.

OREGON'S LEGALIZATION

Over the last two decades, northwestern America has led the fight for death with dignity in the United States, having the headquarters for organizations such as Compassion in Dying. Oregon also led the nation in the late 1980s in initiating town meetings across the state to achieve consensus on what to fund in its Medicaid program for low income people.

Oregon has a means by which citizen-initiated bills may become law by popular referendum. In November 1994, Oregonians approved the Oregon Death with Dignity Act. This Act legalized assistance in dying from a physician by the prescription of drugs.

The day after the Act passed, a local judge permanently enjoined its implementation, concluding that it violated the equal protection clause of the U.S. Constitution. The injunction was appealed to the Ninth Circuit Court of Appeals, which lifted the injunction. It ruled that James Bopp, an advocate for people with disabilities who crusades against such laws and had initiated the suit, did not have standing to sue.[20]

On June 26, 1997, as noted above, the U.S. Supreme Court ruled in two cases that no such basic right to physician-assisted suicide could be inferred from either of the Constitution's clauses about due process or about equal protection. What this meant was that, unlike in *Roe* v. *Wade,* no essential Constitutional right was found in this area of personal liberty such that all state laws violating this right would be thrown out. However, to say that there is no inherent right in the Constitution to something does not imply that a particular state cannot grant that right, and the Supreme Court indicated that a state such as Oregon could do so if it wished.

After this ruling, and surprisingly—to the irritation of Oregon's voters—the Oregon legislature *repealed* the very Act which its citizens had passed 19 months before. An intense argument ensued in the state's media, like similar battles before in the northwest. The Catholic church again lobbied heavily against legalization, spending $2 million for television ads. This time, billionaire and libertarian George Soros intervened on the other side. (Soros had already funded a project designed to improve the way Americans die.) Altogether, $4 million was spent against legalization, $1 million in favor.

Neil Adkins, the son of Kevorkian's first patient, Janet Adkins, participated in an ad against legalization, saying, "I will probably die with this inside me, with this question: Could I have prevented my mother from dying?"[21] Boston-based physician-ethicist Linda Emanuel came out strongly against legalization, saying, "In organized medicine, there is a strong and growing awareness that a policy in favor of assisted suicide will not work." She suggested that experience in Holland showed that some percentage of attempted suicides wouldn't be successful.[22] The Oregon Medical Association opposed legalization, where previously it had remained neutral. Nevertheless, in the previous November in 1996, 60 percent of 2,700 physicians in Oregon who replied to a survey said they were not morally opposed to physician-assisted suicide.[23]

Voters appeared unfazed by predictions of lack of success, abuse, and slippery slopes. They seemed especially irritated at their politicians' attempt to revoke an

Act that they had passed. One popular ad said, "Not one time in all of Oregon history has the Legislature had the arrogance to try to appeal a voter-passed initiative."[24]

The previous referendum had narrowly passed 51 percent to 49 percent. This time, in November 1997, Oregonians approved the measure 60 percent to 40 percent. (One poll even found that 50 percent of Catholics voted for it.)

Despite the dramatic appeals on both sides, the Act's restrictions made few people eligible. Patients not only had to be (1) clearly competent, (2) dying of a terminal disease (defined as having less than six months to live, as confirmed by a primary physician and a second, consulting physician), but also (3) endure a 15-day waiting period after the initial request in case they changed their minds and to avoid impulsive decisions. Physicians are not allowed to administer the fatal dosage, only to prescribe it.

For the first five months after suicide became possible, no patients availed themselves of the option—to the surprise of both supporters and opponents. With such a change, some glitches and controversies were to be expected in the implementation. At the urging of socially conservative Congressmen Orin Hatch and Henry Hyde, DEA agents briefly threatened to go after physicians prescribing lethal dosages of morphine, until Attorney General Janet Reno stopped them. Oregon Medicaid officials announced they would reimburse physicians for counseling and aiding the dying. Some pharmacists refused to handle the relevant prescriptions.

In 2001, Bush Attorney General John Ashcroft, after swearing to the Senate that he would not let his conservative personal values influence his enforcement of the law, instructed DEA agents to go after physicians in Oregon who prescribed lethal prescriptions to terminal patients, as allowed by Oregon law. Patients in Oregon appealed for an injunction, which was granted by a federal judge.

Ashcroft's authority to pursue this line of action was shaky. States define murder and exceptions to it, not the federal government. No national law exists defining murder or exceptions to it.

After the bombing of the World Trade Center on September 11, 2001, Ashcroft developed new priorities, and prosecution of Oregonian physicians ceased to be the subject of his press conferences.

On March 26, 1998, the first known legal suicide occurred by a woman suffering from terminal breast cancer who had been given less than two months to live.[25] According to Compassion in Dying, an Oregon-based advocacy group, the woman died about 30 minutes after taking the medication. By July 1998, two more cases had occurred. Four terminal patients who made a request to use the new law died before they could be helped during the 15-day waiting period.

As Oregon goes down this new road, three practical issues have become important. First, is alternative care—such as palliative care and referrals to hospice—adequately encouraged? Data indicate that the answer is positive. Surveys always show that most people prefer to die at home or in a homelike setting, not a hospital. Oregon has the lowest in-hospital mortality rate, suggesting a good level of referrals for home health care and respect for advanced directives.[26]

Second, as more people use their freedom to die under the new law, will there be many botched suicides where people end up in long-term comas? Opponents of legalization claim this happens 25 percent of the time in Holland with attempts at physician-assisted death.[27]

Although the figure of 25 percent is too high, some assisted deaths do have complications, as borne out by the experience of the Hemlock Society. (see below) Moreover, virtually no physician has received training in how to manage a certain, dignified, painless death. In Holland, in 21 of 114 cases where the physician intended to watch a patient kill himself, the physician had to intervene to cause death. Overall, around 6 percent of cases of both assisted suicide and euthanasia had some problem.[28]

This is a strange argument by opponents for several reasons: It is a complaint about the "how to" part of the argument, asserting that the present law isn't good enough to guarantee death. Such a claim will be correct for some patients. Previous experience with AIDS patients attempting assisted suicide at dosages recommended by the Hemlock Society showed that some patients had high tolerances to massive dosages of central nervous system depressants, and hence, did not die easily or quickly, sometimes ending up in vegetative comas.

To avoid this possibility, the patient needed to ask a friend to be present to possibly help at the end by attaching a large plastic bag over the patient's head and securing it with duct tape, such that the patient could suffocate to death. (This is what critic Nat Hentoff calls an "Exit Bag," sarcastically referring to the efficient, self-administered form of it with velcro straps that can be ordered from the Hemlock Society.[29]) Use of such an "Exit Bag" subjects a friend to the charge of murder, and as such, leaves many dying patients faced with the tragic dilemma of either dying alone (with a possibly botched effort) or asking a friend to risk prosecution for murder.

However, the logical implication of this argument is not to rescind the Act but to go one step further and allow physicians to administer a fatal dosage. This suggests the Act is at present an ill-advised political compromise that may have morally bad effects in leaving patients with the above dilemma.

A third problem under the new law concerns financial resources. People with Medicare, with Medicaid, or with good private medical insurance can use the law, but what about the many working people who lack medical insurance? In particular, will the working poor need to forgo hospice care because they have no insurance, and thus be led to choosing assisted suicide? To its credit, Oregon has tried to address this measure by its groundbreaking Oregon Health Plan, where most of the previously uninsured, terminally ill citizens now have access to hospice programs. As with Holland's experience, this suggests Oregon's experience should not be generalized to states with poorly funded state Medicaid plans, and might put patients at risk of dying early for lack of money.

What about managed care organizations subtly pushing early death to save money? One misperception is that hospice and palliative care are cheap. A 1998 study showed that physician-assisted death might make a difference in only one-half of 1 percent of costs at the end of life.[30]

Finally, an old-fashioned way of dying still exists, especially where physicians are trained well and respect patient's wishes.[31] That way, simply put, is that a competent patient can decide to die by not eating and not drinking. It is not generally painful to do so. Although it takes some determination, it may help the family as it indicates a firm resolve and no ambivalence. One woman went 11 days without fluids and 51 days without food before she died this way.[32]

Physician Susan Tolle adopted an "it's here, it's legal, let's deal with it attitude," producing the *Guidebook for Health Care Providers* to help practicing physicians.[33] This book emphasizes the impact on the family of a dying patient's decision to have assistance in dying as well as on the health professionals involved, and for those the patient chooses *not* to have involved. Family members and health professionals kept in ignorance of the patient's decision may experience unresolved grief and anger, and hence, the *Guidebook* recommends that a patient involve everyone in his decision.

Of course, no doctor or nurse can be forced against his or her conscience to participate in such a death, but the issue becomes complicated because a physician cannot *abandon* the patient (this word has special connotations in medicine, as patient abandonment is illegal). Somewhat controversially but pragmatically, the *Guidebook* says that a physician who objects to participating in the death "must transfer care so that the needs of the patient can be met" and "must not hinder the transfer."[34] Psychiatrists and psychologists must evaluate the patient if a physician suspects a treatable depression led to the decision to die, but such mental health professionals have their own problems when they are morally opposed to such deaths. In this case, "they may have difficulty objectively evaluating patients and should consider declining. [They should also] disclose personal biases to the attending physician at the time of the referral."

Numbers of Patients Requesting Death from Physicians in Oregon and Numbers actually using prescriptions to die[35]

1998	24 Rx, 16 deaths	6/10,000 deaths in Oregon
1999	33 Rx, 27 deaths	9/10,000 deaths in Oregon
2000	39 Rx, 27 deaths	9/10,000 deaths in Oregon
2001	44 Rx, 19 deaths	7/10,000 deaths in Oregon*

*33 physicians participated in writing these prescriptions.

The *Guidebook* encourages physicians to obtain the drugs for the patient, keep them until the time of death, and be there with the patient in her home as she takes them.[36] Details have been thought out: The physician should insist on an advanced directive specifying a "do not resuscitate" order for emergency response personnel, counsel the family that the death may not be immediate but may take hours and have complications, be ready to administer antiemetics and analgesics, counsel and support the family during and after the death, sign the death certificate and sign other papers required by the Act, and arrange transfer to a funeral home. (One can see why such services should not be reimbursed!)

Should physicians actually attend deaths in this manner, it would be an extraordinary return to home visits and to the ancient tradition of physicians "being with" patients at the bedside as they die. Surely this will be the new Rorschach test in medical ethics, with one side viewing such aid as barbaric and the other, as humanistic.

ETHICAL ISSUES

Overview: Direct and Indirect Arguments

Two very different kind of arguments occur about the ethics of physician-assisted dying. The first kind focuses directly on the morality of such assistance, either arguing it is intrinsically wrong or arguing that it is intrinsically right. The other kind grants that such assistance in a few rare cases may be justified, but opposes legalization based on the bad indirect effects of such legalization. These will be called direct and indirect arguments for and against physician-assisted dying.

Use of this distinction will further conceptual clarity about exactly what is being claimed on each side, and such usage will help us keep the arguments in order. The main direct argument against physician-assisted dying is that it is always wrong to kill, and the two main countering, direct arguments are that such assistance is required by recognition of the values in our culture of personal autonomy and mercy. Most of the typical arguments against physician-assisted dying are indirect and involve predictions about the slippery slope. Many variations of "slope" claims about legalization are possible, appealing to changes in the role of physicians, undue influence of reimbursement, effects on the poor and disabled, and risk of errors and abuse. Many slope predictions involve, as we shall see, a particular kind of claim about opening up the dark side of human nature.

DIRECT ARGUMENTS ABOUT PHYSICIAN-ASSISTED DYING

The Wrongness of Killing

The most general, direct argument against physician-assisted dying is that it is a kind of killing of innocent humans, conjoined with the more general claim that it is wrong to kill humans. Any time one human being consciously acts to end the life of another, a terrible evil is committed. Such an action, it is said, violates the will of God.

This argument does not argue that what is wrong about killing is that it can become uncontrollable after a few justified cases, but that any killing is *intrinsically wrong*, no matter what the circumstances. The most ancient justification of this claim is based on religious metaphysics: that a God exists, that Scripture correctly reveals his laws for humans, and that one such law is for humans never to kill each other. Based on this view, some Christians and some orthodox Jews are complete pacifists, preferring death to self-defense.

Chapter 3 noted that Scripture really bans "unjustified" killings, and hence, just wars and the death penalty for murderers are seen as permissible. The question at issue here concerns whether helping a terminally ill patient die is "unjustified killing." After all, God presumably allows the person to experience the disease and no one escapes the final end of death.

More important, we need to examine the background conditions for why the rule against killing has been important throughout the millennia of civilization in the West. Throughout this history, most people have wanted to live as long as possible. That fact is less true today. Why?

The answer is that our view of dying is different now because of the successes of medicine over the last 50 years. Medicine has now largely advanced the cures for the old, acute diseases that killed swiftly, and left us with chronic diseases that kill slowly, such as cancer and heart disease. In the past, people tried to live as long as possible because most never experienced the disability and dysfunction that came with chronic diseases, but now most people realize that one can live so long that quality of life becomes miserable. For most people, what counts is quality of life, not the quantity of days lived.

Now consider the rule against killing and physician-assisted dying. When you help me accomplish what I want to do, you do a good thing, and morality encourages you to help me. When you prevent me from doing what I want to do, you hurt my interests and me, and your actions are probably immoral. Whether or not dying assisted by physicians is good or bad may depend, not on what has been traditionally judged moral or immoral, but on the wishes of the dying patient. Specifically, whether physician-assisted dying is moral or immoral would not seem to depend on whether it promotes or hinders mere life or death (the traditional view), but on whether the dying patient desires it.

Of course, critics can object that helping me do what I want to do is not a good thing if I want to do something immoral such as steal my neighbor's car. And, they say, helping people die is immoral.

But why should we allow this objection? Why should we accept the underlying premise that "helping dying people die is immoral" unless some *further reason* is given? To simply assert this objection is to beg the question. It is not an *argument against* a position to assume that it is wrong.

In sum, to argue that "assisting the dying" is morally equivalent to killing is misleading because killing almost always refers to, first, taking the life of a person who does not want to die, and second, someone who is not a dying patient. Whether the traditional role of physicians is special, such that it forbids killing as specified in the Hippocratic Oath, is a different argument—an indirect one—that we'll consider later.

Killing vs. Letting Die

There has been a debate in medical ethics for several decades now about whether there is a morally significant difference for physicians between killing and letting die. Perhaps the best way to understand this debate is as a variation of the above claim that it is wrong to kill directly. What has been accepted for a long time in medicine is that it is sometimes permissible to allow patients to die by ceasing medical treatments, but never permissible to take more active means to bring about death.

Chapter 2 describes how medical practice in the United States evolved to a point where most physicians feel ethically comfortable with forgoing or withdrawing treatment—including artificial nutrition—to hasten death in a terminal patient. However, intentional termination of a dying patient's life is still considered unethical by the AMA and is also, of course, illegal in every state except Oregon.

According to one bioethicist, Jack Kevorkian's assistance to Janet Adkins raised the question "whether there is any clear distinction between assisted suicide and active euthanasia." In assisted suicide, as the term was being used in that passage, the patient ends his or her own life; in active euthanasia, the physician's action is the immediate cause of death. A leading physician in medical ethics has admitted, "I have had occasion to give a patient pain medication we both knew would shorten her life."[37] Is this much different from killing the patient? Most physicians now respect a patient's request to withdraw nutrition or hydration, but most would still resist doing anything directly to cause the death of the patient. This asymmetry assumes a profound difference between acting to withdraw treatment (with the intention of hastening death) and acting to actually cause death (with the same intention). Is there really any difference? Is the difference only semantic?

As noted, the U.S. Supreme Court in its *Quill* v. *Vacco* ruling asserted that there was a moral difference for physicians between killing and letting die, although it did so without any argument (and it had so much help! Over a hundred *amicus* briefs were filed, with distinguished ethicists on each side.) Such a distinction, it asserted, was neither arbitrary nor unreasonable.

In 1975, in a famous article in the *New England Journal of Medicine*, the philosopher James Rachels attacked the distinction between "active" and "passive" euthanasia.[38] Rachels argued that this distinction, though still dominant in modern medicine and law, has no inherent moral value and that—when it is erroneously taken for anything more than a shorthand pragmatic rule—leads to decisions about death based on irrelevant factors.

Rachels's logic cuts two ways: First, letting a vegetative patient die is just as bad (or good) as killing him; second, killing a vegetative patient is just as good (or bad) as allowing him to die. There is nothing moral or immoral in the act of passive or active euthanasia itself; rather, morality or immorality is determined by motives and results in the context of that act. Focusing on whether an act is active or passive, he argued, may confuse our judgments, leading us to think that passively allowing people to die slowly and horribly is morally superior to actively bringing about a quick, painless death.

Rachels's position was controversial. Is intending death by removing a respirator equivalent to suffocating a patient with a pillow? If a patient is allowed to die, isn't that patient killed by the disease? But if someone acts directly to bring about dying, isn't that human agent the cause of death? One critic argued:

> What is the difference between merely letting a patient die and killing that patient? Does it depend upon activity or passivity? Does it depend on an agent's intentions? I think that neither of these factors is relevant. What is relevant is the cause of death. When the cause of death is the underlying disease process, the patient is simply allowed to die.[39]

In support of Rachels, it can be argued that in practice the line between active and passive is hard to draw. In some cases, not acting can be considered active; one example might be not giving antibiotics to Karen Quinlan to treat the pneumonia she developed in her final weeks. The neurologist and medical ethicist Ronald

Cranford sees no great difference between letting die and killing and argues that "most medical professionals are just wrong on this issue." Cranford also holds that if the physician's motive is to relieve suffering in a dying patient, it is permissible to kill.[40] However, this does not imply (as is sometimes feared) that there is no difference between killing and assisted dying; as Jean Davies argues, just as "rape and making love are different, so are killing and assisted suicide."[41]

Meanwhile, a consensus has emerged that most deaths of dying patients in America today are managed deaths. A survey by the American Hospital Association found that 70 percent of deaths in hospitals involve some decision by a physician or relative to cease treatment.[42] Although many people worry that Oregon's legalization of prescriptions for the dying will result in a slippery slope, critics such as bioethicist Dan Brock worry that "the covert managing of death" is just as dangerous, if not more dangerous.[43]

Mercy, Compassion, and Relief of Suffering

One of the most persuasive arguments for physician-assisted dying is the appeal to mercy. Observing another human being in untreatable pain, howling like a wounded animal, can move even the most callous of us to tears. The most natural response is to end such suffering. We do this for our pets; why can't we do the same for humans? Moreover, the suffering of terminal patients is not confined to physical pain, as bad as that is: It also involves helplessness, stress, exhaustion, terror, loss, and other experiences that are difficult even to imagine.

Mercy means different things to different people, however, and if we intend to be merciful, we will need to understand what each individual patient wants. To some patients, mercy may mean being helped to die. To others, mercy may simply mean relief of pain. To still others, it may mean reassurance—relief from the fear of becoming incompetent, or of living hooked up to machines, or simply of dying in a hospital. And it should be remembered that to some, mercy may mean being supported and encouraged in their efforts to live—being offered treatment as long as there is a chance of survival.

A big issue here has to do with relief of pain. Is it possible to relieve all pain and make dying patients completely comfortable? Joanne Lynn, a physician and hospice director, believes that no patient need die in pain:

> [Lynn] has cared for over 1,000 hospice patients, and only two of these patients seriously and repeatedly requested physician assistance in active euthanasia. Even these two patients did not seek another health care provider when it was explained that their requests could not be honored. New patients to hospice often state they want to "get it over with." At face value, this may seem a request for active euthanasia. However, these requests are often an expression of the patient's concerns regarding pain, suffering, and isolation, and their fears about whether their dying will be prolonged by technology. Furthermore, these requests may be attempts by the patient to see if anyone really cares whether he or she lives. Meeting such a request with ready acceptance could be disastrous for the patient who interprets the response as a confirmation of his or her worthlessness. Future research should systematically document the number of patients who

prefer voluntary active euthanasia even in the supportive environment of hospice.[44]

Similarly, the physician Cicely Saunders, who founded St. Christopher's Hospice in London, says that patients there need never suffer pain. She gives these patients Brompton cocktails—a powerful brew of morphine, heroin, alcohol, and cocaine. (Note that British physicians do not worry about making terminally ill patients "drug addicts.")

On the other hand, Derek Humphrey of the Hemlock Society argues that "it is generally agreed that 10 percent of pain cannot be controlled. That is a lot of people."[45] It is also true that not everyone experiences pain in the same way, and a condition which would be acceptable to some patients might be intolerable to others.

A related question is not simply whether or to what extent pain can be relieved but what the cost of relief might be, and what costs are acceptable. In this context, we are not talking about financial costs: The issue is the cost to the patient's well-being. Powerful narcotics such as Brompton cocktails numb consciousness and can reduce patients to a vegetative state during their last months of life.

Dying patients must make a tradeoff between consciousness and relief of pain, and not every patient considers that tradeoff acceptable. For some patients, being conscious and able to talk to relatives and friends is more important than avoiding pain. Here again, autonomy becomes relevant. What counts as a benefit or a harm must be defined within each patient's own value system, and who else but the patients themselves can make judgments about this tradeoff?

A wider question, as noted above, is what relief of pain implies about physician-assisted dying. As we saw earlier in this chapter, leaders of the hospice movement believe that few if any patients would ask for assisted death if they were aware that hospice care could keep them free of pain. However, advocates of physician-assisted dying argue that pain is only one aspect of suffering and therefore that relieving a patient's pain does not necessarily relieve his or her suffering. *Pain* is physical; *suffering* is a broader and more personal matter.

Peter Admiraal, a physician and one of the leaders of assisted dying in the Netherlands, agrees that uncontrollable pain is rarely the only reason for wanting death:

> There is severe dehydration, uncontrolled itching and fatigue. These patients are completely exhausted. Some of them can't turn around in their beds. They become incontinent. All these factors make a kind of suffering from which they only want to escape. . . .
>
> And of course you are suffering because you have a mind. You are thinking about what is happening to you. You have fears and anxiety and sorrow. In the end, it gives a complete loss of human dignity. You cannot stop that feeling with medical treatment.[46]

The main arguments against this is that in almost all cases aggressive treatment by physicians trained in palliative care can reduce such symptoms. But such care is expensive and such specialists are rare—raising the issue of whether America commits enough resources to dying well.

Patient Autonomy

One significant issue in physician-assisted dying—as in assisted suicide—is patients' autonomy. Autonomy was an important concept for John Stuart Mill, who argued in his *On Liberty* that "over his own body and mind, the individual is sovereign." Mill believed that government should not impose on individuals its view of when and how they should die.

One way to put the argument for patients' autonomy with regard to assisted dying is to compare a person's life to a business: If I own a business that is making money, it makes sense for me to keep it open; but if the business is losing money, I would be imprudent to wait until there was no money left at all before closing.[47] Similarly, a terminally ill patient owns his or her body and need not "stay in business" till the very end.

One issue that involves autonomy concerns several questions about risks that are important issues in physician-assisted dying: Who is best qualified to assess the danger of dying too soon? What degree of risk is acceptable? Who should determine acceptability? How does the risk of dying too soon compare with the risks entailed by alternatives?

Physicians usually believe that they are best qualified to assess risk, and they're right as far as statistical risk is concerned. But *acceptable* risk is evaluative as well as statistical, and many patients want the right to make their own judgments about what is acceptable risk.

It is important to realize that when terminal patients make such evaluations, their concern is more than just fear of pain. Derek Humphrey of the Hemlock Society has written, "It isn't just a question of pain. It is a question of dignity, self-control, and distress. If you can't eat, sleep, or read, and the quality of life is so bad, and there is a certainty that you are dying, it is a matter of dignity" to be able to end your life.[48]

It is also important to emphasize that in order to make the best decisions about acceptable risk, patients and their families need information. University of Utah philosopher Margaret Battin holds that physicians rarely discuss options with dying patients.[49] She believes that patients' informed consent should be sought not only for medical research but also for ways of dying. Especially when experimental drugs and surgery are involved, terminal patients should be informed about different outcomes and different ways of dying so that they can choose "the least worst death." At present, however, adequate information is rare, and thus genuine choice by patients is also rare. For Battin, the right to control the circumstances of one's own death was "the most important civil-rights issue" of the 1990s.

INDIRECT ARGUMENTS ABOUT PHYSICIAN-ASSISTED DYING

Empirical, Conceptual, and Financial Slippery Slopes

In discussions about physician-assisted dying, people often made claims about the *slippery slope*, one of the most famous ideas in ethics (also called the thin edge of the wedge—or simply "wedge"—argument). Claims about the slippery slope figure prominently in bioethics at both ends of life: about changing rules about how people die and about changing rules about how it is permissible to create people (discussed in Chapter 5).

Although claims about such slopes are frequently made, the nature of this claim is often vague and ill-defined. Generally, a slippery slope argument asserts that if a preliminary neutral or good step is accepted, a series of other changes will inevitably occur, leading to a final, very bad result. As a metaphor, it often sees society as a teetering ball perched atop a steep slope, but leaning downward, braced by chocks on the ground, preventing it from descending. The chocks are our basic moral principles.

There are two general kinds of claims about slippery slopes, *empirical* and *conceptual*.[50] Claims about empirical slopes assert that once you take the first step, something bad in human nature is unleashed, which will be uncontrollable. Previously, the moral rule held this bad thing in check, but now an exception has been made that sets a precedent, so the absolute moral rule is gone. Pandora's Box is open.

In cases like Janet Adkins's, critics claimed that once one kind of vulnerable, incompetent patient was killed, this precedent would allow a similar kind of killing in other, similar situations. Because of a prejudice against the elderly and loss of intelligence, society would quickly expand the killing of cognitively impaired elderly people. For example, dementia patients and then still a third kind, for example elderly patients in nursing homes with mild cognitive deficit, and so on, down the slippery slope until masses of vulnerable, elderly patients would be killed. This kind of claim is an *empirical* slope prediction.

First, because it says that, once society changes a rule about protecting one class of patient, bad forces will be unleashed that cannot be restrained and kept contained to the original class.

Such claims about empirical slopes are often made about legalizing physician-assisted suicide. Law professor Yale Kamisar observes that "not all people are kind, understanding, and loving. Yet they will be making decisions about the elderly and helpless. A lot of pressure may be placed on people to choose euthanasia when they really don't want it."[51] Norman Fost—a Wisconsin professor of pediatrics and medical ethicist who maintains that in every society where physician-assisted suicide was legal it was applied too broadly and "the situation got out of control"—argues that assisted dying "gives a doctor and the patient an easy out."[52]

Both these men assert that empirical slopes will occur. For Kamisar, there are unkind, nonunderstanding, and nonloving people who will make decisions to let the elderly and helpless die for the wrong reasons if we change. For Fost, history shows assisted suicide cannot be kept within bounds, and in addition, physicians and patients will be cowards and lazy, taking the "easy way out."

A *conceptual* slippery slope asserts that once a small change is made in a moral rule, other changes will inevitably follow, because of the demands of reason for consistency in treating similar cases similarly. At the time of the Karen Quinlan case in 1976, disability advocate James Bopp said that if you "accept quality of life as the standard," then "first you withdraw the respirators, then the food and then you actively kill people. It's a straight line from one place to the others."[53] Bioethicist Daniel Callahan then said that the logic of the case for euthanasia will inevitably lead to its extension far beyond terminally ill competent adults. If relief of suffering is critical, Callahan said, "why should that relief be denied to the demented or the incompetent?"[54] In the claims of both these people, what justifies one kind of case will soon justify another.

Other examples of conceptual slopes are easy to see: First we will allow abortion of a fetus because of Down syndrome, then we will let a newborn with Down syndrome die. In this kind of slope, as opposed to empirical slopes *it is always the demand of reason to treat similar cases similarly that expands the initial change.*

Contrasts may be made among the two kinds of slope claims. The empirical claim is a prediction about unstoppable expansion if some moral change occurs, whereas the conceptual claim refers to a linkage in reasoning once certain premises are accepted. Where the empirical slope says one small change will create many others because of something bad in humans, the conceptual slope says the same kind of change can occur because of something higher in humans, namely reason's need to treat similar cases similarly.

The primary difference between the two kinds of slopes is that one describes the power of ideas and the other the momentum of change. In a *conceptual* slope, the urge to logical consistency drives the expansion to cover more cases. I find engineers very receptive to this kind of thinking. It's also a kind of thinking with a low tolerance for ambiguity and shades of meaning over different cases.

In an *empirical* slope, it's not logical consistency driving the change, but merely the fact of change itself. As one man once said, "Once I'm off my diet, something is unleashed and it's hard not to eat more and more." Another example: once you get away with a little cheating on your taxes, it's hard not to cheat more and more. In all these cases of empirical slopes, something bad inside people is kept in check by an imposed morality or regimen.

In September 2000, physician Michael Swango was arrested as a serial killer of patients. Charged and convicted with killing three patients in New York State, Dr. Swango was estimated to have killed at least 60 patients, possibly hundreds, starting in Zimbabwe in the early 1980s and moving around the world (when arrested, he was on his way to Saudi Arabia for a new job).[55] His diary, used to convict him, revealed that he killed for the "thrill" of the power to kill and "the sweet, husky, close smell of an indoor homicide." It is just such malice in human nature that people assert could be unleashed with legal, physician-assisted deaths and the existence of such a "thrill" is one desire grounding claims about empirical slippery slopes.

It is perhaps unfortunate but historically true that slippery slope claims are associated with the mass killings by the Nazi SS and German physicians earlier this century. In the article by Leo Alexander mentioned previously, we can see examples of both claims. First, Alexander mentions an empirical slope:

> All destructiveness ultimately leads to self-destruction; the fate of the SS and of Nazi Germany is an eloquent example. The destructive principle, once unleashed, is bound to engulf the whole personality and to occupy all its relationships. Destructive urges and destructive concepts arising therefrom cannot remain limited or focused upon one subject or several subjects alone, but must inevitably spread and be directed against one's entire surrounding world, including one's own group and ultimately the self.[56]

Once the rule against killing innocent citizens was broken, Alexander asserts, the SS and Nazi physicians knew no bounds.

Alexander also wrote:

> The beginnings at first were merely a subtle shift in emphasis in the basic attitude of the physicians. It started with the acceptance of the attitude, basic in the euthanasia movement, that there is such a thing as life not worthy to be lived. This attitude in its early stages concerned itself merely with the severely and chronically sick. Gradually the sphere of those to be included in this category was enlarged to encompass the socially unproductive, the ideologically unwanted, the racially unwanted and finally all non-Germans. But it is important to realize that the infinitely small wedged-in lever from which this entire trend of mind received its impetus was the attitude of the nonrehabilitable sick.

Once physicians may kill one kind of patient because quality of life was so low as to make "life not worthy to be lived," they not only *may* use similar reasoning in other cases, but (reason says) *they should.*

In practice, few people separate empirical from conceptual claims about slippery slopes, but that does not mean that we should not. By noting exactly what is supposed to drive the expansion, we can more accurately verify if such predictions came true in the past.

Slope predictions have been made with increasing frequency about legalization of physician-assisted dying.[57] For example, in the votes and referendums in Washington and Oregon, such claims were the major weapon of opponents of legalization.

Claims about slippery slopes are difficult to evaluate because the predicted, final bad event is so often far in the future. However, there are three such claims from the past that we can evaluate now: one about the *Quinlan* case, one about Holland's experience, and claims about Oregon's new law. Claims about the first two have been made by nationally syndicated columnist Nat Hentoff.

Hentoff is a disability rights advocate who opposes abortion and any kind of euthanasia or assisted suicide. In 1987, he expressed his concerns about the implications of the *Quinlan* decision.[58] Supporters of physician-assisted dying usually say that they are seeking this option only for patients who are adult, rational, dying, and in voluntary cases, but Hentoff emphasized that in 1975 Karen Quinlan met none of these criteria. Later, in 1992, and believing that we are already on the slippery slope, he described Jack Kevorkian's actions and the decriminalization of physician-assisted dying in the Netherlands as a "reckless cheapening of life."

> The September 1991 official government Remmelink Report on euthanasia in that country revealed that at least 1,040 people die every year from involuntary euthanasia. Their physicians were so consumed with compassion that they decided not to disturb the patients by asking their opinion on the matter.[59]

What can we say about these claims? First, it is certainly true that the Quinlan case did not start with the obvious case of assisted dying by competent adults who could clearly and repeatedly express their wish to die, but a very complex case where the wishes of the young woman were unclear. Nevertheless, we would have expected the precedent of the Quinlan case to first, make it very easy for competent patients to die, and second, to generalize to other kinds of incompetent patients, such as senile, demented patients in nursing homes. Yet neither happened. It took 22 years after the *Quinlan* decision before the first terminal patient died legally in Oregon in 1998 with the help of a physician, and many patients like Karen Quinlan are still maintained in institutions across the country—hardly a slippery slope.

As mentioned, supporters and critics see the results in Holland in opposite terms: Some see the glass as half full, others as half empty. There is no doubt that some cases in Holland violated the guidelines. Certainly the original supporters did not forsee requests by depressed mothers and anorexic young women, and it does seem true that some horribly deformed newborn babies were allowed to die. Certainly 1,000 cases of physician-assisted death, for patients who did not document their competence and requests, goes beyond the guidelines.

Nevertheless, these abuses seem like aberrations, not the crushing, unstoppable downward momentum of a real slippery slope. As said, nearly 99 percent of the patients killed had cancer or terminal AIDS. As said, most of these patients had a physician who knew them intimately and who had treated them for years, such that even if they became unconscious before they could make (and repeat) their request for assisted dying, these physicians knew the wishes of these patients. And the Dutch still trust their physicians much more than Americans.

Moreover, as we shall study in detail in Chapter 8, some cases occurring in the 1970s where babies with Down syndrome and spina bifida were allowed to die did not result in a slippery slope. Instead, the Americans with Disabilities Act made it very difficult to kill such babies. At least in Holland and North America, some predicted slippery slopes about euthanasia did not occur.

•

An important claim about an empirical slope from legalizing physician-assisted dying is the argument that *financial motives are most important* in predicting human action. Some people were shocked when Oregon made it possible for a physician to not only help a patient die, but paid her for so doing. For them, once we allow physicians to make money on assisted death, Pandora's Box is really open.

In North America in traditional medicine, the more procedures a physician did on a dying patient, the more money the physician made. New systems of managed care give the physicians all their money at the beginning of the year, and if they go over that allotment, they lose, whereas if they have underspent, they get a bonus (or their group does). In the old, fee-for-service system, physicians had a financial motive to keep a dying patient alive as long as possible. In the new system, the motives are reversed.

The claim about an empirical slope here is that the cheapness of families and the avarice of physicians will conspire to speed sick patients to an early grave. It is not a claim about a conceptual slope because reasoning is not seen here as the driving force and, indeed, is seen only as a mask of the real motives, which concern money.

Is this claim true? The honest answer is that we don't know. North Americans are largely untested in these areas. They are used to some third party paying for the expensive medical bills of their dying relatives and few people ever have to pay such bills themselves. Physicians, too, are used to aggressively treating patients and being well paid to do so, especially in certain specialties such as oncology, cardiac surgery, and cancer surgery.

One nagging worry is that some historians think that the ultimate reason for the rise of Nazi Germany was economic. After losing World War II, the Germans were made to pay huge war reparations, which caused great harm to the German economy and created much ill will. Since World War II, and especially in the last two decades, North America has experienced an unparalleled economic boom. What will happen when times turn bad again and families must choose between grandma's care in a long-term nursing home and a child's college tuition?

It is odd that in formal discussions of ethical issues in medicine, money rarely plays any but an abstract role. One emergency room physician, Norman Paradis, raised this issue publicly in connection with the death of his own father, a surgeon, who was diagnosed with pancreatic cancer, the most lethal and swift of all cancers.[60] Paradis's father told him that he had seen "physicians torture dying patients" and insisted that he wanted neither surgery nor chemotherapy. Paradis assured his father that, as a physician, he knew what to do. He was sure that his strong, direct, professional-to-professional communication with his father's physicians was unequivocal: Make my father comfortable; do no more.

As soon as he left, however, his father was taken to surgery. Why? Because, Paradis says, "consulting surgeons get paid thousands of dollars an hour when they 'decide' to operate." When the younger Paradis called to refuse his consent for further surgery, he was told that his decision was "mistaken." His father underwent further, massive surgery and died the next day. Medicare paid more than $150,000 for these operations. When Paradis objected to Medicare officials, claiming that his father's physicians had proceeded without consent and had violated proper procedures, he was told that there were so many cases of fraud over $1 million that they could not be bothered with his case. Paradis concludes, "Our health system is structured to meet reimbursement rather than patients' needs."

Perhaps the surgeons in this case were genuinely convinced that surgery was an acceptable risk and in the patient's best interest, but perhaps they were guilty of a conflict of interest. If it is fair to argue against physician-assisted dying by pointing out that some families and institutions may seize the advantage to save money, it is also fair to note that some physicians and institutions make millions by maintaining the status quo. Isn't it possible that some specialists could lose enormous amounts of money if assisted dying were practiced? And if so, might they not have a conflict of interest in opposing assisted dying?

In most areas of life, we assume that people work for money, and we give them monetary incentives to work harder. When it comes to physicians, we assume that they will be moral and will not recommend treatments only to make money. Perhaps most of them don't. However, when a reasonable case can be made for denying treatment, treatment is often administered anyway—and the physician makes more money. Is this just a coincidence, or is there some connection?

In any case, this argument cuts both ways. If money motivates everything, then patients are kept alive and "tortured" so physicians can make more money. Which is worse? Such torture or early deaths?

Mistakes and Abuses

People who are opposed to physician-assisted dying often point out that there is almost always some risk of error: That is, a patient who is helped to die may in fact have been able to survive, at least for some time. In other words, there is a danger of dying too soon and losing valuable months or years.

The surgeon Christiaan Barnard recalls a young woman with ovarian cancer who repeatedly begged him to kill her painlessly with morphine.[61] Aware that her condition was terminal—and hearing her screams at night—Barnard decided that he should help her die. When he came into her room with a syringe loaded with morphine, she was quiet, and he thought at first that she was in too much pain even to scream. Then he realized that she was in a state of semiconsciousness, apparently beyond pain, and at the last moment he changed his mind. The next morning, the woman felt better; soon she was in remission, and she lived another few months. Stories like this abound in medicine.

In the Netherlands, some critics of the guidelines for assisted dying claim that physicians are often mistaken about what is "intractable and unbearable" suffering and imply that some physicians are sending patients to needlessly premature deaths. In Janet Adkins's case, many people were quick to say that physicians aren't infallible diagnosticians and that patients sometimes defy a dire prognosis.

Let us put this point differently. In bioethics, many discussions begin with a phrase like, "If a patient has a terminal illness. . . " Notice the word *if*. In presumably terminal illnesses, there are actually few absolute facts until the patient's very last days. Before then, how "terminal"—how close to death—the patient actually is may depend on many factors that are not easy to assess precisely: the patient's attitude, the family's attitude, the attitude of staff members, the quality and level of care, and so on. Moreover, some supposedly terminal patients have been misdiagnosed altogether and have recovered with different treatment. Physician-assisted dying may allow mistakes of this kind to pass too easily. Once physician-assisted death has taken place, there is no appeal.

There are also risks in waiting. The wife of a former secretary of Health, Education, and Welfare "waited" (as some critics contend Janet Adkins should have done) and then spent "much of the last 5 years of her 14-year bout with Alzheimer's in a nursing home as a near vegetable"; her husband wrote that her death at age 80 "was a very delayed blessing."[62]

Slope Claims about the Roles of Physicians

Some critics fear that physician-assisted dying may create a dangerous new role for physicians, conflicting with their traditional role as healers. Boston University law professor George Annas, for one, has said that Jack Kevorkian is "on the lunatic fringe" and that it would be very difficult "to find one other doctor in the country who would support" him.[63] The physician and bioethiaist Leon Kass has said of Kevorkian: "I feel the deepest shame for my profession that he should be counted a member."[64] As an expert witness on medical ethics, Arthur Caplan testified against Kevorkian in a Michigan court.[65] The philosopher Daniel Callahan said that Kevorkian's assistance was:

> a dangerous and wrong thing to do. I can't think of a single way to defend him. [Legalization of euthanasia] would add a whole fourth new category where private individuals would, in effect, be licensed to kill one another to relieve suffering. We don't want to expand the category where one could kill even in the name of mercy. It would change the nature of medicine and open the way to abuse. We are better off without such a law.[66]

Some critics see physicians as arrogant and as having too much control over their patients' lives and deaths; they argue that giving physicians the option to kill would vastly increase their power. Some physicians themselves think that medicine as a profession has difficulty controlling excesses by its members and that it would also have difficulty preventing abuses of assisted dying.

Such objections, however, are essentially practical rather than theoretical. It can be argued in response that, given adequate safeguards, these considerations would not necessarily compromise the role of physicians as healers.

Part of the real debate here is about the question, "What is medicine *for?*" Patients reply, "To help patients as they require help." Physicians may reply, "To heal," and they may add, "To advance the ideals of the profession of medicine and to uphold its professional norms." Patients' and physicians' replies can lead to the same results in some cases, but not all. If one ideal of medicine is the sanctity of life, for example, that might conflict with helping terminal patients die.

Here one can ask, Why aren't physicians "patient advocates"? Whose side are they on, and why aren't they on the side of their dying patients? Why can't medicine ensure that patients will die as they want? If a patient cannot die painlessly, who is to blame? If a physician doesn't keep a patient free of pain, isn't that patient abandonment? Why are so many patients afraid to enter a hospital? Why is there no guarantee of continuity of care? Why don't hospitalized patients trust their physicians to help them have a "good death"?

Questions like these arise because every month seems to bring a new case where physicians overrule the expressed wishes of a patient or family, and usually the patient and the family end up traumatized. Let us consider some of the factors involved in the issue of physicians as patient advocates.

With regard to hospital care, for example, even if a patient has signed an advance directive and has designated a proxy, a relative can challenge the patient's decisions. Also, the hospital's risk manager as well as the patient's own physician will be expected to take steps to avoid lawsuits brought by family members. Additionally, a member of the nursing staff may oppose a decision to let a patient die. In many cases, the easiest thing for medical professionals to do is let the process of dying take its course, even though that may be precisely what the patient didn't want.

The general public, of course, wishes that physicians and hospitals would worry less about litigation and allow the patient to make his or her own decisions.

Most people feel that if the patient is a competent adult, the physician should do what the patient wants—no matter what that may be. They would like the physician to say, "After we've discussed these matters, I'll follow your wishes exactly, even if I personally don't agree with your decision and even if one of your family members threatens to sue me. My job is to do what you want and to respect your trust in me and the medical profession. I'll keep you free of pain, in control as much as possible, and if it comes to it, I'll help you die peacefully—even if it means taking somewhat active means. Even if I have to go to court, even if I need to fight my own hospital, and even if I must fight your family's lawyers, I'll be on your side."

These people also argue that physicians do not necessarily know best. Fifteen years ago, almost all physicians were as staunchly opposed to removing respirators as they now are to assisted dying: The medical profession held that removing a respirator would compromise the physician's role and violate medical ethics. A few years later, the profession said the same thing about withdrawing nutrition and hydration. Could it be that physicians do not understand what their role should be and when they should change it in regard to dying patients?

On this issue, medical opinion clearly differs from public opinion. Although physicians acknowledge the needs and suffering of dying patients, most of them resist any changes that would expand the physician's role to "patient advocacy" if that entailed killing. Part of their argument is that physicians should "do no harm," but this begs the question of what constitutes harm. If a patient requests assistance in dying, refusing to give that help may itself be harm.

Another factor in physicians' opposition seems to be reluctance to give up or share control. One physician reviewer expresses a complaint by physicians that the public wants to "wrest control of the dying process from the healing professions." This is perhaps unfortunately worded; it sounds as if a hypothetical physician is saying something like: "It is better for you, the dying patient, to die according to the natural processes of your disease than for me to change my role, because I am most comfortable with my role as it is now." An argument which would be at least more tactful is that physicians feel responsible for their patients and are disturbed by the idea of abdicating that responsibility.

On the evidence, it seems safe to conclude that most laypeople do not accept any of these arguments by the medical profession and would like to see physicians act more as patient advocates. Public opinion in general seems to be that the professionals who know the most about disease and dying should assist in death, that it is physicians who know most about disease and dying, that it is the job of physicians to help patients, and that therefore, physicians should help terminally ill patients die as they wish.

With regard to the general debate over the role of physicians as healers or patient advocates, two final points should be noted. First, in Oregon where the law allowed physician-assisted dying, no physician in the United States must assist any patient who wants to die. As with abortion, only a small percentage of physicians are actually involved in assisted dying.

Second, the controversy about the role of physicians in assisted suicide has focused too much on Jack Kevorkian and not enough on the larger picture. Every year, over two million Americans die. Most of us will die of cancer, coronary artery disease, stroke, or one of the degenerative diseases. Despite all the newest drugs and all the medical advances, some of us will have a very bad death that medicine cannot do much to alleviate. On any given day—while people write articles about the pros and cons of physician-assisted dying and while the AMA resists it—hundreds of people are dying in a way they hate.

FURTHER READING AND RESOURCES

Margaret P. Battin and Arthur G. Lipman, eds., *Drug Use in Assisted Suicide and Euthanasia* (Monograph published simultaneously as the *Journal of Pharmaceutical Care in Pain & Symptom Control*) (Haworth, 1996).

Kathleen M. Foley and Herbert Hendin, eds., *The Case Against Assisted Suicide: For the Right to End-Of-Life Care* (Johns Hopkins University Press, 2002).

Derek Humphrey, *Final Exit: The Practicalities of Self-Deliverance and Assisted Suicide for the Dying*, 2nd Rev edition (DTP, 1997).

Sherwin B. Nuland, *How We Die: Reflections on Life's Final Chapter* (Vintage Books, 1995).

Classic Cases about the Beginning of Life

Part II Overview

Abortion, Assisted Reproduction, and Cloning

Although controversies about death and dying rocked the world in the last three decades of the twentieth century, most of the battles between prochange and antichange advocates had shifted by 2000 to issues about creating human life. The first chapter in this section discusses issues about abortion, which suddenly became legalized throughout America in 1973, and focuses on a controversial abortion in 1973 by physician Kenneth Edelin in Boston, Massachusetts, as well as on some controversial medical experiments then on live-born fetuses.

The following chapter reviews what happened next, starting with controversies in the early 1970s and exploding with Louise Brown's successful birth from in vitro fertilization in 1978. It also describes developments such as the Baby M case involving surrogate gestator Mary Beth Whitehead, recruitment of young women for compensation to be egg sources for infertile women, and the dangers of multiple gestation in cases such as the McCaughey septuplets.

The last two chapters in this section describe the many issues that orbit around various forms of cloning, such as stem cell research from human embryos, the creation of cloned embryos of a patient as possible self-medication, and the explosive issues of reproductive cloning. Announcement of the cloned sheep Dolly in 1997 sparked many controversies about cloning.

It is also true that a failure to achieve a national consensus over abortion in America (legal since 1973), as well as the growing attention to ethical issues surrounding assisted reproduction, had already led social conservatives to feel that medical developments at the beginning of life "were moving faster than our wisdom." Hence, the intensity of the fight over all forms of cloning today can be seen in part as a backlash by people who felt their views had not been heard in the previous legalization of abortion or in social acceptance of new forms of assisted reproduction.

So the following four chapters provide a web of issues surrounding the ethics of the creation (and termination) of early human life by physicians and scientists. Logically, it made sense to start with embryos and assisted reproduction, move to abortion and surrogacy, and end with cloning, but this sequence ignores the history of what actually happened in bioethics, with abortion being legalized first in 1973, followed by Louise Brown's birth in 1978, followed by two decades of tumultuous stories about assisted reproduction, followed by creation of Dolly in 1996. Thus the sequence of these chapters provides a historical context in which to understand today's issue about stem cell research and cloning.

CHAPTER 5

Abortion

Kenneth Edelin

This chapter discusses abortion, its history prior to its legalization by the U. S. Supreme Court in 1973, the controversial trial of physician Kenneth Edelin for the death by abortion of a late-term fetus, subsequent legal developments, and the ethical issues on all sides of the continuing debate over abortion. It also discusses controversial fetal experiments in the 1970s and subsequent issues about fetal and fetal-tissue research.

THE LANGUAGE OF ABORTION

This book will use medically accepted terms for the stages of a human life, so after sperm meets egg and conception occurs, an *embryo* results, which after 9 weeks until birth is called a *fetus,* which at birth is called a *baby.*

Definitions of these terms have legal and ethical consequences. For example, a baby can be the subject of a homicide charge, but not a fetus. Critics of abortion object to the connotation of "fetus" as a being containing less value than a baby and refer to the growing fetus as a baby. Critics of cloning, such as Bishop Drennen of the National Council of Catholic Bishops, constantly speak of "the embryo/baby" and "embryo/fetus" on national television. Speaking this way is to assert the absolute value of the new human organism from embryohood to birth.

This text will not speak that way because to do so is to beg too many questions at the start. Instead it will follow the commonly accepted medical definitions above.

BACKGROUND: HISTORY, SHERRY FINKBINE, *HUMANAE VITAE, ROE* V. *WADE*

Historical Overview

Many Christians and Jews believe that the Bible or the Torah forbids abortion. In this regard, however, a British professor of church history writes:

> The Bible certainly teaches the value of human life, and forbids the murder of any human being (Psalm 8). But life, in biblical terms, commences only when the breath

enters the nostrils and the man or woman becomes a "living being" (Genesis 2:7). . . . Consequently in biblical terms the fetus is not a person. This is brought out clearly in the laws relating to murder. For though the Ten Commandments in Exodus state clearly, "You shall not murder," the text goes on, in the following chapter, to differentiate between causing the death of an adult human being and causing the death of an unborn human fetus. For whereas "whoever hits a man and kills him shall be put to death" (Exodus 21:12), " . . . if some men are fighting and hurt a woman so that she loses her child, but is not injured in any other way, the one who hurt her is to be fined." There is no suggestion in the Old Testament law, as there is in a comparable Assyrian one, that "he who struck her shall compensate for the fetus with a life." Indeed, the biblical text does not ever regard the loss of her fetus as causing the woman "harm," for it goes on to specify what should happen "if any harm follows." At no point is any consideration given to the notion that the fetus itself might have rights. And this absence of concern for the fetus is also implied by the imposition of the death penalty on women who conceive out of wedlock, without any consideration being given to the fact that this killed both the fetus and the woman (Deuteronomy 22:21, Leviticus 21:9, Genesis 38:24).

. . . Turning to the issue of abortion as such, I am somewhat puzzled that biblical fundamentalists, who oppose abortion so strongly, should pay so little heed to the silence of the Bible on this issue. . . . Whether this silence is significant or not, the fact ought to be faced that whatever views one many hold about abortion, no straightforward appeal can be made to the teaching of the Bible, for the Bible simply does not discuss it.[1]

Moreover, Jesus does not speak against abortion anywhere in the New Testament.

If abortion is not condemned in the Old Testament or in the Gospels, why have so many Christians, in particular, come to believe that it is immoral? An answer to this question can be given in historical stages, focusing on the Catholic church as an example.

The Old Testament took its final form during the fifth century before the Common, or Christian, era (B.C.E.) and the New Testament around the year 200 of the Common era (C.E.)—the time when Christianity began as an organized religion. As a formal, organized religion, Christianity has always opposed abortion, but its view of what constitutes abortion has changed significantly over the nearly 2,000 years of its existence.

By the fourth century C.E., Christian teaching about sex was in crisis. Celibacy was the Christian ideal; but there were two problems with that ideal. On the one hand, Christianity would die out if too many Christians took celibacy too seriously (much later, the Shakers held to the ideal and did die out). On the other hand, as a practical matter lifelong celibacy was impossible for most people. Consequently, Augustine revised Christian teaching to allow sexual intercourse in marriage, but only if the intent was to have children.[2] It follows from Augustine's doctrine that abortion must be sinful, because it thwarts the only permissible purpose of sex.

In the twelfth century, Christian doctrine began to separate abortion from homicide by distinguishing between "formed" and "unformed" embryos—a concept that had to do with the soul rather than with physical development. In the thirteenth century, Thomas Aquinas held that God "ensouled" male embryos at 40 days of gestation and female embryos at 90 days. Aborting a male embryo at

40 days was thus punished more severely than aborting a female embryo at the same age, since the male was formed by then but the female was still unformed. Although any abortion at any time was considered sinful, the penalties (penance, etc.) increased when the fetus was "formed."[3]

During the nineteenth century, science and religion began to conflict in many areas, and scientific evidence began to discredit the Thomistic concept of ensoulment. In 1870, Pope Pius IX reacted against the general conflict between religion and science by convening the First Vatican Council, which declared that his edicts and those of future popes would henceforth be "infallible." The meaning of papal infallibility was unclear at the time and is still debated by Catholic theologians today,[4] but the general reaction of the Catholic church was clear: it moved toward faith and away from the claims of science. As the church retreated from science during the period from about 1869 to 1900, it encouraged attention to Mary (who had been neglected), supported "creationism" against geological explanations of the origins of the universe, emphasized miracles (the miracle of Fatima was recognized shortly after the First Vatican Council), and vigorously attacked Darwinism. Protestant Christianity generally held the same views about abortion.

Beginning in the mid-nineteenth century, then, the popes denounced abortion in increasingly absolutistic terms. During this time, Catholicism came close to teaching that personhood began at conception, a view it called *immediate animation*.[5] In an earlier era, as we have seen, the church had differentiated between formed and unformed fetuses, but Pius IX essentially drew no such distinction: the prohibition was the same for almost any woman who had any kind of abortion. This official Catholic denunciation of abortion has, of course, continued throughout the twentieth century.

However, the Catholic doctrine of *double effect* allowed two exceptions: abortion was permissible in cases of ectopic pregnancy (in which an embryo grows in a fallopian tube) and uterine cancer (in which uterus and fetus must be removed together). According to the doctrine of double effect, an action having two effects, one good and the other evil, is morally permissible under four conditions: (1) if the action is good in itself or not evil, (2) if the good follows as immediately from the cause as from the evil effect, (3) if only the good effect is intended, and (4) if there is a proportionately grave cause for performing the action as for allowing the evil effect. Under this doctrine, exceptions to the general prohibition of abortion were made for ectopic pregnancy and uterine cancer because in both cases the purpose of an abortion was to save the life of the mother.

•

Historically, legal restrictions on abortion were far more lenient than Catholic doctrine. During the seventeenth century, European common law did not consider aborting even a "quickened" fetus an indictable offense. In 1803, an English statute made abortion of a quickened fetus a capital crime; however, it continued to use quickening as a dividing point, and it imposed lesser penalties for abortions before quickening. From the seventeenth through the nineteenth centuries, American law followed English common law: Abortion before quickening was only a misdemeanor or might even be legal if it was done for therapeutic reasons on the recommendation of two physicians. In 1973, in *Roe* v. *Wade*, the

United States Supreme Court reviewed the legal background of abortion and concluded:

> It is thus apparent that at common law, at the time of the adopting of our Constitution, and throughout the major portion of the 19th century, abortion was viewed with less disfavor than under most American statutes currently in effect. Phrasing it another way, a woman enjoyed a substantially broader right to terminate a pregnancy than she does in most States today. At least with respect to the early stage of pregnancy, and very possibly without such a limitation, the opportunity to make this choice was present in this country well into the 19th century. Even later, the law continued for some time to treat less punitively an abortion procured in early pregnancy.[6]

In the United States, this leniency changed after the Civil War, when most states made abortion illegal, stipulated firm cutoff points, and imposed stiff penalties. The American medical profession was also opposed to abortion in the period from 1870 to 1970. Feminist historians argue that this legislative trend and the stance of the medical profession both reflect paternalism and misogyny:

> Anti-abortion legislation was part of an anti-feminist backlash to the growing movement for suffrage, voluntary motherhood, and other women's rights in the nineteenth century. The prevailing public prudery and anti-sexual moralism condemned feminism and considered sex for pleasure evil, with pregnancy as punishment.[7]

These feminists point out that before the Civil War, most babies had been delivered by midwives, who competed with physicians for clients; thereafter, physicians took over, and almost all physicians were men.

Modern Developments

Before abortion was legalized (or perhaps more accurately, relegalized) in the United States, an abortion was likely to be a horrifying experience. Physicians who performed abortions often did so only for the money and sometimes treated their patients badly. Some physicians demanded sex from their patients as part of the price of an abortion. Other physicians accompanied the abortion with a lecture to the woman on her "promiscuity." Some of the specific medical procedures were meant more to protect physicians from the law than to help patients. Though abortion is a painful process, anesthesia wasn't used; and no explanation was given beforehand of what would happen and why. If there were any adverse effects, the woman had no legal recourse. Frequently, the woman did not even know the physician's name and had been forbidden to try to make contact again. Furthermore, as bad as they were, illegal abortions by physicians were also very expensive. Thus such an abortion was beyond the reach not only of poor women but also of teenagers who might be from well-off families but who couldn't or wouldn't tell their parents.

Despite all this, hundreds of thousands of illegal abortions were performed in the United States during the 1950s and 1960s. Many women died as a result of abortions: 193 women died in 1965 alone, and over 1,000 died during the decade of the 1960s.[8] Because what they had done was illegal, victims of botched or unsanitary abortions came into emergency rooms only at the last possible moment, when they were desperate. Many of these women died of widespread abdominal infection, and those who recovered often found themselves sterile or chronically ill. Poor women ran the greatest risks from illegal abortions, and in 1965, 55 percent of abortion-related deaths were among nonwhite women.

1962: Sherri Finkbine   In 1962, Sherri Finkbine was living with her husband and their four children in Phoenix, Arizona,[9] and she was pregnant with a fifth child. During her fifth month of pregnancy, she took thalidomide tranquilizers. Thalidomide is a teratogen ("monster former"), often producing babies with missing arms or legs—a fact that is now well known but in 1962 was just becoming apparent. It had been tested on animals, but it was not tested on the appropriate species of *pregnant* animals until it had already caused numerous human tragedies.

A "therapeutic" abortion was requested, ostensibly for Sherri Finkbine's health, and was scheduled at a local hospital. A local district attorney threatened to prosecute, however, and the Finkbines had to go to Europe at their own expense to seek an abortion. The severely deformed fetus was aborted in Sweden, where therapeutic abortion had been legal since 1940.[10]

1968: *Humanae Vitae*   On July 29, 1968—5 years before *Roe* v. *Wade*—Pope Paul VI stunned liberal Catholics around the world by emphasizing in an encyclical called *Humanae Vitae* that the Roman Catholic Church would not accept any form of artificial birth control. What perhaps made this ruling particularly startling was its timing: It came during a period of enormous worldwide social change, associated significantly with young people (there were student uprisings in the United States and elsewhere—notably Paris—against the Vietnamese war), and marked by increasing tolerance toward sexual relations outside marriage, partly because unwanted pregnancies were increasingly avoidable.

Humanae Vitae drove many American Catholics to open defiance of official church teachings. In 1993—over 25 years later—though Pope John Paul II had by then made the defense of this encyclical a pillar of his own papacy, 90 percent of American Catholics disagreed with the church's position and believed they were free to make their own moral decisions, even if those decisions contradicted church doctrine.[11] The encyclical also had another unintended effect: it drove many Catholics out of the priesthood and out of Catholic universities. Some of these apostates became founders of the new field of bioethics.[12]

1968–1973: Steps toward *Roe* v. *Wade*   As a result of social changes, and of cases like Sherri Finkbine's, American culture had come to accept the concept of legalized abortion before *Roe* v. *Wade* in 1973. In the 5 years just preceding *Roe* v. *Wade*, 18 states, with 41 percent of the American population, liberalized their own abortion laws; 67 percent of Americans, then, lived either in those states or within a 100-mile drive of one of them. The first state to legalize abortion had been Hawaii (in 1970), followed by New York, Colorado, North Carolina, and California. (Ronald Reagan, who was then the governor of California, signed its bill into law!)

If *Roe* v. *Wade* had not eliminated the need, more states would have followed suit. It is noteworthy that if the United States Supreme Court should ever make abortion a "states' rights" issue, most American women could still have abortions because most of these liberalized state laws are still on the books.

In other words, it is not true that *Roe* v. *Wade* suddenly occurred and that thereupon many people suddenly changed their ideas about abortion. Rather, many Americans had already changed their views, and *Roe* v. *Wade* reflected this new reality.

Also true is the fact that many people had *not* changed their views about abortion and hated the 1973 *Roe* v. *Wade* decision. These opponents felt that such changes should have occurred legislatively in states or Congress, where views on both sides could be argued openly, even passionately. But that did not occur, leaving critics of abortion angry and feeling disenfranchised in national public policy about personal reproductive values.

1973: *Roe* v. *Wade*   The decision of the United States Supreme Court in *Roe* v. *Wade* (1973) concerned "Jane Roe," a woman from Dallas, Texas, whose real name is Norma McCorvey. ("Wade" was Henry Wade, district attorney of Dallas County.) In March 1970, when the events in the case began, Texas had a law criminalizing all abortions; Norma McCorvey wanted a safe, legal abortion by a physician and challenged the constitutionality of the Texas law.[13]

The Supreme Court had already decided in *Griswold* v. *Connecticut* (1965) that a right to "privacy"—the legal equivalent of personal liberty—is implied by the Constitution and had therefore allowed couples to receive birth control pills (the point at issue in *Griswold* was whether a state might forbid such contraception). In *Roe* v. *Wade*, the Court decided that privacy also implies the right to have an abortion.

This right was not unqualified, however: a woman's right to terminate a pregnancy was balanced against the rights of the fetus, which increase as gestation time increases. The Court emphasized that religious and philosophical views about fetal development and personhood differ greatly, but for legal purposes it drew the line at *viability*. After viability, states could make abortions illegal; before viability, they could not.

The Court defined *viability* as the point when a fetus is "potentially able to live outside the mother's womb, albeit with artificial aid. Viability is usually placed at about 7 months (28 weeks) but may occur earlier, even at 24 weeks." The Court summarized its trimester system, in which viability divides the second and third trimesters, as follows:

> A state criminal abortion statute of the current Texas type, that excepts from criminality only a *life-saving* procedure on behalf of the mother, without regard to pregnancy stage and without recognition of the other interests involved, is violative of the Due Process Clause of the Fourteenth Amendment.
>
> (a) For the stage prior to approximately the end of the first trimester, the abortion decision and its effectuation must be left to the medical judgment of the pregnant woman's attending physician.
>
> (b) For the stage subsequent to approximately the end of the first trimester, the State, in promoting its interest in the health of the mother, may, if it chooses, regulate the abortion procedure in ways that are reasonably related to maternal health.

(c) For the stage subsequent to viability, the State in promoting its interest in the potentiality of human life may, if it chooses, regulate, and even proscribe, abortion except where it is necessary, in appropriate medical judgment, for the preservation of the life or health of the mother.

This trimester system for allowing states to legalize and regulate abortion became the subject of great discussion over the next two decades. Justice Rehnquist immediately called it a "Procrustean bed," and Justice Sandra Day O'Connor predicted that it would inevitably be revised.

Note that a state "may" forbid ("proscribe") abortion. It need not. A state could legalize abortion at any time up to the actual birth. Note also that a state may pass a law allowing abortions in the third trimester not only to preserve the *life* of a mother but also to protect her *health*. Antiabortionists argue that this constitutes a loophole justifying almost any abortion, because two physicians can almost always be found who will say that continuing the pregnancy would endanger the mother's health. Indeed, *health* is a vague term and can be used in many ways. In the 1960s, for instance, Alabama law permitted abortions only for the health of the mother, but some physicians interpreted the word quite broadly and performed first-trimester abortions on any woman who decided to terminate her pregnancy.

•

Legalized abortions throughout the 1970s and 1980s hovered around 1.5 million in America, but in the 1990s started to decline. By 1997, about 900,000 abortions occurred and in 1998, that figure dropped to 884,000.[14]

About a fifth of such abortions were performed on teenage girls under age 19. From 1988 to 1997, about 7 women per year died from these legal abortions, which were almost always performed in out-patient clinics, not in hospitals.

Of women and girls who have abortions, less than 1 percent are under age 15, though older teenage girls account for about 24 percent; women in their twenties have 55 percent of abortions; women in their thirties, 18 percent. Married women have nearly 20 percent of abortions. Minority women are more than twice as likely as white women to have an abortion, although many minority women today do choose to bring the fetus to term.[15]

THE EDELIN CASE

The Legal Environment: Experiments on Aborted Fetuses

The case of Kenneth Edelin began in Boston in October 1973, and to understand the legal environment, it is necessary to look at a key episode that had taken place several months earlier, in the first quarter of 1973—just after the decision in *Roe* v. *Wade.*

This earlier event involved two experiments that had been performed on aborted fetuses at Boston City Hospital, where Edelin was a resident. Some physicians reasoned this way: since aborted fetuses were going to die anyway, why not use them in experiments to help other fetuses? This particular research was designed partly to prevent cases like Sherri Finkbine's, in which substances ingested by the mother might harm the fetus: to determine which drugs would cross the placenta, the physicians in the study gave antibiotics to women undergoing abortions and then examined the aborted fetuses. One of the findings was that clindamycin crosses the placenta and becomes concentrated in the fetal liver; this showed that syphilis in the fetus could be treated with clindaymycin if the mother was allergic to penicillin.

In one of these studies designed to test an artificial womb, eight fetuses were aborted by hysterotomy (essentially a cesarean delivery). They weighed between 300 and 1000 grams. Fetuses weighing 1000 grams today are often viable when placed in neonatal intensive care units. The large, 1000-gram fetus was placed in a warm saline solution mimicking the amniotic sac and researchers described it in their article as making frantic "gasping" and as using its arms to clutch objects as it slowly died.

Another such experiment on late second trimester fetuses studied the effects of lack of glucose on the brain (a condition arising, for example, when a diabetic pregnant woman goes into shock). After injecting potassium chloride to stop hearts of the fetuses, but before anoxia damaged their brains, the 12 fetuses were decapitated and the brains removed. The researchers said the brains were successfully maintained with artificial replacements for glucose.

Although these experiments were performed in 1973, it was not until 1975 that the public took notice, and then the sky fell. Maggie Scarf's "The Fetus as Guinea Pig" appeared in a fall 1975 issue of the *New York Times Magazine* and shocked everyone when it accurately described the above experiments (this magazine is very influential because many of the news editors for television shows and magazines live in New York City and read it).[16] In the same year, social conservative and Yale theologian Paul Ramsey published *The Ethics of Fetal Research,* in which he called such experimentation evil exploitation and "unconsented to research on unborn babies."[17]

These experiments, as well as research on embryos for "test-tube babies," outraged Congress and directly led to the ban on use of federal funds for research involving human embryos. The exact date in the late 1970s when this ban took effect is unclear, but it continued until President George W. Bush in the summer of 2002 allowed a small window of research to open with federal money (more on this in Chapter 6).

This study caused a considerable furor. An article describing it appeared in the *New England Journal of Medicine,*[18] and copies were sent to certain Boston Catholics, who were infuriated. When a councilman held a hearing on September 18, 1973, to investigate fetal experimentation at Boston City Hospital, antiabortionists packed the auditorium. One of the witnesses they heard was Mildred Jefferson, an assistant professor of surgery at Boston University who was not only an antiabortion physician but also an African American physician. (Later, Kenneth Edelin's lawyer had no doubt that Jefferson had been asked to testify precisely because she was black and staunchly opposed to abortion.) Jefferson testified, perhaps correctly, that some of the women undergoing abortion who were involved in the study were too young to consent legally and in any case had not given their written consent. If the researchers had indeed failed to obtain genuine consent, they would technically be open to charges of "grave robbing," illegally procuring bodies for medical experimentation.

Kenneth Edelin and "Alice Roe"

In 1973, Kenneth Edelin was 35 years old, and he—like Mildred Jefferson—was African American. (When he became the first physician prosecuted for performing an abortion after *Roe* v. *Wade,* many observers would wonder if the fact that he was black had something to do with it, though the district attorney, Newman Flanagan, denied any link.) Edelin, the son of a postman, had grown up in a poor section of Washington, D.C. He did his undergraduate work at Columbia University, received his M.D. from Meharry Medical College in 1967, interned in Ohio, and then served for 3 years as a United States Air Force physician (with the rank of captain) in England. In 1971, he began his residency at Boston City Hospital, which Bill Moyers called the "city hospital in the Boston ghetto" in a documentary on the case. (It was also the model for a later television series, *St. Elsewhere.)* Edelin was in his third year as chief resident in obstetrics when he was assigned to perform an abortion on "Alice Roe."

"Alice" was a 17-year-old, black, West Indian student. She remained anonymous throughout the case, and little is known about her personally or as a patient. She had been examined by Edelin's faculty supervisor, Hugh Holtrop, who estimated that she was 22 weeks pregnant. She was also examined by Enrique Giminez, a first-year resident from Mexico, who later testified against Edelin, giving a different estimate of 24 weeks; and a third-year medical student who assisted during the abortion agreed with Giminez's estimate. At the time, the hospital (which was poor) had no ultrasound machine and so could not reach a more precise estimate of gestation. In either case, however, it was a very late, second-trimester abortion.

Even though Holtrop had admitted Alice Roe, and even though a late second-trimester fetus was involved, Kenneth Edelin was assigned to the abortion. It is true that as a third-year resident, Edelin carried out substantial work at the hospital; it is also true that attending obstetricians like Holtrop all had private practices and actually spent little time at Boston City. Moreover, Holtrop later said that he had admitted Alice simply because he was the only obstetrician on duty when she arrived. However, Edelin disagreed, claiming that Alice Roe had originally been Holtrop's patient; and the surgeon William Nolen, who wrote a book reviewing the case (Nolen is also the author of *The Making of a Surgeon),* concluded that Holtrop had dumped the case on Edelin.[19]

To complicate matters, Holtrop had obtained Alice's and her mother's permission for Alice's participation in another preabortion experiment to see if aminoglutethamide would increase the hormone output of the placenta. Accordingly, the substance was given to Alice intravenously and her urine was analyzed over the next 24 hours; this study took place on October 1 and October 2, 1973.

Edelin planned to abort Alice Roe's fetus by injecting saline solution into the amniotic sac, but when he inserted a needle on October 2 to sample the amniotic fluid, he drew blood. This indicated that the patient had an anterior placenta (that is, a placenta attached to the front wall of the uterus); thus a saline solution injected into the placenta could travel from there into her bloodstream, where it could be lethal.

The abortion was therefore rescheduled as a hysterotomy and was performed on the following day, October 3, 1973. A hysterotomy is essentially abortion by cesarean surgery; it involves cutting through the lower abdominal wall. Instead of Giminez (the resident who estimated gestation time as 24 weeks), Edelin chose as his assistant Steven Teich, the third-year medical student mentioned earlier. However, Giminez watched the hysterotomy anyway (he was uninvited, and where he was when he observed the procedure became a matter of dispute).

What happened next is controversial. Giminez would later testify that Edelin made the cesarean section, reached in, cut the placenta from the abdominal wall, then waited perhaps 3 minutes, and after this interval removed a dead fetus. If such a wait took place, that would be important, because a baby cannot breathe on its own inside the uterus: It begins breathing (if at all) only when it is brought out. Edelin would later be charged with "neglecting" the baby by not removing it immediately, thereby causing it to suffocate.

Afterwards, the fetus was taken to the morgue, where it was preserved in formalin, as required by hospital policy for aborted fetuses weighing more than 600 grams. This later meant that the district attorney had a "body," and photographs of the "body" were eventually shown to the jury.

One fact about this case merits repeating here. Edelin had originally intended to abort the fetus by saline injection, and if the position of the placenta had been different, he would have been able to do so legally. It was for the safety of the mother that he performed the abortion by hysterotomy, leaving himself vulnerable to the manslaughter charge.

The Case in the Courts

Edelin's Trial and Conviction   A grand jury decided that enough evidence existed to indict Edelin. Some legal strategists believe that Edelin seriously erred by testifying at the pretrial hearing and not invoking his Fifth Amendment right against possible self-incrimination. Holtrop, in contrast, invoked his right against self-incrimination and was not indicted. After the hearing, Edelin changed lawyers.

The actual charge against Edelin was manslaughter, defined in Massachusetts as "wanton, reckless" omission or commission of an act which causes death; Massachusetts law further defines "wanton, reckless" conduct as "the legal equivalent of intentional conduct" and as "disregard of the probable consequences to the rights of others." The trial judge gave the following description: "The essence of wanton or reckless conduct is the doing of an act or the omission to act where there is a duty to act, which commission or omission involves a high degree of likelihood that substantial harm will result to another."[20]

The principal participants in the trial were Newman Flanagan, the prosecuting district attorney (described as "witty, flamboyant, competent, and tough"); Edelin's trial lawyer, William Perkins Homans, Jr., a well-born Boston lawyer who often defended unpopular causes; and the presiding judge, James McGuire. The jurors—selected after much wrangling between the lawyers—were mostly white; three of them were women and 13 were men; 10 were Catholic. (A study had predicted that jurors likely to convict Edelin would be blue-collar Catholics over 50 years old, who had dropped out of Catholic high schools, and who regularly read Catholic newspapers.)

Massachusetts did not pass an abortion law until August 1974 (22 months after *Roe* v. *Wade*), and in the absence of a specific state law, Judge McGuire instructed the jury that *Roe* v. *Wade* was "absolutely controlling." Since *Roe* v. *Wade* equated personhood with viability, this meant that the jury would have to determine whether or not this specific fetus had been "viable." Remember that the Supreme Court had said only that viability is "usually" placed at 24 to 28 weeks, not that viability necessarily falls within that range; more important, the Supreme Court had not specified how to determine whether or not viability fell into the range. In the Edelin case, if the fetus was *not* viable, no "person" had been killed; and if no person had been killed, Edelin could not be guilty of manslaughter.

Edelin testified that the procedure he performed on Alice Roe had seemed long to Giminez because at this stage of pregnancy the thick abdominal muscle wall was not yet stretched enough to be cut easily. Edelin also said that he had made a Pfannenstiel ("bikini") incision because he considered it safer than a vertical incision and because it would leave less of a scar. The surgeon William Nolen later agreed that making such an incision would take awhile, especially for a resident who had never done one before, though he said that it would certainly not take 3 minutes (as Giminez had testified);[21] however, Edelin's testimony implied that Giminez had confused the initial abdominal incision with the second incision detaching the placenta.

As noted above, the fetus had been preserved, and the prosecution introduced a picture of it ("the deceased") as evidence, over the angry objection of the defense attorney, Homans, who argued that the picture would be "inflammatory" and would tell laypersons nothing about fetal age or viability. Judge McGuire allowed one picture to be shown but charged the jury not to view it "from any emotional point of view."[22]

When the district attorney, Flanagan, summed up, he argued, first, that the fetus had been a "person" when the placenta was cut; second, that Edelin had indeed waited 3 minutes and that this delay constituted "wanton, reckless conduct"; third, that legal abortion was intended to end a pregnancy, not to produce a dead fetus—and therefore that Edelin should have helped the fetus (which Flanagan said had been live-born) before cutting the placenta.

Judge McGuire specifically instructed the jury that an unborn fetus was not a person and could not be the subject of a manslaughter indictment. Such an indictment could refer only to a "person," defined by Massachusetts law as a being who has been born. Birth was the key event, and the judge instructed the jury: "You must be satisfied beyond a reasonable doubt . . . that the defendant caused the death of a person who had been alive outside the body of his or her mother."

Thus the jury had to decide two points: (1) Had Alice Roe's fetus been alive outside the mother's body? (2) If so, did the fetus (who would then be called a *baby*) die as a result of "wanton, reckless conduct" by Edelin? The jurors said "yes" to both points and convicted Edelin of manslaughter. Edelin was later sentenced by Judge McGuire to 1 year of probation.

The Edelin trial was followed intensely by the media and the public. Proabortion groups supported Edelin, as did some antiabortion physicians who hated prosecution of physicians more than legalization of abortion. Medical journals also strongly supported Edelin. Antiabortion groups saw Flanagan, the prosecutor, as their knight: Edelin had stepped over a legal line, they said, and had to be punished. A few months later, as described in Chapter 2, Karen Quinlan's physicians would take notice.

When the verdict was announced, liberal Boston media implied that a black man in an abortion case in Boston couldn't get a fair trial from white Catholics. Even the conservative William Buckley said, "The case can be presented as the lynching of a black Marcus Welby by a bigoted community."[23] The foreman of the jury, however, retorted passionately that the aborted fetus was also black and that the jury had also been concerned about its life.

Appeal and Acquittal: The Higher Court's Decision   If the conviction by the trial court had stuck, Kenneth Edelin could have lost his medical license. He appealed, however, and the Massachusetts Supreme Court agreed to hear the case on direct review. He was also given, almost immediately, a vote of confidence by the trustees of Boston City Hospital, who offered him a permanent position.

In December 1976, more than 3 years after the abortion itself had taken place, the Massachusetts Supreme Judicial Court overturned Edelin's conviction, declaring that no evidence of criminal negligence had been presented at the trial. The higher court said, "In the comparative calm of appellate review, the essential proposition emerges that the defendant had no evil frame of mind, was actuated by no criminal purpose, and committed no wanton or reckless act in carrying out the medical procedures on Oct. 3, 1973."[24] Notice that for its own reasons—possibly because commentaries by its own judges indicated deep divisions and confusion—the higher court did not require a new trial for Edelin but simply acquitted him.

The Aftermath

After the decision, Edelin was described as "jubilant" and said he felt "terrific" about the verdict, saying, "It's great to be able to smile again after 2½ years."[25] He said that the reversal was a victory for all physicians regardless of whether they performed abortions. He also said that the decision upheld the principle of nonprosecution of physicians who acted in good faith and who followed accepted medical standards.

In his television news program on the evening of December 17, 1977, Walter Cronkite triumphantly announced that Edelin had been acquitted of "manslaughter by abortion."[26]

William Nolen, the surgeon who later carefully examined the evidence in the case, argued that the fetus had not been outside the womb, had thus not been technically "born," and was thus not a person;[27] hence, he concluded, there could have been no manslaughter and Edelin could have broken no law. Nolen's conclusion was particularly interesting not only because he himself was a surgeon but also because he was opposed to abortion. Nolen believed that Edelin had intended the abortion to kill a very late second-trimester fetus but had been surprised to find, once the patient was opened, that the fetus was viable. Nolen doesn't say that Edelin actually suffocated the fetus; but he does say that whether a newborn has a will to live ("that spark") can be known only if it is taken out of the womb, slapped, and helped to breathe:

> What is disturbing in the Roe case is that, by his own admission, Edelin made no attempt to see if the child had that spark. As [Jeffrey] Gould [another physician who testified] said, the will to live isn't always immediately apparent; it becomes obvious only if "the physician will try to stimulate, will try to give a little bit of oxygen, and look for a favorable response." . . .
>
>   The Roe baby wasn't given this bit of provocation that might—just might—have shown it had the will to live. Why? The answer is distressingly simple. No one wanted the Roe baby to live.[28]

In 1993, Newman Flanagan was still Boston's district attorney. Kenneth Edelin had a private practice in obstetrics and gynecology in Boston until 1996, when he became Associate Dean for Students and Minority Affairs at the Boston University School of Medicine, where he is a professor of obstetrics and gynecology, and where he continues to teach and practice today.

ETHICAL ISSUES: FROM PERSONHOOD TO VIABILITY

Final Basic Concept: Personhood

What is a *person?* In the context of abortion, some philosophers, especially woman philosophers, draw a distinction between a person and a human being. They argue that although a fetus is human, it does not meet certain criteria of personhood; and that since a fetus is not a person, it does not have a right to life. In this sense, *human* is a factual term whereas *person* is an evaluative term, implying a right to life.

The most famous and intuitively plausible of these arguments is probably Mary Anne Warren's. Warren offers a *cognitive criterion* of personhood[29] and holds that a fetus does not meet this standard. According to Warren, to be a person is to be able to think, to be capable of "cognition." What separates a normal, adult person from, say, a rat, is certain capacities—for reasoning, reflective self-awareness, communication, agency (motivated action), and consciousness of the external world. Warren does not think that any one of these capacities alone is sufficient for "cognition"; rather, these capacities define the core criterion as a group. A being lacking all of these capacities does not meet the cognitive criterion, and hence cannot be a person.

Let us examine some issues concerning this cognitive criterion. To begin with, it can be objected that the criterion does not represent an adequate definition because it both includes some "nonpersons" and excludes some persons. The cognitive criterion does seem to admit to personhood some beings that we don't naturally regard as persons; there is good evidence, for instance, that apes communicate and are conscious, and there is some evidence that they may reason and may be self-aware, yet we don't usually consider them persons. Moreover, the cognitive criterion seems to suggest that there is no reason, morally speaking, to protect vulnerable human beings whose cognitive capacities are absent, have been lost, or are as yet merely potential, such as patients in the late stages of Alzheimer's disease, comatose patients, or newborn babies. If a fetus can be aborted (and thus killed) because it fails to meet the cognitive criterion and therefore is not a person, why wouldn't these others also fail to meet the criterion, and why wouldn't it also be permissible to kill them?

Suppose, moreover, that we accepted the cognitive criterion. In that case, another problem would arise. If what makes people valuable is cognition, then isn't it wrong to deprive beings of *potential cognition?* And wouldn't deprivation of potential cognition make abortion wrong? In this regard, the philosophers Don Marquis and Warren Quinn offer two premises: first, what is wrong about killing a person—a college student, for example—is depriving him or her of future cognitive experiences;[30] second, what is wrong about killing an adult person is also what is wrong about killing a human fetus.

Marquis and Quinn's argument is an interesting one, and indeed many people would accept their first premise, at least after some reflection. Other explanations of why it is wrong to kill a person—that killing violates a person's rights, for instance, or that killing is against God's will—seem to beg the question: It can be argued that phrases such as *violation of rights* and *against the will of God* are simply other ways of saying that an act is wrong.

However, Marquis and Quinn's second premise may be more vulnerable. It can be argued that a being without an already existing self or personal identity cannot have a personal future to be deprived of. Consider an analogy: Imagine an omnipotent deity—God—who creates a universe, then considers creating a second parallel universe, but then decides not to create the second world. Now imagine a powerful evil force—Satan—who wants to destroy the existing universe. It seems, intuitively, that destruction of the existing world by Satan would be wrong; but it does *not* seem wrong for God to refrain from creating a second world. Although God has not allowed a second universe, and thus has disallowed a vast amount of cognitive experiences, he has neither done any wrong nor wronged any person.

Another argument against Marquis and Quinn is analogous to a strategy that is used to dissolve the "paradox of harm": the *baseline* concept. This concept requires a starting point (baseline) from which an adverse change is plotted; i.e., it requires an existing being who is made worse off. We could, then, posit a baseline concept of personal identity and argue that without some baseline of existence as a person, one cannot be harmed. On the other hand, though, the *normality* concept of harm would tend to support Marquis and Quinn's reasoning: this concept requires a norm of development which is not met; and on a normality concept of personal identity, one could be harmed by not existing (because nonexistence deprives a being of any chance to obtain normality).

A different type of argument based on potentiality suggests a *genetic criterion* for personhood: to be a person is to have the unique genes of a specific human being. In the Edelin case, for example, even if Alice Roe's fetus wasn't yet a person, it was certainly a potential person; shouldn't it therefore have been treated as a person?

It may seem, at first glance, as if this argument would imply that contraception, or even masturbation, is wrong, since either of these might prevent potential persons from coming into existence; but this kind of reasoning is a *straw man*—a "false opponent," too easily refuted. No antiabortionist wants to produce billions of extra people; antiabortionists merely see each *particular person* as valuable from conception. John Noonan, who advocates a genetic criterion, argues that when sperm and egg meet and merge genes, a genetically unique individual is created (unless, of course, the zygote divides into identical twins)[31]: The resulting embryo has all the potential in its DNA to be a full person, provided that it finds a nurturing uterus. However, having the potential to become a person is not being a person, as we realize when we consider the thousands of frozen embryos stored around the world. Another problem with the genetic criterion is that it collapses the distinction between being human and being a person—as we realize when we consider that a dead human has a unique set of genes. These implications seem to constitute a *reductio ad absurdum* of the genetic criterion.

A third possible criterion for personhood (in addition to the cognitive and genetic criteria) might be called the *neurological criterion.* This is actually a minimal version of the cognitive criterion; it defines a *person* as a human being with a detectable brain wave. This simple standard would be applicable across many issues of medical ethics; it would, for instance, recognize as persons both quasi-anencephalic babies and adults in PVS. With regard to abortion, the neurological criterion would consider a fetus a person when it developed brain waves, but not before (a fetus develops brain waves at about 25 weeks of gestation).

It should be noted that criteria of personhood become relevant in many other issues in medical ethics. For example, the cognitive criterion has been proposed in issues involving patients in PVS, impaired newborns in so-called "Baby Doe" cases, and primates in medical experiments.

Viability   *When* does a human fetus become a person with a right to life? With regard to this question, personhood has become closely linked with *viability*—the ability to survive as an independent entity.

In *Roe* v. *Wade,* the Supreme Court said that a state could ban abortion after viability, implying that viability is the key event—the development which separates nonperson, nonprotectable second-trimester fetuses from third-trimester fetuses, who are protectable persons. However, the concept of viability is vague, and the Court did nothing to clarify it. (A *vague* concept is one with no sharp boundaries, e.g., "baldness.") When does viability begin? In *Roe* v. *Wade,* as we have seen, the Court said only that viability is "usually placed" at about 28 weeks but "may occur earlier, even at 24 weeks," leaving the matter otherwise indeterminate.

In Kenneth Edelin's trial, the district attorney, Newman Flanagan, seized on this vagueness to try to establish that Alice Roe's fetus had been viable. One antiabortion physician testified that a baby could live outside the womb after as little as 12 weeks of gestation. But for how long? Only a few minutes, the physician testified, though maybe for longer. However, the defense attorney, William Homans, counterpunched by asking the physician how he defined viability; the physician said that viability was "capacity to survive [outside the womb] even for a second after birth." As Homans questioned several other physicians who were testifying as expert witnesses for the prosecution, he got each of them to admit that he had never known a fetus to survive for even a few days outside the womb after less than 24 weeks of gestation.

In general, Edelin's critics argued that they knew exactly what was meant by viability: ability to survive independently of the mother. In reality, some fetuses who are born early are not viable: they will die no matter how hard physicians try to keep them alive. Others will survive, though, and neonatologists usually know which is which. (Ultrasound tests can often indicate probable viability.) To Edelin's opponents, the point was that he had never tried to find out if the fetus was viable; he just assumed it wasn't. His supporters replied that of course neither he nor anyone else had tried to determine viability, since the point of abortion is to kill a fetus. The point is not to look inside the uterus, see if the fetus is "viable," and save it if it is; the intention is to kill it, regardless.

Other Arguments about Abortion

The Argument from Marginal Cases   In the Edelin case, one question that arose was, "Where do you draw the line?"—that is, the line between fetuses which may and may not be aborted. Reasoning based on this kind of question is called the *argument from marginal cases,* and it is one of the most widely used ideas in ethics. With regard to an issue like abortion, the argument from marginal cases is as follows: Beings at the "margins" of personhood cannot be nonarbitrarily distinguished from those at the "core," because personhood and nonpersonhood are linked by a continuum. (The argument from marginal cases often appears in other issues as well, including animal rights—where it is based on the continuity of primates and human beings—and individual versus collective responsibility.)

The argument from marginal cases is related to the problem of jumping the fact-value gap, since another way of expressing this argument is to say that when marginal cases exist, there is no factual point or marker which could serve as a nonarbitrary (true) connecting premise between facts and values. That is, the question "Where do you draw the line?" implies that in certain moral issues, any candidate for a fact-value connecting premise will inevitably jump the fact-value gap. Consider this argument about abortion:

1. A human with a brain wave is a person.
2. Killing a person is morally wrong.
3. Therefore, killing a human with a brain wave is morally wrong.

In this argument, premise 1—which combined the evaluative definition of a *person* with a factual statement about fetal brain waves—is offered as the connection between facts and values; but according to the argument from marginal cases, that premise is arbitrary. Why? Because any other factual event in fetal development might equally well be chosen. Moreover, it is held, any other premise we might suggest to serve in this way would also be arbitrary.

Antiabortionists say that fetal development is smooth and continuous: there are no quantum leaps. Thus there is no specific, identifiable point of "ensoulment" or "personhood" or even "viability." No matter what week of gestation is considered, it seems arbitrary to make *that* week the marker of personhood or viability, because the fetus of a week earlier has almost the same qualities. Whatever time or marker is chosen, someone can always plausibly ask: Why not choose some other time or some other marker? For example, why not choose the preceding week?

Is the argument from marginal cases a good one? People who argue for abortion rights sometimes draw an analogy with the color spectrum: although each shade in the spectrum does resemble the shades next to it, colors that are more widely separated—and of course the colors on the two ends—are clearly distinguishable. Another analogy might also be made: a full-grown oak tree, or even a sapling, differs clearly from an acorn, even though the process by which an acorn becomes an oak is smooth and continuous. Similarly, then, we can in fact distinguish a newborn baby, and even a late-term fetus, from an embryo despite the continuous development from embryo to newborn. In other words, the existence of marginal cases does *not* make all distinctions impossible.

In practice people make such distinctions all the time, despite the fact that many marginal cases exist. Aristotle, for one, recognized that we habitually make these kinds of distinctions, and he observed that people with education, intelligence, and good judgment—not surprisingly—do this best.

Thomson: A Limited Proabortion View   Suppose that the fetus in the Edelin case *was* a person. Does it logically follow, then, that killing this fetus is immoral? The philosopher Judith Jarvis Thomson has argued that it does not.[32]

Thomson asks you to imagine that you have been admitted to a hospital for an operation, and that after the surgery you awaken to find yourself hooked up to a famous violinist whose kidneys have failed and whose blood is entering and leaving your body through tubes; your kidneys are being used without your permission to keep the violinist alive. Thomson argues that it is immoral for the hospital to force you to keep the violinist alive by using you in this way without your permission (although presumably you might be used *with* your permission, and it might be saintly of you to volunteer).

Thomson grants the antiabortionists one crucial premise: that the fetus is a person with a right to life. She sets up this hypothetical situation, however, to argue that even so, not all abortions are immoral. In her imaginary situation, the violinist cannot demand as a right that you keep him or her alive by allowing your kidneys to be used. Similarly, Thomson argues, a fetus cannot demand as a right (or its champions cannot demand this right for it) that a woman must keep it alive by carrying it to term. For Thomson, the most telling case is rape, because (by definition) a rape victim has not consented to sexual intercourse and therefore has not consented to conceiving a child; if conception occurs as a result of rape, the rapist's fetus, in particular, has no claim on the woman's body. Similar arguments might apply when a woman has used contraception responsibly but the contraceptive fails.

Thomson's view is relevant in the Edelin case because there was a possibility—a hint—that Alice Roe's pregnancy had resulted from incest. It was rumored that Alice had waited as long as she did before seeking an abortion because she didn't want to acknowledge what had happened to her, or because she didn't want her mother to know. If Alice was in fact a victim of incest, then Thomson's argument would allow the abortion, even if the fetus was by then a person. However, if Alice had simply been careless about contraception, Thomson's argument would not justify an abortion.

Thomson's argument is an example of reasoning *by analogy*. Here, an analogy is being drawn between the patient who is being used involuntarily to keep the violinist alive and a woman who is involuntarily pregnant—for instance, the violinist's dependence on the other patient is said to be analogous to the fetus's dependence on the mother. When anological reasoning is used in this way, the strength of the argument depends on how appropriate the analogy actually is: the closer the "fit" between the two things that are said to be analogous, the more strongly the inferred conclusion is supported.

In this case, critics of Thomson's argument, such as Francis Kamm, have objected that the analogy breaks down. They argue, for instance, that the patient who is being involuntarily used can simply unhook himself or herself, and that detaching a cannula from one's vein is not really like killing a fetus by abortion. Since something "active" must be done to end a fetus's life, these critics maintain that to make the analogy exact, the violinist would have to be doing something like blocking the other patient's way out of the room, so that the other patient could escape only by, say, cutting the violinist up.[33] (To grasp the idea of this criticism, try imagining a gigantic baby blocking the way out.)

It is interesting to note that both Thomson's original argument and this critical response suggest a concept of abortion as "self-defense." This concept is by no means new, however; it goes back at least as far as the sixteenth century, when the theologian Thomas Sanchez argued on this basis that an embryo could be aborted in an ectopic pregnancy.[34] Sanchez, using Augustine's doctrine of "just war," identified an embryo growing in a fallopian tube as an "unjust aggressor" against the life of the mother and maintained that a mother could legitimately kill such an embryo in self-defense.

Feminist Views   Certain worldviews support certain moral premises, and some feminists believe that most of the premises in arguments about abortion are ultimately determined by whether a worldview embraces or attacks feminism. Here, *feminism* pertains to the right of a woman to make her own choices and lead her own life in equality with, not under the control of, the men in her life. (This is, of course, a broad, rather loose definition.) Many feminists hold that differing moral opinions about abortion involve not the metaphysics of personhood but the roles of women or women's sexual and economic liberation.

One feminist writer argues that the key question about abortion is whether women should be forced to bear children in a way in which men are not. If an embryo is a person who has a right to life at the mother's expense, then women will always be potential slaves of biological reproduction:

> With all the imperfections of our present-day attitudes, I'm still a lot better off in terms of the sexual choices I have than women of my mother's generation. I was a lot better off after the sixties than I was before them. What sexual freedom I now have has been very hard-won. I wouldn't give it up for anything. . . . There's a larger crisis, one that has to do with the tensions between feminism and the backlash against it. On the one hand, society is encouraging sexual freedom; on the other hand, it's punishing people for indulging in it and not emotionally preparing them for it. Both women in general and teenagers in particular are caught in the middle.[35]

Conservative Religious Views   We have already noted the religious argument that personhood begins at conception. A related idea is that each human pregnancy happens for a divine reason, and this may be the basis for an argument commonly called the *sanctity of life*. People who believe in the sanctity of life assume that a particular being, which has been conceived, has survived to implant itself in the uterine wall, and has been growing inside a woman since then, was *meant by God to have been created at this place and time*. It follows that any interference with the growth of this being would thwart God's plans. In the language of laypeople, this is sometimes expressed as, "God must have meant for me (you, her) to become pregnant, or else I (you, she) wouldn't be."

Two replies can be made to this kind of conservative religious view. First, such a view is very fatalistic in terms of one's personal relation to God, and it seems reasonable to ask, "*Why* must I (you, she) accept everything that happens? If everything comes from God, doesn't the choice to have or not to have an abortion also come by God? Why make the fatalistic assumption that one can follow God's will only by accepting pregnancy? Why can't a reasoned choice to have an abortion also reflect God's will?"

Second—and this reply is logically prior to the first one—how does a woman (or a couple) know what God's will about a particular pregnancy might be? Unless God speaks to us directly, revealing his wishes, how can we assume that planning whether and when to have children is not best for us? How do we know that God does not want us to do what we believe will be best for us?

A Final Consideration: Abortion as a Three-Sided Issue

Many of us in North America are so accustomed to living in a tolerant democracy, where individual liberties are respected, that we sometimes fail to understand how we got where we are or what the larger, worldwide picture is. In the United States, we can easily forget that our historical policy of individual rights and liberty represents a hard-won victory which citizens of many other countries have never achieved. Millions of women in China, for instance, were forced to undergo abortions if they became pregnant before their mid-twenties or after they already had a child: the Chinese government imposed a limit of one child per family. In Romania under the long (and only recently ended) dictatorship of Nicolae Ceausescu, millions of women were denied contraception or abortions: the Romanian government wanted to increase the population and forced women to have as many children as possible.

Perhaps it is this kind of forgetfulness that explains why our media sometimes present abortion as an issue with two sides: antiabortion versus pro-choice. In fact, the global picture of abortion in recent history is most accurately portrayed as a *three-sided* issue involving two extremes and a compromise between them—forced birth versus forced abortion versus individual choice:

- *Forced Birth.* Extreme (example, Romania)
- *Forced Abortion.* Extreme (example, China)
- *Individual Choice.* Compromise (example, United States)

In other words, the idea of leaving decisions about abortion up to the women affected is, in terms of the world as a whole, not one of two sides but rather a compromise between two extremes.

RELATED ISSUES

The Antiabortion Movement

Efforts to overturn *Roe* v. *Wade* have taken various paths since 1973. Some have, of course, involved legislation, but probably the most prominent antiabortion activities have taken the form of protest.

Some of the protest has been violent, and the violent elements of the movement invoke a higher, special "antiabortion morality." During the 1980s, protesters bombed many abortion clinics. Two men from Texas who attacked several abortion clinics in Florida were sentenced to 30 years in prison; among other crimes, they had kidnapped a physician who performed abortions. In 1984 alone, there were 24 arson or bombing attacks on abortion clinics. One bombing—in Pensacola, Florida—took place on Christmas morning and was described by one of the conspirators as a "birthday present to Jesus."[36] A few weeks earlier, a bomb at a clinic in a suburb of Washington, D.C., had almost killed a guard.

By the end of the 1980s, public opinion had turned dramatically against antiabortion violence. As a result, the vast majority of the antiabortion movement used the kind of nonviolent protest mounted by Operation Rescue, an organization founded by Randall Terry in 1988. Modeling themselves on the nonviolent demonstrations (such as sit-ins) that had taken place in the south during the civil rights movement, these protesters practiced civil disobedience in front of abortion clinics; they hoped, by their example, to prick the conscience of the nation. Some leaders were fined and jailed for blocking traffic and other minor infractions of the law.

During the 1990s, however, the protest movement targeted physicians who performed abortions as the "weak link" in the chain; these physicians sometimes found protesters outside their homes on Saturday mornings. It was such campaigns of harassment that may have led, in March 1993, to the point-blank murder of the physician David Gunn as he was leaving an abortion clinic in Pensacola, Florida. Dr. Gunn had been performing abortions once a week at the clinic, and his picture had been posted across northern Florida by antiabortionists on the kind of "WANTED" sign used by the FBI for fugitives from justice. Spokespersons for Rescue America and Missionaries to the Unborn announced that Dr. Gunn's death had saved numerous babies from abortion; later, one of these spokespersons "rejoiced" when the Pensacola clinic found it difficult to replace Dr. Gunn.

On July 29, 1994, at another abortion clinic in Pensacola, a second physician—John Bayard Britton—was killed by an antiabortion leader and former minister named Paul Hill. Dr. Britton and his volunteer security escort, James Barrett, were both fatally shot, and James Barrett's wife was wounded; Dr. Britton had been wearing a bulletproof vest, but Hill (who would be convicted in November 1994) was said to have aimed the shotgun directly at his head. That same night, an abortion clinic in Virginia was bombed, though there were no injuries.

In January of 1998, on an otherwise peaceful morning, the campus of the University of Alabama at Birmingham was rocked by an explosion at an abortion clinic across the street from a Ronald McDonald House and a block away from student apartments, where windows were shaken by the blast. An off-duty Birmingham policeman was killed when he touched the package, which had a steel plate as a backing, designed to ricochet the hundreds of nails inside into the people who found the bomb. Emily Lyons, a nurse at the clinic was severely maimed, but survived after intensive efforts by physicians at UAB Hospital, a few blocks away. Police searched for the alleged bomber, Eric Rudolph, for months in the hills of North Carolina. As of the printing of this book, Rudolph is still wanted by police.

In the fall of 1998, a sniper killed an upstate New York physician who performed abortions after the physician returned home with his wife and four sons from synagogue. During the previous four years, snipers had shot and wounded three Canadian physicians and a physician practicing near Rochester, NY. Dr. Barnett Slepian was shot and killed in his kitchen by a gunman firing through a window and crouching behind his backyard fence. Slepian had been targeted by antiabortion groups since the 1980s and had vowed not to let the groups deter him from providing abortions.

In June of 2002, James Charles Kopp was extradicted from France for the murder of Dr. Slepian. Known as "Atomic Dog" for his antiabortion fanaticism, Kopp admitted in late 2002 that he had intentionally shot Dr. Slepian. Also charged were two New Yorkers, whom the FBI said funneled money to Kopp and harbored him from police.

In 2002, antiabortion activists began to use digital video cameras to photograph women entering abortion clinics and to post their pictures on the Internet. (They had already done so to physicians performing abortions.) Abortion rights activists vehemently protested such tactics.

Access to abortion continued to be a major issue in rural states such as North Dakota where abortion clinics have been closed because of lack of support of the medical community. (Consider that the three visits required of RU-486, for a college student living in Grand Forks, means three long trips to Minneapolis and back.) Because physicians doing abortions are targeted, residency programs sometimes offer no training in doing abortions. Some residents in obstetrics have had to demand training in abortion.[37]

Attempted Abortions Resulting in Live Births

Attempts to abort late-term fetuses have sometimes resulted in live births. In 1977, a physician, Ronald Cornelson, testified in a California criminal court that after a botched saline abortion resulted in a live-born 2½-pound baby, his colleague William Waddill had choked the infant and had also suggested injecting potassium chloride to kill it. (It can be noted that a 2½-pound baby may well be viable; this was the birthweight of the jockey Willie Shoemaker, who was born prematurely and was kept warm in a shoebox in an oven.) Waddill was tried twice for murder, but both juries were deadlocked.[38] In 1979, at the University of Nebraska Medical Center, another 2½-pound baby was born alive after an attempted abortion, was purposefully left unattended, and died after a few hours.

Because of such cases, physicians today will rarely perform an abortion after 23 weeks of gestation; and there are some newer techniques for preventing abortions that would produce live births. For example, use of prostaglandins to induce abortion is now avoided, since prostaglandins, although safer than suction or surgical techniques, resulted in 30 times more live births. For first-trimester abortions, the most typical technique was formerly injection of hostile fluids (saline or urea), followed by dilatation and curettage (scraping), a technique called *D and C*; but D and C has been replaced by suction curettage or uterine aspiration. For late-term abortions, dilatation and evacuation—*D and E*—is used: the fetus is cut into parts and removed in pieces. To ensure that all the pieces have been removed (since any fragments left behind would produce infection in the mother), the dismembered fetus must be reassembled outside the womb. Late second-trimester abortions use hysterotomy, as in the Edelin case.

Fetal-Tissue Research and RU-486

Tissue from aborted fetuses may help patients with neurological disorders such as Parkinson's disease. The tissue required for such neurological research must be adrenal tissue producing dopamine; and it must be obtained from fetuses whose gestational age is 8 to 11 weeks, since after 12 weeks the tissue begins to differentiate into the normal cells and structures of the brain and thus loses its elasticity. Treatment consists of a drug (dopamine) delivered as (fetal) cells: In the operation, a small hole is drilled through the patient's skull and fetal cells are dripped directly into the devastated area of the brain. (Note that this is in no sense a "brain transplant" but simply a tissue transplant.)

A panel of the National Institutes of Health (NIH) studied this issue and concluded that even if abortion may be immoral, fetal tissue obtained from abortions can be ethically used for research if the woman's decision to donate tissue is made separately from, and after, her decision to abort.[39] On January 22, 1993—the twentieth anniversary of *Roe* v. *Wade*—the newly elected President Clinton lifted a 4-year ban on fetal-tissue research.

RU-486, mifepristone, the "morning after" abortion pill, was tested on millions of women in China, Sweden, Britain, and France. It became legal in France in 1987 and in 2000 became a standard item in health clinics in French high schools. Its introduction into America was fought for a dozen years by groups calling it "chemical warfare on the unborn" and who boycotted drugs made by its manufacturer Hoechst AG of Germany.[40]

Mifepristone works by having the woman come to a doctor's office and taking the pills, which block the action of progesterone. Two days later at home, she takes misoprostol, a prostaglandin that makes her uterus contract. This drug combination, taken in this way, causes heavy bleeding and cramping which lasts from one to two weeks (in rare cases, a month) and which causes the embryo to detach from the uterine lining. Two weeks later, the woman returns to the doctor's office to make sure the embryo has been aborted. In 5 percent of cases where it fails, surgical abortion must then occur.

On September 29, 2000, the FDA approved it for use in America during the seventh week of pregnancy, but in the years since, it has not proved popular, in part because abortion clinics charge $100 more for a pill-introduced abortion than a D and C, in part because of a 24-hour rule about informed consent in some states (making the need for three visits, not two).

Emergency Contraception

In 1997, the American Medical Association, Federal Drug Administration, and Planned Parenthood publicized a method of controlling unplanned pregnancy that had been known for over 25 years. That method is called *emergency contraception* and consists of doubling up on birth control pills within 72 hours of an act of unprotected sex in which a woman thinks she may have become pregnant, followed by a second dose 12 hours later.

Such pills work in several ways. Use of pills containing estrogen and progesterone block the release of the egg from the ovary, block the movement of the embryo down the fallopian tube, or prevent implantation of the embryo in the endometrium.

This method is a "days after" and "just in case" strategy. If the woman waits until a pregnancy test reveals she is pregnant, it is too late because her urine does not chemically change until after embryonic implantation. This method also requires either a woman to have birth control pills on hand, even if she is on some other method of birth control or her partner uses condoms, or that she be able to obtain such birth control pills very quickly.

For the latter reason, some physicians in some cities—especially at women's medical clinics—began to advertise that they would prescribe such pills on request. They also said they would implant IUDs for similar reasons, which can be done up to a week after possible conception but which are more costly. Emergency rooms are also supposed to offer victims of rape such preventive measures.

Because of difficulties surrounding RU-486, advocates for family planning promote Plan B, a way to get emergency contraception over the Internet (www.GotoPlanB.com) without seeing a physician (and directly, in some pharamacies in the Northwest).[41] Plan B promotes Previn, which contains high doses of ordinary birth control pills and which lacks the nausea and 2-week routine of RU-486 (Previn is taken once, then again 12 hours later). Previn has been in use for years in Canada, Africa, Asia, and South America.

The phrase "emergency contraception" masks a fact that is objectionable to conceptionists, namely, the fact that an embryo is being destroyed. Champions of emergency contraception say that the word "abortion" should only refer to termination of an embryo that has already implanted.[42] The reason for defining this process as "contraception" appears to be the desire to give women, parents, and participating physicians a way to not think of themselves as being involved with abortions. Nevertheless, there is no doubt that these measures deliberately intend to terminate the growth of a human embryo that otherwise might be gestated to a human baby.

Another advantage of emergency contraception is that it reduces the number of fetal abortions. Holland, where emergency contraception has been available and encouraged for decades, has the lowest rate of abortion and teenage pregnancy of any westernized country.[43] A disadvantage of emergency contraception is that it does not prevent sexually-transmitted diseases.

As this practice grows, and it is indeed growing, it will make many physicians rethink their views on termination of pregnancies. Previously, physicians could distance themselves from abortions, which were almost exclusively done by abortion specialists in clinics that were free-standing places unconnected to hospitals and the group practices of physicians. With this new option, the most likely physicians who will get requests for emergency prescriptions for birth control pills are those who would normally see young women or their parents, that is, those in family medicine, gynecology, adolescent medicine (even pediatrics), and internal medicine. As such, being for or against termination of unintended pregnancies will become less abstract for such physicians, as their own patients and their families come to them with requests.

The general problem of unintended pregnancies is unlikely to go away simply with education. For the last 25 years, over 1 million teenage American girls have gotten pregnant each year and about half of all American pregnancies are unintended each year.

One reality check is whether physicians and parents are prepared to give young girls birth control pills in advance. In an excellent study published in 1998, a thousand young women were studied for a year.[44] In the treatment group, half were given such pills in advance; the half in the control group had to call a physician to get a prescription. As might be predicted, 180 women used postcoital contraception in the first group, but only 87 in the control group, showing that ease of access is important in preventing unintended pregnancy.

Maternal versus Fetal Rights

The issue of maternal versus fetal rights has developed new aspects during the years since the Edelin case. This general issue, of course, includes abortion, but not all cases of conflicting rights actually involve abortion; some have arisen when pregnant women were willing to continue pregnancy.

A famous case that did involve abortion occurred in 1989, when Nancy Klein, who was in her twenties, went into a coma at an early stage of pregnancy because of head injuries in an auto accident. Her physicians wanted to abort the fetus: they believed that an abortion might bring her back to consciousness; they also felt that an abortion would be in her best interest because certain drugs that she should receive could not be given while she was pregnant (these drugs might injure the fetus), and because her cerebral blood volume would increase once she was no longer pregnant. Antiabortionists went to court to try to block the abortion, while Nancy Klein's husband, Martin, pressed for it. Martin Klein prevailed and the abortion was performed (amid protests). Nancy Klein emerged from the coma after 11 months and now lives a normal life.

Two well-known cases have concerned cesarean section. The earlier of these took place in Washington, D.C., in June 1985, when Angela Carder ("Angela C") and her 26-week-old fetus died shortly after undergoing a cesarean section ordered by a judge for the sake of the fetus. Angela Carder was dying of a rare form of cancer and had evidently requested chemotherapy and resisted the operation, although some witnesses said that she was so confused and dulled that her real wishes could not possibly have been known. The baby was delivered alive but died 2 hours later; Angela Carder herself died 2 days later.[45]

The second of these cases took place in Illinois in late 1993, when the physicians of a pregnant woman referred to as "Mother Doe" sued in court to force her to undergo a caesarean section. The fetus in this case was becoming oxygen-starved, and the physicians wanted to deliver it at once by cesarean section because they felt that if they waited for a full-term delivery, the baby would be born retarded or even in PVS. Mother Doe, on the other hand, was a religious woman who believed that God would miraculously protect the fetus until a healthy infant could be delivered through natural childbirth. The basic issues at odds in this case were whether the fetus had a right to normality at birth and whether a competent woman can ever be compelled to undergo surgery in the interest of a fetus. The Illinois Supreme Court upheld the mother's right to refuse surgery. The status of the baby at birth is unknown.

An unfortunately common issue that has developed in cases involving maternal versus fetal rights has to do with substance abuse by the mother. In cases like these, the mother typically intends to carry the fetus to term, but because of her abuse of drugs or alcohol, it is likely that the baby will be born impaired. Between 1987 and 1992, 160 women in 24 states were charged with injuring a fetus during pregnancy by taking drugs such as cocaine.[46] Such a case often arises in the third trimester, when the fetus is obviously viable and thus would be considered a person, or at least a near-person, by most people. The conflict then is between a vulnerable fetus, whose interests are served by coming into life unimpaired by alcohol or drugs, and a drug-dependent mother who often can barely cope with her pregnancy, let alone with her life.

It should be noted that the problem of substance abuse during pregnancy affects not only women and fetuses but society as a whole. Fetal alcohol syndrome, for instance, is often cited as the leading cause of mental retardation.[47] Many people are disturbed that government, through the offices of local district attorneys, can intervene in pregnant women's lives for the sake of fetuses; for other people, however, the prospect of babies—and communities—needlessly harmed by preventable retardation or congenital drug dependency is equally disturbing. There may also be an element of class conflict here, since critics opposed to intervention say that almost all the women who are prosecuted are drug abusers rather than middle class alcoholics; and it is true that far more babies are harmed by alcohol than by cocaine.

Finding a broad, consistent policy about conflicts between maternal and fetal rights is difficult. It is possible, of course, to conclude simply that no interference with competent pregnant women should be allowed. However, such a conclusion would seem incompatible with a consensus that has become clear in medicine regarding an issue raised by Jehovah's Witnesses. The medical profession holds that a pregnant Jehovah's Witness can be forced to accept blood transfusions to save the life of a third-trimester fetus; the rationale for this policy is that while the woman could be allowed to decline a transfusion for herself, she should not be allowed to decline it for a fetus, who as an adult might not choose to become a Jehovah's Witness. It is sometimes argued that this medical policy also justifies intervening with pregnant substance abusers. (On the other hand, though, the Jehovah's Witness in this example is hospitalized, whereas the substance abuser may not be.)

In moral issues, there are sometimes true tragedies—situations in which, no matter what is done, there can be no good outcome. Cases of maternal-child conflict may be among them.

The *Whitner* case tilted state protection towards the fetus, reversing a decades-long emphasis on maternal autonomy and rights, and hence, distressing advocates for women's rights. On April 7, 1992, Cornelia Whitner, a 28-year-old, African American woman, was found guilty under a South Carolina law charging her with failing "to provide proper medical care for her unborn child by using crack cocaine while pregnant." The controversial law required physicians and nurses to notify the district attorney when women seeking parental care were discovered to be abusing drugs harmful to their fetus, making health professionals agents of drug and law enforcement. The law also required that a "viable fetus" in the third trimester of pregnancy should be offered the same protection as a child, thus equating such fetuses with full persons.

In practice, the South Carolina law made such mothers choose between mandatory drug rehabilitation while pregnant and, if they continued using drugs, jail. Most such women chose rehab. Critics said such a policy would deter drug-using women from seeking medical treatment during pregnancy, that black women using cocaine were prosecuted but pregnant white women drinking alcohol were not, and that harm to the fetus of using cocaine during pregnancy had been exaggerated. (Some babies gestated by mothers using cocaine appear to be normal children.)

Defenders of the law cited the estimated 70,000 American women using cocaine while pregnant and the fact that society could not turn a blind eye to the harm of nearly a million children over the next dozen years. They also agreed that white women or pregnant women abusing alcohol should be similarly prosecuted.

In June of 1998, the U. S. Supreme Court declined to review the South Carolina law, which had been twice upheld by that state's supreme court, thus letting the law stand.

LEGAL TRENDS AND DECISIONS

Viability

In 1983, Justice Sandra Day O'Connor predicted that medicine would push viability "further back toward conception" and that the trimester system established in *Roe* v. *Wade* would be "clearly on a collision course with itself."[48] Her prediction has not come true. Although medicine has made intense efforts to treat premature babies more effectively, in 1992 the consensus in neonatology was that "before 23 or 24 weeks, [the fetus] simply cannot survive. And nothing that medical science can do will budge that boundary in the foreseeable future."[49] The problems— apparently unsolvable—are that earlier than 23 or 24 weeks of gestation, the fetal lungs are simply too immature to function, even with a respirator; and that certain essential organs, such as the kidneys, do not develop early in pregnancy.

This recently acknowledged fact weakens one argument against abortion. Clearly, the argument from marginal cases must lose some of its force, since *lung viability* now serves (and has served for over 25 years) as a practical indicator of viability and thus, in fetal development, can be offered as a marker of personhood.

A number of legal developments will be discussed in the following section, but there have also been at least two with regard to viability. In 1979, in *Colautti* v. *Franklin,* the United States Supreme Court gave physicians broad discretion in determining viability. The decision said that "the determination of whether a particular fetus is viable is, and must be, a matter for the judgment of the responsible attending physician," apparently precluding the possibility of another case like Kenneth Edelin's. However, in 1989, in *Webster* (possibly referring to the Edelin case), the Supreme Court allowed a state to require a physician to check after abortion for viability of the fetus.

U.S. Supreme Court Decisions

In the two decades since *Roe* v. *Wade,* abortion-rights advocates have pressed for broader protection and antiabortion forces have mounted legal challenges. A culmination came in 1992, with the Court's decision in *Planned Parenthood* v. *Casey* (widely known as the "Pennsylvania decision"): The Court reaffirmed the "essential holding" of *Roe* v. *Wade,* including "the right of a woman to choose to have an abortion before viability and to obtain it without undue interference from the State."[50] (Note in particular the phrase *undue interference.*) A few months later, in December 1992 (this was the month before President Clinton's inauguration)—as if to say that it had taken its stand on abortion law and would not budge in the future—the Court turned down a request to review an appellate decision voiding severe antiabortion restrictions that had been legislated in Guam.

During the last two decades, however, the Court has been willing to fine-tune certain details of *Roe* v. *Wade,* and to these we now turn.

Consent of Fathers

The 1976, in *Danforth,* the Court invalidated state laws requiring a woman to get consent for an abortion from either the matrimonial or the biological father. The Court held that such consent amounted to giving these men a veto over the woman's decision, and because the woman "is the more directly and immediately affected by the pregnancy," she should not be subject to any such veto.

Consent or Notification of Parents

The *Danforth* decision also said that a state cannot pass a law giving parents of teenage girls a veto over the decision to have an abortion. In 1979, however—in *Bellotti* v. *Blair*—the Supreme Court said that although a state may not give parents an absolute veto over a minor daughter's decision to terminate a pregnancy, the state may require a minor to obtain the consent of one or both parents if it provides her with an alternative to having to consult or inform the parent or parents. Another decision held that a state law was legal if it merely required a clinic to inform or notify a parent before a teenager's abortion. By 1992, 35 states had laws requiring a parent's consent or notification when minors sought abortions, although only 18 states actively enforced such laws.[51]

Informed Consent of Patients

During the 1980s, the Supreme Court struck down laws in Ohio and Pennsylvania that required, before an abortion, the patient's informed consent, a 24-hour waiting period, or discussion of alternatives by the physician with the patient. The language in these "informed consent" statutes had been, in fact, dissuasive rather than informative. In its "Pennsylvania decision" in 1992, the Court reversed itself on this point, ruling that informed consent and a 24-hour waiting period did not constitute "undue burdens" on women seeking abortions. This change brought abortion into line with informed-consent requirements for other medical procedures of equal risk.

Government Support

Several other decisions concerned whether the federal government or state governments could be required to fund abortions for women who are unable to pay for them. In *Harris* v. *McRae* (1980), the Supreme Court held that although a woman has a right to an abortion, she does not have a right to a *free* abortion at the expense of federal or state government. Congress passed laws banning use of public funds for abortions for women unable to afford them, and many states followed suit. The *Webster* decision in 1989 also said that states may ban public employees or public hospitals from performing abortions.

Partial-Birth Abortions

Frustration with U.S. courts also led antiabortion advocates to focus on the kind of abortion most vulnerable to prohibition, so-called "partial-birth abortion." Such advocates claimed that abortion could be performed right up to birth, even though a fetus could survive outside the womb. Defenders of abortion rights insisted that only prevention of grave harm to the mother ever justified such abortions. The first Partial-Birth Abortion Ban Act in Congress defined such procedures as where "the person performing the abortion partially vaginally delivers a living fetus before killing the fetus and completing the delivery."[52] This bill was vetoed by President Clinton in 1996, as was a similar bill in 1997. By the end of 1998, state laws outlawing partial-birth abortions had been struck down by federal courts 18 out of 19 times.[53]

UPDATE

As the 21st century began, it became more and more apparent—in its *Pennsylvania* and *Guam* decisions, and in its refusal to hear any more challenges to *Roe* v. *Wade*—that the U.S. Supreme Court was going to let abortion remain legal in America. As some predicted, such closure of the judicial route, combined with successive failures in the U.S. Congress to pass a Constitutional amendment barring abortion, led some antiabortionists to conclude that peaceful means had failed and that violent means were now justified. As we move into the third millennium, and after 25 years of legalized abortion, passions about the ethics of abortion still run hot in American society.

After reviewing the account of this case, Kenneth Edelin wants to emphasize that Alice Roe was the first person in her family to go to college and that a pregnancy would have prevented her from attending college or becoming financially stable.

FURTHER READING

Francis M. Kamm, *Creation and Abortion*, Oxford University Press, New York, 1992.

Don Marquis, "Why Abortion Is Immoral," *Journal of Philosophy*, vol. 86, 1989, pp. 183–202.

Warren Quinn, "Abortion: Identity and Loss," *Philosophy and Public Affairs*, vol. 13, 1984, pp. 24–54.

Michael Tooley, *Abortion and Infanticide*, Oxford University Press, Oxford, 1983.

Mary Anne Warren, "On the Moral and Legal Status of the Fetus," *The Monist*, vol. 57, 1973, pp. 43–61.

CHAPTER 6

Assisted Reproduction

Louise Brown and Beyond

*D*uring the last two decades, one of the fastest growing and most exciting fields of medicine has been (what is called) "assisted reproduction technology" or ART. This field has raised many ethical issues about whether and how children should be created.

This chapter begins by discussing the events surrounding the birth in 1978 of Louise Brown, who was called the first "test tube baby," and the ethical controversies that preceded and followed her birth. The second half of the chapter describes developments and issues in the use of ART since Louise Brown's birth.

"Test tube" conception is less emotionally called in vitro fertilization (IVF). (*In vitro* means "in glass".) It involves fertilization outside the womb, in a Petri dish, and it is part of a new field called assisted reproduction. As some wit remarked about IVF, people already knew how to have sex without making babies, and they now have discovered how to make babies without having sex.

BACKGROUND: IN VITRO FERTILIZATION

In this chapter, key terms are necessarily but perilously defined, because battles between opposed positions in reproductive ethics often occur by using evaluatively (or nonevaluatively) defining key terms. (The fact–value gap, discussed in the last chapter, can be crossed or finessed in defining key terms such as *embryo* or *baby*.)

Conception takes place when a sperm fertilizes an egg. A fairly common but mistaken belief is that conception happens in the woman's vagina or uterus. In fact, sperm move up the vagina, through the uterus, and into the narrow fallopian tubes. The two fallopian tubes, which are the size of a straw, normally carry one egg a month from the ovaries to the uterus. Conception occurs in the upper third of a tube when the first sperm penetrates the egg.

In human embryology, a successful union of sperm and egg is called a *zygote*. After conception, a zygote immediately begins dividing: It first divides into two cells, which then divide to form four cells, which then divide to form eight cells, and so on. At the stage when this organism travels down the fallopian tubes to the uterus, it is called an *embryo*.

Conceptionists, who believe personhood starts at conception, do not refer to this organism as a zygote but as an embryo. They also reject the term *pre-embryo* for an embryo that has not attached to the uterine wall.

In an ectopic pregnancy, the embryo does not reach the uterus but instead starts to grow in one of the two fallopian tubes; for the mother, this is a life-threatening condition. Surgery to remove the threatening embryo is required; this is a paradigm of where the doctrine of double effect would allow an abortion to save the life of the mother.

A woman has all her eggs at birth, but during a woman's regular ovulatory cycle, only one egg is normally primed each month for conception. Drugs such as Clomid and Pergonal stimulate the ovaries to release more than one egg (a process called *superovulation*).

After fertilization, the zygote or embryo descends the last two-thirds of the tube on its way to the uterus. Three days later, it tries to implant itself on the uterine wall.

In at least 40 percent of pregnancies (and possibly as many as 70 percent), the embryo aborts, probably because half or more of all embryos have some chromosomal (genetic) irregularities. More commonly, the mix of hormones from the woman is not quite correct that month to be supportive of gestation.

From 9 weeks of gestation until birth, the organism is called a *fetus.* A newborn human being, alive outside the womb, is by custom and law called a *baby.*

About one married couple in 12 cannot conceive a child after 1 year of trying. Infertility stems from many factors, including the woman's age at the first attempt to conceive (older women are more likely to have difficulty conceiving), damage from pelvic inflammatory disease (PID), previous abortions, uterine abnormalities, and (on the part of the man) a low sperm count. Infertility is often blamed on the woman, but men actually account for 50 percent of it.

Women today anguish as popular reports emphasize that only 7.8 percent at age 42 will be able to have children because 90 percent of their eggs will be abnormal. Because of assisted conceptions to celebrities, such as singer Celine Dion and model Cindy Margolis, young women often believed falsely that they had decades to become mothers, when in fact their fertility declines markedly at age 27.

LOUISE BROWN'S BIRTH

Lesley Brown, the mother of the first child conceived in vitro, grew up unhappily, without much of a family. Her father had left when she was born, and her mother placed her in a state home at an early age. She grew up in Bristol, a port on England's western coast with severe unemployment and widespread illiteracy. In 1963, like many other British teenagers, Lesley dropped out of high school and took a job in a factory. Later laid off, by then she had met her future husband, John Brown. After a few months, they were living together. Lesley had a new job in a cheese factory, and John drove a truck.

Five years older than Lesley, John had a previous wife who had run off with another man, leaving him with a daughter and reluctant to remarry. Lesley wanted children, however, and when she and John decided to have a child, John said that, if she became pregnant, he would "do the right thing." Despite some rocky episodes, they were married; but after 9 years of trying, Lesley never became pregnant. The couple tried to adopt a baby, but babies were scarce.

Several years before, Lesley Brown's fallopian tubes had been severely damaged by ectopic pregnancies. When told of this, like many such women, she blamed herself.

Depressed when other women talked about their children, Lesley saw a future of "years of just weighing and packing cheese and coming back to a quiet, empty flat." Their infertility didn't matter to John, but it did to Lesley, so much that she said that she wouldn't blame him if he left her for a fertile woman.

Then Lesley Brown became a patient of Patrick Steptoe. The Browns traveled to Oldham, the small, bleak city in northern England where Steptoe practiced, and not the kind of place where medical breakthroughs might be envisioned:

> Early the following morning, we walked up the hill that led to Oldham General Hospital. It was winter in a strange bleak town and no one was about. We passed open spaces, with buildings flattened by bulldozers or bombs, and great empty mills, still standing, with their windows smashed, leaving dark, gaping holes like wounds.[1]

Newsweek described the hospital as a "cluster of Victorian buildings that were originally a Dickensian workhouse."

The first conception of a human baby by in vitro fertilization did not happen without years of preparatory work and ethical controversy. Two decades of research preceded the birth of Louise Brown, beginning with work by Robert Edwards, a physiologist at Cambridge University.

Edwards worked with mice in the 1950s and learned how to control the time of ovulation in females by a long trial-and-error process of precisely balancing hormones, resulting in the Fowler-Edwards method for induced superovulation. In America, Min Chang in 1954 at the Worschester Foundation in Massachusetts achieved what most physiologists dreamed about at the time: the first in vitro fertilization in a mammal and proved her feat by having a white female rabbit deliver a litter of black pups.

In 1965, 13 years before the birth of Louise Brown, Edwards first tried to fertilize a human egg. Interestingly, Edwards faced barriers so enormous that many scientists thought that a birth through in vitro fertilization was technically impossible, much the same way that reproductive cloning is thought about today (see next chapter). As with cloning, Edwards also faced the task of achieving his experimental goal without harming the mother or the fetus.

Edwards needed to overthrow established laws and facts of his time, such as the view that gonadotrophic hormones could not make a mammalian ovary release eggs. Having already done so with mice, Edwards balanced progesterone and estrogen in women (which the ovaries normally release to thicken the lining of the uterus to receive a fertilized egg).

At the time, scientists believed that human sperm had to be (what is called) capacitated for conception; that is, chemicals had to be removed from the head of a sperm that inhibited penetration of an egg. Most scientists believed that capacitation occurred in only one way, by exposure to uterine secretions, but Edwards proved this view incorrect.

Adding his own semen one night to a ripe human egg in a dish, the next morning Edwards unexpectedly discovered that, in a test tube, he had created the first human embryo.

Did Edwards know that he had thereby unleashed some of the greatest fears of ordinary people about science? The image of Robert Edwards was that of a scary science fiction movie: lone scientist late at night in lab artificially creates human life, stealing mystery from life's conception.

Perhaps he realized how people would be frightened by his feat. In any case, he soon destroyed the embryo. Later, when he tried to repeat his accomplishment, he could not. Nor did he announce what he had done, partly because he could not repeat it and partly to avoid negative publicity. Nevertheless, a human life had been created outside the womb.

From whatever way we look it, this was truly a seminal experiment.

Although getting women to produce extra eggs and at the right time was an initial goal, and the next was to fertilize them outside the womb in a Petri dish, the real problem was getting enough eggs in the first place. To do so, obviously, the eggs had to be removed—a fact that presented an enormous problem in the mid 1960s.

Eggs are stored in the two ovaries and, normally each month, one is released. If it meets a sperm and conception occurs, the embryo travels down the fallopian tubes to the uterus where—if hormones are correctly receptive—it implants and gestates. For fertilization outside a woman's body, lots of eggs are needed, such that sperm can be introduced to many eggs, and only the healthiest embryos are reintroduced into the woman's body.

Enter now another interesting development, the role of outsiders in medical breakthroughs. Established medical science frowns on people at its fringes. Yet occasionally, those seen as quacks and as fringe scientists turn out to be visionaries.

In this story, Patrick Steptoe, an obscure gynecologic surgeon practicing in a small hospital near the industrial city of Manchester, became the key partner whom Edwards needed for eventual victory. In the mid-1960s, scientists in France and Germany used newly developed fiber optics to create a *laparascope,* a long thin tube containing a lens with a light. Steptoe published a paper describing how he made an incision near the navel and with the laparascope could see the reproductive organs and eggs.

Edwards realized the potential for removing eggs created by superovulation and proposed a partnership. Interestingly, Edwards' academic colleagues at Cambridge thought his partnership was a bad idea. As Joseph Goldstein remarked on the occasion of awarding Edwards one of the most prestigious awards in medicine in 2001 (the Lasker Award), "Edwards' colleagues in Cambridge raised their academic eyebrows, thinking he was mad to hook up with a nonacademic surgeon in private practice in a backwater hospital who was fiddling around with a dangerous foreign device that should never have been allowed into England in the first place."[2]

Edwards's collaboration with Steptoe began in 1968 and it took a decade of failed attempts to produce Louise Brown. Amazingly, roads were so poor on the east side of England that the trip between Cambridge and Manchester took 8 hours (Edwards also worked in a lab at Cambridge which lacked running hot water!). In 1969 and 1970, the duo successfully harvested eggs from infertile women and created embryos under glass.

The next decade saw Olympian attempts by Edwards and Steptoe to achieve an IVF pregnancy, attempts indicative of much medical research today where one breakthrough comes on the backs of a thousand failures. In the first phase, only after 41 tries did they get an embryo to implant but it failed to travel down to the uterus and started to grow in a fallopian tube. Called an *ectopic pregnancy,* this is a dangerous condition which potentially can kill the mother if the embryo is allowed to gestate, so the embryo had to be removed.

Over the next decade, they recruited over a hundred infertile women, who volunteered for their experiments in their quests to have a baby. They changed from implanting the embryo in the fallopian tube to implanting it directly in the uterus, where they finally succeeded on the 102nd attempt. The key? The same as with the mice: getting the hormone balance right. That "102nd attempt" was the birth of Louise Brown.

With Lesley Brown, Steptoe slipped the laparascope through a small slit at her bikini line and guided it into her ovaries, where he searched among the hundreds of eggs for the one being primed for ovulation. Searching for it was difficult enough; but when he found it, he had to insert another thin tube and suction it out. Without Steptoe's perfection of this delicate procedure, IVF would have been impossible.

Steptoe began his treatment of Lesley Brown by removing an egg from her ovaries. Then John Brown's semen was introduced to Lesley's egg in a Petri dish containing a culture fluid of salt, potassium chloride, glucose, and a bit of protein. Examination by microscope revealed that a sperm had penetrated the ovum. After being cultured for two days, the resulting embryo was mixed with supportive fluids, put in a syringe that looked something like a turkey baster, and squeezed through Lesley's dilated cervix into her uterus.

In late 1977 Dr. Steptoe told Lesley she was pregnant. Now a long wait began to see if Lesley would lose her fetus. Before this, many women had had eggs successfully fertilized in vitro; a smaller number had had eggs implanted with a resulting pregnancy. But of the few who had become pregnant, each had lost the embryo or fetus. But Lesley made it to 5 months, when amniocentesis showed a normal pregnancy.

Lesley Brown developed some minor problems during pregnancy: She had a mild case of toxemia (a metabolic disturbance caused by absorption of bacteria at the laparascopy site); also, the fetus was small (today we know this is both normal for IVF babies and a risk to their health). She spent the last month of her pregnancy at Oldham Hospital, by then under siege by the media.

The baby, a girl, was delivered by cesarean section on July 25, 1978. (After the amniocentesis, Steptoe had known that the fetus was female, but the Browns had chosen not to know its sex.) To protect the family's privacy, the delivery took place at night (slightly before midnight), with only a few people present. A BBC film team in Oldham was still negotiating with the hospital when Steptoe announced that the birth would occur in minutes. By this time, Lesley Brown had begun to realize how special her child's birth was going to be. She left her hospital room in darkness; nurses held flashlights as she walked to the delivery room. "Dozens of policemen and security officers lined every corridor as I walked along. It felt as if I was moving in a dream."

The Browns called their baby "Louise Joy." She weighed 5 pounds 12 ounces, was entirely normal, and was described as "beautiful, with a marvelous complexion, not red and wrinkly at all."[3] Immediately after her birth, John Brown said, "For a person who's been told he and his wife can never have children, the pregnancy was "like a miracle." I felt 12 feet high."

The day after Louise Brown's birth, the London newspapers had huge banner headlines: "IT'S A GIRL!" "THE LOVELY LOUISE!" "BABY OF THE CENTURY! JOY TO THE WORLD!" and the *New York Times* gave the story front-page coverage for 3 days. Behind these exuberant headlines, media coverage of this story had some disturbing aspects.

One disturbing development was the intensity of the coverage. Months into Lesley Brown's pregnancy, word had leaked out that a "test tube" baby would be born in Oldham. Interest in the story was to be expected, but during the last weeks of the pregnancy, and as the birth approached, the integrity of some journalists vanished. One American reporter telephoned a fake bomb threat to the hospital, hoping that it would force Lesley Brown outside; in the ensuing evacuation, a pregnant woman went into labor. Another reporter disguised himself as a priest and approached John Brown, asking to be admitted and offering to comfort Lesley. Throngs of Japanese photographers constantly photographed anyone—man or woman—who left Oldham Hospital, on the off chance that someone might be Lesley Brown.

When someone at the hospital revealed that the birth was imminent, six reporters for the *National Enquirer* left Florida and within 24 hours were at Oldham Hospital trying to buy worldwide rights to the Browns' story from Steptoe; a bidding war started among English tabloids. The *Enquirer* also tried to bribe an administrator, offering $100,000 for details about the birth. After the birth, daily headlines spread rumors ("TEST TUBE BABY ALMOST DIES"). Urged not to watch television or read newspapers, Lesley was told not to go near the windows to escape the scrutiny of telescopic lenses.

Another disturbing aspect of the coverage was its sensationalism and inaccuracy. Steptoe and Edwards had refused to be interviewed by reporters. (Although everybody wanted to know the Browns' identity and background, Steptoe had initially protected their anonymity. He did not want Lesley Brown to be upset; he also wanted to act as a go-between to get the Browns a trust fund for their baby, as he eventually did—reportedly $100,000 for an exclusive story.)

This silence on the part of Steptoe and Edwards frustrated reporters, some of whom took liberties in their stories or simply guessed at the facts. *Newsweek* said, for instance: "Steptoe, 65, is a flamboyant and somewhat mysterious figure; he declines to discuss his origins (reported to be in Eastern Europe)."[4] In fact, Steptoe was born in Witney (near staid Oxford), had been educated in London at King's College and St. George's Medical School, was married, and had two children. The "flamboyant" physician lived the life of an overworked obstetrician at a county hospital in an English industrial city.

Newsweek also wrote that Edwards often commuted "in the company of a rabbit that was serving as traveling receptacle for an egg under study." But Edwards himself wrote that:

> We transferred some fertilized human eggs into rabbits to see if they would grow there, but they didn't. This brief episode with rabbits led to all sorts of rumors in the press and elsewhere, and to a description of me taking hundreds of embryos to Cambridge, and of Patrick driving his Mercedes through Oldham with a rabbit in the seat next to him![5]

Scientific Reaction to the Birth

Not all medical researchers greeted Louise Brown's birth with jubilation. Two contradictory forms of criticism were, on the one hand, that IVF was trivial; and, on the other hand, that it was dangerous. There were also some procedural questions.

The director of one fertility program characterized Steptoe's achievement as merely "a cookbook thing." Another critic said that it was mundane and called the birth a "cheap stunt." Richard Blandau, a well-known fertility researcher, criticized Steptoe for not revealing how many failures had preceded this one success and thus for giving "false hope to millions of women."[6] Blandau also said that Steptoe had violated medical ethics by selling his story to the *National Enquirer* instead of publishing it in a medical journal.

There was some resentment here, because a self-described "county doc" in a small city hospital with poor research facilities had surpassed institutions with enormous budgets. Moreover, some of the criticism was unfair. For instance, Steptoe had sold the story to the *Enquirer* not for himself but for the Browns; and Blandau missed the point that the significance of Louise's birth was not its probability or improbability, but rather that IVF could be done at all.

Blandau's skepticism was understandable in the light of earlier claims. In the 1940s, the physician John Rock had announced a successful IVF but had been unable to prove it. The Italian researcher Petrucci (also in the 1940s) claimed to have fertilized a human egg in vitro, grown it for 29 days, and then destroyed it because it was becoming "monstrous—a story that fueled later fears about "monsters," though Petrucci had never provided any evidence for it.[7]

As events in recent years have shown, ART carries the potential for fraud, and to counter skepticism, Steptoe needed to prove that Lesley Brown's fallopian tubes had indeed been irreparably damaged; otherwise, many critics were ready to say that an egg could have "sneaked down" and been fertilized in the normal way. This explains why he delivered Louise by cesarean section and why he filmed Lesley Brown's damaged tubes.

Media Reaction to the Birth

Sensationalistic reporting had harmed Edwards before the Brown story. (One reason why he refused interviews was his belief that he had been harmed by British television when his work was discussed on a documentary that opened with pictures of an exploding atomic bomb.)

In previous years, Edwards had worked on infertility at the National Institute for Medical Research in London, experimenting with surgically excised ovaries, which he bathed in hormones in an attempt to induce the release of eggs. After an alarmist report on a television show, to avoid controversy the institute suspended his funding. Edwards claims that his scientific supervisor, who had herself frozen sperm, flatly told him his work was "unethical";[8] when asked "Why?" she would say only, "Because it is."

Edwards then left for Cambridge University, where he worked partially on a Ford Foundation grant to study population control and fertility. In 1974, the Ford Foundation stopped funding Edwards's work; the official reason was that his work did not promote population control, but Edwards claims that it was also because his work offended some people.

The press incorrectly called Louise Brown a "test tube baby." This term implied to many people that something bizarre had occurred—that a baby had been created without egg or sperm. Later, when Lesley Brown took her baby outside, neighbors who had absorbed this impression of IVF from the media would peer into the carriage, expecting to see something abnormal, a little monster.

In fact, from the beginning of its coverage of the Browns' story, the press had tended to equate any new means of overcoming infertility with "genetic manipulation" and had worried about the creation of mindless slaves and dangerous superhumans. The chief editor at the *London Times* equated in vitro fertilization with state-controlled eugenics.

In contrast, Louise Brown's father, John Brown, saw in vitro fertilization merely as "helping nature along a bit."

Countless articles and television reports about "genetic manipulation" appeared; and Aldous Huxley's novel *Brave New World,* written in 1932, was constantly cited by journalists as having predicted the kind of results they were now deploring—a future in which governments would use technology to control reproduction. This view of *Brave New World* was somewhat muddled: The controls Huxley had imagined were based mainly on psychological conditioning and need to be seen in the context of behaviorism, a school of psychology which was then as feared and misunderstood as IVF seemed to be in 1978. The extension of Huxley's fictional ideas about psychological manipulation to "genetic manipulation," and then to IVF (which is not genetic manipulation at all) is misleading. Moreover, there was an ironic aspect to these citations of *Brave New World,* since Huxley had described the devastating consequences of loss of choice by individuals, and media citations of this novel usually were done in ways to question whether couples should have such choices.

The media and journalists often consider themselves guardians of the public interest, but in the case of Louis Brown, many of them did not distinguish themselves. *Quis custodiet ipsos custodes?* (Who guards the guardians?)

ETHICAL ISSUES: FROM MEDIA SENSATIONALISM TO HARM TO EMBRYOS

IVF as a Religious Issue

Scientists see infertility as due mainly to problems of mechanics (blocked tubes) and chemistry (hormones). However, some people feel that infertility is a punishment for sin, imposed by God. Abortions and sexually transmitted diseases contribute to infertility, as well as professional women who delay first attempts at conception into their thirties. From these facts, some people claim that God is punishing infertile women and men for their aberrant behavior. Similarly, scientists may see IVF as a medical treatment like any other, whereas religious observers take other viewpoints.

Let us now look at some religious—specifically, Christian—views on this issue: those of the Vatican, Augustine, Joseph Fletcher, and Paul Ramsey. These views differ radically on the ethics of assisted reproduction and exemplify the difficulty of discovering "the" Christian position on any issue in medical ethics.

Catholic Views: The Vatican and Augustine   In 1978, the year of Louise Brown's birth, the Vatican condemned in vitro fertilization; one Catholic priest in New York feared that humanity had slipped from "doctoring the patient to doctoring the race." Lest that condemnation be thought of as merely the hasty reaction of just one clergyman, note that after nine years of study, the Vatican Instructions of 1987 equated IVF with "domination" and "manipulation of nature."[9] One bishop said: "The Christian morality has insisted on the importance of protecting the process by which human life is transmitted. The fact that science now has the ability to alter this process significantly does not mean that, morally speaking, it has the right to do so."[10] The official position of the Vatican in 2002 is that sexual intercourse between husband and wife is necessary for moral conception; IVF is condemned because it takes place without intercourse.

Nevertheless, many American Catholics reject this condemnation. They see nothing immoral in helping infertile couples have the children they want. Ironically, these Catholics may be closer to historical Church doctrine than the modern Vatican is.

For 1,500 years, Christian theology accepted the views of Augustine, a fourth-century philosopher and theologian who taught that the desire for intercourse (or "concupiscence") was evil. To Augustine, marriage was the only context in which this desire could permissibly be fulfilled, and even then, only for the purpose of having children. For Augustine, having children within a marriage was a license to sin; and once a marriage had produced enough children, that license was revoked. Augustine specified that original sin expressed itself in lust, and that sin was transferred through intercourse from generation to generation, and Christian doctrine thereafter followed his views.

All of which is to say that there is a certain irony in the claim by the Catholic Church that its theological teachings build directly on the teachings of patriarchs such as Augustine. The modern Church says IVF is wrong because no sex act was involved in creating a child, but Augustine said that such a sex act was inherently evil and, if possible, to be avoided at all costs.

Two Protestant Views: Fletcher and Ramsey   During the 1970s, the Protestant theologian Joseph Fletcher defended IVF as permissible for Christians. Fletcher favors any way of helping infertile couples have children:

> It is depressing, not comforting, to realize that most people are accidents. Their conception was at best unintended, at worst unwanted. There are those who are so

bemused and befuddled by a fatalist mystique about nature with a capital N (or "God's will") that they want us to accept passively whatever comes along. Talk of "not tinkering" and "not playing God" and snide remarks about "artificial" and "technological" policies is a vote against both humanness and humaneness.[11]

For Fletcher, each kind of case should be considered on its own merits to see if it would help or hurt humanity; society must not be locked into antiquated religious prohibitions that take no account of consequences to human beings. Religion is best when it is "pro people," not when it worships abstract "thou shall not's":

> The real choice is between accidental or random reproduction and rationally willed or chosen reproduction . . . Laboratory reproduction is radically human compared to conception by ordinary heterosexual intercourse. It is willed, chosen, purposed and controlled, and surely those are among the traits that distinguish Homo sapiens from others in the animal genus, from the primates down.[12]

Paul Ramsey, on the other hand, was one of the most eloquent Christian critics of IVF. Ramsey, a conservative Protestant theologian at Princeton University, equated IVF with genetic manipulation and predicted that it would lead to societal horrors. In 1970, in *Fabricated Man*, he implied that if physicians could find a tiny egg and fertilize it, why couldn't they alter its genes?[13] He predicted that if they could, they would; and he held that if they did, they would be sinful.

Ramsey came up with some provocative phrases suggesting vague but disturbing harms to society: "test tube babies," "dial-a-baby," "playing God." He was especially good at creating neologisms for rhetorical effect: "mercenary gestation," "supermarket of embryos," "spare-parts man" (a hypothetical cloned twin grown for this purpose and kept unconscious), "celebrity seed" (sperm banks), "human species suicide" (eliminating genetic diseases).

When Lesley Brown was several months pregnant, Robert Edwards attended a symposium on the ethics of IVF at Washington's Kennedy Institute for Bioethics, at the invitation of Sargent Shriver. While senators, national columnists, and other scientists listened, Ramsey condemned IVF and Edwards. As Edwards described it:

> He had to be seen and heard to be believed. I had to endure a denunciation of our work as if from some nineteenth-century pulpit. It was delivered with a Gale 8 force, and written in a similar vein a year later in the *Journal of the American Medical Association*. He doubted that our patients had given their fully understanding consent. We ignored the sanctity of life. We carried out immoral experiments on the unborn. Our work was, he thundered, "unethical medical experimentation on possible future human beings and therefore it is subject to absolute moral prohibition." I was as much surprised as made wrathful by this impertinent scorching attack. He abused everything I stood for.[14]

Ramsey's view of IVF was not based on its presumed consequences to the child, to the parents, or even to society. Rather, it was based on his idea of an embryo as a person. IVF is wrong in itself, he held, because it is "unconsented-to experimentation" on a "person," the embryo.[15]

IVF and Harm to Louise

Many critics predicted that the first baby born after in vitro fertilization might be defective. One obstetrician emphasized that severely defective babies could be created, and that "the potential is there for serious anomalies should an unqualified scientist mishandle an embryo."[16] Another obstetrician said, "What if we got a cyclops? Who is responsible? The parents? Is the government obligated to take care of it?"[17]

Leon Kass, who would later be appointed by President George W. Bush in 2002 as chair of his bioethics commission, argued strenuously that babies created by artificial fertilization might be deformed. "It doesn't matter how many times the baby is tested while in the mother's womb," he averred, "they will never be certain the baby won't be born without defect."[18] Kass clearly implied that without the certainty of a normal baby, experimental modes of conception were unethical.

Nobel Prize winners were surprisingly afraid to condone experimental methods of assisted reproduction. James Watson feared that deformed babies would be born and that they would then have to be raised in custodial homes or killed.[19] Max Perutz, who was a colleague of Edwards's at Cambridge, also condemned IVF research:

> I agree entirely with Dr. Watson that this is far too great a risk. Even if only a single abnormal baby is born and has to be kept alive as an invalid for the rest of its life, Dr. Edwards would have a terrible guilt upon his shoulders. The idea that this might happen on a larger scale—new thalidomide catastrophe—is horrifying.[20]

In 1977, in *Who Shall Play God?* the sensationalistic writer Jeremy Rifkin began many decades of self-serving opposition to all new reproductive techniques. Rifkin decried any kind of assisted reproduction as evil, as "genetic engineering," which he defined as "artificial manipulation of life." Before Louise Brown's birth, he revved up the fear that Louise might be psychologically "monstrous":

> What are the psychological implications of growing up as a specimen, sheltered not by a warm womb but by steel and glass, belonging to no one but the lab technician who joined together sperm and egg? In a world already populated with people with identity crises, what's the personal identity of a test-tube baby?[21]

Socially conservative, pioneering bioethicist Dan Callahan argued that the first case of IVF was "probably unethical" because there was no possible guarantee that Louise Brown would be normal, though it would be ethical to proceed with IVF after this first healthy birth; he added that many medical breakthroughs are actually "unethical" because we cannot know that the first patient will not be harmed.[22]

These arguments do not seem very compelling, What these critics overlooked was that no reasonable approach to life can avoid all risks. Moreover, they demonstrate a psychologically normal but nevertheless illogical tendency to magnify the risk of a harmful but unlikely event. A highly unlikely result, even if that result is very bad, still represents a very small risk. For instance, an anencephalic baby is an extremely bad but unlikely result, but that possible result shouldn't deter people from having kids.

Paradoxes about Harm and Reproduction

Whether children can or cannot be harmed by in vitro conception is a philosophically interesting consideration. The theologian Hans Tiefel writes, "No one has the moral right to endanger a child while there is yet the option of whether the child shall come into existence."[23] But can a "being" be harmed who may or may not exist?

This is an example of (what will be called) *the paradox of harm,* the seemingly self-contradictory idea that someone can be harmed by being born. This idea appears to be morally paradoxical because, first, it seems queer to say that we can harm a being by bringing it into existence; but second, it seems equally odd to say that a mother who could have prevented but did not prevent some harm to her child did no harm by that omission.

A *paradox* results when two different meanings of a key term are used simultaneously. Paradoxes can be dissolved by carefully specifying the different meanings in each part of the paradox and deciding which meaning applies best to each. With the paradox of harm, any approach to dissolving it must distinguish between different meanings of the word *harm.* Like the concept of good, the concept of harm covers a broad range of meanings. In law school, such meanings are covered in one of the major courses, *torts.* For our purposes here, two very broad ways of thinking about harm can be distinguished.

In the first way of thinking, both a baseline and a temporal (time) component are necessary, so that a change occurs which makes someone worse off. In this baseline concept, harm requires an adverse change in someone's condition. With the baseline concept, someone who doesn't yet exist cannot be harmed, because there is no baseline from which change can occur. (Consider the old Yiddish joke: 1st—"Life is so terrible! Better to have never existed." 2nd—"True, but who is so lucky? Not one in a thousand.")

In the second way of defining "harm," harm involves comparing a present deficient condition with what normally would have been. In this normality concept, someone can be harmed by being brought into existence with some defect that could have been avoided by taking reasonable precautions. With the normality concept, the event or omission that causes the defect is the cause of harm. The normality concept underlies the belief that women should do everything possible to have healthy, unimpaired babies; that anything less than the maximal effort is blameworthy; and that it is wrong for a woman to take risks with a future person's intelligence or health. To sum up these two concepts of harm:

> *Baseline Concept.* Requires a starting point (baseline) from which an adverse change is plotted; that is, it requires an existing being who is made worse off.
>
> *Normality Concept.* Requires a norm of development that is not met, for example, because of a woman's actions or omissions while carrying a fetus.

In *wrongful life* cases in the courts, it is claimed that the lives of some children are so miserable that their very existence is a tort. In *wrongful birth* cases, the claim is not that the child's life is totally miserable but simply that the child has been damaged by being born less than normal. Wrongful birth suits appeal to the normality concept. The courts have rejected wrongful life suits by assuming the baseline concept; that is, they have assumed that preventing a birth or killing a baby cannot possibly be a benefit, even to prevent or end a life of total harm.

These two concepts of harm can be applied to IVF. According to the baseline concept, a person created by IVF cannot thereby be harmed because otherwise that person wouldn't have existed. According to the normality concept, IVF could harm a baby if it caused some defect or deficiency that a normal baby would not have had.

UPDATE

Patrick Steptoe died at age 74 in 1988, just a week before he was to have been knighted at Buckingham Place by Queen Elizabeth II. The same week, Robert Edwards became a Fellow of the Royal Society, one of the greatest awards of the English scientific community. As noted, Edwards received the Lasker Award in 2002 for medical achievement.

Edwards today champions greater public support for assisted reproduction and urges England and America to follow the example of Australia, Germany, and France, which support cycles of in vitro fertilization. He also believes, predictably, that children will be safely created one day by cloning and that such origination poses no deep moral problems.

Louise Brown's mother chose to have a second child, Natalie, by IVF in 1982. In 1993, the three female Browns appeared on American television shows to support ART research. At age 15, Louise was a quite chubby girl whose friends teased, "How did you ever fit into a test tube?"

On July 25, 1998, Louise celebrated her twentieth birthday in London at the House of Commons, along with other adults created through IVF. Louise today works in a day care center in Bristol and enjoys going to pubs, playing darts, and swimming. Although she understands the media's interest in her, she now says she just wants to fade into the background and enjoy the life of any 20ish woman at the local pub.

DEVELOPMENTS IN ASSISTED REPRODUCTION

Numbers of Children Created and Rates of Success

Through the use of assisted reproduction, many babies have been born in the United States. The first IVF baby, Elizabeth Carr, was born in America on December 28, 1981. According to the CDC and ASRM websites, between 1981 and 2002, over 50,000 babies were born through AR techniques in America. (Figures lag because it takes 9 months from conception to produce a baby, because some conceptions take place in late December, and because the CDC audits the self-reports of ART clinics to verify numbers, so figures for, say, 1999, don't come out until 2001.)

Less than 50 percent of babies conceived by ART are a result of IVF. Most babies are created by less dramatic techniques such as egg stimulation and insemination of sperm.

In the United Kingdom, one industry source says 50,000 babies have been created by assisted reproduction.[24] In Germany, France, and Australia, where national medical services pay physicians for ART, probably another 100,000 babies have been born. Adding ART births from Scandinavia, Mediterranean countries, and others, the worldwide total may approach a million babies.

Unfortunately, in most of the 1990s and still today, about 80 percent of couples who tried IVF, and who spent at least $10,000 and up to $100,000, go home without a baby. In 2002, fertility clinics claim that about 23 percent of attempts at IVF allowed couples to take home baby, although the actual figures may be more like 20 percent.[25] Chances worsen for women over 40, and drop with each unsuccessful attempt, from 13 percent on the first to 4 percent on the fourth.[26]

Egg Transfer

Australia's Carl Woods created the first human pregnancy from an egg transfer in 1983. In the same decade, scientists began gamete intrafallopian transfer (GIFT), which unites sperm and egg not in a Petri dish but inside a fallopian tube, approximately where normal conception takes place.

By the 1990s, egg retrieval no longer required surgery; it could be done by tubal aspiration using ultrasound imaging. Researchers now try to insert embryos not in the uterus but in one of the fallopian tubes. In the 15 years between Carl Woods's first egg transfer in 1983 and 1998, about six thousand middle-aged women gave birth using eggs from young women.[27]

Previously, it was thought that the age of the sperm or the age of the gestational mother was the key cause of infertility. However, it turns out that, although these two factors contribute to infertility, they can be overcome. The real absolute barrier to successful conception and implantation appears to be the age of the egg, with rapid drop-offs of eggs of women over age 40.

Older men are luckier than older women. A Belgian group in 1993 succeeded in using a single sperm to fertilize an egg, a process called "intracytoplasmic sperm injection" (ICSI) making it possible for the sperm of older men to be used.[28] However, women over 40 can still gestate embryos created from eggs of other, younger women, giving the gestational mother a biological connection to the child.

About 10 percent of IVF attempts today use eggs of younger women. This is therapeutic for women who have many genetic diseases in their families, who have eggs damaged by chemotherapy or poisoning, who have had several miscarriages, or who suffer from premature menopause.

Young eggs in older surrogates make a big difference. Using egg transfer, the success rate for taking a baby home was higher, about 30 percent, and more important, *it was 30 percent regardless of the age of the female gestator,* making egg donation the hope of last resort for many infertile couples. These discoveries explain why fertility doctors need the eggs of young women.

Freezing Embryos

In October 1997, the first birth occurred using previously frozen human eggs; the child was born at an Atlanta AR clinic run by Dr. Bruce Tucker.[29] Four months later, the world first heard about a birth from a frozen human embryo. In 1990, two

embryos were created from different eggs at a California clinic.[30] One was implanted and became a baby; the other remained frozen. Seven-and-a-half years
later, the second embryo was implanted and became a male fraternal twin to his
7-year-old brother. Researchers said it was nothing out of the ordinary. While the
California story was being discussed, the Pennsylvania Hospital in Philadelphia
said a baby had been born there the previous December who had grown from an
embryo frozen for nearly 8 years. (They had not called a press conference because
they regarded it as no big deal.)

In 2002, a California clinic began to freeze eggs of young women about to undergo hysterectomy but who wanted to later become pregnant.[31] Whether these
eggs will be viable after thawing is questionable.

As with freezing and thawing of sperm for insemination, freezing and thawing of embryos screens embryos because those incapable of successful implantation do not survive this process. Normal, sexual reproduction also screens embryos because 40 to 60 percent of embryos fail to implant, in part because half are
chromosomally (genetically) abnormal.

When embryos and sperm are stored and frozen, mishaps may occur. In the
1990s, a white Dutch couple had nonidentical twins, one of which was black
(the black couple who created the embryo decided to adopt the baby). In 2002,
a white couple in London had black twins because the wrong embryos had been
implanted.

On the criminal side, IVF pioneer Cecil Jacobsen, who practiced in the Virginia
suburbs of Washington, D.C., was sent to jail for mixing his own sperm to create
embryos for implantation in dozens of cases. In southern California, Ricardo Asch
was charged with using embryos of other couples to increase rates of success in his
ART clinic and, when charges were filed against him, fled to South America.

ETHICAL ISSUES ABOUT COMMERCIALIZATION

Over the last two decades, much attention has focused on whether payment for egg
transfer or surrogacy is wrong. Sensationalistic stories decry ads offering $50,000
for a tall, healthy woman with SAT scores above 1450. Yet such stories rarely provide any historical context for the new development, nor do they compare the new
wrinkle with traditional practices. To counter these problems, this section gives
some history of innovation and commercial reproductive services and then compares payment for eggs and surrogates to payment for sperm and adoption.

Historical Background: Paying for IVF

For reasons that will be explained in the next chapter, during the 1970s the United
States instituted a ban on federal funds for experimentation on embryos. Since
90 percent of experimentation in the United States is federally funded, this ban
effectively stopped most American research on assisted reproduction.

What this meant for the commercialization was that if ART was going to flourish in America, it would have to be in private clinics that accepted no federal funds.
Furthermore, since few states required insurance companies to cover ART, clinics
had to subsidize any research they did from fees paid in cash by private clients.

At the time, critics doubted that couples would actually pay much for such services, especially if their chances of achieving a baby were not high. The last two decades have proved such critics wrong, with perhaps a million American couples paying for some form of assistance in ART clinics.

An unintended but foreseeable by-product of the federal funding ban on human embryo research in such clinics, with the resulting reliance on funds generated from their paying patients, is that research in these clinics is not regulated by the NIH or IRBs. In other words, new forms of ART can be attempted without going through the cumbersome process of NIH or FDA approval.

Surprisingly, this process has created one of the fastest-growing and most controversial areas of medicine with some stupendous breakthroughs, fueled in part by competition between ART clinics for success in creating babies, as well as some new ethical issues.

Historical Background: Transferring Sperm

The history of helping infertile couples by artificially inseminating sperm of a husband (AIH) is instructive. Around 1850, physician J. Marion Sims, while practicing in Montgomery, Alabama, artificially inseminated 55 infertile wives with sperm of their husbands.[32] He produced one pregnancy (but it later miscarried). He was forced to stop because of strident condemnation of his work.

Later in the 1890s in America, Dr. Robert Latou Dickinson was vilified for practicing AIH, although he persevered. Dickinson was accused of abetting "adultery."[33] Indeed, it took nearly a hundred years after Sims's first inseminations for people to accept artificial insemination of donor sperm (AID). That is not very progressive. Had Sims *paid* his first sperm donors, his critics would have been legion.

The net result? Hundreds, maybe thousands, of couples in America and Europe remained infertile, blaming each other for being barren, going childless not by choice but by fate, and not having heirs. Thus, thousands of kids who might have been born today might have had hundreds of thousands of descendants.

At the end of the twentieth century, insemination of sperm has mostly been accepted. Indeed, Americans have gone from accepting (1) injection of a husband's sperm into the wife's womb, to (2) injection of another man's sperm into a wife's womb, to (3) paying a man for use of his sperm to create a pregnancy, and finally (4) injection of anonymous donor sperm (AID) into unmarried women who wish to become pregnant. Today, couples and single women can select sperm from men at about four hundred sperm banks, where donors receive between $50 and $75 per visit.

Notice that the media's radar screen has scarcely noted that men have been paid to donate sperm for decades, even though, genetically, sperm do not differ as gametes from eggs (in other words, sperm and egg do not differ in their genetic contribution to the child). Once sperm goes outside the womb, many ethical issues arise, but do the issues differ just because women recently have been involved and are also paid for their gametes?

Looking back, people in the past were scared because insemination of sperm sundered creation of children from the sex act, and they feared that such creations would generalize too rapidly, harm the children created, and harm the family by creating children of unknown genetic fathers. None of these fears came true because sex was too much fun and because babies are created (perhaps too!) easily by sex. Danger never existed that sperm transfer would create even 1 percent of a country's births.

Payment for Adoption

Because roughly one out of twelve couples in North America are infertile after 2 years of trying to conceive, and because in vitro fertilization only works for eighty couples out of a hundred, demand is great for healthy, adoptable babies. Furthermore, because most couples in North America are white and want a child of the same ethnic background, the demand for healthy, white babies has skyrocketed.

Such demand led many adoption agencies to charge substantial fees for their services, and the average couple in 2002 seeking to adopt a baby pays agencies nearly $20,000. Some couples pay over $100,000 in their desperate quest to find a healthy toddler.

Like transfer of eggs or organs, agencies do not technically sell babies, which is illegal. But a new industry has sprung up that first connects couples to pregnant women and, second, that recruits women who might carry their fetuses and later put their babies up for adoption. According to one investigative journalist, "That has left only the thinnest line between buying a child and buying adoption services that lead to a child."[34] The doubling of licensed child placement has jumped adoptions in North America in the last few years to nearly 2,000.

Some agencies spend half a million dollars a year just on advertising. Their fees vary according to where the baby comes from and its color: $20,000 or more for a healthy, white baby, $22,000 for a Vietnamese baby, $17,000 for a Chinese baby, and $8,000 or less for a black baby.[35] Agencies that specialize in "closed adoptions" (where the mother never knows the adopting couple) of white babies charge over $100,000 for a successful adoption. Louisiana allows agencies to fly in out-of-state pregnant women and house them during pregnancies, and allows large payments to facilitating agencies (and, some charge, surreptitious payments to the young women).

In 1993, Russia had no foreign adoptions, but in 1997, it placed more children in America than any other country. Many adoptions also come from Romania, the Balkans, Vietnam, and China.

Although black critics have recently decried the differential payments that seem to demean black babies, virtually no one has condemned payment itself. Similarly, virtually no one has criticized "pregnancy counseling centers" that encourage pregnant girls not to abort and to give up their babies for adoption, while charging lucrative fees to couples who adopt the babies.

Paid Surrogacy: The Baby M Case and its Aftermath

Fertilization of embryos outside the womb made it possible for another woman to gestate that embryo to birth, creating so-called "surrogate mothers," either for pay or altruistically.

Several hundred women had helped infertile women create babies when in 1986 biochemist Bill Stern and pediatrician Elizabeth Stern hired Mary Beth Whitehead for $10,000 to bear a child created by his sperm and Whitehead's egg through artificial insemination. At birth on March 27, 1986, in Monmouth County Medical Center in Long Branch, New Jersey, Mrs. Whitehead "bonded" with the Baby M, also known as Melissa Stern, and refused to give her to the Sterns. When Mr. Stern threatened legal action, Mrs. Whitehead fled to Florida with the baby, but was discovered and returned to New Jersey.

At the lower court trial in 1987, Judge Harvey Sorkow upheld the legality of the contract, said it did not constitute baby selling, required Whitehead to hand over the baby, awarded Whitehead $10,000, and decided it would be best for the baby never to see Mrs. Whitehead again. On appeal in 1998, the New Jersey Supreme Court unanimously reversed his decision, declared Mrs. Whitehead the legal mother with full visiting rights, and invalidated surrogacy contracts.

Mrs. Whitehead became a well-known critic of surrogacy and was supported by feminists who believed not only in bonding, but also that women were naturally superior to men in nurturing children. Such feminists are sometimes called *social feminists*. For their part, traditional or *merit feminists* sided with Elizabeth Stern and thought that women should be held accountable for contracts they signed. Ironically, merit feminists saw social feminists as sexist.

Six states (Michigan, New York, Washington, Utah, Arizona, and New Mexico) reacted to the Baby M case by criminalizing commercial surrogacy. Arkansas, Florida, Ohio, Virginia, Nevada, New Hampshire, and California legally recognized paid surrogacy. In many states, laws about surrogacy either do not exist, are based on one particular case, or are even contradictory.

Controversial cases make news; successful cases do not. Jaycee Buzzanca, "the child with 5 parents," was born in March 1995 from a paid surrogate and became embroiled in a divorce between the parents who hired the surrogate. Jaycee was conceived from sperm and egg other than from the parents who hired the surrogate. A California Appeals court ruled in 1998 that the parents who had hired the surrogate were legally responsible for him.

Because laws in most states are unclear or nonexistent, problems sometimes arise, not only of enforcing contracts, but also about the name on the birth certificate. In a 2001 case of paid surrogacy, the Cullitons in Massachusetts successfully sued to have their name on the birth certificate (the surrogate supported their suit).

In England, Claire Austin agreed to be inseminated and bore two female twins for a couple living in France, but the couple wanted her to abort because they wanted a male child. The surrogate refused, flew to California, and the girls were adopted in 2001 by a lesbian couple living there. Also in England in 2000, a woman rendered infertile sued not only for monetary damages for her distress but also for money to hire a surrogate. The court awarded the former but not the latter.

Compensating Egg Donors

Because so many women in North America are childless, and because eggs of young women increase chances of successful in vitro fertilization with a husband's sperm, it has become necessary to pay young women for transfer of their eggs.

Originally, volunteers supplied eggs, but altruism doesn't come close to meeting the demand. The whole practice is called "egg donation," and donors receive variable amounts of money. In 1993, the American Society for Reproductive Medicine (ASRM) suggested a flat fee of $2,500, but payment has long since gone beyond that figure.

Women get paid more than men because egg retrieval is more complicated than obtaining sperm. A woman takes drugs daily for a month or more to induce superovulation, after which eggs are aspirated with a long thin needle inserted through the vagina into an ovary and guided by ultrasound imaging. According to one such woman, each time an egg is sucked from an ovary, "it feels like someone kicked you there."[36] Some people claim that the drugs increase risk of some cancers over the life of the woman, but a 1999 study seems to have disproved this claim.[37]

Europeans find the argument against sales compelling. Mark Sauer, a leading American researcher in AR, relates, "While attending the World Congress [in 1996] of in-vitro fertilization in Vienna, I was impressed by the almost universal criticism leveled at practitioners in the U.S.A. by colleagues abroad with respect to the payment of [egg} donors. Allegations of "pimping" for patients in need of eggs seemed a rather cruel accusation, . . . "[38] Yvon Englert, a Belgian researcher was convinced that "U.S. ooycte donors come from the middle and poor classes of American society" (false, most are solidly middle class) and that with payment, "the risks for both donors and receivers not to observe sanitary norms are much higher, oocyte donors being interested in hiding possible health problems."[39] Yet European researchers at this Congress lamented the lack of egg donors in their countries.

What really ticked off critics was not only payment per se but payment that advertised for specific qualities in women. Indeed some well-publicized advertisements (*ads,* not cases!) put critics into froth and created media frenzy reminiscent of the birth of Louise Brown.

In the winter of 1998, a New Jersey AR clinic advertised that it would pay young women $5,000 for a month's worth of eggs. This was double the approved rate of $2,500. A year later, an ad ran in a newspaper at Princeton University and at other Ivy League universities, stating that an anonymous couple was offering $50,000 for a "woman over 6 feet tall and with SAT scores over 1450 who was willing to sell her eggs."[40] The conjunction of the amount of the money, the targeted campuses, and the desire for two specific qualities made the ad a subject of national news. A spate of articles appeared across the country in venues such as the *New York Times* to the *Bioethics Examiner of the University of Minnesota Center for Bioethics* to *Boston Magazine* and *The New Yorker.*

Every one presented the information to the public in condemnatory, sensationalistic terms leaving the impression that paid assisted reproduction was an out-of-control juggernaut. Typical was the blurb beginning the article in *Boston Magazine:* "Ivy League coeds have been offered as much as $50,000 to "donate" their eggs to infertile women. When one desperate couple bought another woman's eggs, they entered a brave new world of egg harvesting, where biology, technology, and the marketplace collide, raising disturbing questions about breeding for perfection and profit."[41]

ETHICAL ISSUES INVOLVING PAYMENT FOR ASSISTED REPRODUCTION

One of the pressing ethical issues is whether the market should govern the transfer of human sperm, eggs, surrogacy, and adoptable babies. If so, how much should the government regulate in order to protect prospective parents and resulting children?

Is Commercialization Itself Wrong?

Some critics believe that egg transfer should only be done for altruistic, noncommercial reasons. Such critics see the phrase *egg donor* as masking the essential nature of the transaction, which is the sale of a human egg. In efforts to be consistent, they may even agree that purchasing and transfer of sperm should be illegal, and of course, most such critics would ban commercial surrogacy.

These critics believe that such sales are wrong in two different kinds of ways: intrinsically wrong and indirectly wrong. The first charge may appeal to religious or Kantian premises about the inherent value of humans being incompatible with being priced in the market. It may also look at the larger structure of society and claim that some relationships between people should not be subjected to the tyranny of money. The other kind of objection is that commercialization is not in itself wrong but is wrong indirectly because of the bad consequences it inevitably creates. This is an empirical claim, capable of verification or falsification by social scientists. One kind of bad consequence is the slippery slope, where critics say that commercialization of sperm, eggs, and gestation will spread to other areas, such as selling of organs or sexual favors in prostitution.

Defenders of payment retort that the wrong assumption here is the simplistic, either-or categorization. Indeed, perhaps the really exploitive argument is to say that only good, unpaid, altruistic women should be allowed to be surrogates—what is often called the *compassion trap*. This is the false first step of casting all surrogates as either whores or Madonnas: a woman must either be a bad surrogate and earn money, or be a good surrogate and earn no money. The compassion trap also insidiously implies that women who bear children for others in return for money aren't compassionate, just greedy.

Defenders of payment also ask whether enough young women will go through egg donation for altruistic reasons? Voluntary donation has failed to deliver enough blood for operations and has never become adequate to meet the need for transplantable organs. Ditto bone marrow for dying leukemia patients.

The major problem here is that if you don't permit monetary compensation, you don't get young eggs and hence you don't get wanted babies. Second, if you compromise to permit compensation but don't permit a market, many problems also arise. Finally, if payment for ART is intrinsically wrong, why isn't payment for adoption? If payment for ART is not for babies but for "services," why isn't the same also true of adoption?

Payment as Exploitative and Coercive

In April 1998, the New York State Task Force on Life and Law issued a *Report on Assisted Reproductive Technologies* and attempted to set a standard fee.[42] The approach they adopted in suggesting a set fee mirrors the dangers of central planning in planned, socialist countries such as Cuba and China. The fee is supposed to reimburse donors for their time and effort, not their eggs. Since the time and pain for egg donation should be roughly the same, the Commissioners reasoned, it should be easy to set a standard fee for all donors. In this way, they hoped to avoid the bidding up of eggs from women with desirable traits.

In practice, however, this regulatory solution leaves everyone attempting to do what bureaucrats in planned countries have never been able to do: understand all the complexities of human beings and set a fixed price in advance of what a given service should sell for. The Commissioners were forced into this box because they didn't want the fee to be set so low as to be exploitative of poor women nor so high as to be coercive of the same. They are thus in the business of gazing into crystal balls and second-guessing the inner springs that move women to do reproductive work. They are also mistakenly judging that the same fee will be exploitative or coercive for all women—an obvious falsehood. In this regard, the complicated reasons women have for engaging in such new reproductive work need more careful examination.

Market advocates say we don't want to regulate the price of something that, in truth, only a real market can correctly gauge. Whether it is worth $10,000 or $30,000 to a woman be a nanny, surrogate mother, or assembly-line worker will depend on dozens of factors about each women—factors that will change from year to year even for a particular woman. Only a variable payment will accurately reflect variable mixes of such factors.

Advocates also argue that experience has shown that, because of the travails involved and if they are not paid, too few people will emerge to offer the human tissue or services necessary to create or sustain human life. If one accepts the premise that creating wanted human life is a primary good, and one believes that choice about such lives should be up to humans, then society should allow payment for such services.

Sometimes objections about exploitation masquerade as objections to commercialization. The mask is lifted when one asks, "Well, then, just how much would an egg donor (sperm donor, surrogate, potential adopting mother) have to be paid for it *not* to be exploitation?" If the interlocutor cannot come with any sum, the true objection surfaces.

The Catch-22 faced by the New York State Task Force in trying to navigate these waters in regulating payment for eggs can be illustrated another way about surrogacy. Suppose someone suggests that paying a surrogate a million dollars would surely disqualify an arrangement from being categorized as exploitative. But people then object, "That is such a vast amount of money that it distorts the arrangement. People shouldn't be tempted so greatly to commercialize something private and personal." In this case, the proponent of commercialization can't win at any amount—be it low or high!

Sometimes these objections also imply that men are exploiting surrogates. Certainly from reading interviews with paid surrogates, nothing could be further from the truth.[43] Paid surrogacy seems to mainly empower the women who do it, making them special and contributing real money to the family's income. A surprisingly large number do it *despite objections from husbands,* or must battle husbands who want to keep the baby. Anthropology Researcher Helen Ragone discovered no case of a woman being a surrogate *and* being exploited by a man.

Does payment for assisted reproduction lead to exploitation of the poor by the rich? Advocates of payment say this tired argument shouldn't be used to pick on surrogacy or egg donation. Is this a service that rich people can buy that poor people can't? It ignores that some middle-class people will value a particular service so much that they will forgo normal middle-class desires and thus buy a service that "only rich people" can afford.

Exploitation is about not having any choices. Paid surrogacy, egg donation, and gestation-to-adoption expands the definition of what society values about women. To defenders of payment, this does not sound like exploitation of women.

Good of the Child

Critics of payment argue correctly that we can't just look at the issues from the viewpoints of childless couples because children have rights, too. Indeed, too many stories about assisted reproduction focus on would-be parents and very few focus on the good of the child.

Some critics today claim that to be created by sperm from an anonymous male donor harms the resulting child. Advocates for such practices retort that it's difficult to see how babies can be harmed by being created this way, because they never otherwise would have existed (baseline concept), they are healthy as ordinary babies, and they are very much wanted by the previously infertile family. Defenders of assisted reproduction retort that some life is better than none. A child can't be "harmed" by being brought into an existence it otherwise would have lacked. Sometimes such defenders retreat by asserting that, as long as the adult doesn't later want to kill himself, or the baby's life is not one of total pain ("wrongful life"), it's better off existing than not.

However, we must tread carefully here, because "good of the child" is a loaded, ambiguous phrase. The usual assumption made by conservative critics of assisted reproduction is that the ideal way to be born is to be a child of married, heterosexual parents who carefully plan the pregnancy. Any deviation from this idea, say, by introducing a third party as a sperm or egg donor, or surrogate, is held to harm the resulting child.

Both views of harming children contain problems. According to the first, most of the children born on the planet are "harmed" in their conceptions because their birth isn't planned or their parents aren't married. If the only moral way to produce a child is the ideal way, *most conceptions are immoral.* (Indeed, until the eighteenth century, people with money mainly married to secure property rights and a third of children were born bastards.[44]) On the other hand, the second view implies that a child can be very less-than-normal (e.g., suffer from fetal-maternal alcohol syndrome) and not be harmed because otherwise he wouldn't have existed. This also seems far-fetched, especially if the parents or society could have exercised precautions to make the child normal.

Previously in this chapter, the normality conception of harm was distinguished from the baseline. To this we now add a new definition of harm: less than ideal conception. And in truth, it is possible to argue that some children are harmed by nonideal conception. On the other hand, because most children are not created under ideal conditions, this conception implies that most children are harmed in being created. That seems like a reductio ad absurdum conclusion.

Perhaps the solution is to define *harm* neither as a departure from the ideal nor as avoiding the worst outcome ("any life is better than no life") but as a departure from the average. A child born from assisted reproduction would then only be harmed if he is less healthy than the average child born of traditional coitus (remembering that about 1–2 percent of such traditionally conceived children have some kind of defect).

This normality conception of harm implies that most children conceived from anonymous sperm donors, egg transfers, or carried by surrogates are *un*harmed by their unique origins. So if we use the best-interests-of-the-child criterion, almost all births from assisted reproduction are morally permissible.

Another common objection to paid surrogacy is that it's wrong because it's not best for the child. This objection holds that it's wrong to deliberately bring a child into the world where the rearing mother does not do the gestational work. Paying for gestation is inherently wrong because having a confused identity with at least three, and maybe five, parents harms a child.

As time passes, I think we will come to see this objection as the same as saying that it's wrong for a woman to have a child whom she doesn't rear herself and instead uses day care, public schools, and baby-sitters. In past centuries in wealthy families, children had nannies and au pair girls who did much of the real work of day-to-day child raising. Long ago, we handed over home schooling to professional teachers. Whether such arrangements are best for the child largely depend on the details of the case and the motives of the parties. Properly done, such arrangements need not be bad for the child, whether it be a method of reproduction or a method of rearing a child.

Harm by Not Knowing One's Biological Parents?

A major question raised with assisted reproduction is whether children created by AID, anonymous egg donation, or gestated by surrogates can be harmed by not knowing the characteristics of their genetic ancestors and being debarred from ever having a relationship with such ancestors. One compromise nicely solves this problem.

The reasonable solution is to allow gametic donors or surrogates to be *confidential* but not *anonymous*. In this practice, names and identities of donors are kept from children created from gametes of men and women, but these men and women are allowed (or encouraged) to update their files every 5 to 10 years so that their biological children can know about genetic diseases and their lives. This practice protects the desire of some donors and some surrogates not to have contact with children created from their gametes, while also giving them the chance to change their minds.

Surprisingly, many sperm and egg donors, or surrogates, do not mind maintaining such records and express a desire to know about the lives of such children.[45] It is mainly the parents who adopt the donated sperm, egg, embryo, or child who object to children knowing such donors.[46] Thus, making such knowledge optional would not seem to discourage people in the future from donating sperm and egg, or from being surrogates, and would allow children later to find out who else created them and why.

Harm to the Family?

Many of the criticisms against new forms of assisted reproduction, or of paying for reproductive assistance, assume that the ideal nuclear family is the one pictured in old television comedies such as *Leave It to Beaver* or *The Donna Reed Show.* Although students know that such perfect families rarely exist today, most falsely believe that something like these nuclear families actually did exist in the past. They think that only recently did the nuclear family decline, due to working mothers, high rates of divorce, feminism, or lack of religious schooling.

In her masterful surveys of American family life over the last centuries, historian Stephanie Coontz contradicts these widespread beliefs. In *The Way We Never Were,* she writes,

> . . . the middle-class Victorian family depended for its existence on the multiplication of other families who were too poor and powerless to retreat into their own little oases and who therefore had to provision the oases of others. . . . For every nineteenth-century middle-class family that protected its wife and child within the family circle, then, there was an Irish or a German girl scrubbing the floors in that middle-class home, a Welsh boy mining coal to keep the home-baked goodies warm, a black girl doing the family laundry, a black mother and child picking cotton to be made into clothes for the family, and a Jewish or an Italian daughter in a sweatshop making "ladies" dresses or artificial flowers for the family to purchase.[47]

So the family pictured on *Leave It to Beaver* did not exist for most Americans at most times in history.

Professor Coontz also relates a study where researchers tracked kids to adolescence and predicted which kids would be happy, which unhappy, based on their childhoods and parenting. The researchers were wrong two-thirds of the time, worse than if they had guessed randomly. They vastly overestimated the trauma resulting from the typical stresses of childhood, while they underestimated the lack of maturity that resulted from having a protected, stress-free adolescence.

Today, it is really a strict taboo to acknowledge any evidence that goes against the prevailing wisdom about the family and child development. In 1999 "family values" conservatives attacked psychological studies showing that sexual abuse of adolescents and children is not universally damaging and that some adults emerge unscathed.[48] Similar studies in 1999 showed that most children do fine in homes without live-in fathers. Rather than being seen as good news about the resilience of children, or the effectiveness of therapy, conservatives attacked messengers, vowing to revoke any federal funding of such psychological studies.

Little real empirical research exists about what forms of child raising harm children, in part because we cannot experiment on children or put them in controlled studies. This point is important to keep in mind when conservatives claim that new forms of child creation harm children. Being raised on a kibbutz, in day care, or being gestated by a surrogate, may not be harmful at all. Speculation about harm to teenagers when they discover that their conception or gestation differed slightly from traditional conceptions is likely just that, speculation.

Only Perfect Babies?

At some AR clinics, researchers store extra eggs for later use with infertile couples. Pictures of the women from whom the eggs were taken are available to be shown to prospective parents, and indeed, private egg brokers may arrange a meeting between prospective buyers and sellers.[49]

Some critics argue that allowing any selection by prospective parents is wrong, and that such parents should be forced to accept the first available embryo, or that embryos should be randomly assigned. This argument was also once used against use of in vitro fertilization, where critics said all adoptable babies should be placed before new reproductive techniques are allowed.

Such restrictions would likely be unacceptable to many prospective couples, however, because most want to maintain the semblance of an ordinary pregnancy and childhood, which means that they select an embryo from parents who will be racially and ethnically as close to them as possible. (And people who want a child of their own may not be willing or able to adopt a special-needs baby or baby of a different race.) Also, many infertile foreign couples come to American physicians for AR either because their own countries do not offer such services or because there are few suitable egg and sperm donors in their own countries. As such, they are only interested in a very specific kind of donor, e.g., Japanese American for prospective Japanese parents.

It is true, however, that in a small number of AR clinics in America, couples may select already-existing embryos at a cost ($2,750) much less than what it would cost ($16,000) to create an embryo from people selected in advance. Those embryos are created when one couple changes its mind after contracting for an egg donor. When that happens, the young woman has already taken fertility drugs for a month and her ovaries are full of ripe eggs, so the clinics remove the eggs and fertilize them with a variety of different sperm, keeping records of each embryo created. Couples may then select an embryo from this woman's eggs (seeing a picture and description of her) that was fertilized by sperm from a man whose picture they see and whose life they read about.

Will such choice lead to desires for only perfect babies? This is a large question, one that we will discuss later in the chapter on genetics. But we note here that many people believe that it is permissible to use such techniques to let infertile couples choose *against* diseases that embryos might carry. Sensationalistic stories imply that allowing preimplantation (genetic) diagnosis (PID) will lead to a society that encourages eugenics. Is this fear and that of desires for only perfect babies realistic?

One reason to think it is not realistic is the fact that the cost of screening for a single disease can be as much as $20,000, which most insurance companies will not pay.[50] Thus, the idea that a couple will screen out hundreds of embryos and only implant the perfect one is ridiculous because few couples have the millions of dollars to pay for such batches of tests.

What worries critics is that if couples already want to try to influence traits of their future babies, and if there is market for sperm and egg sellers, then couples will select traits in ways the critics don't like. That is, they will select traits of men and women that the purchasing couple deems desirable. As one such critic put it in discussing a market for egg donors, "this approach is harmful not only because it serves to reinforce social prejudice but also because it fragments women as persons by commodifying their characteristics, which seems at least as harmful as commodifying their eggs."[51]

The view's implications for denial of personal choice are staggering. The dangers to personal reproductive liberty come from both choice-restricting liberals and social conservatives, and we certainly see that here.

Such critics never think of themselves as prejudiced (and hence, don't want their own range of choice restricted) but always worry about the prejudiced choices of other people. Second, what is the alternative to allowing choice? A set product? Only choice within a certain range? To do so would be like requiring people only to buy cars rated highly by *Consumer Reports.*

Moreover, the same critics who decry selection of traits in embryos always ignore adoption. Why is selection by ethnicity or race bad in one case but permissible in the other? Why is both selection by ethnicity and race plus large payment permissible for adoption but not for eggs or embryos or surrogates?

Finally, the critic forgets that there is a whole range of choice in life where people make selections based on what they value in others: in fraternities and sororities, in country clubs, in hiring and firing, in dating, in choosing a person to marry and have children with, in making friends, in deciding where to live, and in choosing whom to hire. Many of these choices reinforce social prejudice, but the government does not ban them.

Comparing Payments for Kinds of Reproductive Assistance

American society now permits payment for adoption, sperm donation, surrogacy, and egg transfer. Europeans regard such practices as rampant American commercialism. England bans most of them.

At the very least, we should have a consistent policy of payment for services leading to creation of human life. If payment is banned for egg donation, it should be banned to facilitate adoption. If payment is allowed to a pregnant woman to support her gestation for later adoption, similar payment should be allowed when a couple contracts with a woman for gestation.

Multiple Births

The number of multiple births worldwide has soared as a result of implantation of multiple embryos through IVF, and as a result of the introduction of Clomid and Pergonal, drugs that produce superovulation.

The multiple pregnancies that frequently result from assisted reproduction have created ethical issues as well. In a multiple pregnancy, nutrients and oxygenated blood in the womb become a scarce resource; and to prevent disabilities resulting from deprivation in utero, physicians recommend "selective reduction" of all but one or two embryos. In 1985, a Mormon couple, Patti and Sam Frustaci, conceived septuplets but refused to have such a reduction performed. Four of their seven babies died, and the three survivors had severe disabilities, including cerebral palsy. The Frustacis sued.[52]

Multiple birth babies are often premature (they may weigh less than two pounds), are three times as likely as single babies to be severely handicapped at birth, six times as likely to have cerebral palsy (which may not show up for a year or more), and may have to spend many months in neonatal intensive-care units (NICUs). Nevertheless, in France—where pregnancy is sometimes pursued with an almost religious zeal, and where each new baby means a bonus from the government,—the number of triplets has increased tenfold since 1982 and the number of quadruplets has increased thirtyfold.

In 1996 in England, and after taking the fertility drugs Merton and Pregnyl for two days, Mandy Allwood released seven eggs (unknown to her) before she had sex with her lover. All of them conceived. Four months later, she was offered a large cash bonus by London tabloid for exclusive rights if all made it to term. So Mandy announced she would not reduce any and would go for maximal births. As a result, she lost all seven. In 1997, Denise Amen and her husband were offered the chance to reduce five growing embryos but refused. One of their quintuplets was born blind and others are "developmentally slow."[53]

Ten years before in 1987, Ron and Roz Helms of Peoria, Illinois, had quintuplets with the help of a fertility drug Pergonal, after taking Clomid to no effect for 5 years. Warned that Pergonal might produce multiple births, they went ahead. One child spent a year in a NICU, another had seizures, and a third has mild cerebral palsy. Medical bills for the quints were nearly $3 million for their first decade.

In 1997, an Iowa couple, Bobbi and Kenny McCaughey, used Pergonal to conceive seven embryos, refused to reduce (abort) any, chose to risk having one or more severely disabled babies, and said that any results were "God's Will."

The appeal to God and the role of human choice in multiple pregnancies has become a national controversy. To say "it's up to God" how many babies come about is misleading since humans took drugs to artificially stimulate release of many eggs, something that wouldn't have happened naturally. (Another problem with attributing too much to God is seen in the case of a Pentecostal woman named Jane Simeone who prayed that all her triplets would survive like the McCaughey's but who felt like a failure in God's eyes when two of her babies immediately died.)

Couples who very desperately want to conceive often pray intensely for pregnancy and consider any reduction to be a violation of that prayer. Even though they are often given a choice of how many embryos to implant, they often maxi-mize the number implanted to maximize chances of any success, taking multiples as a bonus. They do not perceive such a choice to be choosing to risk having a dis-abled child in order to maximize their own chances of having any child. (It appears that the McCaugheys were not given a choice by their two physicians, i.e., after seven eggs released, they were not told, "Since you don't believe in reduction, it might be better to wait until next month when so many eggs aren't released.")

Critics of the decision by the McCaugheys said that if God was clear about any-thing in this case, it was that the McCaugheys were not intended to have kids. They also said that if a couple takes a fertility drug, and it results in too many conceived eggs, they should be willing to reduce the embryos for the good of the children born. In other words, a couple shouldn't run the risk of severely disabled kids and say it's "God's will" if it happens.

New York City's Major Guiliani was on a call-in radio show in late 1997 when an Orthodox Jewish woman with five little babies (three of them identical triplets) said she felt like killing herself because her multiple babies were driving her crazy. Although the Mayor quickly got her help (he was running for reelection!), what about all the other parents who don't get such help? At the time of the McCaughey case, Jacqueline Thompson, a black mother of sextuplets, and her husband Linden were living exhausted in Washington, D.C., without help or support, until the McCaughey case came along and officials felt embarrassed by Thompson's lack of help.

After the above cases, the media in 1998 followed a black couple named Chukwu in Texas who had octuplets (one died at birth) at a cost of $2 million, while largely ignoring a white couple in the same state giving birth to septuplets and, later, a black Alabama couple in 2002 with septuplets (after the McCaughey seven and the Chukwu eight, six didn't create much media interest). In Mexico City, a woman thought to be carrying seven fetuses delivered only six babies, and up north in San Diego, a woman old enough to be a grandmother at 55 gave birth to quadruplets.

Going back, the year 1996 set a record for births of multiples with 6,000 babies born in groups of three, four, or more, a 20 percent jump from the previous year. Why did that happen then?

For most couples without reimbursement for in vitro fertilization, the easiest way to overcome infertility was to first take the drug Clomid; if that didn't work, they could turn to Pergonal or Metrodin to stimulate the ovaries to release many eggs at the same time. The problem is that introduction of sperm can create one, two, or even eight embryos. In vitro fertilization in contrast allows physicians to control how many embryos are introduced.

At their fourth birthday in 2001, the McCaughey septuplets lagged in devel-opment behind normal children (true for all preemies) and were not all potty trained.[54] Joel has suffered seizures, for which he is on medication. Nathan has a form of cerebral palsy called spastic diplegia that requires botox injections (to par-alyze spastic muscles) and orthopedic braces. Alexis has a different form of cere-bral palsy, hypotonic quadriplegia, which results in weak muscles. Alexis also has had trouble walking and learning to talk. In addition, for 4 years she has had an indwelling feeding tube. Another child, Natalie, also has required a feeding tube during these years. Although Bobbi and Kenny McCaughey are home schoolers, the task of home schooling Nathan and Alexis, who are developmentally delayed, was too great, and the two children attend a public school for such children.

After spending a year on the road on a self-reported "lucrative" speaking tour, requests for talks fell off, so Kenny stayed at home for a few months, helping Bobbi with the kids. But then he grew restless and wanted a job outside the home. Explaining why he wanted to leave, he said that, "It goes back to biblical times, you know, when the man went out, did hunting; they did their things to supply the bread for the family." So he took a job on an assembly line producing metal parts.

Today, fertility doctors realize that chances of damaged children vary almost directly with the number of embryos allowed to gestate. In other words, if six are implanted, one is almost certain to be born with cerebral palsy or blind.

By 2002, the American Society for Reproductive Medicine (ASRM) had *not* reached a consensus on how many embryos to implant to reduce the risk of creating damaged children. The probability of an impaired baby varies directly with the number of embryos implanted. Unfortunately, the chance of having any baby at all also varies directly with the number of embryos implanted (hence, the ethical dilemma of how many embryos *should* be implanted). The ASRM suggests implanting no more than two embryos for women with good prognoses, no more than three for women with above-average prognoses, and "no more than five good-quality embryos" for women with below-average prognoses.[55]

ART physicians may be torn between wanting to achieve high rates of pregnancy per number of couples attempting pregnancy versus low rates of multiple births and impaired newborns. Gladys White, a bioethicist specializing in reproductive ethics, suggests clinics may be biased in favor of the first.[56]

ART and Justice

Most couples using IVF pay cash. The average cost of a cycle of IVF is $8,000. Such private payment causes little controversy, and almost no one thinks that government has any right to ban the pursuit of babies by couples using ART. Couples who spend their own money to create families don't excite many zealots.

Indeed, a *Constitutional right* may exist to noninterference by government for couples who use ART. In his comment about *Eisenstadt v. Baird*, Supreme Court Justice Brennan said, "If the right of privacy means anything, it is the right of an individual, married or single, to be free of unwanted government intrusion into matters so fundamentally affecting a person as the decision whether to bear or beget a child."[57]

The New York Commissioners also put themselves in a box by worrying about whether AR services would be equally available to all women. This is like banning women from working on a Mercedes assembly line because they will never be able to afford such a car. Should we also ban work as nannies unless a woman can afford a nanny herself?

As with paid organ donation, there is a frustrating tendency of people to pick on new reproductive options for their egalitarian intuitions. But we always need to ask, not just of new reproductive advances, but also of any new advance in medicine, why should it be made equally available to all? There is a distressing lack of understanding among many people that a medical system can be just without subsidizing equal, maximal benefits to all.

But *subsidized* ART becomes controversial. Most insurance companies cover costs of buying and giving fertility drugs such as Clomid, and many cover surgery to diagnose or repair damaged fallopian tubes. But most states do not require, and hence most insurance companies do not cover, reimbursement for cycles of IVF.

Infertile people claim infertility is a disease, and that IVF procedures should be covered by insurance like any other disease. On September 1, 2001, New Jersey became the fifteenth state to mandate that insurance companies pay for infertility treatments, including IVF.[58]

Insurance companies decried the law, saying that "pregnancy is a lifestyle choice," not a disease, and predicted higher premiums to consumers. The Massachusetts Association of Health Maintenance Organizations estimated that its members pay $40 million more in premiums to cover infertility treatment for two thousand couples. A 1994 study estimated the cost (including occasional premies in NICUs) to be between $67,000 and $800,000, and$114,000 for couples aged 45 and older.[59]

The New Jersey law covers egg retrieval and, after less costly options fail, cycles of IVF. Women under 35 must fail to conceive for 2 years to be eligible, but only 1 year is required for women over 35.

Dorothy Roberts, a law professor at Northwestern University School of Law, sees such laws as requiring blacks to subsidize treatment that may help white couples conceive, while other laws discourage black women from conceiving (especially poor black women on public assistance). Twenty states enacted laws recently denying benefits to mothers if children are conceived while the mother is on public assistance.

So the objection that coverage for IVF is racist amounts to this: first, white people disproportionately use IVF and, second, coverage for IVF reflects distorted priorities about health care funding, which should be redirected toward providing basic care for everyone.

Perhaps the greatest injustice is requiring workers to subsidize ART, even though some such workers will later (when they change jobs) lack even basic coverage. Many people who cannot work are not old enough for coverage by Medicare (which begins at age 65) but not so poor that state Medicaid programs would cover them.

In countries such as France, Germany, and Australia, where national health services finance IVF or at least give free cycles, some critics claim that governments shouldn't fund ART until services for people with disabilities are adequate.

The beginning of this section noted that people pursuing children with ART and paying cash caused little controversy. As the next chapter discusses, that is true so long as parents don't pursue techniques such as cloning.

Older Parents

One of the consequences of using eggs of younger women, and ICSI, is that more older people can create their own children. In 1980, an Australian team led by Carl Woods was criticized (ironically by Steptoe and Edwards!) for accepting a

42-year-old woman as their first IVF candidate because of the increased chances of birth defects. Her baby was born without defects. In 1993, a 59-year-old business-woman in England gave birth to twins gestated by her from eggs, fertilized by her husband's sperm, which had been donated by a woman in her twenties.

Two births in 1997 pushed this debate into public consciousness. In the first, a 63-and-two-thirds-year-old woman named Arceh Keh gave birth to a healthy baby girl in March 1997. The following month, actor Tony Randall, age 77, fathered a healthy baby daughter.

Most AR clinics cut off age limits at 55, and the clinic in Los Angeles believed Mrs. Keh was 55. IVF was used with sperm of her husband, 60 at the birth of the baby, and a donated egg from a younger woman. After birth she breast-fed her baby. The reason for the cutoff was that physicians believed that postmenopausal women did not have a healthy uterus, or hormones, to gestate a baby. They were proved wrong, at least in one case. Physicians also worried that the stress of pregnancy on an older woman's body might harm the woman. In this case, as well as a previous case in 1994 where a 62-year-old Italian woman gave birth using similar methods, no harm to the mothers has been reported.

Of course, the question for public policy was whether society wants to encourage older people to have children when they may be senile or dead when their children are in college.

In 1990, one-third of American AR clinics excluded women over 40. By 1998, the new practice of using eggs of younger women has removed such limits, especially for couples willing to pay the extra money to young women to donate.

THE ETHICS OF GENDER SELECTION

Gender selection has brought about a new problem in countries such as China, the Republic of Korea, and India. For years in these societies, females have often been neglected and seen as inferior to males. The strong preference for a male child leads many families to abort females after determining the sex of a fetus by the use of a sonogram. Thus, high rates of female abortions have led to an extreme shortage of females and a highly unbalanced male to female ratio.

Women are in demand in China, where 20–44-year-old never-married men outnumber their female counterparts 2 to 1, who are often kidnapped and sold into marriage. *Science* magazine predicts that in the year 2020, 1 million "excess" Chinese males will enter the matrimony market.[60] Despite laws that ban sex-determining testing in India and China, at least 60 million females are "missing."[61]

Recently, a new technique called Microsort has been developed to distinguish sperm by gender. The sorting relies on the fact that X chromosomes are heavier than Y chromosomes because they carry more DNA. By using a modified flow cytometer instrument the heavier sperm can be separated from the lighter sperm producing 90 percent accurate results.[62] Although officially intended for use in preimplantation genetic diagnosis, Miscrosort may be used by people in countries such as China and India to select only male babies, thus making gender selection less expensive and more easily available to millions of couples.

BACK TO THE FUTURE: UNSTIMULATED IVF

Louise Brown was born from "unstimulated IVF"; that is, her mother, Lesley, took no drugs to create release of extra eggs.

Because of the risks to children from multiple births, researchers around the world are very interested in unstimulated IVF.[63] Improvements in ultrasound scanning, egg collection, and embryo culture may mean that just one embryo will be enough for a successful conception. If perfected, unstimulated IVF could really improve the experience of IVF for women who attempt IVF.

Unstimulated IVF could provide substantial benefits. Because it avoids the use of drugs, women undergoing treatment are not exposed to the risk of hyperstimulation syndrome. Using just one embryo for transfer also means that the risk of multiple pregnancies is removed. Probably more significantly, unstimulated IVF would cut out the cost of the drugs, thereby reducing the expense of IVF significantly.

Unstimulated IVF also has disadvantages. It won't work for all women, particularly those who aren't ovulating properly. It will also mean that no spare embryos will be available for freezing after the IVF cycle, meaning that patients will need to undergo further cycles, stimulated or unstimulated. Finally, it's not entirely clear that success rates of unstimulated IVF will be as high as those associated with stimulated IVF.

CHAPTER 7

Battles over Embryos and Stem Cells

*T*his chapter discusses issues associated with research on embryos, including cloning embryos for medical research. We shall call this *embryonic cloning* (in the literature, it is also called *therapeutic cloning*). The next chapter focuses on cloning to produce children, or *reproductive cloning*. Since the announcement of the cloning of the sheep Dolly in February 1997, anything to do with reproductive cloning has created controversy, and embryonic cloning has links with both reproductive cloning and abortion.

This chapter also discusses issues about adult stem cells (cells created without creation of human embryos), and the history of controversies about embryos and medical research.

HISTORICAL BACKGROUND: EMBRYO RESEARCH

As discussed, *Roe* v. *Wade* made abortion legal in all states in 1973. This judicial fiat in some ways circumvented democratic consensus and legislation, which in most states had not jelled to permit abortion.

Two years later in 1975, the public became aware of two experiments in 1973 that studied an artificial womb and the effect of deprivation of glucose on the fetal brain by experimenting on twenty live-born, but dying, human fetuses. Maggie Scarf's "The Fetus as Guinea Pig" in the *New York Times Magazine* and Yale theologian Paul Ramsey's *The Ethics of Fetal Research* introduced Americans to these shocking new developments in medical research.[1]

What was shocking was that, almost as soon as abortions were permitted, researchers had *legally* experimented on live-born fetuses. Such research seemed to substantiate fears about slippery slopes.

Three years after *Roe* v. *Wade*, in 1978, "test tube baby" Louise Brown was born, again without consensus and without any approval of an ethics committee or national oversight. As discussed in the last chapter, Steptoe and Edwards did create and destroy human embryos to perfect their techniques, and then as today, creation of babies by IVF had the foreseen but unintended by-product of sacrificing many human embryos.

In 1979 obstetricians Howard and Georgeanna Jones established the first American IVF clinic at Eastern Virginia Medical School (EVMS) and in 1981 achieved the first American baby born via IVF, Elizabeth Carr.

Given such developments, the Catholic Church and conservative Christian groups in North America saw IVF as something alien and suspect, i.e., as a medical technology out of control and at war with nature. Followers of such religions came to think that natural motherhood and natural conception were under attack.

Thus began in America the politics of the embryo, which have intensified over 25 years. In 1977 Congress created the *Ethics Advisory Board* (EAB) to decide which federally funded research on embryos and fetuses might be done. At the time, creation of the EAB was seen as a way for Congress to fund such research without taking any criticisms from antiabortion groups, who had already linked opposition to abortion with opposition to medical research involving human embryos. The EAB eventually concluded that some research on assisted reproduction with embryos was morally permissible, but as we shall see, these recommendations were never enacted. The EAB would never take up the separate issues of what specific research with embryos could be federally funded.

The Rios Case   In 1981 Mario and Elsa Rios, a wealthy American couple, died childless while their IVF-created embryos existed in a frozen limbo. Their story made headlines because neither the Rios nor the infertility clinic had provided for this contingency. Several ethical questions arose. Could the Rios embryos simply be destroyed? If they were implanted in surrogate mothers and carried to term, could the children later sue in American courts for an inheritance from the Rioses? Should the anonymous donor, whose sperm had been used with Elsa's egg, be consulted about his wishes?

An ad hoc committee of the Australian government required that the embryos be preserved until each of them could be adopted. They never were, and over the years, the embryos deteriorated from the effects of freezing, making the issues moot.

The Demise of the EAB   Before the EAB could take up issues about which kinds of research with embryos could be federally funded, the Reagan administration (1981–1989) came to Washington, D.C. Believing that destruction of embryos was linked to destruction of fetuses in abortion, both the pro-life Reagan administration and the subsequent Bush administration (1989–1993) did not renew the EAB's charter, which ended in 1981. Hence, no federally funded research involving human embryos was ever approved.

In other parts of the world, the English and Australian governments allowed public monies to fund medical research using embryos up to day 14 of the embryo's life. As a result, Australian infertility companies began to license breakthroughs to American physicians.

The Davis Case   In 1990 Mary Sue Davis and Junior Davis of Tennessee divorced and fought for custody of seven embryos frozen in their IVF clinic. Both had remarried and after her remarriage, Mary Sue Davis wanted the embryos to donate them to another infertile couple. In 1992 the Tennessee Supreme Court decided that Junior did not have to become a father against his will, and after that, a lower Tennessee court later ruled that Junior could destroy the embryos, which he did.[2]

The False Cloning Alarm   In 1993 people became alarmed when researcher Jerry L. Hall "cloned" human embryos in a laboratory. What he had really done was to twin an existing human embryo.

Twinning human embryos had several advantages for medical research. First, it produces more embryos for infertile couples who, for various reasons, have difficulty producing enough for their cycles of IVF. Second, twinning is useful in the diagnosis of genetic disease by the method of testing one cell of an eight-cell embryo. If many tests needed to be done, having many embryos is beneficial. Emphasizing the distinction between a born baby and a 14-day-old mass of cells (an embryo), the least harmed babies are created by permitting genetic testing on twinned human embryos.

The Human Embryo Research Panel, January of 1994   In June 1993, with a more sympathetic Clinton administration (1993–2001), Congress revoked the regulations requiring EAB approval of embryo research. The Clinton administration also soon allowed federal funds for research in experiments using tissue derived from aborted fetuses.

Skeptical about its new freedom because of the growing clout of antiabortion politicians in Congress, the NIH formed a new oversight committee in 1994, the Human Embryo Research Panel. This Panel consisted of four bioethicists, two lawyers, seven scientists, and six members of various other backgrounds.

The Panel was asked to divide possible research with human embryos into three categories: acceptable for federal funding, unacceptable, and warranting further review. When the Panel found itself forced to hold its meetings in public, it was surprised to find itself targeted by antiabortionists.[3] Members of the Panel received in the mail graphic pictures of decapitated, mature fetuses. During the hearings, passionate antiabortionists created a hostile environment, seeking control and a platform.

Under these circumstances, the Panel concluded that federal funding of research with embryos would improve the success and safety of procedures to reduce infertility, and that the present situation, where such federal funding was prohibited, would lower the quality and ethical oversight of such research. More important, such research could help physicians understand how pediatric and adult cancers developed. The Panel also concluded that parthenogenesis, where an egg is stimulated to begin dividing without fertilization, might offer insights into ovarian cancers.

Embryos created specifically for research are called *research embryos*. Embryos left over after IVF are customarily called *spare embryos*. The Panel rejected the compromise that research could proceed on spare embryos so long as new embryos were not created to be destroyed by medical research. Why? It said that embryos available from couples attempting IVF have higher rates of genetic abnormalities, so basic research needed original, healthy embryos from young couples.

The Panel also rejected as too controversial what Jerry Hall had done, the *twinning of human embryos* before implantation, as well as cross-species fertilization.

Despite the expectations of the Panel's members, who thought themselves politically savvy and hence thought that their recommendations would be accepted by Congress, their recommendations were rejected in 1995 because legislation about partial-birth abortions unexpectedly preoccupied Congress. After that, most Congressmen did not want to push legalization of research allowing destruction of human embryos.

The Dickey-Warner Amendment (1996)   Indeed, in January 1996, conservative Congressmen successfully added a clause to NIH's appropriations bill stating that, "None of the funds made available in this act may be used for . . . research in which a human embryo or embryos are destroyed, discarded, or knowingly subjected to risk of injury or death greater than allowed for research on fetuses in utero."

NIH now saw the writing on the wall. Previously, it had tried to get around the federal ban on embryo experimentation by interpreting some medical research as not putting embryos at risk, such as genetic screening of embryos for hereditary disease. But what about the embryos not implanted after such screening? That was a flash point.

The Hughes Incident (1997)   The Dickey-Warner Amendment nixed the research of geneticist Mark Hughes. Hughes had made *Science* magazine's list of scientific breakthroughs for 1992, being cited for his work in genetics on human embryos. He had pioneered a technique for taking DNA out of a single cell of a human embryo and testing that DNA for cystic fibrosis (CF). Taking one cell from an eight-cell embryo with undifferentiated cells does not do any damage to the embryo, but such testing does mean that embryos with CF will be destroyed and not implanted.

Although the ban on federal funds had stayed in effect, research on embryos to prevent genetic defects was possible with private funds, such as from Planned Parenthood. In 1997 Hughes had both private funds to pursue embryonic screening and much larger federal funds to pursue other genetic research not involving embryos. Yet Hughes lost all his federal funding for his other work because federal funds had paid for a small refrigerator (used to store embryos) in his private lab.

Dolly Is Announced (1997)   On February 24, 1997, every newspaper in the world carried huge headlines proclaiming that a lamb named Dolly had been created by cloning, a technique previously thought to be impossible and known only by the scary scenarios of science fiction. Almost everyone speculated that humans would be next and also condemned the possibility. (The next chapter discusses such reproductive cloning in great detail.) Dolly's birth by cloning also galvanized interest in embryos, especially embryos created asexually through cloning or thereafter twinned.

Immortalized Human Stem Cell Lines Created (1998)   In late 1998, John Gearhart of Johns Hopkins University and James Thomson of the University of Wisconsin discovered how to create immortalized stem cell lines. Gearhart had started with tissue from aborted fetuses; Thomson had dissected human leftovers left over after assisted reproduction (spare embryos).

What are stem cells and why are they important? Stem cells are marvelous, primordial cells that have the potential to develop into any kind of differentiated cellular tissue: bone, muscle, nerve, and so forth. In theory, they could be grown into replacements for almost any part of the human body. Found in embryos and the umbilical, stem cells also exist in our body to help us grow new cells when we are injured. If we are hurt and lose blood, stem cells are activated to make new blood. If these primordial cells can be controlled by scientists, in theory they could be directed to form new bones, neural cells, cardiac tissue, and, thus, to cure many diseases.

The remarkable achievement of Gearhart and Thomson was to discover how to create a biological factory for continually producing stem cells, rather than tediously deriving minute amounts from embryos and fetuses.

But they did so using private funds. Now a larger issue loomed: given that the National Institutes of Health and its funding mechanism was the world's treasure of scientific talent, should such a treasure be allowed to work with this new discovery?

ACT Uses Cow Eggs to Grow Human Embryos   On November 12, 1998, Advanced Cell Technology of Massachusetts announced it had made differentiated human cells revert to a primordial, pluripotent state by fusing them with cow eggs. That is, they made human stem cells out of normal human cells in the "Petri dish" of a cow's egg. Although the cow's egg, from which the nucleus was removed, was just the medium for the nucleus of the human cell, the procedure worried critics who sounded alarms about human/cow hybrids. President Clinton and NBAC immediately condemned any attempts to create children out of such hybrids (although no one was suggesting such a thing might be tried).

NBAC Backs Research on Embryonic Stem Cells   Although it had condemned reproductive cloning in 1998, The National Bioethics Commission (NBAC) concluded that the government should fund research on stem cells created from human embryos. That recommendation never was accepted by the more conservative Congress.

Adult Stem Cells Discovered   Physicians already knew that the body has stem cells that are needed to grow new kinds of cells, but they had no easy way to grow such cells until Thomson and Gearhart did so from human embryos. In the summer of 2001, scientists discovered stem cells not only in bone marrow but throughout the human body. Over the next year, a series of reports gave researchers hope of creating biological factories (cloned cell lines) to grow stem cells without initially sacrificing human embryos. Two years later in 2003, the ease of growing so-called "adult stem cells" was still being debated, as was the issue of whether they were as valuable in medicine as embryonic stem cells.

President Bush's First Press Conference   On August 11, 2001, President George W. Bush announced his policy on federally funded research on embryos. He rejected use of such funds to create embryos for research, but said he would allow such funds for research on 60 stem cell lines created from spare embryos. The announcement occurred on television in prime time, signaling a new national emphasis on bioethics.

A year after this press conference, the actual number of sources of stem cells appeared to be quite small, less than a dozen, and scientists questioned whether the policy was really working to get scientists the biological material they needed.

SHOULD EMBRYOS BE USED IN MEDICAL RESEARCH? FOR AND AGAINST

Arguments for and against use of embryos in medical research have been passionately made for several years now. The remainder of this chapter explores those arguments.

Valuable from Conception

For Church Father Thomas Aquinas in the thirteenth century, ensoulment was said to occur at 60 and 90 days for male and female fetuses. Later, in 1869, Pius IX eliminated the phrase *ensouled fetus* in announcing that abortion of the entity at any stage resulted in excommunication.[4] Since then, Catholic teaching has emphasized the value of human life "from the moment of conception." So it was no surprise that in 1982, Pope John Paul II said to a group of scientists,

> I condemn, in the most explicit and formal way, experimental manipulations of the human embryo, since the human being, from conception to death, cannot be exploited for any purpose whatsoever.[5]

Potential for Personhood

Many scientists say that, before 14 days, the human embryo has no human form and cannot experience pain. Why then give it value? One reply is that, despite the fact that some zygotes become pathological tissue and despite the fact that some zygotes twin, the embryo is what Jesuit Richard McCormick calls "powerfully on its way" to development as a person. Even though it may later twin or even become diseased tissue (and hence, not implant), it is seen by conservative believers as a member of the human family.

Why is that? As McCormick writes about the human embryo:

> . . . it remains [as having] potential for personhood and as such deserves profound respect. This is *a fortiori* weighty for the believer who sees the human person as a member of God's family and the temple of the spirit. Interference with such a potential future cannot be a light undertaking.

Slippery Slope

In addition to asserting the intrinsic value of the embryo, McCormick worries about what will happen if human embryos are regarded as mere commodities for research. (In this passage, "preembryo" refers to the embryo before implantation on the uterine wall.)

> If we concluded that preembryos need not be treated as persons, would we little by little extend this to embryos? Would we gradually trivialize the reasons justifying

preembryo manipulation? . . . Furthermore, there is uncertainty about the effect of preembryo manipulation on personal and societal attitudes toward nascent human life in general. Will there be further erosion of our respect? I say "further" because of the widespread acceptance and practice of abortion.[6]

Here we have a new kind of slippery slope argument. It is not that experimentation on embryos would be the first step down an unstoppable slippery slope. Rather, McCormick claims, we are already way down the slope with legalized abortion and shouldn't take any extra steps to make the top of the slope more slippery. Like all arguments about the slippery slope, McCormick assumes agreement about what counts as a bad result, in this case, legalized abortion.

Reductio ad Absurdum

Many commentators, however, think that treating the embryo as valuable because it is a potential person can be refuted by a *reductio ad absurdum*: a line of reasoning, i.e., one which shows that some logical implication of an idea is absurd and thus casts doubt on the idea itself. In this instance, consider that if a woman starts procreating (as is often possible) before her teens and continues throughout her fertile years, she may easily produce a dozen or more children. If each potential person is valuable, then we ought to actualize the greatest possible number of potential persons; but given the consequences of overpopulation, this conclusion hardly makes sense. Also, there is clearly a philosophical difficulty in claiming a right to life for a frozen embryo when no particular woman has a duty to gestate it.

If embryos are persons, it also follows that all the following are killing persons: creating embryos for in vitro fertilization, for freezing for later use, for preimplantation genetic diagnosis, or for medical research. Similarly, intrauterine devices (IUDs) that prevent implantation of embryos kill persons; it is also true for them that dislodging an implanted embryo by dilation of the cervix and curettage or by scraping of the uterine lining (D and C) is killing a person or murder. Clearly all these claims are silly and false. Clearly, then, the premise that generated these claims is false, and that premise is that human embryos are persons or "almost persons" and cannot be destroyed.

Just Tissue

A human embryo is not a person but only human tissue. A human embryo has no more moral status than a pint of human blood or a severed appendix. What gives the human embryo value is a decision by a woman to let it use her body for nine months in gestation, and if this occurs, the embryo can be gestated, be born, and become a baby with moral value. But embryos themselves have no more value than acorns or any other kind of seed.

The Interest View

New York (Albany) philosopher Bonnie Steinbock argues that value is created when something has an interest. Generally speaking, a necessary condition of having an interest is being able to desire something. One of the most basic desires is to avoid pain. We don't think vegetables feel pain, so we don't think they have desires. We do think cats and dogs feel pain, so we think they have an interest in avoiding pain.

The law makes a great deal of interests, conflicts among them, and how to resolve conflicts of interest. As such, the concept of interest covers a lot of intellectual territory.

As for embryos, it is commonly accepted that before the emergence of the primitive streak at 14 days, there is no possibility of any neural development such that any being could be "there" to feel pain. The human embryo at this stage is still more like a blackberry than a tadpole.

As such, Professor Steinbock argues, the embryo has no interests and has no cares or desires about what happens to it. So, Steinbock argues, it does not matter whether an embryo fails to implant in the uterine wall, whether it is dislodged by an intrauterine device (IUD), or whether it is used in research. It only begins to matter when neurons form to create *sentience,* the ability to feel pain.

Potential Value Is Not Value

Although embryos have the potential under ideal conditions to become persons, such potential in itself confers no moral value. The goods in a lumber store have the potential to build a dozen houses, but when the store burns down, we do not say that a dozen houses were destroyed, nor do insurance companies reimburse for that larger amount.

Let us put this point a different way. As mentioned, fertilization during superovulation results in the availability of more than one fertilized egg, or embryo. Not all are usually implanted, so what is the ethical status of the remaining embryo when they are frozen for future use? In North America alone, about two thousand spare embryos exist at any one time in frozen nitrogen. If all these embryos were destroyed tomorrow, it is not like a mass murder of two thousand people occurred. Indeed, does it make any difference to the reader whether two thousand or twenty thousand embryos exist now or were destroyed? What difference to anyone the reader knows would it make, either way?

Finally, a Roman Catholic physician, M.V. Viola, wrote in 1968:

> A significant number of fertilized ova (some estimate one in three) never implant in the uterus under normal conditions. If in fact these are lost souls, the Church should be consistent and make efforts to administer baptism to them.[7]

But no one is going to baptize embryos that fail to implant because, among other reasons, no one really believes them to be persons or even "deserving of respect."

Potential Value Is Symbolic

Ah yes, perhaps that's true, but that raises just the problem at hand, namely, our growing insensitivity to death and the destruction of human lives. Exactly the same argument could be made about death from a mass killing in a country on the other side of the globe and one might ask similarly, "Indeed, does it make any difference to the reader whether two thousand or twenty thousand people exist now or were destroyed? What difference to anyone the reader knows would it make, either way?"

But is this the moral ideal we want to hold up to our children? To move toward? Isn't the opposite better, where we strive to make each human life valuable? Even if we usually miss that ideal, isn't positing it better than succumbing to the opposite view, that no one matters except those within a mile of me?

Potentiality and Cloning

The strongest argument of opponents of embryo research is the potential of the human embryo, given the right conditions, to become a person. But they have forgotten one thing: what cloning shows is that any cell of the body can become a person. The nucleus of any differentiated cell can be put into an enucleated human egg, a spark applied, and (with luck) a new embryo formed that is a near-copy of the genetic ancestor.

The revolutionary aspect of cloning is that it makes not just embryos special because of their potential for personhood but *any human cell* whatsoever. Maybe that's why opponents of embryo research so vigorously attack all forms of human cloning, because they know that it is the death blow to the argument-from-potential to protect embryos.

Embryos Must Be Treated with Respect

Bioethicist David Ozar argues that although an embryo may not be a person, neither is it just a pebble or tissue.[8] Embryos are not simply the property of an owner; they deserve respect in view of their potential as persons. What does *respect* mean? Well, for one thing, they should not be eaten, nor should they be put in tiny bottles and used as earrings. Gene Outka claims that respecting embryos also means that they could not be substituted for the eyes of rabbits in testing cosmetics.

Another way to put this point is to emphasize that a large amount of bodily products, such as bone, cartilage, blood, and tissue can be legally sold from cadavers. Large firms specialize in such sales and broker them to research institutions and medical schools. Respecting embryos would include banning them from being bought and sold this way.

Respect Is Compatible with Research on Embryos

It is possible to be a good scientist and treat valuable sensitive material with respect in medical research. One might make an analogy with animal experimentation. We must harm animals to test new forms of heart surgery or new kinds of lenses for human eyes. But in using animals for our benefit this way, this does not mean that we should not minimize their pain, psychological terror, or in any way make fun of them.

In the same way, researchers who have the privilege of using human embryos could be taught, required, and legally enjoined to treat them with the greatest respect. To make another analogy: physicians and medical students should treat the newly dead with respect, and not practice intubation or spinal taps or surgery on such neomorts without the family's permission, for to do so is to offer no respect to the life just expired or those who loved the patient. In the same way, one could argue that human embryos should be treated carefully in view of the persons that— under different circumstances—they could have become.

What's So Special about an Embryo?

Princeton bioethicist Peter Singer asks us to imagine a sperm and an egg on two sides of an IVF slide. Case 1: Just before the joining of sperm and egg, the couple change their minds, so sperm and egg are washed down the drain. Case 2: Same as case 1, but the couple change their minds one minute after the sperm and egg have been joined. Again, the material is washed down the drain. Case 3: Same as case 1, but the technicians discover that the drain is blocked; the sperm and egg may thus have united in the drain, and if not retrieved immediately, the resulting embryo will die of exposure. Singer argues that these three cases do not differ morally, and that none of these embryos has a right to life.

The Semantics of the Embryo?

As mentioned in the last chapter, conception takes place when a sperm fertilizes an egg, usually in a fallopian tube. In human embryology, a successful union of sperm and egg may be called a *zygote,* a preembryo, or an embryo. After conception, this entity immediately begins dividing: It first divides into two cells, which then divide to form four cells, which then divide to form eight cells, and so on.

During the 1980s, pro-choice theologians and bioethicists referred to this organism as a preembryo, reserving "embryo" for when it attached to the uterine wall. This was a semantic attempt to divest the embryo of any moral value. In the same way, "therapeutic cloning" is an attempt to put a pro-research twist on this kind of cloning, emphasizing benevolent intentions (although most researchers regret ever publicizing the word *cloning* as applied to creation of cell lines).

In the 1990s, antiabortion speakers took the opposite tact, speaking of the "embryo/fetus" or even "embryo/baby," deliberately running together the ends of a long spectrum of gestation. Another expression used is "embryo/child."

The Indeterminacy Argument

Although Father McCormick does not assert that human embryos are persons, he thinks we should treat them as if they were persons because we are unsure when personhood begins. To use his analogy, if the hunter is not sure whether what is in the bushes is a deer or a human, he should not shoot into the bushes.

By the same token at the other end of life, if we are unsure whether a patient will emerge from a coma, shouldn't we wait as long as possible before declaring that person dead? Isn't that the minimum we owe one human being?

A more subtle objection emphasizes the indeterminacy of the boundaries of sentience. Well-publicized stories have taught us that patients can hear and perceive when under sedation for surgery. Other patients have been declared dead and then awakened, recalling jokes made in their presence and procedures done on them (an important argument for not allowing medical students to train on the newly dead). Similarly, we are not sure exactly when the embryo develops sentience. Perhaps the most rudimentary form is like phototropism when a plant bends towards light. Even so, when any doubt exists, we should be cautious, and in couples with a general principle of respect for embryos, such caution entails not subjecting any such being to any unnecessary medical research.

What Is an Embryo?

As a result of scare tactics, some opponents of embryo research conceive of the embryo as a very tiny baby, one small enough to fit inside a test tube. Aristotle incorrectly thought that such a tiny sperm was transmitted in the sex act via ejaculation to the womb, where human embryogenesis merely consisted of a tiny human stretching out and growing.

In medieval philosophy, the seat of the soul was conceptualized as being occupied by a *homunculus*, a tiny person. It is likely that some opponents of embryo research conceive of the embryo as just such a homunculus, rather than more correctly as a small blackberry. If so, they agree with Steinbock's view that embryos only count morally when they can perceive pain because they think of the human embryo, like Aristotle, as a tiny baby from conception. For them, it would be wrong to subject such a tiny baby to painful procedures in medical research.

More substantially, just when does an entity become an embryo? If no medical research or contraception is to be allowed after the entity becomes an embryo, then the point of demarcation is very important. Traditionally, some groups have claimed such status from the moment of conception, but biologically just when is that moment?

The following passage from Ronald Green illustrates this problem:

> Some believe that the embryo exists at the moment that the sperm comes into contact with the egg. At that time, they reson, two separate sex cells cease to be and the embryo (or zygote) begins to develop. But what does "contact" mean here? It has recently been found that the egg emits chemical signals that serve to attract sperm when the sperm are still relatively far off in the uterus and even before they have entered the fallopian tubes. Do these "chemoattractant" signals amount to "contact"?
>
> A better candidate for the fertilization "event," and, hence, the "beginning" of the embryo, might be the penetration of the egg's tough outer membrane (zona pellucida) by the sperm. This triggers a host of chemical changes that cause the sperm to undergo what is known as the "acrosome reaction." At this time the genetic package carried in the sperm's head separates from the remainder of the cell body and passes through the zona into the egg's cytoplasm. This sets off a cascade of electrochemical reactions that are now being closely studied by reproductive biologists. Within seconds, signals pass to the zona that normally render it impenetrable by other sperm. If we think of fertilization as the beginning of a unique individual, the acrosome reaction might be a good candidate event, because from this time onward the product of conception usually results from only one sperm and one egg. But things are not quite that simple. Sometimes more than one sperm penetrates the egg, which results in polyploidy, an excess number of chromosomes in the zygote. Although this condition usually prevents further development or results in stillbirth, sometimes the embryo is able to correct the problem by ejecting

the excess chromosomes. This highlights the fact that the new diploid genome remains unstable for a considerable period of time after sperm penetration of the egg. Should we perhaps say that fertilization has occurred only after all these possibilities have been eliminated?

Or should we stipulate that fertilization occurs at an even later time? Once inside the egg, the remaining parts of the sperm trigger further events. The egg itself now completes sexual division. It extrudes half of its forty-six chromosomes to form a "polar body," a small sphere adjacent to the egg proper. The egg's remaining twenty-three chromosomes migrate to the cell's center, where, eighteen to twenty-six hours later, they line up with the twenty-three chromosomes from the sperm. This is syngamy, literally, the "spouses joining together." In biological terms, if we think of a new individual as coming into being with the appearance of a cell having a new "diploid" genome, a full complement of forty-six chromosomes, syngamy would seem to be a good candidate for a starting point. This is the moment that the "zygote" is said to come into being. Some legal jurisdictions that ban embryo research and that must therefore define when the embryo comes into being have chosen syngamy as the defining event.

However, there are some problems with viewing syngamy as decisive. Biologists usually describe the cells of an organism as having the full range of cellular structures, including a single cell nucleus that contains DNA within its own nuclear membrane. But at syngamy the zygote has no definitive nuclear membrane. Up to this point, the genetic material is contained in the two "pronuclei" of the male and female gametes that have begun to break down and blend together. A distinctive diploid cell nucleus does not make its appearance until the two-cell stage, after the zygote undergoes its first cell division, which may occur anywhere from twenty-four to thirty-six hours after sperm penetration. Is the zygote, then, not the start of the embryo? Must we await the appearance of a two-cell entity following the first cleavage division?

Further complicating matters is the fact that the twenty-three paternal chromosomes apparently do no work at all during the first few cell divisions. In human beings, the earliest developmental process, at least until the eight cell stage, seems to be entirely governed by egg cell structures and the maternal chromosomes. This is why a parthenote (or parthenogenote), an egg that has never been fertilized but that has been stimulated electrically or chemically, can be made to cleave for several divisions. During the earliest phase of its development, when only maternal chromosomes are active, the parthenote looks and behaves exactly like an embryo, although in humans its growth inevitably stops at the four- or eight-cell stage, when the presence of paternal genetic material is needed for further development. In human beings, a working set of forty-six chromosomes is necessary for new human cells to exist, but such chromosomes do not appear until the four- or eight-cell stage of development. Thus, we haver a number of equally compelling candidate events for the start of an embryo, events spread out over a period of perhaps twenty-four to forty-eight hours. This indicates how misleading it is to speak of "the moment of fertilization." Instead, as one recent embryology textbook puts it, "fertilization is a series of processes rather than a single event."[9]

The Opportunity Cost of Missed Research

We are accustomed to hearing a lot of hype about new medical advances, and such exaggeration makes us falsely believe that medical advance is relentless, proceeding on many fronts. This is more public relations than fact.

Few really major breakthroughs occur in medical research in any one decade. The creation of immortalized stem cells from human embryonic and fetal tissue was one such breakthrough. To not allow this line of research to be aggressively pursed would be a major tragedy.

Nor is it enough to let private companies or other countries do the research. America's National Institutes of Health (NIH) are the crown jewel of the world's scientific treasure, and it would be a tragedy if such a resource could not pursue this new avenue of investigation. Moreover, by having NIH federally funded studies, one insures the highest level of peer-reviewed, objective research—the kind that is most beneficial in the long run to patients.

Therefore, banning use of embryos in federally funded NIH research deprives millions of people of new medicines that, without this research, might not be discovered for another hundred years. That would be sad for the patients who need these new medicines.

Not "Just Tissue," *My* Tissue!

One of the well-known problems of transplants of foreign organs, blood, and tissue into a patient's body is rejection of the foreign material when recognized by the immune system. Drugs that suppress the immune system to allow acceptance of foreign tissue may cause cancer after decades of use. So ideally, it would be much better to grow bone, blood, organs, or particular masses of cells from one's own body for that body's future use.

That is where creating embryos from the reader's own cells could be used to grow tissue for the reader's future medical needs. By using donor eggs (perhaps even cow eggs, as ACT did), embryos could be created by somatic cell nuclear transfer (embryonic cloning) that were nearly identical, genetic copies of the reader's basic genetic structure (or *genome*).

Libertarians argue vehemently here that what an individual does with his or her body should be up to him or her. A federal ban on storing "self-made" medicine from one's own embryos seems to make Big Government too intrusive into personal liberty. At its most extreme, it seems to make all citizens potentially live less (by denying them new medicines) to value embryos.

Embryo Politics as an Issue of Religious Power

As Dartmouth bioethicist Ronald Green observes, the politics of embryo research have become a litmus test of the power of the religious right over American medical research.[10] One may question why this is so, and why they did not choose to focus on starvation or housing or medical coverage for the poor.

One may also question whether they really respect the beliefs of others when they try to impose their religious beliefs on national policy about medical research. After all, it is one thing to say that "I refuse to participate in, or benefit from, research performed on embryos," but it is quite another to say, "No one should do so."

The involvement of such groups in bioethics raises interesting questions about separation of church and state in North America. This is especially complicated when such groups do not reveal their religious premises in public debate.

CONCLUDING COMMENT: THE POLITICS OF EMBRYOS, THE POLITICS OF BIOETHICS

A member of the 1994 Embryo Panel, University of Wisconsin law professor Alta Charo, once remarked that, at least in the case of human embryos, "logical arguments are only rationalizations for gut feelings or religious viewpoints."[11] She decided then that, for government commissions, "I don't think we can make good suggestions unless we understand what is compelling for the public." It is likely that her view influenced her later colleagues on NBAC, on which she also served.

One thing is for sure: bioethics has entered the national political agenda, and in particular, the bioethics of medical research on embryos and material derived from them. Whether or not this is good or bad for bioethics, only the future will reveal.

FURTHER READING

Ronald M. Green, *The Human Embryo Research Debates: Bioethics in the Vortex of Controversy,* Oxford University Press, New York, 2001. The best overall source; includes history of the debates in public policy in America, the work of various commissions, and scientific background.

S. Holland, et al., *The Human Embryonic Stem Cell Debate,* Bradford/MIT Press, Cambridge, Mass. 2001.

In 1991, the *Kennedy Institute of Ethics Journal* had exchanges between Jesuit Richard McCormick and secular law professor John Robertson on the moral status of embryos in research. See Volume 1. In 2001 and 2002, Volumes 11 and 12 had several articles on the same topic.

CHAPTER 8

Reproductive Cloning

Should We Clone Humans?

O n February 24, 1997, the Rosalind Institute near Edinburgh, Scotland, announced that 7 months before it had brought to birth a lamb named Dolly originated by cloning, a feat previously thought impossible (the Institute had waited 7 months to make the announcement until authorities approved its applications for patents on various cloning processes).

Alarmists predicted that these cloning techniques might be applied to humans because a mammal is a mammal is a mammal. Such predictions resonated against a background of 50 years of scary tales about human cloning in science fiction, television shows such as "The X Files," medical thrillers, and novels of fantasy and horror. No wonder that 97 percent of people polled had an immediate reaction of "yuk" to human cloning.

Since that day in 1997, cloning has not gone away. Indeed, cloning humans became the biggest issue in bioethics in decades, so much so that religious conservatives constantly talked against it and any linkage with it doomed other issues such as stem cells from cloned embryos. President George W. Bush's first prime-time television address to the nation in the summer of 2001 indirectly concerned reproductive cloning, which he declared to be absolutely wrong, echoing the sentiments of a vast majority of both ordinary Americans and American bioethicists.

A 2003 group, a UFO sect called the Raelians, claimed they had cloned human babies, but produced no babies, no scientists, and no evidence for their claim. Nevertheless, and perhaps there was no other news for about a week around the world, the story received daily coverage. The story was a hoax.

And yet another side of the story existed. Some of the things most people believed about human cloning were false. Second, because human cloning was linked by opponents to abortion and cloning of embryos, the topic became politicized and hence, facts about it became politicized. Scientists and drug companies wanted to exploit the new techniques to make better drugs and livestock, and were more than eager to let human cloning be made into a federal crime if it would leave them free to pursue their own ends, even if the new crime had little Constitutional basis and was founded on misperceptions.

On March 4, just a few days after the announcement of Dolly, President Clinton asked a little-known commission to make recommendations in 90 days about whether human cloning should be a federal offense. This National Bioethics Advisory Commission (NBAC) recommended making creation of a human by cloning into a federal crime, presumably with jail sentences to enforce it. In so doing, it went well beyond the previous ban on federal funding of research on embryos and proposed a vast new area of federal intrusion into the reproductive life of couples seeking services in what had hitherto been a hands-off area of private infertility clinics.

A year after the announcement of Dolly's birth, rough-hewn Chicago physicist and sometime fertility researcher Dick Seed (whose name was no Hollywood caricature) announced in 1998 that he wanted to clone his genes and produce a child, creating a universal sense of repugnance. His announcement revved up politicians into a heat of anticloning speeches and introductions of countless state bills to ban cloning.

THE SCIENCE OF CLONING

While attending a scientific meeting in Ireland, Ian Wilmut of Scotland's Rosalin Institute heard colleagues describe how Danish scientist Steen Willadsen, working at Grenada Genetics in Texas, had created a lamb clone by enucleating an egg's nucleus (i.e., removing the nucleus from the egg) and fusing what was left with the nucleus of a cell from the genetic ancestor of the sheep they wanted to re-create.

What Ian Wilmut later did with an adult lamb was to create the lamb Dolly from differentiated, specialized cells of her adult ancestor, a feat previously thought to violate a law of nature.

In his first three attempts, another researcher, Steed Willadsen, had actually succeeded in producing a live lamb, and in other (unpublished) work had done far better, having cloned cells from embryos that had 120 cells, in contrast to the usual 8-celled embryo.[1] In other words, the 120-cell embryo had already started to create differentiated cells, so Willadsen's results created new, undifferentiated embryos from these cells and were the base upon which Wilmut worked.

When Wilmut heard rumors of Willadsen's work, it was enough to draw him into similar work for the next decade. The rest of the world went in a different direction, pursuing basic research in the new field of molecular biology rather than (what was thought to be) outdated embryology.[2]

To understand Wilmut's achievement and what it means for human reproduction, it is also important to understand some background. *Cloning* is an ambiguous term, even in science; it may refer to molecular cloning, cellular cloning, embryo twinning, and somatic cell nuclear transfer (SCNT). Only the latter is what occurred in Dolly and the latter is what most people care about regarding human cloning. In molecular cloning, strings of DNA-containing genes are duplicated in a host bacterium. In cellular cloning, copies of a cell are made, resulting in what is called a *cell line*, a very repeatable procedure where identical copies of the original cell can be grown indefinitely. In embryo twinning, an embryo that has already been formed sexually is split into two identical halves. Theoretically, this process could continue indefinitely, but in practice, only a limited number of embryos can be twinned and retwinned.

Finally, there is the process of taking the nucleus of an adult cell and implanting it in an egg cell where the nucleus has been removed. A variant of this process called *fusion* (which was actually done to produce Dolly) is to put the donor cells next to an enucleated egg and fuse the two with a tiny electric current. A blastocyst (aka *blastomere*), an embryo of about a hundred cells or less, starts to develop because the pulse that produces fusion also activates egg development. In fusion, mitochondria from both the donor and the egg recipient mix, whereas in strict transfer of a nucleus, mitochondria are only present in the enucleated egg.[3]

At a 1997 conference on mammalian cloning, Wilmut stressed that present techniques were inefficient: he started with 277 sheep eggs and got only one live lamb. Nevertheless, his statement has been widely misunderstood, partly because he has emphasized how many eggs he started with and not how many fetuses resulted in live births. The actual statistics were: 277 eggs fused in oviducts with sperm, 247 recovered from oviducts, only 29 of which were transferred at the stage of morula or blastocysts, which created 13 pregnancies in lambs, three of which came to birth, and one of which was healthy and lived, Dolly.[4]

Myths about Cloning

Cloning Does Not Reproduce an Existing Person   Reproductive cloning recreates the genes of the ancestor, not the ancestor himself. That is, cloning recreates the genetic base of a person, some of which is genetic, but other parts of which stem from nongenetic sources, such as environmental input into the body (e.g., kind of food and drugs ingested), subjective experiences (forming peak experiences and character), and personal decisions based on free will. None of the latter would be re-created by reproductive cloning.

As such, many of the portrayals of reproductive cloning in movies convey falsehoods. A child with the genes of an ancestor would not have any memories of the ancestor, as does the character Ripley in the movie *Alien Resurrection.*

This also means that you can't reproduce yourself. Narcissistic people, who think cloning a baby with their genes will do so, are mistaken. Cloning reproduces about 99.8 percent of the ancestor's genes (the other .2 percent come from mitochondrial genes in the host egg), but even such a small percentage of different genes as .2 percent can be significant. Identical twins have small differences in random inactivation of the X chromosome and, as such, differ in personality and traits as adults.

Of course, the main difference is that a resulting child would not have the memories of the adult ancestor. Nor would it necessarily have the personality, outlook, or drive of the ancestor, because these qualities depend in part on early childhood experiences, chosen acts that mold character, schools the child attends, and the people who mentor the adolescent.

Any elderly narcissist who originates a child by cloning to re-create himself will be disappointed at the result. Unfortunately, he or she will be unlikely to realize their disappointment since it will take twenty years for the child to grow to adulthood, and by that time, the narcissist will likely either be dead or suffering from a chronic neurological disease.

Cloned Humans Would Not Be Drones but Persons   A child created by reproductive cloning would need to be gestated by a human female for 9 months, and his birth would be like that of any other child. He would have no distinguishing marks on him to indicate his origins. As such, he would feel, sense, think, and hurt like any other human child.

Today, we do not believe that a child's origins affects his status as a person—it does not matter whether your parents were married, of different races, gay or lesbian, or whether you were conceived in a test tube. As such, children created by cloning would be, ethically, persons with all the rights of other persons.

Some widely quoted authors such as Leon Kass have questioned this, implying that not he, but prejudiced others, might treat cloned children as less-than-human. If this were so, it might not be in the best interest of a child to be originated this way.

But notice that the same logic implies that it might not be best to be created as a child of an interracial couple because "other people" might be prejudiced against such marriages and children. The effect of such reasoning is to strengthen prejudice, not to weaken it, and to give it too much weight in what, after all, is supposed to be *moral* reasoning. The way to combat prejudice is to expose it and combat it with knowledge and reasoning, not give in to it.

For this reason, we must be careful when we speak of children originated by cloning. To call them "clones" is to be prejudicial because that word is now so negative, so pejorative, that it connotes bad things about such children and people who created them. Similarly, to imply that children created by cloning would be raised in batches connotes all kinds of bad, silly things, such as seeing them as zombies, as sources for harvesting of organs for genetic ancestors, and, in general, as less than human.

Cloning Would Have No Effect on the Gene Pool   One sometimes hears the objection that cloning will decrease the diversity of the human gene pool. Diversity in such a pool is good for the human race because unknown diseases may appear in the future, against which idiosyncratic genes may offer the best defense to the minority of humans who have them. In this way, it is hypothesized that blacks with genes for sickle-cell disease escaped early death from malaria in Africa and whites with genes causing cystic fibrosis escaped lethal airborne diseases caused by viruses (cystic fibrosis creates excess mucus in the lungs, eventually killing patients, but perhaps protecting young people from infection of viruses long enough to reproduce).

Behind this objection is the idea that characteristics of children originated by cloning would not be individually chosen by parents but stamped out, machine-like, in vast, uniform quantities. A variant of the objection is that prospective parents are so easily influenced by a few cultural stereotypes that millions would choose genotypes of famous movie stars, in the same way that names such as Heather and Jennifer became suddenly popular 20 years ago among white parents.

Even if all the above were true, which is very doubtful, originating children by cloning this way would have little or no effect on the human gene pool. A few facts explain why. First, originating a child by cloning requires in vitro fertilization, which is unsuccessful 75 to 80 percent of the time and which in over 35 states must be paid for by the prospective parents at nearly $8,000 per attempt. Furthermore, of the people who use IVF, only a tiny percentage would consider cloning. So the numbers of children originated by cloning are going to be small, not vast.

A little math here goes a long way. Around 2000, the planet held over 6 billion people, and by 2010, that number will probably be at 6.5 billion. Even if a million people were originated by cloning, their genes would have little influence on the 6.5 billion—especially because each person will have free will, grow up, probably fall in love with a person not originated by cloning, and create children sexually with mixed genes. There is no reason to think that people originated by cloning will need this procedure to reproduce or prefer it over sexual reproduction (which is more fun!).

For this reason, it would be very difficult to elevate the quality of the human gene pool by either cloning or any kind of eugenic-parental selection of traits. In the same way, worries about the deterioration of the human gene pool are also misfounded, as the next generation will mix "inferior" genes with other genes, resulting in new combinations.

The above reasoning illustrates a law in population genetics called *the law of regression to the mean*. What this means is that if you have a very big population, for example, 6 billion people reproducing, then over time, abnormal values will be normalized. The crushing weight of the numbers stabilizes the mean.

When you understand this, you see that the human gene pool is actually very stable. Even a billion superior humans originated by cloning would reproduce with the other 5 billion normal humans, and within two or three generations, the superior genes would be diluted. But creating a billion humans by cloning is impossible now, as it would require 5 billion attempts through IVF at creating babies.

At bottom, worries about effects of cloning on the human gene pool all mistakenly assume mass production of humans from a cookie-cutter mold. But this assumption is no more true for cloning than it was for debates about test-tube babies 30 years ago.

Lack of Informed Consent of Children Created by Cloning   One sometimes hears that attempting to originate a child by cloning would be an unethical experiment on the resulting child because such a child could not give informed consent to the experiment. This objection rests on a misconception.

The misconception is not that it wouldn't be an experiment to create a child this way, for that would be true. The misconception is first, the idea that any child can consent to any experiment before birth, and second, that to be ethical, such an experiment would require such consent.

Both of these conditions are false. If the second were true, virtually every improvement in the neonatal nursery or pediatric surgery would be unethical. And thousands of experiments have in fact been done on babies to improve their health and to fix congenital defects. Medical progress depends on them.

It might be countered that such experiments are designed to improve the health of the baby, whereas cloning is not, being merely designed to gratify the ego of narcissistic parents. But that counter begs the question about the motives of parents who would use cloning.

Commodification   Originating babies by cloning is often held to be making babies into "things" or commodities, not Kantian "ends-in-themselves" or persons, because it is assumed that the babies are only created for very specific qualities and that such creation for such reasons might be imitated by thousands of other people (*Newsweek* cover story: "Thousands of parents clone Michael Jordan and Brad Pitt").

As we saw in previous chapters, such objections forget that prospective parents make similar choices now in pursuing adoption of babies of a certain race, gender, ethnicity, or health status. As we saw, substantial amounts of money exchanges hand to facilitate adoptions. And yet no one considers the babies adopted to be "commodities" or the parents to be bad for pursuing, say, healthy female Chinese babies.

The objection also makes the usual mistake of assuming bad motives in parents utilizing a new method of conception. This history of reproductive ethics, going back to artificial insemination and amniocentesis, shows that each new option will be greeted with this objection.

Brave New World   Conservative Leon Kass believes that originating humans by cloning is the essence of the destruction of our human essence by evil medical technology. He and others cite Aldous Huxley's futuristic novel *Brave New World* as an argument against going in this direction.

But such citation is misguided. *Brave New World* is about the dangers of mass-conditioning society through behavioral techniques. Only the beginning example is about assembly-line reproduction of prechosen genotypes (admittedly, this is a powerful scene). Ironically, the main message of *Brave New World* is the danger of the state taking away choice from parents about ways of creating children. Yet opponents of cloning cite this novel to do exactly that!

Moreover, people have been so powerfully conditioned to reject anything associated with the word *cloning* that they rarely think for themselves about this topic. So there is a double irony in citing *Brave New World* to oppose cloning, both for the misunderstanding about choice and for the other misunderstanding about how conditioning can wipe out real thought.

Scientists Are Not Frankensteins   Dr. Frankenstein in Mary Shelley's novel of the same name is the archetype from which most future scary pictures of scientists are drawn. Arrogant, unfeeling for his creation, working in an isolated lab, seemingly spouseless and childless, this mad scientist is meant to be inhuman and scary.

Mrs. Shelley wrote this book to scare people, to make money, and to become famous. She was not a sociologist who did a careful survey of the qualities of working scientists, and she was not a scientist herself. Nor had she ever worked with scientists.

In fact, most scientists are pretty normal, with kids and spouses, who share our fears about runaway technology and dehumanizing medical tools. Given this fact, it is important not to impute bad motives to scientists without evidence.

Remember that the scientists who get the most attention from the media—Richard Seed, Panos Zavos, and Raelian Brigitte Boisselier—are not in laboratories actually working but constantly working their cell phones to make appearances on television and radio. These people seek not to help infertile couples, but publicity. They should not be confused with all the real scientists working diligently, and ethically, in their offices and labs.

ARGUMENTS FOR AND AGAINST HUMAN CLONING

Moral arguments against human reproductive cloning divide into two kinds, the first arguing that such cloning is *intrinsically wrong,* the second arguing that, while not intrinsically wrong, it is *indirectly wrong* because of undesirable things associated with such cloning or undesirable things that would be the inevitable results of such cloning. We will first consider arguments that human reproductive cloning is intrinsically wrong.

As said, these arguments are *moral* ones, in the domain of ethics, so they are not *legal* ones. A different kind of argument about reproductive cloning occurred in the United States about constitutionality of making reproductive cloning a federal crime. This was the intent of the Human Cloning Prohibition Act of 2001, which passed the House of Representatives in 2001 but did not pass the U.S. Senate in 2002, so it did not become law.

The legal argument against this bill is that the Bill of Rights or U.S. Constitution does not give Congress the right to make laws about how Americans originate children, choose not to originate children (contraception), or choose to stop children from growing inside them (abortion). While states may do so as a way of regulating medical practice and of protecting children, this is not a power reserved for the federal government.

Direct Arguments Against Human Cloning

Against the Will of God   Many clergy believe that originating children by cloning is not God's will. God ordained in Genesis that humans will reproduce as did Adam and Eve, man and woman begetting children, and that is God's Plan for Humanity.

To deviate from the plan is wrong. Just as gay men and lesbians were not meant in this Plan to have children, so children were not meant to be created asexually. (Indeed, cloning would commit two sins at once if the genetic ancestor was a gay man.)

Notice that this argument is an inference about God's will. No-where in any scripture does it say that medical science should not use reproductive cloning to produce children. Notice too that most advances in the history of medicine have been greeted by the same argument that the change is against God's will, based on the interpretation of that will of that time.

The Right to a Unique Genetic Identity   With Dolly's birth and the real possibility emerging of cloning a human baby, various people began to assert that what was wrong with cloning a human baby from a genetic ancestor's cells was that it would violate the right of each person to "a unique genetic identity." Some theologians at the Vatican made this claim (although they had never made it before Dolly's birth).

An initial problem about this argument concerns twins. Since identical twins share 99.9 percent of their genes, isn't their right to a unique identity violated by being a twin? Certain techniques of assisted reproduction, such as implanting many embryos, drastically increase the likelihood of such twins. Are they therefore wrong?

A bigger problem with this objection is the assumption that one's genes are one's identity. This reductionist line of thinking in modern genetics lies behind similar objections that a child created by cloning would not have a soul because it shared the same genes as the ancestor. Both objections assume that genes make the person, the self, the identity, and yet we know that is incorrect because environment also contributes to personhood (and also, possibly, so does free choice).

Unnatural and Perverse   Why would anyone want to originate a child by cloning? Why not use the fun method of sex? If a couple is unable to have a child through sex, why not adopt?

Sexual reproduction is natural. Cloning, or asexual reproduction, is unnatural. What is good for plants or animals should not be used for humans.

People who want to originate babies by cloning have something wrong with them. They are either narcissistic or so desperate—after all other methods of having children have failed—that they will subject their future child to a perverted experiment in which his very personhood will be at risk when he later learns that he is "just a clone."

In reply, it should be noted that this objection begs a lot of questions. First it assumes that what is primitive or "natural" is always best. That is certainly not true for a man and woman who are naturally infertile. Second, it assumes that the new way of making babies is "perverse" and therefore wrong, a charge that created many other new ways of making babies in the past. Finally, it assumes bad motives on the part of would-be parents, and why assume them?

The Right to an Open Future   Critics claim that parents choose a certain genotype, say, athlete Michael Jordan's or actor Brad Pitt's, for a reason and with certain expectations. After their investment in in vitro fertilization (required to create a child through cloning), they would expect the resulting child to have qualities similar to Jordan or Pitt. Moreover, they would expect the child to become rich and famous through being, respectively, a professional basketball player or actor.

But, so the argument goes, this is unfair to the child. At birth, a whole universe of careers should be open to every child. It is wrong for tennis mothers to impose their wills on their children in their hell-bent determination to make them into tennis stars; it is wrong for East Asian parents from an early age to push their children into premed careers, and it is wrong for soccer dads and little league coaches to push their children into athleticism.

Why is this so? The heart of the objection about a closed future lays in explaining this answer. At bottom is the premise that parents should not have children to fulfill their own needs, desires, or fantasies, but instead simply for the good of the child. In this sense, parenting should be Kantian, not egoistic or egotistic.

It is certainly not in every child's best interest to have a pre-conceived career foisted on him or her by parents regardless of that child's abilities and, perhaps more important, his or her own free decision. More than one child has felt the agony of being pushed into a Procrustean bed where he or she does not fit, while desperately trying to gain the love and respect of parents who only define success as fulfilling unrealistic expectations.

If parents create children expecting very specific traits (basketball skills, acting talent), the objection continues, then children can be damaged psychologically when they cannot, or choose not to, fulfill such expectations.

The argument above is part of the widely heard objection about "designer babies," i.e., that it is "just wrong" for parents to try to create children with "blue eyes and blonde hair" and with a strong interest in music and tennis. Instead, parents should accept whatever God or nature gives them.

The most dangerous idea of all is that parents should be free to reject, or not love, babies who lack the qualities they want. Already a dangerous tendency has started among some parents to not aggressively treat impaired babies suffering from genetic diseases at birth, followed by equally dangerous practices of death-by-abortion after sonogram has determined that you are a female fetus. If we add to this the possibility of using pre-implantation diagnosis during in vitro fertilization to not implant any embryo with cystic fibrosis or Down's syndrome, we are already halfway to the bad place of parents rejecting children in the nursery when they emerge with the wrong genes.

The whole point of this reduction is to challenge the premise that parents should be able to accept or reject babies based on qualities they have or lack. That is to be denied. Since it is to be denied, any practice that would further this is also to be denied, such as the practice of trying to create children with certain specific qualities.

(This objection will be countered in the section below entitled, "Closed Future?")

Indirect Arguments Against Human Reproductive Cloning

Abnormalities   At present, a high rate of abnormalities plagues efforts to create primates by somatic cell nuclear transfer. Any such conception of a human baby by cloning would be an experiment on a child, and no such experiment is justified without a compensating, likely benefit for the child. Such a benefit does not now exist. As such, attempts are wrong to create a child by cloning the cells of a human ancestor and gestating it to birth.

Indeed, because a child is likely to be born with some genetic defect, conceiving a child from cloning might now even be considered a form of child abuse. If the motives of the parent were bad, then deliberately creating a child who was likely to be genetically defective would be like deliberately choosing to implant an embryo with cystic fibrosis rather than a healthy one.

Notice, however, that this objection is very dependent on the existing state of scientific knowledge. If scientists learned to originate baboons and chimpanzees by cloning without defects, and if they learned how to originate safely by cloning all other mammals, then the chances of a defective cloned baby would drop drastically and the force of this objection would correspondingly diminish.

Notice, too, that when we discuss abnormalities, we need some baseline for comparison. Over 50 percent of embryos created sexually do not implant successfully in the human uterus and are lost, half of which are chromosomally abnormal. About 2 percent of live-born babies have some genetic defect. Millions of babies are born after the mother smoked or drank during their gestation, yet we do not criminalize such smoking and drinking during pregnancy. (Perhaps we should, but the point is that the press focuses on the sensationalistic, remote cases of cloning and ignores the obvious harm all around.)

Deep Inequality   Many people are aware that some people start out in life much better than others, through no merit or fault of their own. Some children get two parents, four grandparents, lots of gifts at holidays and birthdays, special preschool and afterschool tutoring, and attend the best private schools and universities. On the surface, it seems unfair and unjust that some children get so much while others get so little.

Over the last centuries, civilized societies have mitigated some of the more extreme effects of this *environmental inequality:* estate taxes have reduced how much can be inherited from parents, income taxes have redistributed money from high earners to those on disability and public assistance, and expanding economies have created new opportunities for hard working, talented people to get ahead.

Even so, the gap between rich and poor across the planet is astonishing, especially when the life of a well-off North American is compared to a poor, starving African. Much remains to be done to increase the minimal well-being of the world's peoples, most of whom are poor and short-lived.

Given that background, reproductive cloning is the start of a new kind of *biological inequality,* much deeper than our hitherto environmental inequality. Because reproductive cloning would normally involve a conscious choice to clone the genome of one person rather than another, it is likely that rich families so choosing would choose genomes of very good qualities. If safe and successful, such families could create strong, clever, talented, energetic dynasties that outstripped normal humans. It would be a biological case of "the rich get richer, the poor get poorer."

This really is something new in human evolution. Sexual reproduction randomly exchanges genetic material, making sure that the great genetic norm of human nature never rises or falls too much. But in a single swoop, particular families single-mindedly devoted to raising their genetic stature over generations could biologically outdistance normal humans and even their past ancestors.

As such, reproductive cloning poses a grave new danger to social justice. Moreover, because this danger is "written into biology," it would be much harder to undo. People without superior genes would find it much harder to compete against such superior people, even when the competition was completely fair.

But is this the way we want the advanced countries of the world to go? Toward a deeply stratified society that divides into Superiors, whose genotypes were chosen by committed families bent on superiority, and Normals, whose genotypes were randomly assigned by the spin of the genetic roulette ball in sexual reproduction?

(Of course, one problem with this line of thinking is the assumption that families could strictly force their children to use cloning to create future children.)

Direct Arguments for Reproductive Cloning

Good of the Child   Almost all ordinary discussions of cloning beg two important questions: they assume bad motives on the part of parents or scientists involved in creating a child by cloning, and they assume the child would be harmed by knowing he was created this way.

We can see just how much is begged or assumed when we counter these assumptions. First, a child created through cloning would know that he was very much wanted by his parents. After all, creation of such a child would require in vitro fertilization, which at best is successful only 25 percent of the time. Thus, prospective parents probably would have to try several times to create a baby this way, and pay real money for their efforts.

In contrast, all that many people know about the wishes of their parents is that their parents had sex and did not abort. They have no clear evidence that their birth was wanted or planned. This fact especially applies to children created before *Griswold* v. *Connecticut* in 1965 made it legal for physicians to give contraceptives to patients.

To give this argument some play, let's assume that technical difficulties are overcome about reproductive cloning and that children produced this way are safe. Besides knowing he or she was wanted, is there anything about being originated this way that could be in the interests of a child?

Well, for one thing, few parents would knowingly re-create the genotype of an adult with a congenital disease such as blindness, deafness, Down syndrome, or cancer. In so far as possible, parents would choose children who would be, at least because of their genes, as healthy as possible.

This in itself will be a great good for the child. Placing aside for the moment worries about eugenics, it is hard to ignore the good of a life where one is not constantly challenged by hurdles from physical or mental disabilities.

Next, consider that certain traits might be genetically based. We already know that, to an extent, looks and physique are, because we see resemblances in a family. Suppose, too, that intelligence, wit, temperament, sociability, verbal ability, mathematical ability, and analysis are somewhat genetically based. Suppose, again, to give the argument more rope, that parents could choose children increasing some of these traits in resulting children above the norm. Would doing so be good for the child?

Other things held equal, it is hard to see why they would not. Although it may not be politically correct to say it, all other things being equal, it is better to live life as a beautiful, smart, healthy person than the reverse, and it is hard to see why such a life is not in the interests of the person so created.

Of course, opponents will say that such a person has been created as a purchased "commodity," as an "object," and subject to the unrealistic expectations of the parent. We will consider the objection about expectations below, but for now, notice that this general line of objections applies to any service that parents buy for present children with the same goals in mind, such as sending children to elite private schools. Yet no one considers the latter to be bad for the children; in fact, the reverse is true.

Finally, we should notice that there's a dilemma that proponents of reproductive cloning encounter in which either way they lose. If cloning is unsafe, then it hurts the child, and therefore it's wrong to do. If cloning is safe, then it improves the child and is eugenic, and therefore wrong to do. Obviously, trapped in this false dilemma, the proponent of cloning can never win.

At bottom, what may scare opponents of reproductive cloning the most is the possibility that it will work, be safe, and be in the best interests of the children created. Then some children really will have more, biologically, than others, and some families may create "biological dynasties." But be that as it may, these are not objections about the intrinsic evil of cloning, but indirect ones, focusing on harm to equality (which we considered above).

Only Way to Have One's Own Baby   One of the main legitimate reasons to produce a child is to have a child with (half) one's own genes. Whether it's to have one's family line continue or "a bit of me going into the future," no one questions the soundness of this parental motive.

Now in some rare cases, asexual reproduction will be the only method by which a parent can have a genetic connection to a resulting child. Men who are azoospermatic (producing no sperm) or women whose eggs are too old to conceive often still want a child who is genetically related to them. Reproductive cloning would allow each parent to have a child (assuming two children) with a strong (99.9 percent) genetic connection to the respective parent.

Although men with very low sperm counts could have a child asexually through intracyptoplasmic sperm injection (ICSI) into a donated egg, there is no option for a man who lacks sperm and a woman who lacks good eggs and who also want a genetic connection to a child. For either parent, the only route to a genetic connection to a child is the asexual one of using a cell from a nucleus of, say, a skin cell, and using the genes inside it via cloning to create a human embryo.

The combination of two forces makes this a much stronger argument than might at first appear. First, many women delay age of pregnancy as they pursue careers and are disappointed when they marry late that they cannot conceive. One recent study emphasized that less than 10 percent of women have healthy eggs at age 42. That is, over 90 percent will fail to have a child with their own egg, meaning that whatever child they adopt or create with donor eggs will have no genetic connection to the mother.

Second, the force of the urge to be genetically connected to a child has usually been vastly underestimated by intellectuals, bureaucrats, and politicians. When government and private insurance refused to pay for in vitro fertilization in the late 1970s, everyone thought that few parents would pay cash for the experimental procedures, much less that struggling college professors with little money would forsake cars and a house in attempts to have a genetically related baby. But forsake them they did, and a $4 billion industry was born.

Hence, the millions of couples with women in their forties who are trying to conceive a child, either in a first marriage or later one, and who strongly desire a genetic connection to a child or two, will be the prime movers in the quest to originate children by cloning. Hence, this argument will appeal to more people, and for different reasons, than might at first have been thought.

Stronger Genetic Connection   A child created by cloning would have *all* the parents genes, not just half, right? So he or she would have not the usual 50 percent genetic connection to a parent, but nearly 100 percent. But if half a genetic connection is good, why isn't double that also good?

See this as an onus of proof argument. Since people and courts assume in public policy that a biological (genetic) connection makes for a better, stronger bond between parent and child, why wouldn't a stronger bond be just as good or better? Whatever it is that makes genetic bonds good for children, isn't a stronger bond also good? If not, why not? If it's just the novelty of a stronger bond, that is not an argument against the bond, just a new item for empirical investigation.

Do our law and courts see the genetic connection this way? Indeed they do. In a dozen cases around the country after a dispute arose, a baby who was adopted and who spent several years with an adopted family was returned to a parent with whom he shared a genetic connection. The point here is not to judge the merits of the final resolution of custody of the child (some of which may not, in fact, have been in the best interests of the child) but to emphasize how much weight our society and law puts on binding a parent to a child through transfer of genes.

In another context, countless talk shows feature unmarried women who have had sexual relations with more than one man, each of whom could be the father of the child. On these shows and often in life, the men say that, "If it's mine, I'll support the child." And the law agrees, assigning paternity and requirements of child-support if a DNA test identifies a particular man as the father. All of these cases point to the power we assume of the genetic connection to the child.

But those are sexual connections, where only half a parent's genes are bequeathed to a child. Imagine a total, 100 percent genetic connection. Wouldn't that bind males to sons in an incredibly strong way? Couldn't that be a good thing for some sons, to have fathers so tightly bound to them? Or for a girl, to have a mother so tightly bound?

Indirect Arguments for Reproductive Cloning

Closed Future?   Opponents argue that children created by cloning will have a closed future because parents will expect, say, tennis stars or professional basketball players. Explaining why that is false gives some important insights into who people created by cloning really be.

First, any adult created by cloning will have free will. Too often in discussions about nature versus nurture, or genetics, people talk as if college students and adults are not responsible for their sexual choices, health behavior, grades, choice of mates, and choice of careers. No parent or script can negate free will or take it away.

One reason so many people forget about free will, when it comes to reproductive cloning, people still accept the old science fiction idea of clones as zombies. When a person created by cloning is thought of as a drone or zombie, it is easy to forget about free will. Indeed, the word *clones* (as in "an army of escaping clones") seems to denote beings lacking such free will.

Second, many parents have expectations of children, even before birth. But almost all parents love their children and realize that they cannot go against a child's unfolding nature or desires. No matter how much a parent might want his child to become a physician, if the child hates science, the parent's wish is not going to come true. And most parents understand the wisdom of not subjecting their children to unrealistic expectations. So, too, would parents of cloned children behave this way.

Opponents retort that parents using cloning will be a special subset of parents, much more likely to impose their expectations on resulting children. Even if this is so, what should we make of it? Notice that it is not always bad for parents to have high expectations of children. Too many parents have low or no expectations of their children. Having expectations per se is not a bad thing.

The best retort to this objection is that, at bottom, it assumes bad motives on the part of parents. Why should we assume this? Why shouldn't the onus of proof be on those who want to see such parents as bad? Indeed, this author suspects that when originating humans by cloning becomes safe in the future, we will be in for some surprises. For example, suppose that a child is created from the genes of a girl who was an all-state champion swimmer in the breast stroke and who had very high ability in math, scoring in the top 1 percent of standardized tests and excelling in AP math classes in high school. But what is often overlooked is the role of supportive parents in such achievements. Now suppose that the child cloned never learns to swim and is never exposed to math, and doesn't develop these abilities (assume she's now 24 years old and that it's too late then to develop these abilities). In that case, we will learn, perhaps painfully, that parents of children cloned for certain abilities cannot just sit back and wait for the abilities to unfold but will need to be just as involved as the ancestor's parents, and if they were not, it will be easy to see where the blame should go.

Liberty   Those wishing to curtail reproductive cloning because it might increase social inequality need to put their cards on the table and not hide behind subterfuge. They rarely say exactly what they want to do and that is to decrease the liberty of the average person to have children and to create a family.

Now the liberty to create children and a family is not absolute and may be outweighed by a much greater social good. But in the rest of our lives, we prize liberty very highly, especially when it comes to creating families and what goes on inside them.

Notice that we are not willing to curtail our personal liberty to create more social-political-economic equality in most areas of our personal lives. For example, we could make private schools illegal and require all children to attend public schools. This would get the best parents involved in PTAs and community boards, which in turn would raise the level of all public schools, thereby helping equality. In the South, where private academies continue the vestiges of racially segregated schools, and in general, where elite preparatory schools create a class of highly privileged students, equality is not furthered by giving the best students the best resources.

But few people favor mandatory public schools because it would take away so much freedom from parents about how their children are educated. It is for this reason that some people hate busing, because it forces some children to be bused across the city in the name of furthering equality.

The point is not about busing and public education but about how it is easy to pick on reproductive cloning, sacrificing it to equality, because so few people want to exercise this liberty. But the principle is the same: sacrifice liberty for equality, and what justifies the sacrifice in one area of reproductive live may be extended to another. For example, if only well-off people can afford in vitro fertilization or surrogate gestation, shouldn't it be banned too, in the name of equality?

A Rawlsian Argument for Cloning and Choice   A surprising number of people are against any attempt to improve the genetic qualities of the human race, labeling such attempts "eugenic" (and hence, wrong). But one argument of recently deceased philosopher John Rawls may counter this sentiment.

Justice, according to Rawls, applies not to acts between individuals but most fundamentally to the basic structure of society. Rawls argues famously in his *A Theory of Justice* that the principles of justice that apply to the basic structure would be chosen in a hypothetical social contract where parties choose under a "veil of ignorance" about their position in society when the veil rises. Now consider the following passage from Rawls.

> I have assumed so far that the distribution of natural assets is a fact of nature and that no attempt is made to change it, or even to take it into account. But to some extent this distribution is bound to be affected by the social system. . . . it is also in the interest of each to have greater natural assets. This enables him to pursue a preferred plan of life. In the original position, then, the parties want to insure for their descendants the best genetic endowment (assuming their own to be fixed). The pursuit of reasonable policies in this regard is something that earlier generations owe to later ones, this being a question that arises between generations. Thus over time a society is to take steps to preserve the general level of natural abilities and to prevent the diffusion of serious defects. These measures are to be guided by principles that the parties would be willing to consent to for the sake of their successors. I mention this speculative and difficult matter to indicate once again the manner in which the difference principle is likely to transform problems of social justice. We might conjecture that in the long run, if there is an upper bound on ability, we would eventually reach a society with the greatest equal liberty the members of which enjoy the greatest equal talent.[5]

To the argument that we should not attempt to improve the human race, Rawls provides a framework for a cogent reply: if we were in the social contract—taking the long view of millions of people over many generations—and we did not know which generation we would inhabit when the veil lifted, wouldn't we choose to make the later generations as genetically talented as possible, compatible with the equal liberty of each to procreate in preceding generations? Reasonable people would certainly think so.

It cannot be stressed too much that, on Rawlsian principles, state coercion has no place in improving the genetic heritage of the human race. For Rawls and most members of democratic societies, the first principle of civilized life is protection of our basic civil liberties. Any attempt to impose a procreative program on us violates such liberties. Equally, when the state says we can not reproduce in certain ways, it also violates our liberties.

Under the veil of ignorance, it is in the interest of future children to allow our parents to create each of us with as much natural talent as possible, with the best genes, and with the best chance at a long, healthy life. One could even argue that, although this is controversial, that under this intragenerational veil of ignorance, famous theory of justice, people are not just permitted to improve the genes of future children, but are *obligated* to do so. Why? Because it is wrong to choose lives for future people that makes them much worse-off than they otherwise could have lived.

Politicization of Facts about Cloning   Feminists have noted that gender bias may infect how scientists see the facts: women and men approach a context with different interests and backgrounds, and as such, may have different filters that interpret data differently to generate "the" facts.

Certainly there are areas in science where worldviews affect how people see the facts. Perhaps most famously, Creationist scientists dispute that humans evolved over millions of years by evolving from chimpanzees, and Intelligent-Design-theorists (the new version of creationism) dispute the age of the earth and the molecular origins of life from a molecular, God-less soup.

There are many other controversial areas of science where the facts are very politicized. Many scientists believe in global warming, as do all radical environmentalists, but Danish researcher Bjorn Lomborg believes that many claims of environmentalists about global warming are false or exaggerated. Claims about genetically modified food are similarly highly politicized by scientists and environmentalists.

Indeed, certain topics generate a lot of heat in science: anything to do with death or the environment, and certainly anything to do with sex, homosexuality, lesbianism, or transgender. Assisted reproduction and parenting are also hot-button topics.

As a general rule, it seems that the more emotion swirls around a topic, the more politicized are facts about it. And certainly reproductive cloning is one of the most emotional, and hence most politicized, topics of the last century. So we would predict, and do find, that even the most respected scientists and physicians are unable to rein in their passions when writing about cloning.

It is often easy to emphasize that the glass is half empty when it's also half full. You can emphasize that Ian Wilmut started with 277 eggs to get one lamb, or you can emphasize that he brought three cloned lambs (one live, named Dolly) to birth from 13 fetuses from 29 implanted embryos. You can emphasize that Dolly in old age has arthritis, and imply that it's from her unique origins, or you can test a thousand lambs of similar age created sexually and describe how many also have arthritis (or use Occam's razor and emphasize that journalists taught Dolly to stand on her hind legs to beg for food, gave treats that made her fat, and may have caused her arthritis).

A BROADER LOOK: LINKS BETWEEN EMBRYONIC AND REPRODUCTIVE CLONING

Fears of slippery slopes of justification abound about research on human embryos. Leon Kass made such fears explicit in an article that appeared just before the announcement of the recommendations of the National Bioethics Advisory Commission. "And yet, as a matter of policy and prudence, any opponent of the manufacture of cloned humans must, I think, in the end oppose also the creating of cloned human embryos."[6]

Because he fears that allowing cloning of human embryos will inevitably lead to implantation of a human embryo originated by cloning, he wants to test physicians and scientists who favor lifting the ban on embryo research by making them endorse "an absolute and effective ban on all attempts to implant into a uterus a cloned human embryo (cloned from an adult) to produce a living child."

To the criticism that the techniques of human asexual reproduction are not that complicated and that someone in the world will eventually originate a living child by cloning, Kass would put the onus of proof on those who would permit the "horror" of such origination: "Perhaps such a ban will prove ineffective; perhaps it will eventually be shown to have been a mistake. But it would at least place the burden of practical proof where it belongs: on the proponents of this horror."

Reverse Linkage Arguments

If it is true that embryonic cloning cannot be divorced from reproductive cloning, then other things also follow. For one thing, if reproductive cloning is not bad, then neither is embryonic cloning. If reproductive cloning is not intrinsically bad, but only bad because of abnormal results, then we should study how to prevent abnormalities by funding research in embryonic cloning.

In other words, the argument above says that because reproductive cloning is evil, we shouldn't fund anything that would help us do it. But if that is false and reproductive cloning is just a tool—just another way to make a baby and help start a family—then we should investigate all possible ways to create such a tool.

Not funding research on cloned embryos, or on ways to prevent abnormalities in reproductive cloning in primates, seems especially perverse. If abnormalities are the major reason for prohibiting reproductive cloning, then surely research to prevent them is justified. But if the real objection is the assumption of the intrinsic evil of reproductive cloning, then we should dispense with the cover of arguing about abnormalities and get to real issue.

THE FUTURE

Reproductive cloning will not go away, especially because it will be difficult to police every top scientist in every corner of the world. (Remember: the techniques involved do not require cyclotrons or great financial investment and might be done by scientists who leave North America to pursue their vision, say, in Bangalore, India.)

Whatever happens in the future, the world will undoubtedly overreact to the nature of the first human baby created by cloning. If the baby is abnormal, in whatever way, the world will rush to make cloning illegal. If the baby is normal, by all apparent means, then much of the hysteria about reproductive cloning will die down, just as it did in 1978 after the IVF birth of Louise Brown.

If babies created by cloning develop into normal children, then the argument will shift to possible dangers to children from cloning, and using cloning might be considered more like drinking while pregnant: bad, but not completely evil.

There is also another possibility that could really change the world: Children created by cloning could be adorable, bright, very healthy, very lovable, and hence, become children that everyone wants. Critics such as Francis Fukuyama will say that such a possibility would change "who we are" and our human essence,[7] but others would see it as a happy fact, a blessing to such children and their families, and an area which should be off-limits to federal government intrusion.

FURTHER READING

Gregory Pence, *Who's Afraid of Human Cloning?* Lanham, Md.: Rowman & Littlefield, 1998.
Human Cloning Foundation, www.humancloning.org.
Francis Fukuyama, *Our Posthuman Future,* New York: Farrar Straus & Giroux, 2002.
Leon Kass, *Human Cloning and Human Dignity: The Report of the President's Council on Bioethics,* New York: Public Affairs Press, 2002.

CHAPTER 9

Letting Impaired Newborns Die

Baby Jane Doe

"Baby Doe" cases arise when parents of impaired neonates or physicians charged with the care of these neonates question whether continued treatment is worthwhile and consider forgoing treatment in order to hasten death. This chapter focuses on the case of Baby Jane Doe, which took place at Stony Brook, New York, in 1983. It also discusses the Baby Doe rules and ethical issues of Baby Doe cases.

BACKGROUND: HISTORY, PRECEDING CASES, AND THE BABY DOE RULES

Historical Overview

In ancient Athens, both Plato (in *The Republic*) and Aristotle (in *Politics*) advocated killing impaired newborns. In ancient Sparta, a cyclops baby (that is, an infant born with a single eye or with the two eyes fused) would be left to die in a country field. Later, in ancient Rome, babies who looked grotesque were discarded in the same way: Roman parents who didn't want impaired babies abandoned them in rural fields to die of exposure. Exposure remained a very common practice during the first four centuries of the Christian, or Common, era (C.E.); such "letting die" was legal and was not considered infanticide. Actual female infanticide was practiced, for most of two millennia, by Bedouin tribes of Arabia, the Chinese, and much of the population of India.[1]

Around the year 300 C.E., the Roman emperor Constantine was converted to Christianity and was persuaded to ban parental infanticide. Christianity strongly condemned both abandonment and infanticide, but the church had neither funds nor people to care for abandoned babies; it did not establish a foundling hospital until the eighth century in Milan. In his *History of European Morals*, William Lecky observes, with regard to the influence of Christianity, that although it was the first religion to value the "castaways of society," its role in protecting infant life "often has been exaggerated."[2]

During the Middle Ages, wet nurses acted as agents for parents wishing to rid themselves of children (a practice that would continue well into the nineteenth century). In the eighteenth century, when the population of Europe was exploding, exposure and infanticide were used as methods of birth control. During the reign of Napoleon, so many babies were abandoned that he established his own foundling hospitals, where parents could deposit a baby on a sort of turntable set into the front entrance, spin it to send the baby inside, and depart unseen. In France in 1833, over 100,000 babies—20 to 30 percent of all newborns that year— were thus abandoned.[3]

A hundred years ago, Thomas Wakley, the founder of the medical journal *Lancet,* campaigned against exposure, infanticide, and abandonment. In 1870, the Infant Life Protection Society was founded to prevent parents from collecting payments for dead babies from multiple life insurance policies.

In the Western world in modern times, "letting die" tends to take place in a different kind of context—the hospital. Neonatal intensive care units (NICUs) were developed during the 1960s primarily to keep premature babies alive, and during the 1970s small respirators and feeding tubes began to be used to save such babies and other infants at risk; these new technologies saved some infants who had been born barely alive. However, caring for infants in NICUs is very expensive, and— although this is often impossible to know from external observation—premature babies have frequently suffered neurological hemorrhages or lung damage from respirators. Both the expense of NICU treatment and the low quality of life that can be predicted for many infants receiving such care have raised ethical questions about which babies should be treated and who should make that decision.

Preceding Cases and Controversies

By 1983, when the Baby Jane Doe case took place, a set of rules known as the *Baby Doe rules* had already been developed as a result of several earlier cases. These earlier cases are described later; the rules themselves are discussed in the following section.

The Johns Hopkins Cases: 1971   Down syndrome is a chromosomal abnormality discovered by Langdon Down in 1866; a person with Down syndrome has 47 chromosomes in each cell rather than the usual 46. The extra chromosome is on chromosome 21; hence the syndrome is also called *trisomy 21* (*trisomy* refers to an extra chromosome). Down syndrome is a genetic condition that always causes retardation and a characteristic facial appearance; it is often accompanied by cardiac or intestinal problems. In the early 1970s—at the time of the Johns Hopkins cases— parents of children with Down syndrome were likely to be told by physicians that although the eventual IQ of a person with Down syndrome could not be predicted at birth, the usual range was between 25 and 60, with some severely impaired individuals below 25.[4] (Whether or not this information was correct will be discussed later.)

In 1971—when NICUs were still relatively new and few impaired newborns were treated aggressively—three babies who had been born with Down syndrome accompanied by life-threatening intestinal defects were patients in an NICU at Johns Hopkins Hospital in Baltimore, Maryland. Two of them were allowed to die.

One of the babies who was allowed to die had duodenal atresia, a blockage between the higher duodenum and the lower stomach that prevents the passage of food and water. The mother of this baby—a nurse who had worked with children with Down syndrome—was told that the infant would die if she did not consent to surgery to open the atresia. She immediately refused to consent, and her husband, a lawyer, agreed with her decision.[5] Pediatric surgeons at Hopkins honored this decision and did not go to court.

A film based on the case of this first baby was made by the Joseph P. Kennedy Jr. Foundation; it is called *Who Should Survive?* and has been shown to millions of undergraduate and medical students.[6] Although the film was meant to raise and discuss the ethical issues involved, it has a serious flaw: It never gives the parents' reasons for their decision. In a commentary accompanying the film, the sociologist Renée Fox mentions that the couple appeared to be "of modest means," suggesting that they had a middle-class income at best, and the lawyer William Curran implies that they let their baby die for purely selfish reasons.[7]

The mother of the second baby who was allowed to die already had children; and according to one of the commentators on this case, the theologian James Gustafson, she explained the decision to forgo treatment by saying, "It would be unfair to the other children of the household to raise them with a mongoloid."[8] (Because of the facial characteristics associated in Down syndrome, it was at one time called *mongolism*.) Gustafson describes this mother's decision as "anguished" but also notes that when she learned that her baby had Down syndrome, she "immediately indicated she did not want the child."[9]

The two babies whose parents refused treatment were not killed; they were simply allowed to die—a course that was thought to be more acceptable morally and less likely to incur legal prosecution. One of these babies took 15 days to die; ordinarily, the baby would have died in about 4 days, but some staff members surreptitiously hydrated this infant.

The parents of the third baby eventually accepted treatment, and this baby lived. This baby's parents had originally been given a pessimistic prognosis for Down syndrome, by an obstetrician who referred them to Hopkins because Hopkins had been willing to allow the other two babies to die. However—and perhaps significantly—the staff at Hopkins then gave them a more balanced view.

Lorber's Criteria for Spina Bifida   In the early 1970s, because of the increasing incidence of cases like the Johns Hopkins babies in NICUs, several well-known pediatricians went public. These included, for example, two pediatricians at the NICU of the Yale–New Haven Medical Center—R. Duff and A. Campbell—who published an article in 1973 in which they admitted frankly that they had accepted parents' decisions to forgo treatment, and that 43 impaired infants had therefore died early.[10] Duff and Campbell's article caused a minor sensation and led to much soul-searching by pediatricians at other NICUs, who were often asking themselves whether they were doing the right thing. Another of the pediatricians who went public was the English physician John Lorber, in 1971—the same year as the Hopkins cases. Lorber wrote an article in which he implied that some babies are so severely impaired or deformed that they are better off being allowed to die without treatment.[11]

Lorber specialized in spina bifida—which, as we will see, was one of the defects afflicting Baby Jane Doe. *Spina bifida* (the term literally means "divided spine") is a hernial protrusion through a defect in the vertebral column, and it is the most common serious neural-tube defect, occurring statistically in 1 in 1,000 live births. It may occur in the form of a meningocele, a protrusion of part of the meninges; or it may take the form of a meningomyelocele, a protrusion not only of part of the meninges but also of the substance of the spinal cord.[12] A baby with spina bifida is almost always paralyzed below the level of the opening and thus has bowel and bladder problems; moreover, the opening makes the baby vulnerable to infections such as meningitis. Quality of life depends on two factors: first, the level of the meningomyelocele; and second, the degree of associated problems such as hydrocephalus—a swelling of cranial tissue that commonly accompanies spina bifida and often causes increased intracranial pressure and decreased blood flow to the brain, resulting in mental retardation. However, the probability of mental retardation can be reduced by aggressive surgical treatment involving tubes called *shunts* to decrease this pressure. (Hydrocephalus was present in Baby Jane Doe.)

Lorber developed criteria to predict which spina bifida babies would die if left untreated: The higher the meningomyelocele on the spine and the larger the affected area of the spine and its coverings, the greater the probability of attendant problems and of death. These criteria were meant to be of practical use, because not all infants with spina bifida die if left untreated, and for infants who live, nontreatment makes them worse off. Lorber's criteria seemed to make it possible to identify babies who *would* die: all those in his lowest category. During the 1970s, criteria like Lorber's were apparently used at Oklahoma Children's Hospital, where it was decided not to treat 24 babies with spina bifida who were in the lowest category and who all subsequently died.[13]

The Mueller Case: Conjoined Twins   On May 5, 1981, conjoined twins, joined at the trunk and sharing three legs, were born in Danville, Illinois, to Pamela Mueller and Robert Mueller.[14] Robert Mueller, a physician, was in the delivery room when their family physician, Petra Warren, delivered the babies, who were named Jeff and Scott. The Muellers and Warren decided together not to treat the twins aggressively, so that they could die. However, other physicians in Danville were deeply divided over the ethics of the Muellers' decision. An anonymous caller alerted Protective Child Services, which obtained a court order for temporary custody of the children.

The Muellers were initially charged with neglect; at a later hearing, that charge was dismissed, but the Muellers were denied custody. In September 1981, they regained custody after pediatric surgeons testified that successful separation was unlikely and the prognosis for the twins was therefore bleak.

It is interesting to note the subsequent events in this case, however. The twins lived, still joined, for about 1 year, at which time they weighed 30 pounds.[15] Shortly thereafter, they were separated in a long operation. Scott, the weaker twin, died; but Jeff, the stronger twin, survived, and later he entered a regular school.

The "Infant Doe" Case: Tracheosophageal Fistula   The "Infant Doe" case in Bloomington, Indiana, took place about 1 year after the case of the Mueller twins, over the course of only a few days—from Infant Doe's birth on April 9, 1982, to the baby's death on April 15. Infant Doe had Down syndrome with tracheosophageal fistula, and once again physicians—and others—were divided over the issue of forgoing treatment.[16]

The prognosis for tracheosophageal fistula, which is more serious than duodenal atresia, tends to depend on the severity of the fistula, or gap. In Infant Doe's case, the gap was fairly small, and an early operation to close it would have had a better than 90 percent chance of success. However, the referring obstetrician, Walter Owens, downplayed this fact in discussing the case with the parents and emphasized his assessment of the problems of Down syndrome itself: He said that some people with Down syndrome are "mere blobs" and that the "lifetime cost" of caring for a child with Down syndrome would "almost surely be close to $1 million." Infant Doe's parents decided not to allow the operation.

In this case, hospital administrators and pediatricians disagreed with the parents' decision and immediately convened an emergency session with a Monroe County judge, John Baker. Testifying at this hearing, Owens repeated his prognosis: that even if surgery was successful, "the possibility of a minimally adequate quality of life was nonexistent" because of "the child's severe and irreversible mental retardation." Infant Doe's father, a public school teacher who had on occasion worked closely with children with Down syndrome, also testified: He agreed with Owens and felt that such children never had a "minimally acceptable quality of life." It is noteworthy that this hearing was held late at night in a room at the hospital where it was not recorded, and that Judge Baker did not appoint a guardian *ad litem* for Infant Doe. Baker ruled that the parents had the right to make the decision about treatment versus nontreatment.[17]

The county district attorney thereupon intervened and appealed the decision to the County Circuit Court—and, after losing there, to the Indiana Supreme Court. Both appeals failed: Each time the court ruled for the parents. The prosecutors then appealed to United States Supreme Court Justice Paul Stevens for an emergency intervention, but Infant Doe died before they arrived in Washington, D.C.

The aftermath of the Infant Doe case is of considerable interest. Owens wrote to the U.S. Civil Rights Commission about his role in the case, maintaining that he was "proud to have stood up for what I and a large percentage of people feel is right"; he also said he was glad that after Infant Doe had died, in only a few days and with little suffering, the parents were able to have another baby—a healthy child who almost certainly would not have been born if the couple had been forced to treat Infant Doe. In 1989, however, reviewing the Infant Doe case and other Baby Doe cases, the commission concluded that Owens's evaluation was "strikingly out of touch with the contemporary evidence on the capabilities of people with Down syndrome."[18]

The Baby Doe Rules

The Infant Doe case was followed intensely by the media and prompted President Ronald Reagan to direct the Justice Department and the Department of Health and Human Services (HHS) to mandate treatment in similar future cases. Reagan, who was opposed to abortion, had appointed as his surgeon general C. Everett Koop, an antiabortion pediatrician who was also opposed to nontreatment of impaired newborns.

Because crimes such as homicide and gross negligence are defined by state rather than federal law, Reagan's Justice Department needed to find an indirect route in order to make nontreatment illegal. The executive branch can set social policy by reinterpreting prior congressional legislation (for example, in the 1960s, laws against racial discrimination began as executive orders by President Lyndon Johnson), and such orders are enforced by threats from the Justice Department that institutions violating them will lose all federal funds. It was through this route that the Justice Department and HHS developed the so-called *Baby Doe rules* requiring treatment of all impaired newborns.

The first step was taken on May 18, 1982 (1 month after Infant Doe's death), when nontreatment was defined as a violation of Section 504 of the Rehabilitation Act of 1973, which forbade discrimination solely on the basis of handicap. This interpretation by the Justice Department created a new conceptual synthesis: *imperiled newborns were said to be handicapped citizens who could suffer discrimination against their civil rights.*

The Rehabilitation Act thus became the basis for an HHS Notice to Health Care Providers that was sent to hospitals, and for large posters that were displayed on the outer glass walls of every NICU:

DISCRIMINATORY FAILURE TO FEED AND CARE FOR HANDICAPPED INFANTS IN THIS FACILITY IS PROHIBITED BY FEDERAL LAW.

A toll-free 800 telephone number was also posted so that anyone around an NICU could report abuses—including concerned nurses, disgruntled parents, ambulance-chasing lawyers, and anonymous cranks. (This "Baby Doe hotline" was despised by pediatricians, who feared it would be used maliciously.) "Baby Doe squads," composed of lawyers, government administrators, and physicians, investigated complaints.

"Interim Final" Baby Doe rules were proposed on March 7, 1983 (about 1 year after Infant Doe had died), and were to take effect in 2 weeks—on March 21. After these interim Baby Doe rules went into effect on March 21, 1983, however, the American Academy of Pediatrics (AAP) sued in a federal district court to stop them. The suit *(Amer. Acad. Ped.* v. *Heckler)* was decided in favor of AAP on April 14, 1983, partly on the basis of procedural issues. In July 1983, HHS proposed new interim rules designed to remedy the procedural problems: These new interim rules became the "Final" Baby Doe rules, announced on January 12, 1984, to become effective on February 12, 1984. However, 10 days after the final rules were instituted, another federal court—the Second Circuit Court of Appeals—issued a ruling essentially making them unenforceable. That ruling came in the famous Baby Jane Doe case, which had started a few months earlier, in October 1983.

Before we turn to the case of Baby Jane Doe, let us briefly consider the Baby Doe hotline and the Baby Doe squads. As long as they existed, the Baby Doe squads were ready on a hour's notice to rush to airports, fly across the country, and suddenly arrive—as a squad arrived one day at Vanderbilt University—like outside accountants doing a surprise bank audit. Records were seized, charts were taken from attending physicians, and all-night investigations took place. The attitude of the squads was that time was of the essence because an innocent baby's life might be at stake. Besides Vanderbilt, the University of Rochester also suffered (in the words used privately by some pediatricians) a "blitzkreig by the Baby Doe Gestapo." Eventually, because of technical objections, smaller signs were placed inside NICUs, where only staff members could read them (the toll-free number remained on the signs, however); and finally, because of the objections by AAP and the national press, the Baby Doe squads were called off.

How were the hotline and the Baby Doe squads able to exist for approximately 19 months (from May 1982 through most of 1983) while the various Baby Doe rules were being contested and struck down? The answer is that they were operated by HHS, probably under its interpretation of the broad authority conferred by Section 504 of the 1973 Rehabilitation Act.

What was the ultimate effect of the hotline and the squads? The answer is probably that although they were widely resented as *methods*, the *concern* they represented found (and has continued to find) a more positive response. In terms of actual numbers, from March 1983 (when the "Interim Final" Baby Doe rules were issued) until the end of that year, the hotline received 1,633 calls; of these, 49 incidents were actually investigated. *Newsday* (a newspaper in Long Island, NY) studied 36 of the investigations and reported the following:

> In some cases, intervention has saved a baby with a fair chance of living a useful life; in others, extraordinary surgical measures have given babies no more than a few extra days of life at enormous financial and emotional costs. In one case, the medical bills mounted to $400,000 for a baby who doctors say "has zero chance for a normal life expectancy." In a few instances, parents had to give up custody of their children to the state after they refused to permit surgery. . . .
>
> Records of 49 cases investigated by the Health and Human Services Department's civil rights office during the last 19 months show that in only six cases has government intervention appeared to have made a difference, with children given operations or treatment they otherwise would not have had. In 14 of the cases, mostly originated by anonymous calls, investigation proved that allegations of insufficient treatment were false or that treatment was medically impossible.[19]

Thus the Baby Doe squads did force more treatment for some infants (such as the six mentioned, who were sick and profoundly retarded), although during their existence the squads discovered no provable violation of federal antidiscrimination laws.[20]

THE BABY JANE DOE CASE

The Medical Situation: Kerri-Lynn

On October 11, 1983, while the Baby Doe rules were being revised, "Baby Jane Doe" was born at St. Charles Hospital of Long Island, NY. Because she had several major defects, she was transferred to a NICU at University Hospital of the State University of New York (SUNY) campus at Stony Brook, for care by its neonatal specialists.

The baby's name was Kerri-Lynn, but she was called Baby Jane Doe by the media and the courts. Her parents—who were known only as Linda and Dan A.—were lower-middle-class people working hard to improve their lives; Linda A. was 23 and Dan A. was 30. They had been married 4 months when Linda became pregnant, and Dan had built two extra rooms onto what has been described as their "modest suburban home" in the "flatlands of eastern Long Island."

Kerri-Lynn weighed 6 pounds and was 20 inches long. According to testimony, she was born with spina bifida, hydrocephalus, a damaged kidney, and microcephaly (small head, implying a very minimal brain or lack of most of the brain). Her defects must have been traumatic for her parents: for one thing, her spine was open with the meningocele protruding prominently.

At Stony Brook, two physicians—the surgeon Arjen Keuskamp and the pediatric neurologist George Newman—disagreed strongly about treatment in a case like Kerri-Lynn's, although it is impossible to say whether their different moral views caused them to see the facts differently or their different prognoses led them to take opposed moral stances. Arjen Keuskamp recommended immediate surgery to minimize retardation by draining the hydrocephalus. When Kerri-Lynn was examined by George Newman, he told Dan A. that Kerri-Lynn could either die soon, without surgery, or undergo surgery that would save her life but would leave her paralyzed, retarded, and vulnerable to continual infections of both bladder and bowels. According to Newman's later court testimony:

> The decision made by the parents is that it would be unkind to have surgery performed on this child. . . . On the basis of the combination of malformations that are present in this child, she is not likely to ever achieve any meaningful interaction with her environment, nor ever achieve any interpersonal relationships, the very qualities which we consider human.[21]

(Keuskamp, who withdrew from the case, did not testify in court.) Newman probably told Dan A. something like this about midnight on October 11, 14 hours after Kerri-Lynn was born.

After a good deal of consultation between themselves and with others, Linda and Dan A. decided not to allow the operation to drain the hydrocephalus. They acted on their understanding of the distinction between extraordinary and ordinary treatment, disallowing surgery but allowing so-called palliative care: food, fluids, and antibiotics. They assumed that Kerri-Lynn would soon die, but 4 days later the baby was still alive. A social worker wrote at this time that Dan A. was in "despair" because Kerri-Lynn had not yet died; she also noted that Linda A. was determined to give Kerri-Lynn "as much love as possible" while the infant was still alive. "We love her very much," Linda A. said, "and that's why we made the decision we did."[22]

Kathleen Kerr broke the Baby Jane Doe story for *Newsday* on October 18, 1983. Kerr, who had numerous "firsts" on the story, was also the first reporter (perhaps the only one) to interview the parents. She described the interview:

> Each time he began a sentence, Mr. A. let out a deep sigh, as though seeking strength to answer. Mrs. A. continually touched her husband's arm and rubbed it soothingly. Mr. A. shed his tears openly. . . .
>
> Mr. A. said, "We feel the conservative method of treatment is going to do her as much good as if surgery were to be performed. It's not a case of our not caring. We very much want this baby." . . .

"We're not being neglectful, and we're not relying on our religion [Catholicism] to give us the answer to what we're doing here."[23]

Kerri-Lynn continued to survive, and—as occurs naturally in some cases of spina bifida—her open spinal wound closed.

Kerri-Lynn's Case in the Courts

On October 18, 1983 (the same day that Kerr broke the story), attorney Lawrence Washburn, acting on a tip from Birthright, a Long Island right-to-life group, filed suit in a state court on Kerri-Lynn's behalf to force treatment. Over the following weeks, the case of Baby Jane Doe proceeded through the courts with enormous speed; everyone seemed mindful of the earlier Infant Doe case, in which the child had died while appeals were still continuing.

An emergency lower-court hearing was held on October 20, with Judge Melvyn Tannenbaum presiding. Because Washburn did not have legal standing to sue, Tannenbaum appointed as Kerri-Lynn's guardian *ad litem* ("for this action or proceeding") another attorney, William Weber. Weber was also temporarily empowered to make decisions regarding Kerri-Lynn's medical care.

At first, Weber supported the parents, but then there was an interesting development. Having talked to Newman, Weber abruptly changed his mind when he read that Newman had written on Kerri-Lynn's medical chart that after surgery, she would be able to walk with braces.[24] Weber concluded that what Newman had written on the chart conflicted both with what he had told the parents and with his testimony in court. On another important point, Newman had testified that the baby had microcephaly and would never be able to recognize her parents. Weber said that this was "A lie. The hospital record shows that the initial measurement of the skull was 31 centimeters (cm), which is within normal limits." A measurement of 31 cm would indicate that Kerri-Lynn had a brain, perhaps even a normal brain. On October 20, therefore, Weber authorized surgery.

The parents' lawyer, Paul Gianelli, then applied to the appellate division of the state supreme court, and on October 21 this higher court reversed Tannenbaum's decision. The justices decided that the law left decisions up to parents when a choice was available between two "medically reasonable" options. This judgment seemed to contradict the legal precedent that to be "medically reasonable," a decision must be not only supported by some evidence but, more important, also in the interests of the child (that is, earlier rulings had required a "medically reasonable option" to be an option in the interest of the child).

Weber, in turn, appealed to another court: New York's highest court, the Court of Appeals. On October 28, Weber lost in this court, which upheld the parents' right to decide. The Court of Appeals noted that this case did not belong in court at all; but that even if there had been neglect of the baby, the parents should have been brought to court by state child-protection agencies—not by unrelated individuals such as Washburn. The appeals court also, emotionally, called Washburn's involvement "offensive" and said that Weber should never have been empowered to make decisions for Kerri-Lynn over the wishes of her parents. It can be noted that, in this decision, the Court of Appeals—along with apparently everyone else in the country who was following the developments—had perhaps become too influenced by the immense publicity surrounding the case. The court seemed to have completely forgotten about the traditional doctrine of *parens patria,* according to which the state protects helpless people against those who might neglect them.

After the decision by New York Court of Appeals, Kerri-Lynn's parents thought they had won. Linda A. said:

> I just want [all this] to end. Just to have a baby like this and deal with it is so much to go through right now. Just let us be with our daughter and leave us alone. . . . If there's hell, we've been through it.

However, by this point action was being undertaken at the federal level, by HHS and the Justice Department.

On October 22, the United States government had informed Stony Brook Hospital that federal investigators were coming to see Kerri-Lynn's medical records. Linda and Dan A. were outraged by this: "They're not doctors, they're not the parents, and they have no business in our lives right now."[25] On October 25, Stony Brook's lawyer announced that the hospital would not let the government examine the records. On October 27, HHS turned the case over to the Justice Department. On October 29, the Justice Department filed suit against the hospital in federal court, charging possible discrimination against the handicapped; and Attorney General Edwin Meese and Surgeon General Everett Koop personally sent Justice Department lawyers to the federal court.

A month later—in late November 1983—a federal judge, Leonard Wexler, ruled that the Justice Department could not have the medical records; Wexler also ruled that the parents had not decided against surgery for "discriminatory" reasons. (It is not clear whether Judge Wexler had himself examined Kerri-Lynn's hospital chart.) Dan and Linda A. were pleased, but by now they were also exhausted: "I'm drained physically, mentally, and emotionally," Dan A. said; "I believed that you couldn't look at what we were doing and say we were wrong."

The case later reached the federal Court of Appeals for the Second Circuit, which—on February 23, 1984—denied the government access to Kerri-Lynn's records. This decision, which would presumably apply in similar cases, had the practical effect of making the Baby Doe rules useless, since if the government could not obtain medical records, it could not enforce the rules. The Justice Department appealed to the United States Supreme Court, but in 1986, in *Bowen* v. *American Hospital Association et al.,* the Supreme Court also held that no records needed to be released.

The Aftermath

As noted, the practical effect of the ruling by the federal appellate court for the Second Circuit in February 1984 was to invalidate the Baby Doe rules. On March 12, 1984—evidently seeking a general ruling—the American Hospital Association (AHA) brought suit in the United States District Court for the Southern District of New York, challenging Section 504 as a legal basis for the Baby Doe rules. Eventually, this suit by AHA and Stony Brook's case were consolidated in *Bowen,* in which the United States Supreme Court ruled in 1986 that because the parents were not "federally funded recipients," Section 504 did not apply. In 1984, meanwhile, AMA had joined pediatricians in seeking an injunction that would prohibit HHS from implementing its final Baby Doe Rules; and in December 1984, the injunction was granted by the appellate court for the Second Circuit.

•

During the court battles over Kerri-Lynn, Linda and Dan A. changed their minds and permitted surgery to drain her hydrocephalus—a decision that became known only months later.[26] In addition, the baby had already been given antibiotics after contracting pneumonia (without these antibiotics, she might have died). Kerri-Lynn continued to live and was taken home on April 7, 1984, at age 5½ months. At the time she went home, one physician predicted that she would "probably always be bedridden."

Nearly 5 years later, she was still living at home with her parents. According to Kathleen Kerr, whose stories about the case won a Pulitzer Prize for local reporting, and who visited with the family over those years, Kerri-Lynn was:

> . . . doing better than anyone expected—talking, attending school for the handicapped, and learning to mix with her peers. She still can't walk and gets around in a wheelchair but her progress has defied the dire predictions.[27]

In 1994, B. D. Colen was Lecturer in Social Medicine at Harvard University. He provided an update on Kerri-Lynn:

> Now a 10-year old, . . . Baby Jane Doe is not only a self-aware little girl, who experiences and returns the love of her parents; she also attends a school for developmentally disabled children—once again proving that medicine is an art, not a science, and clinical decision making is best left in the clinic, to those who will have to live with the decision being made.[28]

In 1998, Paul Gianelli, who represented Baby Jane Doe's parents in their legal battles, told reporters that the child was now 15 years old and still living with her parents, who guard their privacy and hers. "It was a very sad case and yet satisfying," said Gianelli, who ultimately won his cases in court for the parents.[29]

ETHICAL ISSUES: FROM SELFISHNESS TO PERSONHOOD OF IMPAIRED NEONATES

Selfishness

The theologian James Gustafson criticized the parents in the Johns Hopkins cases of 1971, arguing that they had been selfish. Living one's life for others, Gustafson said, is the primary ethical requirement of Judaism and Christianity, and the parents didn't want to do that. C. Everett Koop, who became surgeon general in the Reagan administration, argued similarly in 1979: "Why not let the family find that deeper meaning of life by providing the love and the attention necessary to take care of an infant that has been given to them?"[30]

John Paris, a Jesuit opposed to Gustafson's position, noted:

> That concern, as the spate of press commentaries indicates, finds its roots in a fear
> that the "me" generation is reverting to the ancient practice of exposing impaired
> newborns to the elements, or worse, that a "consumer" society is demanding the
> elimination of its less-than-perfect products.[31]

John Fletcher, an Episcopalian priest and medical ethicist (he was at one time the
chief consulting medical ethicist for NIH), also disagreed with Gustafson, taking a
different view of the religious values involved. Fletcher said that he himself could
"stand by the parents" in such cases and "would not want to come down real hard
on them" for letting a baby die by forgoing treatment.[32] Others who disagreed with
Gustafson asked whether everyone really sees the purpose of life as living for others; it was also asked whether, if living for others is a religious value, nonreligious
people should be forced to adhere to it.

With regard to "selfishness," it can also be pointed out that considering what
is entailed by raising and caring for a profoundly afflicted child is not necessarily
"selfish" but may be simply realistic. For a couple who both work, for instance,
raising a severely disabled child usually means that one parent must give up his or
her job—and that the couple will lose this income. Also, some disabilities are lifelong; people with Down syndrome, for example, now have an average lifespan of
55, and some of them live into their seventies. Is it so "selfish" for parents to decide
that they are not "called" to spend their own lives caring for such a child? (Moreover, parents may well consider that their disabled child might outlive them.)

Disability advocates argue that disadvantaged children cannot be allowed to
die merely because they don't fit into their parents' plans; but if we do not consider
the family's good in some way, aren't we in effect saying that the birth of an impaired child—a random event—must be fatalistically accepted by every family,
no matter what hardships it entails? Families today and the family as an institution
seem shaky enough; how much more stress can most families reasonably be expected to manage? Although we cannot always make the interests of the majority
the determining factor in a decision, surely those interests must be given some
weight, and it can be held that how best to consider them depends on each case and
each family.

If we think, then, not about what people want to do but about what they *ought*
to do, will we conclude that a parent who allows a disabled infant to die lacks
morality or is merely following a different morality? Fred Bruning, a writer for
Newsday, defends the course of leaving parents alone:

> This is a dilemma that transcends politics, or ought to. Who but parents can begin
> to interpret the meaning of a child born with terrible handicaps? Here is a situation
> in which "feelings" alone are inadequate. . . . Nor is sweet reason sufficient ei-
> ther. For every argument, there is a counterargument; for every epiphany, a corre-
> sponding burst of doubt. Everything is right, everything is wrong. Morality has de-
> ceptive moves. . . .
>
> Travelers familiar with Beirut claim it is a city lost to hope because consensus
> is impossible. Perhaps it can be said that parents of severely damaged children in-
> habit a Beirut of the spirit, a place where innocence has no armor, where there is

no distinction between suffering and survival. The rest of us are strangers, and we ought to let the parents consult the doctors, reach their decisions, tend to their babies, grapple with their lives. We ought to respect their heartache and their wishes. We ought to leave them in peace.[33]

Bruning's words are eloquent, but surely there are limits. It would probably seem more appropriate to leave parents alone within certain parameters—if we can decide on those paramaters.

Implications of Abortion

Today, many pregnant women undergo amniocentesis or sonograms, and if the results indicate a fetus with a chromosomal abnormality, many of them terminate the pregnancy and try again for a healthy baby. Such abortions may take place legally even late in the second trimester, when the fetus is large and perhaps at a stage of development where some "preemies" are saved. This practice raises a significant ethical issue.

When amniocentesis indicates spina bifida, for instance, the fetus will almost always be aborted. But if spina bifida justifies abortion, why doesn't it also justify letting a newborn with spina bifida die? Similarly, if an abortion is permissible because the fetus has Down syndrome, why shouldn't Down syndrome justify allowing a neonate to die? Birth, after all, does not change the medical condition: In this sense, it can be argued that the significance of birth is merely symbolic or emotional. Note that this logic is neutral between opposed moral conclusions about nontreatment. That is, if there is *no* good reason why a neonate with, say, spina bifida should be allowed to die, then presumably there is no good reason why a fetus with spina bifida should be aborted.

If parents want to forgo treatment in these cases, then, should they be required to justify the decision, or should they simply be left alone? When a woman decides to abort a fetus (even a healthy fetus), she is not asked to give a "good reason." Why are we so much more concerned when an impaired newborn is involved?

Is there a consistent position—a position that allows us to accept choice with regard to abortion but not with regard to "letting die"? This section also shows the power of conceptual slippery slopes, discussed in Chapter 4.

Nontreatment versus Infanticide

An important moral question is whether it would not be more compassionate to simply kill impaired and imperiled newborns than to let them die slowly by forgoing treatment. Legally, killing such an infant would be homicide, whereas forgoing standard treatment is at worst neglect, and legal experts agree that forgoing entails much less danger of prosecution than killing; but that is not the point here. Nor is the major issue whether forgoing is actually more humane, since that question is at least partly factual. In terms of ethics, the essential issue seems to be whether infanticide and forgoing are really morally different.

In both forgoing and infanticide, the motive—the death of the baby—is the same, and so is the result: In both, the baby dies. If the motive is the same in both decisions, and if both decisions lead to the same result, how can the two decisions differ morally? This might seem to be a matter of simple logic: Whatever makes one decision good (or bad) should also make the other decision good (or bad). If so, the kind of action itself, or its active or passive nature, should make no difference.

Nevertheless, some people do draw a distinction between nontreatment and infanticide. One reason offered for such a distinction—based on the realistic assumption that people are not perfect and make mistakes—is that killing is too quick and too final. Allowing an infant to die, on the other hand, leaves the door open for a while, in case (for example) parents have a change of heart or physicians develop a different diagnosis or prognosis. Another argument for forgoing treatment is that it shows more respect for the value of life: A quick end cheapens life, it is held; but when treatment is forgone, parents and professionals must themselves suffer through a slow death.

Personhood of Impaired Neonates

Before he became surgeon general, C. Everett Koop wrote that allowing brain-damaged infants to die would create an empirical slippery slope: It would lead to killing other impaired newborns and end with killing "all people with neurological deficit after an automobile accident."[34] He argued that "each newborn infant, perfect or deformed, is a human being with unique preciousness because he or she was created in the image of God."[35] On the other hand, the Catholic theologian Richard McCormick argued that an infant can realize some "good" of its own only if it can *potentially form human relationships.*[36] The issue of *personhood* underlies both Koop's and McCormick's arguments.

With regard to personhood, it would generally be accepted that moral decisions about forgoing treatment are different when "persons" rather than "nonpersons" are involved. The vexed question is what factual qualities confer personhood: As is discussed in Chapter 5, the core concept of personhood may be well understood, but marginal cases are problematic. (This issue is also discussed in Chapter 10, on animal rights.) Many good thinkers have been frustrated by the attempt to find a theory of personhood that would satisfactorily explain all our intuitions—our basic moral beliefs—about cases at the margins.

In the preceding examples, Koop is arguing that "each newborn infant, perfect or deformed" is a person, whereas McCormick is arguing that not every infant is a person and is proposing the capacity to form human relationships as a criterion or standard of personhood. Consider an anencephalic infant, for instance (an infant born without a higher brain); according to McCormick's standard, such an infant would not be a person. McCormick's "relationships" standard is probably a reasonable attempt to define or delimit personhood; whatever its theoretical merits, however, there are practical objections to it. For one thing, physicians may not agree about the diagnosis of a condition like anencephaly; in the case of Kerri-Lynn, for example, Newman believed that her small head indicated a state similar to anencephaly and concluded that she would never recognize her parents, but Arjen Keuskamp seems to have disagreed. Moreover, it can be difficult to make accurate or dependable predictions about potential. Associations of parents of babies with spina bifida hold that a person's potential can never be known until his or her life is lived.

Of course, McCormick's standard is by no means the only criterion of personhood that has been offered. For instance, some commentators who are considering impaired newborns in particular have proposed using a *cognitive criterion* of personhood. This cognitive standard is discussed in Chapter 2 and again in Chapter 7: On one formulation, it identifies certain qualities or characteristics having to do with cognition—thought—and assumes that without these qualities, personhood does not exist (the qualities commonly include reason, memory, and self-awareness); another formulation is simply that to be a person is to be able to think. With regard to impaired infants, some people who apply the cognitive standard argue that a newborn is not a person until some time after birth. The philosopher Peter Singer holds that children should not be regarded as persons until "a few months" after birth; the physician and philosopher H. T. Engelhardt once held that they aren't persons until they form a self-concept, around the age of 2; the philosopher Michael Tooley holds that they are not persons until they can use language.[37] For Singer, Engelhardt, and Tooley, newborns fail to meet the cognitive criterion.

How good is the cognitive criterion of personhood? As was noted in Chapter 2, in the context of letting adults die (that is, in the context of brain death), the cognitive criterion, though not a legal standard, is actually used by many families. However, its application to impaired newborns may be more questionable. Allowing parents to forgo treatment for an imperiled neonate is one thing; claiming that a child is not a person until perhaps age 2 seems to be quite another. Someone might, of course, suggest that evaluating the personhood of an impaired infant could be *deferred* for some months or even a year or two; but leaving aside the moral status of such a course, it does not take much imagination to see that the practical and emotional difficulties would be enormous.

The personhood of impaired newborns presents significant problems, then, and these problems are relevant to the debate—which is prominent in such cases—over whether forgoing treatment should or should not be a private decision. Was Kerri-Lynn's case, for instance, a private, personal family decision, or was it a case of neglect that public policy must not tolerate? One member of a group advocating recognition of the sanctity of life in public policy criticized the parents, maintaining that "private individuals and private groups of individuals don't have the right to make life or death decisions in private in an unaccountable manner."[38] On the other hand, many people argued that Kerri-Lynn's parents should be left alone to make their own decisions about her care. Do problems of personhood effectively prevent us from applying Mill's concept of harm in this context—that is, are we in effect unable to distinguish between *private life* and *morality* here? As discussed in Chapter 2, Mill's harm principle calls for government not to interfere with decisions that put no other *person* at risk of harm; but the principle may not help us in these cases, if we cannot agree on whether or not nontreatment will harm a person. In other words, if the issue of personhood remains unsettled, simply applying the principle of harm begs the question.

It seems important to reach some conclusion about personhood, in order to establish limits for public policy. However, if we decide that (as Koop maintained) every impaired newborn is a person, it might follow that no parent could decide to let such a child die, and this would of course severely limit a family's range of choices—a result that many people would consider unacceptable. On the other hand, if we allow the widest possible range of choices, we are in essence allowing each family to decide for itself what personhood is and which beings in the family are and are not persons—and this too might have unacceptable consequences. (In fact, it is not hard to find cases in which limiting the range of family choices about nontreatment might seem permissible or even essential. In July 1983, to take one example, the state of Tennessee intervened to allow chemotherapy for 12-year-old Pamela Hamilton, over her father's religious objections. Another such case occurred in Boston in 1988, when a young child became ill; the child's parents, who were Christian Scientists, called a practictioner instead of a physician; the child suddenly died 5 days later, after apparently improving for a while; and the Boston district attorney Newman Flanagan charged the parents with manslaughter.)

What *can* we conclude about personhood, then? Following is one suggestion.

In moral discourse, we usually seek answers to the question, "What is right?" Sometimes, however, we must admit that with regard to a certain issue we are hopelessly deadlocked: Fundamentally different answers are given. The personhood of impaired newborns may be such an issue: It is possible—perhaps even likely—that in cases like these, involving the margins of personhood, we will never have precise, absolute answers. This does not imply, however, that we must simply give up on morality and resort to arbitrary decisions or force.

When we must acknowledge the existence of fundamentally different answers to a moral question, there is a natural solution: We can shift from *content* to *process*. In other words, rather than thinking of a solution as a specific answer, we can seek a process that will result in the fairest solution. (Trials by jury are one example.) A common problem with the concept of process is that the shift from content to process can be made too soon, before it is really certain that a deadlock has developed; but with regard to the personhood of impaired newborns, it seems clear from decades of experience that many people do disagree fundamentally.

We can, therefore, search for the best *process* to resolve disputes about the personhood of impaired newborns and thus about treatment versus nontreatment. For instance, we can think of such cases not in terms of *what* is decided but rather in terms of *who* should decide. Possible answers would then include parents, judges, physicians, bioethicists, the clergy, and ethics committees; and for many people, the first plausible candidates will be the parents.

Prognoses and Ethical Frameworks

Cases of treatment versus nontreatment are often all grouped together, and sometimes even lumped together with cases of assisted suicide and physician-assisted dying, as "euthanasia." This is confusing and possibly dangerous. It is important to differentiate physician-assisted dying, which involves terminally ill competent adults; from assisted suicide, which involves nonterminal competent adults; it is also important to distinguish both of these from nontreatment of incompetent adults in PVS, and it is important to distinguish all of these from allowing impaired newborns to die.

One reason why such distinctions are important has to do with establishing *criteria* for forgoing treatment. As discussed in Chapter 2, the criteria for nontreatment of "never competent" patients should presumably be much higher than the criteria for competent or formerly competent patients whose own wishes can be known or inferred. With "never competent" patients, it can be argued that the decision to forgo treatment must be based on evidence which is "beyond a reasonable doubt," and this would also be true for patients (such as some infants with spina bifida) who may be "presently incompetent but later to be competent." On this argument, then, the standard of "beyond a reasonable doubt" would apply to forgoing treatment for impaired infants.

In practice, criteria for nontreatment of impaired babies tend to be based on long-term prognoses, and whether such prognoses are "beyond a reasonable doubt" is at least highly questionable. For one thing, medical diagnosis and prognosis are almost always subject to differences of opinion and to outright error. In addition, when impaired babies are involved, physicians' medical judgments seem to be affected by their own ethical outlooks.

Some medical ethicists try to determine permissible nontreatment by considering what kind of neonatal defect is involved, along a spectrum from less to more serious.[39] Babies whose problems are at the "less serious" end of this spectrum should be treated, whereas it would be permissible to let babies at the "most serious" (devastating) end of the spectrum die. However, cases in the middle of the spectrum—cases like spina bifida and Down syndrome with associated defects—become controversial. In such controversial cases, prognosis is far from absolute and may be influenced by moral frameworks.

For example, consider John Lorber's predictive criteria for spina bifida, discussed earlier in this chapter. One very vocal critic of Lorber's approach is a colleague of his at the same hospital, the pediatric surgeon R. B. Zachary. Zachary argues that the only real option for babies with spina bifida is either to kill them or to do everything possible for each one of them; basically, he is saying that there is no category of babies with spina bifida who can be "allowed to die." Lorber and some other pediatricians say that the mortality rate is high for babies they place in the worst category of spina bifida, but Zachary maintains that these physicians do not simply withhold treatment; according to Zachary, they "push the infant towards death" by giving:

> . . . eight times the sedative dose of chloral hydrate recommended in the most recent volume of *Nelson's Pediatrics* and four times the hypnotic dose, and it is being administered four times every day. No wonder these babies are sleepy and demand no feeding, and with this regimen most of them will die within a few weeks, many within the first week.[40]

Differing moral views would seem to be at least one factor in this controversy. It should be pointed out, though, that (as noted earlier) the prognosis for an infant with spina bifida may depend on what kind of treatment is given: particularly, whether hydrocephalus is drained to minimize brain injury. We will return to this point later.

Prognoses about the intelligence of impaired people seem to be especially heavily influenced by ethical views; this may not be surprising, since intelligence is an evaluative concept to begin with. Down syndrome is a good example, especially because of the external characteristics associated with it. Let's briefly consider Down syndrome in more detail.

During the last 40 years, there has been a revolution in thinking about IQ in Down syndrome. Most of the earlier studies were probably prejudiced against people with Down syndrome, because these studies focused on people who were institutionalized—a sampling bias that failed to take into account the possibly higher IQs of people with Down syndrome who lived at home, in supportive families. At present, it seems established that although almost all babies with Down syndrome will have IQs below 70, probably less than one-third of them (some studies say only 10 percent) will have IQs lower than 25 and will thus be "profoundly retarded" and untrainable.[41] This indicates that most people with Down syndrome, especially those who receive good early care, will have IQs above 25; some will have IQs above 50; with the maximum stimulation and support, most will probably have IQs between 30 and 70.

What does this imply about "quality of life" for a person with Down syndrome? IQ is a measure of intelligence, of course, and academics and other professional people tend to associate intelligence with happiness. However, it is an unwarranted assumption to think that people with IQs between about 30 and 70 must be unhappy, unless we simply define unhappiness in those terms. Whether one imagines such an existence by thinking of a 6-year-old or a beloved pet, the conclusion must be that, given reasonable stimulation, love, and supervision, most people with Down syndrome will "have a life." To put it another way, they will have a narrative history, and their lives can go better or worse for them. To put it yet another way, most of them would *not* be better off not existing.

Note, however, the mention of early care, stimulation, and support; as with spina bifida, the prognosis for Down syndrome can vary with treatment: Early intervention can raise IQ, whereas custodial care will lower it. Thus there is no way to predict at birth whether a baby with Down syndrome will be at the low or the high end of the potential IQ range; consequently, the best interest of these babies is served by maximal treatment.

It is interesting to realize that although the ethical frameworks loosely described as *sanctity of life* versus *quality of life* are commonly held to be incompatible, these two standards would agree on the early treatment of most babies with Down syndrome. In fact, a similar conclusion may be possible for most babies with spina bifida. It would seem that a neonate with spina bifida has a good chance of "a life"— that is, neither genetics nor probable IQ predetermines a life of misery. Often, it cannot be predicted at birth whether a child with spina bifida will be in the high, normal, or low range of IQ; but most such children will *not* be profoundly retarded. If we cannot assume that low IQ precludes any happiness in life, it can be argued that such children should live—that an IQ described as "borderline," "trainable," or even "imbecile" does not make life so bad that nonexistence would be better.

However, quality of life and sanctity of life do seem to diverge when a prognosis suggests a life of almost total misery and pain: In such a case, considerations of quality of life or the good of the child would indicate nontreatment. If this outcome can be known in advance (a point that not everyone would grant), it would be immoral, from a quality-of-life standpoint, to save the neonate. It is exactly these cases that traumatize pediatric neurologists and families. Because most of these children die, nontreatment is best—but not all of them die, and those who do not die will be worse off.[42]

Before we leave this discussion of prognoses and ethical frameworks, a related matter should be dealt with. Some commentators raise the point that the prognosis for an impaired neonate has implications for the *family's* quality of life; and some parents do see nontreatment as benefiting the family, since caring for an impaired child obviously imposes enormous burdens. If the quality-of-life standard is applied to the entire family, rather than to the baby ("the good of the child"), it may indeed imply nontreatment; however, this would be a radically different interpretation of the standard. When we think of quality of life in, say, cases of PVS or physician-assisted suicide, we are of course thinking of the *patient's* quality of life. Trying to apply the standard to a neonate's family is analogous to arguing that a patient in PVS should be allowed to die, or a terminally ill patient should be helped to die, not for his or her own good but for *our* good.

The Role of Religion

In 1984, the secular philosopher Peter Singer started a controversy in *Pediatrics* by arguing that society should be more concerned about killing monkeys in dubious experiments than about nontreatment of impaired and imperiled human neonates. In fact, he maintained that society should allow very impaired human babies to die:

> Once the religious mumbo-jumbo surrounding the term "human" has been stripped away, we may continue to see normal members of our species as possessing greater capacities of rationality, self-consciousness, communication, and so on, than members of any other species; but we will not regard as sacrosanct the life of each and every member of our species, no matter how limited its capacity or intelligence or even conscious life may be.[43]

Singer (whose views are discussed in Chapter 10) emphasized what he saw as a dramatic asymmetry between our undervaluation of animals and our overvaluation of humans. His actual point was obscured, however, when *Pediatrics* was inundated with letters from physicians protesting his use of the words "religious mumbo-jumbo."[44]

The pediatricians who wrote these letters of protest proclaimed that religion was at the heart of medicine. For them, medical ethics was a branch of religious ethics; they could make no sense of ethics without religion.

There is an ongoing and often acrimonious debate between religious and non-religious physicians, but in many ways the issue is a red herring. This can be seen when we distinguish claims about the importance of religious *values* in medicine from claims about the truth of a religion. That is, whether or not the metaphysical beliefs of the Islamic-Judeo-Christian tradition are correct, modern medicine has undeniably been humanized by values associated with this tradition: respect for human life, family integrity, unselfishness, humility, equal moral worth, and compassion. Perhaps especially, *compassion*—which literally means "suffering with"—has always figured prominently in Judaism, Christianity, and Islam. Moreover, one does not have to be religious in order to value compassion or many other presumably "religious" values. Some religious people believe or argue that atheists must lack compassion, respect for human life, and so on; but so long as these values are not actually *defined* as religious, the claim that atheists cannot hold them is empirical: It can be tested, and disproved, by experience and observation.

In Baby Doe cases, some members of the clergy and some religious physicians have found it difficult to accept parents' decisions to forgo treatment. To many commentators, this attitude seems to lack tolerance and is therefore itself intolerable. Furthermore, it should be noted that some of the people who would advocate nontreatment—or who would at least advocate choice in this matter—are also religious; thus it is not clear how much this particular issue is really about religious values. The issue may have more to do with differing ideas about relationships between physicians and society, physicians and patients, physicians and families, and so on.

The point that religious values do not necessarily lead to choosing treatment over nontreatment bears repeating. Earlier, two cases were cited in which religious parents of older children objected to treatment, on specifically religious grounds. One of these was a girl whose father did not want her to have chemotherapy; another was a boy who died when his parents consulted a Christian Science practitioner rather than a physician about his illness. In both these cases, moreover, society intervened; the state of Tennessee stepped in to allow the girl's chemotherapy, and the state of Massachusetts stepped in (after the fact) to charge the boy's parents with manslaughter.

With regard to religion, some principle seems to be needed to guide society when the issue of treatment versus nontreatment arises. If we want to let parents decide that an impaired neonate should remain untreated, does this imply that parents may also decide not to treat an older child? If it is argued that "religious values" demand treatment for impaired, imperiled neonates, what does this imply about "religious values" that lead parents to deny treatment to older children? The parents of the two children just mentioned belonged to "minority religions" whose tenets came into conflict with standard medical procedures; does this imply that "minority" religious values can be overridden? In practice—in cases involving children of Jehovah's Witnesses, for instance—the courts have mandated treatment by reasoning, first, that religious freedom does not extend to imposing parents' beliefs on their children at risk of life; and, second, that these children may later, as adults, have different religious beliefs.

The Role of the Media

Some disturbing questions are raised by the reporting of Kerri-Lynn's case in the print and visual media, particularly when we consider that Kerri-Lynn not only survived but was able to live at home and even attend school. All the major media simply accepted George Newman's negative prognosis, and almost all dismissed

William Weber, the child's court-appointed guardian, as a fanatic. The media's stance may have unduly influenced not only the general public but even many physicians and medical ethicists, who also took Newman's prognosis as fact.

For example, after Kathleen Kerr's stories on the Baby Jane Doe case had attracted national attention, the veteran medical reporter and columnist B. D. Colen began to cover the case for *Newsday,* and in one of his "sidebar" articles he painted a grim picture of a case that was supposed to be similar. This sidebar described the grueling life and bitter complaints of a mother whose anencephalic or hydrocephalic baby (coincidentally named Cara-Lynn) had been treated, had not died, and was then 2½ years old. In retrospect, what is most interesting is not this other case as such but the way Colen used it as a basis for drawing conclusions about Baby Jane Doe:

> While Cara-Lynn looks far more grotesque than Baby Jane Doe, whose fate is being argued in the courts, the two mistakes of nature have an almost identical prospect for a life filled with pain and devoid of self-knowledge.[45]

Colen's prediction was essentially the same as Newman's: that Kerri-Lynn would never "achieve any meaningful interaction with her environment, never achieve any interpersonal relationships." In fact, this same assumption had already been made by Kathleen Kerr in her earlier stories.

Why did Newman's opinion prevail? That is an interesting question. A year later, a scathing article about the reporting of the Baby Jane Doe case appeared in the *Columbia Journalism Review,* which is often called the "conscience of the news reporting profession."[46] In this article, by Stephen Baer, it was argued that the press had "egregiously failed to meet" its obligation to report the case accurately. Mary Tedeschi, an assistant managing editor of the conservative journal *The Public Interest,* wrote an article for another journal—*Commentary*—charging that coverage of *all* the famous Baby Doe cases was biased.[47] With regard to Kerri-Lynn's case in particular, Tedeschi noted that Newman had written on the chart that "the prognosis was for probable . . . walking with bracing" (a point that Weber had also stressed). She also cited a pediatric neurosurgeon who had treated over 1,000 patients with spina bifida and who held that children whose heads measured 31 cm (as Kerri-Lynn's did) are among "the very brightest" of such children, presumably implying that Kerri-Lynn's IQ could be normal or better.

Admittedly, Stephen Baer was a publicity agent for a right-to-life organization, and Tedeschi also had an ax to grind—she concluded, as a conservative, that "the Baby Doe cases served as a pretext for liberal elites to attack a popular Reagan administration." Still, they both made some good points. Many errors of omission occurred in the reporting of the Baby Jane Doe case. For instance, the public was not informed that although hydrocephalus generally accompanies spina bifida, it does not necessarily cause retardation if it is shunted immediately. Nor was the public informed that when Stony Brook Hospital resisted Koop's attempt to see the baby's medical chart, its motives might have been not to protect the privacy of the family but rather to protect itself from a court suit. Moreover, beyond doubt, pediatricians *did* radically disagree about what treatment was best for Kerri-Lynn, but the two sides of this medical controversy were never presented by the media. As a result, the public—and evidently even some professionals—came to believe that the case involved only moral questions, when in fact medical questions were also at issue. It is astounding to note that such serious charges of inaccuracy and incompleteness could be raised about a story for which the journalist (Kerr) had won a Pulitzer Prize. It also seems astounding that neither the *New York Times* nor the *Wall Street Journal* (to name just two newspapers other than *Newsday*) had checked Kerr's story independently.

At the time of this case, the momentum of the media in support of the parents—and with it the momentum of medicine and medical ethics—became so strong that any dissent was perceived as bigoted fanaticism. Eventually, people read and heard reports of the Baby Jane Doe case with their minds already made up. The nadir may have been reached in November 1983, when Koop was grilled on *Face the Nation* by Lesley Stahl, whose tone implied that she was interviewing a fundamentalist, parent-baiting Big Brother. From the perspective of today, Koop's answers seem impressive: He said that there were discrepancies in the medical chart and that he wanted to see the records simply to learn what was best for the child. Ed Bradley on *60 Minutes* also did a piece on the case, strongly antagonistic to Koop.

With regard to the role of the media, one of the important lessons of the Baby Doe cases is that problems of medical ethics rarely take place in well-defined, predictable circumstances and rarely have neat, clear solutions—and that real-life outcomes may embarrass those who are too confident about their own conclusions.

UPDATE

Legal Trends

Legal developments since the Baby Jane Doe case have involved both litigation and legislation.

Litigation   Most district attorneys are reluctant to prosecute parents in Baby Doe cases, and this attitude seems to have widespread backing. Still, by state law a baby is a person with rights: to live, to inherit money, not to be abused, and so on. Thus criminal prosecution of parents for neglect does sometimes occur, as in the case of the Mueller twins. Prosecution of physicians is also a possibility in such cases. When neonatologists disconnect respirators to let impaired babies die, they risk being charged with violating criminal laws. Since 1992, another source of potential prosecution is the Americans with Disabilities Act (discussed below).

With regard to civil litigation, parents can sue physicians in civil courts for allegedly causing babies to be impaired. Courts are hearing many such suits, and the possibility of such a suit may be a factor that physicians in Baby Doe cases should consider. In the United States, 3.2 million babies are born per year, of which 42,000 are impaired. Today, few parents simply accept birth defects as "fated" or as "God's will," standards of health continue to rise, and couples expect healthy—even "perfect"—babies. When a baby has birth defects, then, parents often blame physicians. (As a result, we see malpractice insurance becoming more and more expensive, especially for obstetricians; we also see more and more lawyers adver-tising to solicit neonatal suits.) Litigation of this nature against doctors can, theo-retically, take the form of "wrongful life" suits or "wrongful birth" suits, and it will be helpful to review these briefly here.

Both wrongful life and wrongful birth suits fall into the general classification of tort law, and in both kinds of actions compensation is sought. A *wrongful life suit* is brought solely by a child. In such a suit, it is claimed that the child would never have been born if not for negligence or error on the part of the defendant, and that the resulting life is so miserable as to be a legal tort or harm; the plaintiff—the child—seeks punitive damages as a compensation for suffering and also to pre-vent or discourage future errors. A *wrongful birth suit* is brought by a parent or par-ents of a child born with defects or injuries; in a suit like this, it is claimed that a physician has caused the injury or defect and that the harm is abnormal develop-ment (rather than life itself), and thus the parent sues for compensation for care of the child. To put this another way, in a wrongful *life* suit, it is argued that the plain-tiff (the child) would have been better off not existing; whereas in a wrongful *birth* suit, the plaintiff (the parent) argues that because of a physician's error, the child needs some kind of special care.

To understand how such suits have been decided in the courts, it is useful to think in terms of the *baseline* and *normality* concepts of harm. The baseline concept, as the term implies, requires a starting point—a baseline—from which an adverse change is plotted (an existing being who is made worse off); the normality concept requires a norm of development that is not achieved. So far, the courts have re-jected almost all wrongful *life* suits, and these rejections have assumed the baseline concept of harm: That is, they have assumed that life is always a benefit, even if it is filled with pain and suffering, and thus that an infant can never "benefit" by not being brought into existence. (The underlying reasoning here has apparently been that if a child could benefit by not being born, it would follow that he or she could also benefit by actually being killed—a conclusion the courts are not willing to draw. Whether or not that conclusion actually does follow is another matter.) Wrongful *birth* suits, on the other hand, appeal to the normality concept and have been more successful in the courts.

A case that had elements (or "counts") of both wrongful life and wrongful birth was that of Jeffrey Gleitman, in 1967. Sandra Gleitman, Jeffrey's mother, had contracted German measles during the pregnancy; Jeffrey was born nearly blind and deaf, and she said that her obstetrician had failed to warn her of this outcome. She was one plaintiff, suing for the expenses of Jeffrey's lifelong care (this was the wrongful birth aspect); in addition, Jeffrey himself was another plaintiff, and the brief for Jeffrey argued that he was so impaired that he would have been better off not existing[48] (this was the wrongful life aspect). The Gleitmans lost, evidently be-cause of the wrongful life element of the case. The judge found that if Sandra Gleit-man's physician had warned her about probable fetal defects she would have had an abortion, and concluded that Jeffrey "would almost surely choose life with de-fects as against no life at all." The rule established by *Gleitman* is that any child who is born impaired as a result of a physician's bad advice, but who would have been aborted had the advice been correct, is therefore unable to recover damages. Since 1982, courts in New Jersey, Washington state, and North Carolina have agreed that, while life itself can never be an injury, parents may recover damages to pay for care that would not have been required if physicians had not made errors.

There does seem to be one example of a successful wrongful life suit, however: the *Curlender* case, which took place in California in 1986. In *Curlender*, the court recognized a claim against a laboratory which had mistakenly told the parents of a child with Tay Sachs disease that they were not at risk, awarding damages even though the child would not have been born if this mistake had not been made.

Legislation   In 1984, Congress amended its Child Abuse Prevention and Treatment Act of 1974 (not the Rehabilitation Act), to count nontreatment in Baby Doe cases as *child abuse.* These amendments (signed into law by Ronald Reagan in October 1984) circumvented the injunction against the Baby Doe rules. They made states, not the federal government, responsible for such cases—getting Uncle Sam out of the neonatal nursery but also leading to problems of their own.

The only exceptions to the regulations under the child abuse act were (1) when an impaired child is "chronically and irreversibly comatose," (2) when a child is inevitably dying, and (3) when treatment would be "futile and inhumane." These exceptions were often interpreted very narrowly, so as to give parents very few choices. Problems resulting from such narrow interpretation were illustrated dramatically in the *Linares* case, which took place in Chicago in 1989. Dan Linares held a NICU staff at gunpoint while he himself disconnected the respirator of his 16-month-old son Rudy, who had gone into PVS 9 months earlier, after swallowing a balloon at a birthday party; Rudy soon died, and Dan Linares was charged with first-degree murder.[49] (A grand jury refused to indict Linares for homicide; he later received a suspended sentence on a minor charge arising from his use of a gun.) There was no doubt, in this case, that Dan Linares was a caring parent, and some such tragedy might have been expected sooner or later as a consequence of the narrowness and vagueness of the exceptions to the child abuse act.

In 1992, the Americans with Disabilities Act (ADA) went into effect; this act protects Americans with a wide range of disabilities (including HIV infection) from discrimination. The application of ADA to newborns with congenital defects—and thus to Baby Doe cases—is so far unresolved.

By 1994, 16-month old Baby K, an anencephalic infant, had been repeatedly brought to a northern hospital's emergency room when its breathing became labored. The hospital appealed to the court to let it not treat the infant, saying the infant was born dying and that treatment was futile. The case was supposed to be a baseline for subsequent cases of medical futility.

The United States District Court for the Eastern District of Virginia disageed with the hospital, citing the Rehabilitation Act of 1973, the Americans with Disabilities Act, the Child Abuse Amendments of 1984, and the Emergency Medical Treatment and Active Labor Act of 1986 (EMTALA).

The Hospital appealed, but in 1994, the Fourth Circuit Court of Appeals reaffirmed its position on the applicability of EMTALA in *In re Baby K.*[50] This higher court affirmed the decision of the district court. In doing so, it focused on EMTALA and its direction that the hospital stabilize Baby K when breathing became unstabilized. It is still unclear what force the ADA had in this decision, but one thing was clear—no legal baseline was established of pediatric medical futility.

Federal regulations, of course, require hospitals to treat all patients needing care who arrive at ERs; it is because ADA was cited that the Baby K case is of particular interest here. Baby K had been on a respirator since birth. When the case was heard, her physicians wanted to disconnect it and let her die; but her mother insisted on continued care, for religious reasons. At its heart, Baby K's case was about whether or not physicians may, without incurring charges of discrimination against the handicapped, overrule parents' decisions about continuing treatment that seems to be medically futile and very expensive.

Trends in Pediatrics

Within pediatric neurology, opinion about treatment in Baby Doe cases has changed dramatically over the past decades: In the 1960s and early 1970s, the consensus was that many such cases should not be treated; today, all but the most hopeless cases are treated.[51]

For example, Lorber's criteria concerning spina bifida initially swung the pendulum toward nontreatment in many NICUs; but during the 1980s, right-to-life organizations and disability advocates swung the pendulum back toward treatment. Also, breakthroughs were made in urology, neonatology, neurosurgery, and CAT-scan diagnosis, and these not only increased the accuracy of prognoses but also improved quality of life for such children. These changes have led to a new understanding:

> Mild to moderate degrees of microcephaly are compatible with normal or even exceptional intellect. This is particularly true in cases of untreated meningomyelocele in which loss of cerebrospinal fluid through the unrepaired hole in the back may decrease the total mass of the head. . . .
>
> Essentially all children with severe meningomyelocele have hydrocephalus. . . . Children with hydrocephalus who are treated reasonably early and who do not develop meningitis have a better chance than 50 percent of being intellectually normal.[52]

The Spina Bifida Association has stated:

> Since we have found it virtually impossible to predict at birth which infants with meningomyelocele will become competitive, ambulatory, and intellectually able, we have not relied on arbitrary guidelines to determine which children should or should not be treated. On the contrary, we believe that all such children should be treated, and we feel that our data show this philosophy to be correct.[53]

The outcome in Kerri-Lynn's case—which was chosen for discussion here because of its fame but was otherwise typical of spina bifida—makes this statement seem reasonable, at the very least. Moreover, the unexpected outcome of the Mueller case and the newer prognoses for Down sydrome suggest that similar reasoning may be appropriate with regard to other defects.

Outcomes

After two decades of debate about Baby Doe cases, the results are equivocal. On the one hand, some impaired babies who would once have died as a consequence of nontreatment are now undoubtedly surviving to lead meaningful lives. Officially, the right of parents to make choices in cases of Down syndrome with related defects, or in cases of spina bifida, has declined dramatically. As a result of the amendment to the child abuse act, many NICU physicians probably overtreat severely impaired newborns.[54] Ironically, the present federal regulations are more stringent than the guidelines of the Roman Catholic Church: The Catholic guidelines allow treatment to be withheld if its results would be "gravely burdensome."[55]

On the other hand, one of the most complex aspects of this chapter is to explain the exact status of whether not treating an impaired, newborn baby is illegal, or indeed, whether it is illegal at all, and if so, exactly for whom it is illegal and why. The answers to these questions are not simple, and indeed, some law schools use the cases in this chapter as way of teaching the complexity of this kind of case.

The best answer is that federal law does not make it criminal for physicians to withhold treatment from impaired newborns. Rather, it threatens to withhold all funding from a state from the federal funding for their Child Abuse/Prevention programs.

Even under this threat, no state has ever been found to be out of compliance with these regulations by the Inspector General's office. As noted universal of Wisconsin bioethicist Norman Fost concludes, "After a decade of the Baby Doe regs, and additional laws which seem to regulate the treatment of the handicapped infants (e.g., EMTALA), numerous appellate court cases, and decades of malpractice and criminal law suggesting that this is a minefield, there are no reported cases of a physician being found liable, civilly or criminally, for withholding or withdrawing any kind of treatment, including food and water, from any patient of any age for any reason . . . the Baby Doe regs do not apply to {a case of nontreatment of an impaired newborn} unless someone reports it as child neglect. Nor does the law require such reports. The risk of that can be reduced (but never eliminated) by securing consensus from all involved."[56]

In fact, and according to Fost, thousands of such infants have had life-sustaining treatment withheld or withdrawn, contrary to the guidelines in the regulations, with no legal consequences to physicians, hospitals, or states.[57]

Many pediatricians, such as Bill Bartholomene, the narrator of *Who Should Survive?* and a former professor at the University of Kansas Medical Center who died of Cancer in 2001, claim that in the 1950s, it was rare for a baby with Down syndrome to live long.[58] Even after institutionalization, nontreatment intending death was the norm, not the exception. Babies who survived were sent to be "warehoused" in custodial institutions, where they were never stimulated or educated. As such, they almost always became severely retarded.

So over the last 30 years, the ethics pendulum in care of impaired newborns has swung back and forth, from nontreatment to overtreatment, and to now, to somewhere in the middle. How much choice a particular couple has in a relevant case will depend on how well their pediatricians and institution understand this complex history and the particular values that the pediatricians bring to the case.

Further Developments

In 2002 the U.S. Centers for Disease Control and Prevention reported that the life span of people with Down syndrome has doubled since two decades ago. In 1983 the average age of death was 25 but in 1997 it rose to 49. Scientists studied nearly 18,000 deaths of such individuals who died between 1983 and 1997.

Baby K continued to receive treatment for over a year but died sometime in 1995. In a related case 5 years later also in the Washington, D.C. area, a panel of judges of the U.S. Court of Appeals for the D.C. Circuit contradicted the fourth U.S. Circuit Court of Appeals order to Fairfax Hospital in the Baby K case. In the Baby K.I. case, the D.C. court said the Hospital for Sick Children in the District of Columbia, despite the alcoholic mother's plea for such treatment, did not need to aggressively treat a severely impaired infant.[59] So the courts overruled one case of pediatric futility and, 5 years later, upheld one.

Several well-publicized wrongful birth suits by parents against physicians have occurred. In New Jersey, parents of a baby with Down syndrome sued pro-life obstetrician James Delahunty, whom they say discouraged them from pursuing amniocentesis when a sonogram showed a fetus with a thick neck (a possible sign in utero of this condition).[60] The jury awarded the couple nearly $2 million and found Dr. Delahunty guilty of "failing to recognize, appreciate, and discuss the results of the tests, particularly ultrasound" with his patients. The verdict may have stemmed partially from his combative behavior in the courtroom.

At least 27 states allow parents to sue for wrongful birth, although Michigan and Georgia recently went in the opposite direction and disallowed them. In a case in 1999, as well as another case in 1990, the Georgia Supreme Court ruled that a couple with a child born with Down syndrome or other impairments could not sue their physician for failure to perform amniocentesis or other prenatal tests.[61]

In France, uproar occurred when, after 13 years of litigation, a court ruled in 1995 that parents of a child born with German measles and not offered an abortion were entitled to compensation for wrongful birth. In two subsequent cases, damages were also awarded to parents of children with disabilities where parents argued that had they had known prenatally of the disability, they would have aborted.

Various critics in France assailed these results, saying they had established a "right not to born," had begun a new "eugenics" program, and would make malpractice premiums soar. In protest, the national association of OB/GYN physicians held a work slow-down. In 2002, the French legislature responded and made wrongful birth suits illegal.[62]

In a review of thirty years of controversy over such cases, noted University of Wisconsin pediatrician and bioethicist Norman Fost concluded that decades of "serious undertreatment" of impaired infants were followed by "an era of serious overtreatment."[63] Within the last 15 years, ethics committees, the ADA, and advocates for disabled infants have resulted in profound changes: "It is difficult to find a single case of withholding life-sustaining treatment from an infant based on diagnosis of Down syndrome or spina bifida since 1985."

FURTHER READING

Fred Frohock, *Special Care: Medical Decisions at the Beginning of Life,* University of Chicago Press, Chicago, IL, 1986.

Michael F. Goodman, ed., *What Is a Person?* Humana, Clifton, NJ, 1988.

Peggy and Robert Stimson, *The Long Dying of Baby Andrew,* Little, Brown, Boston, MA, 1983.

U.S. Commission on Civil Rights, "Medical Discrimination against Children with Disabilities," September 1989.

PART THREE

Classic Cases about Research and Experimental Treatments

CHAPTER 10

Animal Subjects

The Philadelphia Head-Injury Study on Primates

*T*his chapter discusses the conflict between animal-rights activists and scientists over the use of animals in research. It gives a historical overview of opposition to using animals in such research and takes up philosophical concepts underlying the recent animal-rights movement. The central case in the chapter is the research of Thomas Gennarelli, who between 1970 and 1985 systematically inflicted brain injuries on monkeys and baboons to mimic the effects of such injuries in humans. Publicity about this case permanently changed the way animal research is conducted in the United States.

BACKGROUND: ANIMALS IN RESEARCH

Animals and Pain: Concepts and Conflicts

Human beings have used animals for many purposes since prehistoric times, but experimentation on animals did not arise as a specific issue until the beginning of modern science. The premises for the modern debate were set in the seventeenth century, by René Descartes.

Descartes was not only a mathematician and philosopher but also a physiologist, and he studied the circulation of blood by dissecting live animals without anesthesia (which was not invented until 1847). To understand why he considered that permissible, it is necessary to understand his basic philosophical approach, which is known as the *Cartesian* worldview and has deeply influenced western science and philosophy. Descartes, of course, was the author of the famous argument *"Cogito, ergo sum"*: "I think, therefore I am" (it appears in his *Meditations*). According to Descartes, what distinguishes human beings from other animals—what is essentially human—is *res cogitans,* or "thinking stuff," a substantial mind or soul. For Descartes, this mental substance held together transient mental states such as perceptions, feelings, thoughts, and dreams and served as a ground for free will, reason, and moral values. Animals other than human beings, Descartes believed, have no *res cogitans,* no mind or soul, and are therefore ultimately only *res extensa,* or "extended, physical stuff." Thus in Cartesian philosophy animals were merely fleshy machines; no "soul" was reflected in their eyes, and similarly no real pain was reflected by their apparent "pain behavior."

Descartes's idea that animals lack a soul was not unique, of course: This was also Christian doctrine, and Descartes had accepted the teaching that humans have souls created by God whereas animals do not. But Descartes assumed, further, that *soul* is identical to *mind,* so that if animals have no soul, neither do they have a mind; and that if animals have no mind, they cannot feel pain. For Descartes, in order to feel pain, a mind is needed, and—to repeat—only human beings have a mind (indeed, for Descartes, "to be human" was at least partly "to be able to feel pain"). In Descartes's view, there is no middle ground between a human being, who has a soul and thus a capacity to experience pain, and an animal (*any* animal), which has no soul and thus no capacity to experience pain.

Cartesianism represents an attempt to deal with the tension between science and religion by demarcating proper areas for each: The province of science is the study of matter, mathematics, animals, and the human body; that of religion and the humanities is mind, art, and ethics. Obviously, however, it has not come to represent a consensus, or even a widely accepted solution—even for Christians, who are still struggling with the concept of how mind and soul are related, how they relate to morality, and whether animals count in the grand scheme of things (Protestant ministers, for instance, are often asked whether pets go to heaven).

Among Descartes's immediate followers during his own century were an infamous group of early physiologists and vivisectionists (researchers operating on animals without anesthesia) at the Jansenist seminary of Port Royal. Here is a description of the Port Royalists by an eighteenth-century writer, Nicholas Fontaine:

> They administered beatings to dogs with perfect indifference, and made fun of those who pitied the creatures as if they felt pain. They said the animals were clocks; that the cries they emitted when struck were only the noise of a little spring that had been touched, but that the whole body was without feeling. They nailed poor animals up on boards by their four paws to vivisect them and see the circulation of the blood which was a great subject of conversation.[1]

To some extent, the Cartesian concept of animals has persisted into modern times. Some behavioral psychologists, for instance, argued against assuming that animals (especially rats) are conscious and drew a distinction between "pain behavior" and the actual experience of pain. Cows, say, could exhibit "pain behavior," but whether they had mental states and thus had the experience of pain was another matter.

Descartes, as noted above, saw no middle ground between human beings, with minds and feelings, and animals, with no minds and no feelings. The twentieth-century Christian writer C. S. Lewis, however, tried to find a middle ground; he rejected the assumption that animals feel nothing and argued that animals are, in some sense, aware. To describe in *what* sense animals might be aware, Lewis distinguished between *sentience* (ability to feel pain) and *self-consciousness* (awareness of feeling pain): All animals are sentient, he argued, but only human beings are also self-conscious.[2] According to Lewis, then, animals can feel pain, but not as humans do. A rat receiving three electric shocks feels the pain of each shock—the rat is sentient—but it does not think, "I have had three shocks." The thought, "I have had three shocks," requires what Lewis calls "consciousness" or "soul" (he runs these together). Lewis agreed with the eighteenth-century philosopher David Hume, who argued that self-identity requires a permanent self or mental substance that unites all of a person's thoughts as "his" or "hers."[3] For Lewis, a primate (for example), would have a "succession of perceptions," but not the human experience of pain as "my pain."

Lewis, then, identified awareness with self-consciousness or soul (for which he also used the term "deep self"). Some critics have disagreed with this idea, particularly since Lewis assumed that memory depends on self-consciousness. These critics observe that if self-consciousness were needed for memory, animals would never remember anything, and studies of learning in animals would be senseless; but everyone knows that animals can and do remember—a dog that has been kicked by a mailman remembers when he returns. In defense of Lewis, though, it can be replied that much behavior and learning, even with humans, is nonconscious: in driving a car, there is often no conscious thought, "I will stop at this red light"; and painful events in the past may be remembered without being perceived as "mine." That is, as Hume himself insisted, "self-consciousness" is more than simply "consciousness" and more than mere "memory," which might be built into the brain by evolution.

How much pain do animals feel? To what extent is their pain like our pain? On the ladder of evolution from, say, an amoeba to a baboon, at what point does an organism become sentient? At what point can an organism react to pain? At what point can pain be anticipated? How much "mental" pain can be experienced by fish, cats, dogs, or pigs? When can an animal remember pain as "my" pain? How can we know that an animal is experiencing pain as "mine"? Is there a difference between being sentient and being conscious? (If so, how can we know this? If we can't know, why should we use two different words?) Is there a difference between being conscious and having a mind? Is there a difference between being aware of the capacity to feel pain and being aware of a "self" as the subject of awareness? These are not simple questions; in fact, questions about pain in animals raise some of the deepest problems in philosophy of mind and lie behind many controversies about animal research.

Clearly, with regard to questions like these, philosophy of mind blends into ethics. As is discussed in Chapters 2, 5, and 9, one standard of personhood is the *cognitive criterion*, whereby certain qualities related to thought—cognition—are considered necessary for being a person. How can we apply this criterion to animals? What cognitive capacities might qualify an animal for membership in the moral community? In other words, what qualities does an animal need to count in the moral calculus? (Sentience? Consciousness? A soul?) How can we verify such capacities in a species, especially if those capacities have important ethical implications? As we consider various answers to such questions, do we have, as a species, any conflict of interest? Do we have any bias toward accepting some answers and rejecting others?

Some Trends in Contemporary Animal Research

In 2001, about 2.5 million animals were used in about 2.6 million experiments. The number of animals has dropped in half from the 1970s when twice as many were used. The number of experiments using animals has also been halved over the last

2 decades, due to stricter controls, higher standards, and better understanding of how to do more research with fewer animals.

Forty percent of experimental animals are used in basic and applied research, 26 percent in drug development, 20 percent in safety testing, 8 percent in science and medical courses, and 6 percent in other scientific programs. Animal-rights activists have tended to oppose most strongly three types of research in particular: LD-50 tests, Draize tests, and a number of famous psychological experiments on dogs and primates.

LD stands for "lethal dosage," and LD-50 tests (also called simply LD-50s) determine what amount of a substance is necessary to kill 50 of 100 animals. These tests are done routinely across species for substances ranging from soap to chemotherapies. They have been criticized as crude, blunt measures (one wry critic has said that they tell mice how much of something to take for mass suicide). Largely in response to such criticisms from nonscientists, use of LD-50s has declined 96 percent since the early 1970s; many have been replaced by LD-10s.[5]

The Draize test estimates how much certain products will irritate the human eye; the method is to drip a concentration of the product into a rabbit's eye, which is particularly sensitive. Activists have sought alternative tests using cell cultures and computer models.

Psychological experiments that have drawn severe criticism and even scorn from activists include Harlow's study of baby monkeys deprived of their mothers, and Seligman's research on "learned helplessness" in dogs and monkeys subjected to electric shocks. According to activists, not only are experiments like these extremely painful and stressful, but the results have been trivial. Many psychologists, on the other hand, regard Harlow's and Seligman's work as landmarks.

In the past 20 years, some famous philosophers who defend animal rights have been joined by a number of celebrities, including Loretta Swit, Lindsay Wagner, Clint Eastwood, and Johnny Carson. Game show host Bob Barker fought the University of Southern California Medical School over its primate research program. Other celebrities campaigning for PETA and against use of animals in medical experiments include models Kimberly Conrad Hefner and Pamela Anderson, actresses Charlize Theron and "Golden Girl" Rue McClanahan, singers Bryan Adams, Paul McCartney, Kid Rock, Moby, and Lenny Kravitz. Filmmakers have also become involved: Animal-rights issues have been taken up in movies such as *Star Trek IV* and *Project X*. Some stores now refuse to sell products tested on animals. The Body Shop, an international chain of boutiques selling cosmetics, soaps, and lotions, has demonstrated that people will alter their buying habits, if given the opportunity at a reasonable price.

ALF VS. UNIVERSITY OF PENNSYLVANIA: THE HEAD-INJURY STUDY

On Memorial Day in 1984, five members of the Animal Liberation Front (ALF) quietly entered a building of the University of Pennsylvania Medical School in Philadelphia while the school was deserted for the holiday. They went down to a subbasement and broke into a laboratory where they found—and stole—32 audiovisual tapes covering years of experiments on primates.

Everyone agrees that in stealing the tapes, these ALF members broke the law, but there is disagreement over how much other damage, if any, they did. One university official claimed that they had done $2 million worth of damage; but although *American Medical News* reported this figure prominently, no evidence was offered for the exact dollar amount. Subsequent newspaper reports omitted that claim, and it is not mentioned in the final report to the National Institutes of Health (NIH).

The stolen tapes had been made over the course of 5 years by the neurologist Thomas Gennarelli, who was conducting research that involved trying to produce exact brain damage in primates—adult monkeys and baboons. For this purpose, a device had been developed to make a reproducible model of brain injury: A live monkey or baboon, wearing a helmet, would be strapped down, and the animal's head would be subjected to terrific force at a 45-degree angle. Gennarelli had initially used monkeys in these experiments, but the studies with monkeys failed to simulate human head injuries, and as of 1980 he used baboons. All together, Gennarelli's laboratory studied this topic for over 15 years, 1970 to 1985.

There were about 60 to 80 hours of tape in all; ALF heavily edited them to produce a 25-minute segment that showed only abuses. This edited version, called *Unnecessary Fuss* (a quotation from a defender of the project who had thus described the protests), was distributed widely to television stations. It was wrenching and emotionally persuasive; as a reporter for the *New York Times* said:

> One sequence showed a monkey strapped to a table pulling against its bonds. The animal's head was encased in a steel cylinder [attached] to a pneumatic machine called an accelerator. Suddenly, a piston drove the cylinder upward, thrusting the animal's head sharply through an arc of about 60 degrees.
>
>   . . . In another sequence, as an animal lay in a coma, a researcher's recorded voice was heard saying, "You'd better have some axonal damage, monkey," and calling him "sucker."[6]

As shown on the edited tape, the researchers made derogatory and taunting remarks about the animals; these comments sounded adolescent or macho and were particularly damaging to the researchers' position. There was also a lot of profanity, unsterile surgery, and horribly sloppy care of animals. Moreover, the researchers claimed that the baboons were sedated and thus felt no pain; but, as the quotation above describes, several segments showed baboons twisting and struggling to free themselves just before the pneumatic hammer smashed their heads—another damaging point. (Thomas Langfitt, the principal investigator of the overall head-injury program and chairman of the university hospital's neurosurgery department, maintained that even though the animals moved before the tests, they had been anesthetized; his claim is hard to believe when watching the videotape.) Perhaps most repugnant to many nonscientists were several segments which showed the researchers making fun of injured baboons, holding the animals up by broken arms or laughing at conscious but brain-injured baboons. In fact, the effect of these tapes, which the researchers themselves had prepared, was more devastating than any ALF documentary could have been.

Previously, in 1983, several key members of Congress had opposed a bill to strengthen regulation of animal experiments. In September 1984, an organization called People for Ethical Treatment of Animals (PETA) showed the edited tape in two briefings on Capitol Hill; that same evening, the tape was to be shown on ABC's 20/20. During the briefings, the tape was seen by staffers of Senator Weicker and Congressman Natcher, the chairs, respectively, of the Senate and House committees responsible for the NIH budget.[7] The two chairmen and sixteen other members of Congress decided that the public would not like what it was going to see on television that night, and they sent letters to NIH demanding suspension of Gennarelli's studies.

The broadcast of the tape on 20/20 and on major television networks did indeed create a public outcry that forced Margaret Heckler, Secretary of Health and Human Services (HHS), to review the studies. Officials in Pennsylvania, however, denied that animals were being abused "gratuitously" in Gennarelli's laboratory.

In April 1985, PETA turned the stolen tapes over to NIH for review. This took place, however, only after months of negotiation between PETA and NIH. PETA had feared that NIH, which is the primary funding institute for medical research, would be biased and might suppress damaging material; NIH, for its part, had said that it would be objective but that it would not investigate the charges until it received copies of the tapes.

Meanwhile, in early 1985, the Office for Protection of Research Risks (OPRR), a branch of HHS, had appointed a committee to consider the merits of Gennarelli's research. This committee—which consisted of a neurosurgeon, a veterinary anesthesiologist, and a veterinary pathologist, all of whom used animals in research—issued its report on July 18, 1985. The members assumed that there was nothing intrinsically wrong with injuring baboons in order to study head injuries in humans and did not find fault with the scientific purpose of the experiments: "The research, as proposed, is likely to yield fruitful results for the good of society."[8] However, the committee found Gennarelli guilty of nine (of ten) charges. It noted lack of anesthesia, inadequate supervision, poor training, inferior veterinary care, unnecessary multiple injuries to the same animals, humor, smoking, "statements in poor taste" around animals, and improper clothing: "Taken collectively, these conclusions constitute material failure to comply with the Public Heath Service Animal Welfare Policy." In short, Gennarelli's lab had virtually ignored all the rules designed to protect animals, and the university had developed no mechanism at all to ensure that such rules were followed.

On the same day as the committee's report was released, Margaret Heckler (who had presumably obtained a preview of its conclusions) suspended Gennarelli's research. This was the first time a lab had been closed because of abuse of animals. To Carolyn Compton—a physician, pediatric researcher, and spokeswoman for scientists using animals—the closing was a "tragedy."[9] To ALF, on the other hand, Heckler's decision, and the break-in that led to it, represented a momentous victory. Much of the public and the press, including even the conservative columnist James Kilpatrick,[10] had reacted indignantly to the tapes. As one member of the break-in team (identified only as "Lauren") said at the outset:

> We may seem like radicals to you. But we are like the Abolitionists, who were regarded as radicals, too. And we hope that 100 years from now, people will look back on the way animals are treated now with the same horror as we do when we look back on the slave trade.[11]

Violence against animal researchers continues. In 1997 19-year-old Josh Ellerman was convicted of exploding five bombs at a fur farm in Utah. The same year, the ALF claimed responsibility for burning a slaughter plant in Redland, Oregon. ALF claimed responsibility for burning or firebombing facilities in Olympia, Washington (1998), University of Minnesota (1999), Plymouth, Wisconsin (1999), and at the Rancho Veal Corporation in I Petaluma, California (2000). They also raided research facilities in Orange, California, in 1999 and Stanwood, Washington, in 2000, taking away rabbits and dogs being used in research.

OTHER ALF TARGETS

Six weeks after its Memorial Day raid, ALF struck again at the University of Pennsylvania, this time "liberating" three cats, two dogs, and eight pigeons from the veterinary school. The dean of the veterinary school said that the raid "would set back research efforts, including a study to determine the cause of sudden infant death syndrome."[12] An associate dean said that the stolen cats were being used in studies of breathing during sleep, that one missing dog had a steel plate inserted to study osteoarthritis, that another was being studied for ear-canal infections, and that the pigeons were part of a study of broken bones intended to benefit all birds.[13] With regard to the dogs, he also said that the work would benefit other dogs, adding that it had to be done and that more dogs would end up having to be used as subjects.

In December 1984, ALF struck in California. Two rabbits injected with oral herpes and numerous dogs with cancer were taken, along with 100 other animals, from City of Hope National Medical Center in Duarte. ALF members painted a sign in the lab there: "ALF IS WATCHING AND THERE'S NO PLACE TO HIDE!" Ingrid Newkirk of PETA called City of Hope a "concentration camp" where animals were "being used for painful experiments."[14] The associate director of City of Hope said that the theft of these animals had disrupted $500,000 worth of research on emphysema, cancer, and herpes. In this case, ALF had targeted a study testing tobacco carcinogens in dogs. The associate director refused to comment on whether the abducted animals had been treated cruelly but did say that 36 cancerous dogs, 12 cats, 12 rabbits, 28 mice, and 18 rats had been stolen and added, "We're concerned that very important research work may not now be completed."[15]

In April 1985, in what was its largest animal raid to date, ALF hit the biology and psychology laboratories of the University of California, Riverside. In this raid, 467 animals were taken, including a stump-tailed macaque whose eyes had been sewn shut to study a device to help the blind navigate. PETA charged that these animals had been used in painful, unnecessary experiments, some involving starvation; NIH investigated the charges but found no evidence of abuse. The university claimed that $683,000 in damages had occurred, as well as lost research.

In April 1987, an arson fire gutted the $2.5 million veterinary research animal lab at the University of California, Davis; ALF claimed responsibility.

The Taub Case

Alex Pacheco, the president of PETA, in May 1981, volunteered to work in the primate lab of the psychologist Edward Taub in Silver Spring, Maryland. Pacheco told Taub that he wanted to become a research scientist and needed experience, but his actual intention was to videotape Taub's research on animals for PETA.[16] Taub was studying "somato-sensory deafferentation" in monkeys by surgically cutting all the nerves in one limb and then trying to stimulate regrowth. His hypothesis was that some of the damage was due to "learned helplessness," and the research was intended to benefit the half-million Americans who are disabled by strokes each year. Pacheco entered the lab late one night with an accomplice and succeeded in photographing experiments; as a result, Taub was tried in Maryland on charges of cruelty to animals and was convicted on one charge (failing to provide adequate veterinary care).

The tactics used by PETA in the Taub case were controversial. To obtain evidence for the trial, Alex Pacheco invited activists such as Donald Barnes, John McArdle, and Michael W. Fox to search Taub's lab at night; when warrants were served on Taub shortly thereafter, several television stations recorded the event while PETA leaders distributed press releases outside. During the trial itself, each element seemed to have been orchestrated for the maximum emotional impact in the media—with the predictable result that the media portrayed Taub as another Josef Mengele and PETA as the animals' Robin Hood.

As noted earlier, Taub was convicted of one charge—failing to provide proper veterinary care—which had been based on the fact that he did not bandage the animals' wounds. Taub testified that it was better to leave the wounds unbandaged because many years of experience had showed him that the monkeys would only bite and claw the bandages off, making their wounds worse. Veterinarians could not agree on whether or not Taub was right about this; but eventually Taub was exonerated of any failure to provide adequate veterinary care by the American Psychological Association's Ethics Committee, by the NIH (after his appeal), and by an ad hoc committee of the American Physiological Society. After their own investigation of the charges, the medical school and psychology department at the University of Alabama at Birmingham hired him as a full professor.

In 1991, according to the "story of the year" for ethics in *Discover*, four of Taub's monkeys showed:

> dramatic new evidence of the adult brain's capacity to "rewire" itself, something previously thought to be impossible. And ironically, it was PETA's success at keeping the monkeys away from research for a decade that made the discovery possible.[17]

The 15 surviving monkeys had been transferred in 1986 to the federally funded Tulane Regional Primate Center in Covington, Louisiana. In 1990, in an experiment that PETA opposed, a brain researcher—Timothy Pons—tested Taub's hypothesis by examining the brain of a dying monkey before euthanization. Pons was "flabbergasted" to discover that "the entire patch of the cortex corresponding to the arm—about half an inch wide—had been rewired to receive input from the face." Pons concluded, excitedly, "The results offer hope that the brain can be coaxed into rewiring itself after injury." Data from other monkeys in the study later supported this finding.

In 1997, Professor Taub received the William James Fellow award, the highest honor given by the American Psychological Society (a society of researchers in psychology, not to be confused with the American Psychological Association). His research on learned helplessness has helped to show that, following neurological injury, adult mammals can undergo some cortical reorganization, explaining some aspects of phantom limb pain and many cases of tinnitus.

Breakthrough

CNN and ABC News reported in the summer of 2001 that all stroke patients using Professor Taub's Constraint-Induced Movement Therapy, or CI therapy, improved in function. For an affected arm, 30 percent of patients gain close to normal use.[18]

Professor Taub's treatment builds directly on two of the most criticized experiments on animals in psychology: Martin Seligman's experiments on dogs demonstrating learned helplessness and 20 years of Taub's work on monkeys.

A more controversial part of the research is the claim that the brain has the capacity to reorganize after stroke. Some people think that CI therapy jump-starts self-repair of surviving, healthy cells by the brain and spinal cord. CI therapy tries to "wake up cells that have been stunned," says Taub.[19]

"Right after a stroke, a limb is paralyzed," he says. "Whenever the person tries to move an arm, it simply doesn't work." But often the cells that represent the arm are still alive. Unfortunately, the patient assumes the arm is permanently dead, expects failure from trying to use it, and does not. "We call it learned nonuse," Taub says. The more the patient relies on the good arm, the less likely recovery becomes in the bad arm.

Timing is critical. Immediately after a stroke, if movement is induced in the bad limb, damage increases to the brain. But in the second or third week, therapy can begin.

Requiring scarce rehabilitation therapists trained in the new techniques, the therapy goes 6–7 hours every weekday for two weeks. Patients move around with good limbs tightly bandaged. Because of lack of therapists and space, and with little publicity, most patients seeking the new treatment cannot be accommodated.

To begin to meet the demand, in 2001 UAB opened the Taub Clinic for CI therapy. Although neither private insurance nor Medicare pays for the costs, which run $6,000 to $13,000, over 5,000 stroke patients are on the waiting list. Demand for therapy has also created ethical problems similar to that of Seattle's "God Committee," which struggled about how to allocate scarce, life-saving hemodialysis machines in 1962 (see Chapter 14).

ETHICAL ISSUES: FROM SPECIESISM TO SCIENTIFIC MERIT

Ethical Theory

Before 1975, "animal welfare" groups focused simply on humane treatment of research animals. Until recently, however, most scientists dismissed such groups as "little old ladies" and portrayed them as antiprogress; and such dismissals have pushed reformers toward more radical theoretical positions.

Singer: Speciesism and Utilitarianism   In 1975, the Australian philosopher Peter Singer published *Animal Liberation,* in which he argued that animals must morally count for something.[20] To say that animals do not count because they are somehow inferior, Singer held, is like saying that slaves or women do not count; and just as racism and sexism are evil, so is *speciesism.* According to Singer, every argument that supports equal rights for minorities and women—without begging any questions—also supports animal rights. If our moral concern for children, women, and minorities is based on their sensitivity to pain, family ties, and ability to reason, why wouldn't these factors also be a basis for concern for animals? Such arguments put speciesists on the defensive: if the principle of equality applies to all people, despite their obvious differences in ability and intelligence, why shouldn't it also apply to animals?

Singer also argued that a medical experiment using animal subjects must be speciesist unless humans would be willing to substitute irreversibly comatose human subjects. This is an interesting approach. Most people who accept the idea of using, say, a chimpanzee in medical research would cringe at the idea of using an anencephalic baby (an infant born lacking most of the brain). But if the chimpanzee is active, gregarious, sensitive, and responsive whereas the anencephalic baby is hopelessly mute, comatose, and unresponsive, why should the chimp be the victim? If the answer is simply that the baby is human and the chimp nonhuman, Singer would consider the answer speciesist.

In addition to his argument about speciesism, Singer also used *utilitarian* reasoning—the same kind of secular, results-oriented moral premises that scientists use to defend their research. According to utilitarian ethical theory, right acts produce the greatest good for the greatest number; for instance, research on presently sick patients would be right if it would help a greater number of future patients. Stipulating that the "greatest number" must refer only to humans begs the key question, Singer maintained; and once animals count for something, however small, in utilitarian reasoning, radical conclusions follow: experiments that inflict horrible pain on many animals cannot be justified on the ground that they save a few human lives. Actually, the founder of utilitarianism, Jeremy Bentham, argued during the nineteenth century that animals' suffering should count in the moral calculus; he held that the important question was not whether animals could reason, but whether they could *suffer.* Ingrid Newkirk, the British-born leader of PETA, reasons similarly: "When it comes to suffering, a rat is a pig is a dog is a boy."[21]

Singer's position is open to some of the theoretical and practical objections to utilitarianism in general. For instance, consistent application of utilitarianism would apparently obligate individuals to make great sacrifices to help victims of famine, improve the lives of future generations, and relieve the suffering of animals. It would require a parent, for instance, to donate money for famine relief rather than use that money to send a son or daughter to college: Since many lives can be saved by giving $100,000 to CARE, and since $100,000 would pay for the college education of only one child—who does not, moreover, need college to survive or even to be happy—a utilitarian parent could not consider it justifiable to pay for a college education. Philosophers such as Susan Wolf have therefore argued that although utilitarianism may be a model of moral perfection, it "does not constitute a model of personal well-being toward which it would be particularly good or desirable for a rational human being to strive."[22] To put this another way, consistent utilitarianism requires saintly conduct and total devotion to a higher moral goal, but that would conflict with lesser goals, some of which are outside the sphere of morality—goals like mastering medicine or tennis, reading the great novels, or sending a child to college. To put it still another way, should morality ever require us to choose between family and humanity?

In a sense, this kind of argument against utilitarianism is a *reductio ad absurdum:* the premise "We should act to achieve the greatest good for the greatest number" is said to lead to the absurd or unacceptable conclusion "It is wrong for parents to pay for their children's college education." In the context of animal rights, such an argument would take a premise like "Animals should count in calculations of the greatest good for the greatest number" to an absurd conclusion, such as "A few human lives must be sacrificed to save the lives of many dogs." These conclusions, it is held, are absurd or unacceptable because of what they imply about the scope of utilitarianism. For people who argue this way, utilitarianism does not satisfactorily answer the question, "What is morality *for?*" For them, morality must first consider obligations to an "inner circle"—family, colleagues, friends, etc.— even if fulfilling obligations to those in the inner circle does not contribute to "the greatest good for the greatest number." In the context of animal rights, then, the human species might be represented in the "inner circle."

However, not everyone accepts reductios as conclusive arguments against utilitarianism, for at least two reasons. First, it may be contended that a given utilitarian premise does not necessarily lead to a particular absurd conclusion; second, people may disagree on whether or not a particular conclusion is indeed "absurd" or "unacceptable." For instance, it can be argued, in defense of utilitarianism, that an ethical theory which requires a very high standard of conduct may seem to lead to certain absurd or unacceptable conclusions, but that this result is only apparent: The standard may in practice be unattainable, or virtually unattainable, but it is still valuable as a standard. To take one example, early Christianity defined right conduct in a way that essentially required saintliness—"Turn the other cheek," "Go and sell what thou hast, and give to the poor," and so on—but these precepts are nevertheless valued as ideals.

It can be seen that this debate is partly about hypocrisy. Is it hypocritical to profess an ideal such as utilitarianism or early Christianity but not to practice it consistently in actual life? Probably, most people would agree that professing an ideal and not acting on it at all, or not even trying to act on it, is hypocritical. But is it really hypocritical to act on a professed ideal to some extent while taking practical considerations into account—considerations such as the formation of family ties, the inevitability of human weaknesses, and the existence of personal or nonmoral areas of life? Many people would not call that compromise *hypocrisy*, and probably many people do in fact make such a practical compromise in their general approach to living. Still, to a purist a compromise like this is awkward: It seems to amount to saying that starving people or suffering animals are important only intermittently or fractionally—that they are "worth" only one morning a week, for instance, or only 10 percent of one's income. (Hypocrisy is discussed again later, with regard to ad hominem arguments and testimonials.)

Regan: Animal Rights   Underlying the controversy over Gennarelli's experimentation on primates is a more basic issue: whether scientific research on animals is ever justified. Tom Regan, an American philosopher and animal-rights activist, thinks not:

> I argue that the whole system of animal experimentation [and] the whole system of commercial and sport trapping and hunting are morally bankrupt institutions. The only way you change these things fundamentally is by eliminating them—in much the same way as with slavery and child labor.[23]

Regan argues that human beings have rights because they *have a life.* That is, humans have lives that can go better or worse for them, and this is true for each human being independently of whether or not others value him or her. In other words, people have inherent, not instrumental, value. Peter Singer, as we have just seen, applies utilitarianism to animals as well as to humans; Regan, analogously, applies to animals as well as humans the rights-based idea of treating each life as an "end in itself." Regan maintains that many species of animals, like humans, have lives that can go better or worse for them, and he draws this crucial inference: "They too have a distinctive kind of value in their own right, if we do; therefore, they too have a right not to be treated in ways that fail to respect this value."[24] Regan reasons that if humans "count" in the moral calculus because they possess a certain quality, and if animals possess the same quality, then it is inconsistent not to count animals equally. Anyone who wants to argue that there is some difference here must bear the onus of proving why.

Regan's critics say that his argument runs several unjustified inferences together. First, they ask, if any being (human or nonhuman) has a life that can go better or worse, does that fact give every life a distinctive value? Second, and more important, does "having a life" really give animals a value equal to that of humans? Can't human lives go "better or worse" in more complex ways than lives of cows and rabbits? Note, however, that Regan is careful to include a qualification: He says that animals (like humans) have lives which can go better or worse *for them.* His reasoning is that with this qualification, no real comparison is possible between human and animal lives. If fish in an aquarium "have a life" that can go better or worse *for them,* from that standpoint the fishes' lives become as important as human lives.

Of course, simply being clear about the terms or conditions of Regan's argument does not settle the matter, since his position is in fact extremely controversial. Many animal-rights activists agree with him, and some are even more radical;

Ingrid Newkirk of PETA, for instance, holds that any experiment which does not treat animals and humans equally is speciesist; thus, sacrificing an animal to save a human would not be justifiable. John McArdle, a scientist, also agrees. Suppose that either a dog or a man but not both can remain in a lifeboat: Regan implies that because "animals aren't there to be used as our resources," it is morally wrong to kill the dog to save the man, and McArdle concurs—"I would seriously have to question whether I would allow an animal to die just to protect me."[25] On the other hand, the pediatric researcher Carolyn Compton disagrees: "I love animals, but there's no question in my mind that if I were able to sacrifice an animal life to save a human being, I would do it."[26]

Cohen and Frey: A Pro-Human Approach   Some opponents of the animal-rights movement take the position that the scope of morality should not be expanded to animals. Their reasoning is somewhat similar to the argument that abortion is permissible because the scope of morality cannot be expanded to embryos or early fetuses.

The philosopher Carl Cohen, who teaches at a medical school, defends the use of animals in biomedical research by arguing that animals cannot share in the human community. In an article in *New England Journal of Medicine,* Cohen said:

> Notwithstanding all such complications, this much is clear about rights in general: they are in every case claims, or potential claims, within a community of moral agents. Rights arise, and can be intelligently defended, only among beings who actually do, or can, make moral claims against one another.[27]

For Cohen, animals cannot make moral claims and thus have no rights. He rejects the analogy between racism, sexism, and speciesism: Although racism and sexism are indeed bad, he maintains, speciesism is not. "I am a speciesist," he declares, and he adds, "Speciesism is not merely plausible; it is essential for right conduct, because those who will not make the morally relevant distinctions among species are almost certain, in consequence, to misapprehend their true obligations."

Another philosopher, Raymond Frey, argues that the concept of "animal rights" uselessly adds to the confusion in a moral terrain which is already muddled enough. Tom Regan, as we've seen, holds that animals possess rights simply by coming into existence and being the sort of creatures they are. Frey, however, argues that:

> In the case of intrinsic or fundamental, unacquired moral rights . . . what grip we had on rights has, I think, been lost. Rather, we are at sea in a tide of theoretical claims and counter-claims, with no fixed point by which to steer.[28]

What are the appropriate boundaries of the "moral community"? This is a difficult question, especially if we are trying to develop and apply consistently a reasonable interpretation of the cognitive criterion of personhood. It is interesting to note that many advocates of animal rights are also advocates of parental choice with regard to abortion and forgoing treatment in "Baby Doe" cases; for this reason, people who oppose abortion and nontreatment of impaired newborns charge that animal-rights advocates value animals more than humans. (One student wrote a paper comparing the views of an animal-rights philosopher on abortion and animal research, entitling it, "I'd Rather Be His Pet.") It is also argued that expanding the circle of moral concern to include animals while contracting it to exclude human fetuses and impaired neonates is rather odd. In reply, it can be pointed out that whether moral concern should expand or contract with regard to a particular issue depends on the characteristics of the beings in question (sensitivity to pain, awareness, sociability, etc.); it does not depend on membership in a species.

Testimonials and Ad Hominem Arguments

In informal logic, one common fallacy is what is called an *ad hominem* appeal. *Ad hominem* literally means "to the man"; in an argument, the term means an inappropriate personal reference. For example, in a debate during the presidential campaign of 1988, a reporter made an ad hominem attack on Michael Dukakis, asking whether Dukakis (who was opposed to capital punishment) would want a man who had raped and killed his wife to be executed. Dukakis tried to respond logically, but since the question was based on emotion rather than reason, he was not very successful. In a formal debate, which is a purely intellectual exercise (unlike a presidential debate, which is supposed to be informational), one effective reply would be to point out that the question was not pertinent and had been asked to elicit an inappropriate response; another appropriate and effective counterthrust would itself be emotional, an expression of outrage—"I'd kill the bastard with my own hands." The point here, however, is not how a member of a debating team might deal with an ad hominem argument: For our purposes, the important point is that such an argument is a logical error. Thus it can be held that our position on a moral issue should be affected only by the strength of the arguments, not by the emotional impact of answers to personal questions.

In fact, the debate on experimentation with animals has been characterized by ad hominem appeals, which sometimes take the form of *testimonials:* The personal behavior of commentators is often cited, and the specific issue of experimentation is often placed in a wider context. Many animal-rights activists, for instance, mention that they themselves are vegetarians; and both Peter Singer and Tom Regan criticize circuses, factory farming, eating meat, hunting for sport, and wearing furs, and urge others to avoid these practices.

Intuitively, it may seem that an argument by a philosopher—or anyone else—gains greater force when he or she not only argues for acting in a certain way but also does act that way. On reflection, however, it is unclear why ad hominem appeals and testimonials should carry much, if any, weight. In popular culture, of course, such appeals do influence behavior, but their role in rational argument is more questionable.

Consider that once the door is opened for appeals to personal life, many things can walk through. At one conference about animal rights, the English philosopher Stephen Clark chided his audience for feeding meat to pet cats and dogs. At this same conference, some animal-rights activists followed Albert Schweitzer in revering all life and killing nothing, and some emphasized ecological purity, opposing extinction of any species; they themselves, of course, did not hunt. Some people at the conference were vegetarians; some were "vegans"—eating no animal products, not even eggs (from "captive" chickens). Some refused to buy any animal products at all. Some regarded zoos as demeaning to animals and refused to take their children to such places. The most radical people at the conference condemned even pet ownership; Ingrid Newkirk of PETA described the life of pets as an "absolutely abysmal situation brought about by human manipulation."[29]

Leaving aside the personal danger of developing a "holier than thou" attitude—and the practical consideration that such an attitude is unlikely to win many friends for one's moral position—how legitimate are such testimonials? If they are offered, is it legitimate to argue that they are irrelevant? And on the other hand, is it legitimate for opponents of animal rights to demand them? Scientists, for instance, often ask whether critics of animal experiments are vegetarians; if those critics turn out to be meat eaters, the scientists stand ready to accuse them of hypocrisy.

In this regard, it seems useful to distinguish between our evaluation of *arguments* and our evaluation of *people*. In an argument, it is not always correct or appropriate to ask about personal behavior; when we make ethical judgments about people, however, it is certainly relevant to consider their actual behavior as well as their arguments. If we hear someone decry exploitation of the poor and then discover that this person is a slumlord, we will probably decide that he or she is a hypocrite; on the other hand, this does *not* mean that we ourselves must decide to advocate exploiting poor people. In other words, an argument offered by a hypocrite is not for that reason alone necessarily a poor argument. By the same token, it is true that most activists for animals do not eat "animal flesh," and this may make us respect these advocates as sincere—but respecting someone's sincerity need not necessarily lead us to accept his or her conclusion. When we evaluate *individuals*, then, inquiries into personal behavior are sometimes appropriate; and it soon becomes obvious that because espousing morality is far easier than practicing it, hypocrisy abounds in life. But whether we encounter hypocrisy or sincerity, we need to be able to disregard it in considering an *argument*.

Scientific Merit

Assessing Basic Research   The scientific merit of Thomas Gennarelli's research with primates—a specific issue that will be further discussed—can be put into perspective by considering the extent of *basic research* and why it is valuable. Scientific research might be compared to an iceberg. The results or findings that will be applicable to humans are the tip of the iceberg, visible above the water. This small tip is supported by the much larger part of the iceberg, the part that is invisible under the water; that large invisible portion consists of basic research that goes on quietly in labs and is rarely discussed in national media.

Many animals are used in basic research—far more than most people could possibly guess. For every practical success in human medicine, such as cyclosporin or knee replacement, there are perhaps a dozen failures in studies with human subjects and a hundred failures in studies with animal subjects. To arrive at each success, then, hundreds or thousands of animals are used as "guinea pigs." In the United States alone, there are nearly 130 medical schools and a dozen or so pharmaceutical and research institutions using millions of animals each year—mostly rats and mice, but also dogs, pigs, cats, rabbits, and primates. (Worldwide, of course—in Germany, France, Switzerland, Japan, Canada, and Australia, for instance—scientists also use great numbers of animals.) In one year, 1983, a single institution, the Charles River Breeding Laboratories (called the "General Motors" of the American animal breeding industry), produced 10 million animals destined to be research subjects.

At what point, if anywhere, can we draw a line between basic experimentation on animals that is "useful" or "necessary" (and thus, arguably, acceptable) and "useless" or "unnecessary" experimentation? This is a difficult problem. Few people would advocate stopping basic research that offers direct clinical benefits to humans, and few would even recommend stopping research that offers indirect benefits. What most critics want to stop is "trivial" or "repetitive" research, but when these critics cite specific examples (Harlow's research on maternal deprivation in monkeys, say, or Seligman's research on "learned helplessness" in dogs), the researchers often staunchly defend the importance of the work. If all basic research were stopped, medical progress would also stop. On the other hand, if no basic research can be stopped, animal experimentation would simply proceed as it has always proceeded.

"Stopping" research typically takes the form of cutting off funding, and one suggestion has been that only "worthwhile" research should be funded. This sounds reasonable, but actually deciding what is "worthwhile" is very difficult.[30] In practice, this decision is the job of NIH committees of peer reviewers who consider applications for grants. These reviewers are experts, and if they knew in advance exactly which projects were "worthwhile," they would fund only those—but of course they don't know in advance. Sometimes an apparently insignificant project can yield important results, and sometimes an apparently important project can yield little or nothing of value.

At bottom, researchers have faith that the costs of basic studies—in terms of money, effort, time, and the suffering of animals—will one day be outweighed by benefits. At bottom, animal activists are skeptics who doubt or deny that the benefits to humans outweigh the costs to animals.

Assessing the Philadelphia Study   Assessment of Gennarelli's research with primates has involved not only the scientific merit of the project itself but also the treatment of animals by the researchers. These are separate issues, though it can be argued that they are related.

Let's first consider some commentary on the value of this research as such. A peer committee reviewing Gennarelli's grant said that his research would contribute information about the effectiveness of a drug called *mannitol* in reducing brain swelling after trauma, and about management of metabolic balance in comatose patients. Later, the university's own investigator, Thomas Langfitt, claimed that Gennarelli's research had provided the first evidence that regeneration of damaged nerve cells (the great hope of patients paralyzed by spinal cord injuries) may be possible.[31]

On the other hand, critics called these justifications *ad hoc*—simply a way to paper over a lack of real findings. Nedim Buyukmichi, an activist and veterinarian, argued that Gennarelli's studies were too inconsistent to result in a reproducible model of head injuries and too limited in scope to adequately mimic injuries sustained by human victims of accidents: "After 15 years and $11 million to $13 million, essentially nothing has come out of this research that hasn't already been known from studies of human head trauma."[32] Other critics were unimpressed by the purported findings about regeneration of nerve cells, comparing that claim to the ubiquitous trumpeting of "possible" cures for cancer and AIDS.

Interestingly—even amazingly—in all the commentary on Gennarelli's studies, no one on either side has specifically attacked or defended the hypothesis of his research. The explanation may be that it is unclear whether Gennarelli actually had a hypothesis; he seems to have had no goal other than creating one exact injury in one baboon after another.

Lack of a hypothesis might not necessarily imply that Gennarelli's research was valueless, however. Gennarelli can be described as working at the bottom of a pyramid of basic research on head injury. To him, it may have seemed obvious that the first step in such research would be to produce one head injury precisely and reliably, so that it could be replicated and studied by others. Scientists point out, for example, that knowing how to produce different kinds of burns in animals is the first step in studying the physiology of burns and the metabolism of healing. On the other side, animal activists held that Gennarelli had merely bashed primates' heads for a decade without getting anywhere. They argued that even if he had succeeded in devising a reproducible model of head injuries, such a model would offer little help in actually treating such injuries (an argument that scientists have denied).

A separate issue, as noted before, has to do with Gennarelli's treatment of his animal subjects. In turn, this issue itself has two aspects. First, there is the question of how badly or insensitively the animals were treated. Some of Gennarelli's defenders have said that the apparently insensitive comments and behavior of researchers on the tapes were comparable to the type of cynical humor typical among medical residents; also, as noted before, the university's investigator, Langfitt, said that the animals had been anesthetized. Both of these arguments, of course, have been attacked; and neither of them seems very convincing in light of what the tapes show. Activists argue, further, that the researchers were pursing lucrative grants and professional prestige and may therefore have been blinded to their own insensitivity, and to their subjects' plight, by a conflict of interest.

The second question is this: If the animals were indeed mistreated and the researchers were insensitive, does that necessarily affect the scientific value of the research? In other words, could researchers conduct an excellent project even though they mistreated their subjects? For animal activists, Gennarelli's treatment of his animal subjects in itself proved that his project was immoral and thus unjustifiable. Were they right? Can the scientific value or merit of a study be assessed independently of the researchers' behavior?

Before we leave this question, it is relevant to note that many animal researchers say they treat animal subjects with great respect. Since laboratories are now closed to the public, this is hard to verify. However, reports from some students who work as aides in such labs—and some videotapes like Gennarelli's—indicate that these researchers' claim is at least sometimes false.

Ends and Means: Civil Disobedience and Other Tactics

Tactics for stopping experimentation on animals or shutting down abortion clinics are often debated. One question in this debate is whether illegal, unsavory, or even immoral tactics should be used to attain a higher goal. Does the end justify the means?

In discussions of the strategies of animal-rights activists, the terms *civil disobedience* and *terrorism* are often used. It seems important to distinguish between these two concepts. Civil disobedience—as associated with figures like Ghandi in India and organizations like the Southern Christian Leadership Conference in the United States—involves public but nonviolent violations of the law, for the purpose of protesting policies regarded as evil. According to the philosopher John Rawls (who has developed a famous theory of justice), civil disobedience is *not* terrorism if three conditions are met: (1) It must be public, with the protesters clearly identified (the protesters do not conceal themselves under white sheets). (2) It must be nonviolent (the protesters hurt no one; no innocent bystanders are injured or killed). (3) The protesters must accept the legal consequences of their actions (for instance, children actually went to jail in Birmingham, Alabama, during the "children's crusade"). (4) Protesters break a law only after trying to change the law by all possible legal means. The other side of this coin is that activities which do not meet these criteria *are* considered terrorism; and the point of the distinction is that civil disobedience is justified whereas terrorism is not. According to Rawls's criteria, then, many acts of the antiabortion group Operation Rescue would be justified civil disobedience, and some acts of animal-rights activists—especially in England—would be unjustified terrorism.

Let's consider a few examples of specific tactics involving illegality. In England, the Animals Rights Militia planted bombs outside the homes of four animal researchers as a warning and then alerted the police by telephone; no one was injured. Hunt Saboteur, the most radical English group, has bombed meat-packing factories and butcher shops and has strung metal wires as booby traps for fox hunters; Marley Jones, one of the leaders of Hunt Saboteur, has said:

> In Britain we [animal activists] tend to think that most types of actions [which prevent cruelty to animals], short of killing someone, are morally justified. Physical violence, in my opinion, is justified as a last resort, if all appeals to reason fail and there is no other way to save the animals.[33]

In late 1988, four bombs were set off outside English department stores, including Harrods, to protest the sale of furs; a columnist for the *Times* of London commented vehemently:

> Of all the Single Issue fanatics who increasingly infest our society, with their conviction that nothing matters beside their particular cause and that any action, however violent, dangerous, or criminal, is justified in the pursuit of it, the most monomaniacal are those who claim to defend "animal rights."[34]

Here are some examples from the United States. In California in 1988, ALF destroyed a new building for animal research at the medical school in San Diego and burned down a veal-packing plant in Oakland; masked ALF spokespersons took credit for these attacks in televised interviews, vowing to continue them "until the killing of the innocent animals stops." That same year, in Connecticut, a bomb was planted by Stephanie Trutt outside a company that made surgical staples and used animals to train surgeons in handling them; she was arrested for attempted murder.[35] (Access to American medical schools at night and on weekends was once fairly easy, but as a result of such activities, that has changed: New security systems have been installed, allowing entry only to people with specific authorization.)

Some tactics of animal-rights activists, though legal, are ignoble; like the illegal tactics, these are held to be justified by higher ends. In the controversy over abortion, a former priest named Joseph Scheidler at one time urged antiabortionists to infiltrate and spy on pro-choice groups.

Tactics similar to Alex Pacheco's in the Taub case were also advocated by Donald Barnes, a former Air Force psychologist whose radiation experiments on primates were portrayed in the movie *Project X*.[36] Barnes is an example of a leader who has abruptly switched sides on a moral issue.[37]

Another legal but ignoble strategy is deliberately shoddy or unfair argumentation. Barnes, for example, recommends tricks such as monopolizing all the time in a debate, working up an audience's passions before actually appearing, refusing to talk to researchers in private, and flattering reporters. He urges animal-rights activists not to discuss whether a particular experiment is good science or offers benefits: "As much as possible, avoid getting caught up in 'scientific' arguments which you can't win. Beat a hasty retreat to philosophy and brandish your weapons: Tom Regan's *The Case for Animal Rights* and Peter Singer's *Animal Liberation*." He also says, "Bear in mind that the only rationale for using nonhuman animals in research is that, 'The end justifies the means'" (an especially interesting comment when we consider that he presumably considers his own ends as justifying his own means). Tactics like Barnes's, of course, are not confined to the issue of animal rights: Many leaders of many causes resort to unfair arguments and appeal to our emotions instead of using logic and solid evidence.

The Enemy and the "Algeria Syndrome"

One question about animal rights is, "Who is the enemy?" Answers to that question lead us to some significant considerations, including a phenomenon that can be called the *Algeria syndrome.*

To animal-rights activists, of course, animal researchers are the "enemy"—and vice versa. In this regard, however, it is interesting to realize that the activists and the scientists actually have much in common. For instance, subscribers to leading animal-rights magazines are overwhelmingly white, are mostly nonreligious (65 percent are agnostics or atheists), and tend to hold managerial and professional positions; 84 percent are college-educated; 25 percent have MA and PhD degrees.[38] Subscribers to *Physiologist* are overwhelmingly white, are not very religious, and hold academic and professional positions; most of them have PhDs.[39]

Though science and scientists have been condemned by officialdom or the public at various times in the past (Galileo and Darwin are famous examples), modern researchers have not been accustomed to being seen as an "enemy"; in fact, until quite recently they occupied rather high moral ground, at least among educated people. Today, scientists find themselves accused of irrationality, bias, conflicts of interest, money-grubbing, and even ignorance; with regard to animal rights, they are accused of inflicting pain on animals without guiding hypotheses or controls and for trivial purposes, such as proving what is already obvious. Moreover, most scientists adopted a siege mentality and resisted reforms.

It should be noted, though, that with respect to animals in research today, television and the print media present some contradictory images. On the one hand, there are accounts of "miraculous" research breakthroughs which would have been impossible without using animals; on the other hand, there are also accounts of researchers who abuse animals, and in these stories a stereotype of the "mad scientist"—a Frankenstein or a callous torturer—is frequently implied.

Are scientists really *the* enemy? Are they the only problem or even the primary problem in the issue of animal rights? Scientists are rather remote from nonscientists, and "science" is a rather abstract concept for most of us; and it is often easier to attack what is far away and abstract than to confront what is nearby and concrete. We might call this the *Algeria syndrome*. It is somehow easier to take a position against the specter of "research on animals" than to take a position against, say, our own neighbors who do not spay or neuter their pets. This point is worth considering here.

In the United States alone, 22 million dogs and cats are abandoned, killed, or lost each year by owners who fail to make adequate provisions for their care.[40] Many of these owners will simply replace the lost animal with a new pet, as if it were no big deal. At the same time, only about 180,000 dogs and 50,000 cats were used in medical research, and almost all of the dogs would have died anyway in pounds. In fact, for every dog used in medical experiments, perhaps 100 dogs kept as pets will die because of neglect by their owners. Who is the "enemy": a scientist who uses five dogs in seven years, or our own neighbor whose cat gives birth to unwanted litters of kittens? For utilitarians—and for anyone even slightly sympathetic to utilitarianism—numbers like these should count for something. We fall victim to the Algeria syndrome when we attack the abstract target of "Frankensteins" but do nothing to change the situation next door.

UPDATE

Organizational Responses: IACUCs, Foundation for Biomedical Research, PETA

Several experiments reviewed by NIH in the 1980s fared poorly. Among these were studies at City of Hope Medical Center in Duarte, California, which was fined $25,000, lost $1 million in grants, and also lost its Animal Care Assurance, a semi-legal document in which an institution promises to abide by federal regulations. Columbia University lost all its grants involving vertebrates after ALF released pictures of poor lab conditions and inspectors made an unannounced visit.

In 1986, as a result of such abuses—and Gennarelli's—Congress established Institutional Animal Care and Use Committees (IACUCs) for all institutions receiving federal funds for research on animals. These committees try to reduce the number of animals involved in experiments and the amount of pain to which research animals will be subjected; they also try to have lower species used rather than higher species. Although IACUCs are composed mostly of researchers themselves (not laypeople), they do force experimenters at least to justify their projects to fellow scientists—some of whom can be critical at times. Since the existence of IACUCs is directly attributable to the exposure of Gennarelli's experiments, his work can be called the Tuskegee study of animal research (see Chapter 10).

Animal activists see IACUCs as window dressing and insist that the committees do little real good. They also say that the Department of Agriculture, which is responsible for inspecting labs, has had a traditionally cozy relationship with animal-abusing agribusiness. They emphasize that veterinarians on IACUCs are caught in the middle, charged with protecting animals but salaried by the researchers.

During the 1980s, faced with what they perceived as devastating losses in public confidence, scientists decided that they could no longer ignore animal-rights activists. Accordingly, they established the Foundation for Biomedical Research, which lobbies for 350 universities, drug companies, manufacturers of medical devices, and commercial animal-supply companies. The foundation has a paid staff member in most states that have research institutions; it also maintains many lobbyists in Washington, DC, to counter the equally numerous lobbyists of PETA.

People for the Ethical Treatment of Animals (PETA) is estimated to have 350,000 members and $5 million in annual income. It supported Bill Clinton during his campaign for President and was allowed to sponsor one of his inaugural balls, at which naked bartenders of both sexes wore signs proclaiming, "I'd rather wear nothing than fur."

Claims of benefit from Gennarelli's studies were *never* proven. Gennarelli is back to studying head injuries in mammals—this time with pigs.[41]

Today, scientists are vying with animal-rights activists for young minds through extensive educational outreach programs. The Foundation for Biomedical Research sponsors talks by scientists for science majors, medical students, and graduate students about the necessity of using animals in research. A group called Putting People First was started by Kathleen Marquardt in 1992 after a one-sided presentation by a PETA spokesperson in her daughter's elementary school,[42] Marquardt says that her organization has 35,000 members, 100 chapters in the United States, and a paid staff of six.

Animal Research Facilities Protection Act

In 1992, Senator Howell Heflin (Democrat, Alabama) proposed the Farm and Animal Research Facilities Protection Act, which was signed into law by President Bush in August of that year. The act makes it a federal crime to break into a research facility or the premises of a company that breeds research animals; violators face prison sentences of up to 1 year for illegal entry and fines up to $5,000. A vice-president at UAB Medical Center, which had originated the bill, said that this legislation would protect scientists against "activists who use terrorist techniques to interfere with potentially life-saving research."[43]

The 1993 Federal Decision

In February 1993, animal-rights activists won a significant victory for dogs and primates used in laboratory research. Judge Charles Richey of the Federal District Court in Washington, DC, ordered the Agriculture Department to improve the rules that Congress had asked it to write in the Improved Standards for Laboratory Animals Act of 1985—the act creating the IACUCs.[44] Judge Richey concluded that the Agriculture Department had violated the act by giving all power to interpret it to local IACUCs: He implied that members of such committees, including veterinarians, were almost always employed by the institutions they were supposed to regulate and hence had a conflict of interest; and he ordered the rules to be rewritten in order to give someone else the final say about them.

Richey also criticized the government for taking nine years to implement some of its own rules, and he implied that some of the rules were intended more to increase profitability than to ensure the welfare of research animals.

On the other hand, Richey apparently rejected the argument of activists that "a rat is a pig is a dog is a boy": He dismissed claims that detailed records should be required for the millions of rats and mice used in American research. That is, researchers can treat rats and mice differently from dogs and primates.

During the 1990s, positions of animal activists and animal researchers hardened, with activists seeking to abolish all research using animals and researchers branding activists as sentimental "bunny huggers." In addition, researchers adopted a siege mentality, using electronic surveillance and branding anyone who talked to outsiders as a traitor.

This movement to extremes made it difficult for reformers, such as F. Barbara Orlans of the Kennedy Institute of Ethics at Georgetown University, to accomplish her life-long goal of implementing the "Three Rs" of *replacement* of animals by in vitro methods; *reduction* of their numbers through statistical analysis; and *refinement* of experiments to cause the least suffering.[45] The European Union is far ahead of America in implementing this plan, although Congress directed NIH to do so in 1993.

In the fall of 2000, Judge Ellen Huvelle ruled against Johns Hopkins University and other research facilities, concluding that small animals such as rats, mice, and birds must be included under the Federal Animal Welfare Act. Because rats and mice compose 80 to 90 percent of animals used in research, this decision was viewed badly by the losers, who said it would increase costs, paperwork, and slow down research. Congressmen vowed to delay implementation of the decision.

In the 20 counties in and around Atlanta, Georgia, one hundred thousand cats and dogs were killed in animal shelters in both 1997 and 1999, underscoring the huge numbers of animals killed every year in America who were originally created as pets (or from litters of un-neutered pets).[46]

FURTHER READING

Deborah Blum, *The Monkey Wars,* Oxford University Press, New York, 1994.

Carl Cohen, "The Case for Animal Rights," *New England Journal of Medicine,* vol. 315, no. 14, October 4, 1986, pp. 865–870.

R. G. Frey, *Rights, Killing, and Suffering,* Basil Blackwell, Oxford, England, 1983.

James Rachels, *Created from Animals,* Oxford University Press, New York, 1990.

Tom Regan, *The Case for Animal Rights,* University of California Press, Berkeley, 1983.

Peter Singer, *Animal Liberation,* New York Review of Books, New York, 1975. (This book is an expansion of an earlier article of the same title which appeared in *New York Review of Books.*)

Susan Sperling, *Animal Liberators,* University of California Press, Berkeley, 1988.

CHAPTER 11

Human Subjects

The Tuskegee Syphilis Study

*T*he Tuskegee study of untreated syphilis in hundreds of poor African-American men is one of the most condemned experiments in American medicine. A true understanding of the issues involved requires some historical perspective; but because the study was investigated behind closed doors, its details never became widely known, and it is usually discussed in only simplistic, emotional terms.

BACKGROUND: JOSEF MENGELE, THE NUREMBERG CODE, AMERICAN MILITARY RESEARCH

For centuries, the craft of medicine used trial-and-error methods to develop drugs and remedies, but it was not until the *science* of medicine actually began that experimentation became a major part of it.

In the nineteenth century, some "gentleman physicians" experimented in their leisure time, and some of them became famous. One was William Beaumont, whose experimental subject was a patient named Alexis St. Martin. In 1822, Beaumont treated St. Martin for a bullet wound in the stomach; the patient survived, but the wound healed strangely, leaving a hole. Beaumont then employed St. Martin as a servant in order to observe him, and was able to prove that stomach juices digest food. Even this very early relationship between researcher and subject had its problems: Eventually St. Martin refused to continue and ran away, and Beaumont had him sought by the police.

During the early twentieth century, the work of Koch and Pasteur inspired other physicians to experiment. The germ theory of disease opened a new door in medicine, and some physicians eagerly went through.

In the middle of the century, during World War II, some medical experimentation took disturbing or even horrifying forms. Some questionable wartime research in the United States will be described later. On a far more serious level, Japanese physicians carried out deadly experiments on Chinese prisoners of war, killing over 3,000 of them, mostly at unit 731 in Harbin. These Chinese prisoners were injected with dozens of diseases to study the natural course of anthrax, syphilis, plague, cholera, and so on; in one study of plague, 700 Chinese died.[1] It was Nazi Germany, though, which became—and remained—a symbol of the perversion of medical research.

The Nazis and Mengele: Symbols of Medical Evil

Indeed, medicine in Nazi Germany has come to be almost synonymous with evil-doing in the name of science. "Euthanasia" under the Nazis is discussed in Chapter 4: Physicians sympathetic to Nazi ideology participated in programs in which disabled, insane, and comatose patients were involuntarily killed; and even some of the most prestigious German professors of medicine supported extermination of racially "inferior" people. In addition to "euthanasia," there was also a great deal of experimentation on human subjects, much of which was at least irregular and at worst almost unimaginably savage and brutal.

Research on typhus is one example. From 1943 to 1945, experimental vaccines against typhus were given to prisoners on ward 46 of the concentration camp at Buchenwald: gay men, convicted criminals, Russian officers, Polish dissidents, Jews, and Gypsies. In one experiment, a medical professor from the Robert Koch Institute injected blood infected with typhus into 40 involuntary subjects, who then served as a treatment group. All in all, about 1,000 prisoners were used, and 158 died (high morbidity occurred in unimmunized controls, almost all of whom died). No thresholds of infection were established.[2]

Deliberate harm to subjects also took place in other studies. In experiments at Buchenwald, hormones were implanted to "cure" homosexuality, inmates were shot to study gunshot wounds, inmates were starved to study the physiology of nutrition, and women's bones and limbs were surgically removed to study regeneration. In research on malaria, anopheles mosquitoes were flown in from swamps across the world to transmit malaria to subjects. Ernst Grawitz, Reich Physician of the SS (*Schutzstaffel*, or secret police), infected the lower legs of women subjects with staphylococci, gas, and tetanus bacilli. In some subjects, particles of glass and stone were rubbed into wounds to test the efficacy of sulfa drugs.

Experiments at Ravensbrück by Sigmund Rascher—"the Captain"—a doctor for the Luftwaffe (the German air force), were described later by a ward clerk named Eugene Kogon. To study human survival during rapid changes of altitude, Rascher devised something called a "sky ride wagon" which purportedly simulated such changes: an enclosed box on wheels with monitoring equipment inside. He reported that "the blood does not yet boil at an altitude of 70,000 feet."[3] Rascher also experimented with revival after freezing; in this research, he killed about 70 of 200 involuntary subjects—Jewish and Russian prisoners. These subjects were forced to strip and were then exposed to icy water or blizzards. Kogon wrote, "When their screams created too much of a disturbance, Rascher finally used anesthesia." In the next phase of the experiment, nude Jewish women were used to revive the subjects, and Rascher reported "in detail how revived subjects practiced sexual intercourse at 86 to 90 degrees Fahrenheit." The rationale of this study was supposed to be its application to Luftwaffe pilots downed in icy seas; but since nude women would hardly be available to revive such pilots, the actual point seems to have been little more than degradation of the subjects.

At the concentration camp at Auschwitz, Josef Mengele, a physician who came to be known as the "angel of death," participated in the death of 400,000 victims. Since Mengele is the most infamous of the Nazi physicians, we should consider his career briefly here.

Mengele was the oldest of three sons of a successful manufacturer of farm equipment and was raised as a conservative Catholic. He was above average in intelligence but seems to have achieved success in school more by hard work than by intellectual facility. Because he considered the family business too limiting, he chose medicine. Like many pioneering physicians, the young Josef Mengele was ambitious and sought fame. He studied in Munich between 1930 and 1936, with a special concentration in anthropological genetics; in the 1930s, this was a fashionable field and was part of a eugenics movement that had become influential in Germany and in the United States.

In 1931, Munich was the center of the Nazi party and, as such, a center of the Nazi program of "racial purity." To advance himself with his politically conservative medical professors (in the German context, these were professors who simply accepted whatever power controlled political life), Mengele became a Brownshirt, that is, a Nazi storm trooper. Academically, he cultivated professors favored by the Nazis and oriented his own research to their interests; his doctoral thesis, which was published, was on racial jaw morphologies. His aim in research was to secure a full professorship—a rare, highly prestigious appointment. In 1934, Mengele made another astute move by marrying a professor's daughter. Two of his biographers say, "They made a dashing young pair: Irene—tall, blonde, and good-looking; Mengele—handsome in a Mediterranean way, dapper, and with a passion for fast cars."[4]

In May 1943, Mengele began a 20-month appointment as women's physician at Birkenau. His appalling experiments were conducted at nearby Auschwitz, though he was never officially assigned there. He began by clearing the camp of typhus, an accomplishment he achieved by "triaging" sick prisoners and gassing about 1,000 Gypsies; his superiors admired his methodical efficiency and unsentimental attitude toward the sick. Thereafter, he was able to focus on research that was part of his plan for his future professorship. This work was meant to find a way to overcome the effects of genetics by modifying the environment: more technically, to influence a phenotype to obtain a desired genotype. He wanted to find ways to produce traits such as blue eyes, blonde hair, and a healthy body free of genetic disease. As subjects, he needed identical twins, who would be "natural controls" for environmental differences.

Eventually, Mengele would greet incoming trains of boxcars filled with Jews destined for execution. He would examine them, looking for twins and other usable subjects and signaling his choices by a flick of the wrist. The people he chose would live while they participated in his experiments; the rest would be killed at once.

Mengele's experiments are painful even to describe. He experimented with six children to see if blue eyes could be obtained by injecting blue dye; when this study was finished, he cut out the twelve eyes and hung them on a wall of his laboratory, along with some other human organs. He forced female twins to engage in coitus with male twins to see if twin children would be produced. He interchanged blood of identical twins, to see what would happen; then he interchanged blood between pairs of twins. One pair of fraternal (nonidentical) twins—children—consisted of a hunchback and a normal child; Mengele surgically grafted the hunchback to the other child's back, creating the effect of conjoined twins, and accentuated this effect by also sewing their wrists back to back. A witness, Vera Alexander, reported that when the children came back to the barracks: "There was a terrible smell of gangrene. The cuts were dirty and the children cried every night."[5] Mengele had many of his twins (between 150 and 200) killed; some of them he killed himself. Here is a description by another physician who was present at a series of executions:

> After that, the first twin was brought in, a fourteen-year old girl. Dr. Mengele ordered me to undress the girl and put her head on the dissecting table. Then he injected the Epival into her right arm intravenously. After the child had fallen asleep, he felt for the left ventricle of the heart and injected 10 cc of chloroform. After one little twitch the child was dead, whereupon Dr. Mengele had her taken to the corpse chamber. In this manner, all fourteen twins were killed during the night.[6]

In other research, Mengele tried to establish limits of human endurance by subjecting 75 male and female prisoners to electric shock; 25 of them died immediately. To study sterility, he subjected a group of Polish nuns to high dosages of radiation, burning them severely. At one time, he found a hunchback and the hunchback's son; he had both of them killed, their bodies boiled, their flesh stripped, and their skeletons dipped in gasoline for preservation for his anthropological studies of body types. When he came upon seven dwarfs from a Romanian circus family, however, he kept them alive in order to exhibit them to visiting German physicians.

Although his temper occasionally flared when anyone subverted his plans, Mengele was noted for being cool, impersonal, and detached. When, because of an oversight, 300 Jewish children managed to escape a gas chamber and fled to a nearby field, Mengele had them recaptured, then had a gasoline fire set in a large pit and had the children thrown in. Some of the children, on fire and screaming for their lives, clawed their way over dead bodies to the top, where Mengele and SS men kicked them back in.

As the Russian army approached Auschwitz in 1945, Mengele fled. Almost immediately, he was listed as a major war criminal; but even though he used his real name, he managed to escape to Brazil and Paraguay, where he lived in relative freedom for 40 years, several times eluding Simon Wiesenthal and other Israelis who tried to catch him. Later, in conversations with his grown son Rolf, Mengele never expressed any regret for his actions or even any consciousness of having done wrong. He reasoned that it was not his fault that Jews were to be killed at Auschwitz, and since they were to die anyway, why not use them first to advance medical knowledge, Nazi programs, and his own chance of a professorship? Mengele died in Brazil in the summer of 1985 (the identity of his body was confirmed by matching his DNA with DNA donated by his son).[7]

Mengele's actions are often attributed to a pathological personality, but it must be noted that he did not appear to be a psychopath. Of course, we could define his behavior as pathological: That is, we could say that anyone who behaves this way must be a psychopath. However, this would probably be simplistic, and it would

fail to allow for what the philosopher Hannah Arendt calls the "banality of evil"—
the possibility that ordinary people, in relatively normal circumstances, can do terrible things.[8] That the "banality of evil" may indeed be a reality seems to be strongly
indicated by Stanley Milgram's research on obedience to authority.[9]

The Nuremberg Code

After World War II, at the Nuremberg trials in 1946, German physicians defended
themselves against charges of war crimes by saying that they had merely been following orders, that their experiments had been properly related to solving medical
problems of war, and that what they had done was not substantially different from
research done on captives by American physicians.

Although such a defense would be ludicrous for anyone like Mengele, it might
have some credence for minor figures who may have conducted morally dubious
research or mistreated their subjects without committing actual atrocities. However, a problem faced by the judges at Nuremberg in evaluating defenses, charges,
and evidence was lack of a code of ethics for experimentation on captive populations. The judges therefore referred to 10 principles for permissible experimentation, which afterward came to be known as the *Nuremberg code*. The most important principle of the Nuremberg code was that captives should freely consent to
participation in any experiment.

It is noteworthy that one of the observers at the Nuremberg trials was a young
physician named Leo Alexander. Later, in an article in *New England Journal of Medicine*, Alexander gave shocking details of Nazi experimentation and "euthanasia"
and advanced a now famous "slippery slope" explanation,[10] which is discussed in
Chapter 4.

American Military Research in World War II

As noted above, some research in the United States during World War II was ethically questionable. In 1941, for example, American researchers experimented on
orphans at the Ohio Soldiers and Sailors Orphanage, on retarded inmates at New
Jersey State Colony for the Feeble-Minded, and on patients at a mental institution
in Dixon, Illinois.[11] One purpose of this research was to develop a vaccine against
shigella (a bacterial disease causing dysentery), and researchers injected deadened
forms of shigella bacteria into their subjects. No one died as a direct result, but
many of the subjects got very sick.

Some questionable research used military personnel as subjects. Cornelius
("Dusty") Rhoads, director of the leading American cancer hospital—Memorial
Sloan Kettering in New York City—became head of the military's secret chemical
warfare service. As Robert Bazell, a science reporter for NBC, writes, Rhoads:

> supervised the long secret and now infamous tests where thousands of American
> troops were intentionally exposed to mustard and other poisonous gases. Rhoads
> discovered that the mustard gas killed white blood cells and other cells that divided
> rapidly. After the war he and others began to experiment with mustard gas as a can-
> cer treatment and also to search for other systemic poisons that kill dividing cells.[12]

According to a report by the Institute of Medicine in 1993, in most of the research conducted by the armed forces on the acute effects of these poisonous agents, the subjects were "volunteers" who did not know what they were volunteering for; there was no attempt at informed consent.[13] The testing involved 60,000 subjects, of whom 4,000 to 5,000 were used in tests on mustard gas in gas chambers.

Wartime research in the United States had some significant consequences. One later development was that when subjects of the chemical research applied for treatment at veterans' hospitals, the Veterans Administration (VA) denied that they had been exposed to toxic agents (this scenario would be repeated after the war in Vietnam and again after Operation Desert Storm). Another development was that these same toxic agents would later be used as "chemotherapies" against cancer—an outgrowth of the use of military personnel as "guinea pigs" in World War II.

A third long-term consequence was that World War II institutionalized medical experimentation, including some doubtful practices. The Americans (like their opponents) sought cures for dysentery, malaria, and venereal diseases; and when the war itself came to an end, the fight against diseases in the United States did not. In fact, "the prospect of winning the war against contagious and degenerative illness gave researchers in the 1950s and 1960s a sense of both mission and urgency that kept the spirit of the wartime laboratories alive."[14]

During the war, for instance, Franklin Roosevelt established the Committee on Medical Research, which approached its work with a wartime mentality that carried over into researchers' attitudes after the war: disease was the enemy, researchers were the soldiers, and victory could be won—with enough resources and enough will. Also, while the war was still in process, considerations of ethics and informed consent had carried little weight:

> A wartime environment also undercut the protection of human subjects, because of the power of the example of the draft. Every day thousands of men were compelled to risk death, however limited their understanding of the aims of the war or the immediate campaign might be. By extension, researchers doing laboratory work were also engaged in a military activity, and they did not need to seek the permission of their subjects any more than the selective service or field commanders did of draftees. . . .
>
> In a society mobilized for war, these arguments carried great weight. Some people were ordered to face bullets and storm a hill; others were told to take an injection and test a vaccine. In philosophical terms, wartime inevitably promoted utilitarian over absolutistic positions.[15]

Postwar Criticisms

After the war, it became apparent that some researchers had gone too far in their zeal for results; moreover, by the 1970s, the wartime sense of urgency had begun to be tempered by other voices. Faith in the inevitability of scientific progress was waning, and with it faith in medical research. Rachel Carson's *Silent Spring* described the ravages of pesticides; the Cuban missile crisis showed how close we could come to nuclear destruction; drugs hailed as "miraculous" were found to have dramatically harmful side effects, such as the severe birth defects caused by thalidomide. Thus the use of human subjects in medical research began to be considered more critically.

In 1966, in *New England Journal of Medicine*, Henry Beecher—a medical professor at Harvard—criticized 22 specific medical experiments involving human subjects.[16] All of these studies had been published in medical journals, but none of them had obtained informed consent from subjects, and several of them bordered on abuse. Beecher claimed that these 22 studies were not exceptions but rather represented the norm of medical experimentation. At about the same time, another physician, Henry Pappworth, criticized 500 medical experiments on similar grounds.[17]

In considering such criticism, we need to keep a sense of proportion about abuse of subjects in American research, which of course is nothing like what went on in Nazi Germany. Moreover, the Nazi atrocities stemmed from systematic contempt for "undesirables," whereas abuses in American studies have arisen in a basically different way. In American medical research, mistreatment of subjects has tended to arise from conflicts of three types of goals: helping future patients, advancing the researchers' careers, and protecting the interests of subjects. That is, abuses typically arise when researchers fail to keep their subjects' welfare in balance with their other goals.

THE TUSKEGEE STUDY

The Tuskegee study of syphilis began during the great depression—around 1930—and lasted for 42 years. Because of its long time span, some historical background is important for understanding the many issues raised by the Tuskegee research.

The Medical Environment: Syphilis

Syphilis is a chronic, contagious bacterial disease, often venereal and sometimes congenital. Its first symptom is a chancre; after this chancre subsides, the disease spreads silently for a time but then produces an outbreak of secondary symptoms such as fever, rash, and swollen lymph glands. Then the disease becomes latent for many years, after which it may reappear with a variety of symptoms in the nervous or circulatory systems. Today, syphilis is treated with penicillin or other antibiotics; but this treatment has been possible only since about 1946, when penicillin first became widely available.

Until relatively recently, then, the common fate of victims of syphilis—kings and queens, peasants and slaves—was simply to suffer the sequelae once the first symptoms had appeared. Victims who suffered this inevitable progress included Cleopatra, King Herod of Judea, Charlemagne, Henry VIII of England, Napoleon Bonaparte, Frederick the Great, Pope Sixtus IV, Pope Alexander VI, Pope Julius II, Catherine the Great, Christopher Columbus, Paul Gauguin, Franz Schubert, Albrecht Dürer, Johann Wolfgang von Goethe, Friedrich Nietzsche, John Keats, and James Joyce.[18]

•

It is generally believed that syphilis was brought to Europe from the new world during the 1490s by Christopher Columbus's crews, but the disease may have appeared in Europe before that time. In any case, advances in transportation contributed greatly to the spread of syphilis (similarly, much later, transportation would be a factor in the spread of AIDS). For hundreds of years, syphilis was attributed to sin and was associated with prostitutes, though attempts to check its spread by expelling prostitutes failed because their customers were disregarded. Efforts to eradicate it by quarantine also failed.

In the eighteenth century, standing professional armies began to be established, and with them came a general acceptance of high rates of venereal disease. It is estimated, for instance, that around the year 1900, one-fifth of the British army had syphilis or gonorrhea.

Between 1900 and 1948, and especially during the two world wars, American reformers mounted what was called a *syphilophobia* campaign: the Social Hygiene Movement or Purity Crusade. Members of the campaign emphasized that syphilis was spread by prostitutes, and held that it was rapidly fatal; as an alternative to visiting a prostitute, they advocated clean, active sports (also called "muscular Christianity"). According to the medical historian Alan Brandt, there were two splits resulting from disagreements within this reform movement: once during World War I, when giving out condoms was controversial; and later during World War II, when giving out penicillin was at issue. In each of these conflicts, reformers whose basic intention was to reduce the physical harm of syphilis were on one side, whereas those who wanted to reduce illicit behavior were on the other side.[19]

The armed services during the world wars took a pragmatic position. Commanders who needed healthy troops overruled the moralists and ordered the release of condoms in the first war and penicillin in the second—and these continued to be used by returning troops after each war.

•

The spirochete (bacterium) which causes syphilis was discovered by Fritz Schaudinn in 1906. Syphilis is, classically, described in three stages:

- *Primary syphilis.* In this first stage, spirochetes mass and produce a primary lesion causing a *chancre* (pronounced "SHANK-er"). During the primary stage, syphilis is highly infectious.
- *Secondary syphilis.* In the second stage, spirochetes disseminate from the primary lesion throughout the body, producing systemic and widespread lesions, usually in internal organs and other internal sites. Externally, however—after the initial chancre subsides—syphilis spreads silently during a "latent" period lasting from 1 to 30 years, although secondary symptoms such as fever, rash, and swollen glands may appear. During the secondary stage, the symptoms of syphilis vary so widely that it is known as the "great imitator."
- *Tertiary syphilis.* In the third stage, chronic destructive lesions cause major damage to the cardiac system, the neurological system, or both, partly because immune responses decrease with age. During the tertiary stage, syphilis may produce paresis (slight or incomplete paralysis), gummas (gummy or rubbery tumors), altered gait, blindness, or lethal narrowing of the aorta.

Beginning in the sixteenth century, mercury—a heavy metal—was the common treatment for syphilis; it was applied to the back as a paste and absorbed through the skin. During the nineteenth century, this treatment alternated with bismuth, another heavy metal administered the same way. Neither mercury nor bismuth killed the spirochetes, though either could ameliorate symptoms.

In 1909, after the spirochete of syphilis had been identified, two researchers—a German, Paul Erlich, and a Japanese, S. Hata—tried 605 forms of arsenic and finally discovered what seemed to be a "magic bullet" against it: combination 606 of heavy metals including arsenic. Erlich called this *salvarsan* and patented it; the generic name is arsphenamine.[20] Salvarsan was administered as an intramuscular injection. After finding that it cured syphilis in rabbits, Erlich injected it into men with syphilis. (According to common practice, none of the men was asked to consent.)

At first, salvarsan seemed to work wonders, and during 1910 Erlich was receiving standing ovations at medical meetings. Later, however, syphilis recurred, fatally, in some patients who had been treated with salvarsan; furthermore, salvarsan itself apparently killed some patients. Erlich maintained that the drug had not been given correctly, but he also developed another form, neosalvarsan, which was less toxic and could be given more easily. Neosalvarsan also was injected intramuscularly—ideally, in 20 to 40 dosages given over 1 year.

Though better than salvarsan, neosalvarsan was (as described by a physician of the time) used erratically, and "generally without rhyme or reason—an injection now and then, possibly for a symptom, [for] some skin lesion, or when the patient had a ten-dollar bill."[21] It was also expensive. Moreover, neither salvarsan nor neosalvarsan was a "magic bullet" for patients with tertiary syphilis.

Another researcher, Caesar Boeck in Norway, took a different approach: From 1891 to 1910, he studied the natural course of untreated syphilis in 1,978 subjects. Boeck, a professor of dermatology at the University of Oslo, believed that heavy metals removed only the symptoms of syphilis rather than its underlying cause; he also thought that these metals suppressed what is today recognized as the immune system. He therefore decided that not treating patients at all might be an improvement over treatment with heavy metals.

In 1929, Boeck's student and successor, J. E. Bruusgaard, selected 473 of Boeck's subjects for further evaluation, in many cases examining their hospital charts.[22] This method had an obvious bias, since the more severely affected of Boeck's subjects would be most likely to have hospital records. Despite this bias, however, Bruusgaard was surprised to find that in 65 percent of these cases, either the subjects were externally symptom free or there was no mention in their charts of the classic symptoms of syphilis. Of the subjects who had had syphilis for more than 20 years, 73 percent were asymptomatic.

Bruusgaard's findings contradicted the message of the syphilophobia campaign: They indicated that syphilis was not universally fatal, much less rapidly so. These results also suggested the possibility that some people with syphilis spirochetes would never develop any symptoms of the disease.

When the Tuskegee study began in 1932, Boeck's and Bruusgaard's work was the only existing study of the natural course of untreated syphilis.

The Racial Environment

In the 1930s, American medicine was, and had long been, widely racist—certainly by our present standards and to some extent even by the standards of the time. For at least a century before the Tuskegee study began, most physicians condescended to African-American patients, held stereotypes about them, and sometimes used them as subjects of nontherapeutic experiments.

In the decades of slavery before the U.S. Civil War, southern physicians and white slave-owners only treated medical conditions necessary to protect their investment in human "property."[23] John Brown, a former slave who wrote a book about his life under slavery, described how a physician in Georgia kept him in an open-pit oven to produce sunburns and to try out different remedies.

The best-known account of the racial background of the Tuskegee study is James Jones's *Bad Blood* (the significance of the title will become apparent later in this chapter).[24] In the late nineteenth century, the United States was swept by social Darwinism, a popular corruption of Darwin's theory of evolution by natural selection (see Chapter 16). Some whites predicted on this basis that the Negro race (to use the term then current) would be extinct by 1900: Their idea was that Darwin's "survival of the fittest" implied a competition which Negroes would lose. (It bears repeating that this is a misconception and misapplication of Darwin's actual theory.) According to Jones, this popular belief was shared by white physicians, who thought that it was confirmed by defects in African-Americans' anatomy and therefore became obsessed with the details of such presumed defects. Although comparable defects in white patients went unreported, defects in black patients were described in great detail in medical journals and became the basis for sweeping conclusions; to take one example, genital development and brain development were said to vary inversely.

In addition to social Darwinism, physicians shared many of the popular stereotypes of African-Americans; well into the twentieth century, physicians often simply advanced such stereotypes as "facts." The following example appeared in *Journal of the American Medical Association* in 1914:

> The negro springs from a southern race, and as such his sexual appetite is strong; all of his environments stimulate this appetite, and as a general rule his emotional type of religion certainly does not decrease it.[25]

African-Americans were also seen as dirty, shiftless, promiscuous, and incapable of practicing personal hygiene. Around the turn of the century, a physician in rural Georgia wrote, "Virtue in the negro race is like 'angels' visits'—few and far between. In a practice of sixteen years in the South, I have never examined a virgin over fourteen years of age."[26] In 1919, a medical professor in Chicago wrote that African-American men were like bulls or elephants in *furor sexualis,* unable to refrain from copulation when in the presence of females.[27]

Ideas about syphilis reflected this racial environment. For white physicians at the time when the Tuskegee study began, syphilis was a natural consequence of the innately low character of African-Americans, who were described by one white physician as a "notoriously syphilis-soaked race."[28] Moreover, it was simply assumed that African-American men would not seek treatment for venereal disease.

The historian Alan Brandt has suggested that in the United States during the early 1900s, it was a rare white physician who was not a racist—and that this would have remained the case throughout many years of the Tuskegee study. He writes, "There can be little doubt that the Tuskegee researchers regarded their subjects as less than human."[29]

Development of the Tuskegee Case

A "Study in Nature" Begins   Studies in nature were distinguished from experiments in 1865 by a famous experimenter and physiologist, Claude Bernard: In an experiment, some factor is manipulated, whereas a *study in nature* merely observes what would happen anyway. For a century before the Tuskegee study, medicine considered it crucially important to discover the natural history of a disease and therefore relied extensively on studies in nature.

The great physician William Osler had said, "Know syphilis in all its manifestations and relations, and all other things clinical will be added unto you."[30] As late as 1932, however, the natural history of syphilis had not been conclusively documented (the only existing study, as noted above, was that of Boeck and Bruusgaard), and there was uncertainty about the inexorability of its course. The United States Public Health Service (USPHS) believed that a study in nature of syphilis was necessary because physicians needed to know its natural sequence of symptoms and final outcomes in order to recognize key changes during its course. This perceived need was one factor in the Tuskegee research.

A second factor was simply that USPHS found what it considered an opportunity for such a study. Around 1929, there were several counties in the United States where venereal disease was extraordinarily prevalent, and a philanthropical organization—the Julius Rosenwald Foundation in Philadelphia—started a project to eradicate it. With help from USPHS, the foundation originally intended to treat with neosalvarsan all syphilitics in six counties with rates of syphilis above 20 percent. In 1930, the foundation surveyed African-American men in Macon County, Alabama, which was then 82 percent black; this was the home of the famous Tuskegee Institute. The survey found the highest rate of syphilis in the nation: 36 percent. The foundation planned a demonstration study in which these African-American syphilitics would be treated with neosalvarsan, and it did treat or partially treat some of the 3,694 men who had been identified as having syphilis (estimates of how many received treatment or partial treatment range from less than half to 95 percent). However, 1929 was the year when the great Depression began; as it ground on, funds for philanthropy plummeted, and the Rosenwald Foundation pulled out of Tuskegee, hoping that USPHS would continue the treatment program. (Funds available for public health were also dropping, though: USPHS would soon see its budget lowered from over $1 million before the depression to less than $60,000 in 1935.)

In 1931, USPHS repeated the foundation's survey in Macon County, testing 4,400 African-American residents; USPHS found a 22 percent rate of syphilis in men, and a 62 percent rate of congenital syphilis. In this survey, 399 African-American men were identified who had syphilis of several years' duration but had never been treated by the Rosenwald Foundation or in any other way. It was the identification of these 399 untreated men that USPHS saw as an ideal opportunity for a study in the nature of syphilis. The surgeon general suggested that they should be merely observed rather than treated: This decision would become a moral crux of the study.

It is important to reemphasize that the USPHS research—it was undertaken in cooperation with the Tuskegee Institute and is called the *Tuskegee study* for that reason—was a study in nature. The Tuskegee physicians saw themselves as ecological biologists, simply observing what occurred regularly and naturally. In 1936, a paper in *Journal of the American Medical Association* by the surgeon general and his top assistants described the 1932–1933 phase of the Tuskegee study as "an unusual opportunity to study the untreated syphilitic patient from the beginning of the disease to the death of the infected person." It noted specifically that the study consisted of "399 syphilitic Negro males who had never received treatment."[31]

There are also two important points to emphasize about the subjects of the Tuskegee study. First, at the outset the 399 syphilitic subjects had *latent syphilis,* that is, secondary syphilis; most of them were probably in the early latent stage. During this stage, syphilis is largely noninfectious during sexual intercourse, although it can be passed easily through a blood transfusion (or, in a pregnant woman, through the placenta). However, latent or secondary syphilis (as noted above) has extremely variable symptoms and outcomes; and external lesions, which can be a source of infection during sex, do sometimes appear.

Second, these 399 syphilitic subjects were not divided into the typical experimental and control or "treatment" and "no treatment" groups: They were all simply to be observed. There was, however, another group of "controls," consisting of about 200 age-matched men who did not have syphilis. (Originally, there was also a third group, consisting of 275 syphilitic men who had been treated with small amounts of arsphenamine; these subjects were followed for a while but were dropped from the study in 1936—perhaps because funds were lacking, or perhaps because the researchers were by then interested only in the "study in nature" group.)

The Middle Phase: "Bad Blood"   The Tuskegee study was hardly a model of scientific research or scientific method; and even on its own terms, as a study in nature, it was carried out rather haphazardly. Except for an African-American nurse, Eunice Rivers, who was permanently assigned to the study, there was no continuity of medical personnel. There was no central supervision; there were no written protocols; no physician was in charge. Names of the subjects in the study group of 399 were often mixed up with the "controls." The subjects were not housed at any one location or facility. Most worked as sharecroppers or as small farmers and simply came into the town of Tuskegee when Eunice Rivers told them to do so (she would drive them into town in her car, a ride that several subjects described as making them feel important).

There were large gaps in the study. The "federal doctors," as the subjects called them, returned only every few years. Visits are documented in 1939 and then not again until 1948; 7 years passed between visits in 1963 and 1970. Only the nurse, Eunice Rivers, remained to hold the shaky study together. When the physicians did return to Tuskegee after a gap, they found it difficult to answer their own questions because the records were so poor.

Still, there were some rudimentary procedures. The physicians wanted to know, first, if they had a subject in the study group; and second, if so, how far his syphilis had progressed. To determine the progress of the disease, spinal punctures (called *taps*) were given to 271 of the 399 syphilitic subjects. In a spinal tap, a 10-inch needle is inserted between two vertebrae into the cerebrospinal fluid and a small amount of fluid is withdrawn—a delicate and uncomfortable process. The subjects were warned to lie very still, lest the needle swerve and puncture the fluid sac, causing infection and other complications.

Subjects were understandably reluctant to leave their farms, travel for miles over back roads to meet the physicians, and then undergo these painful taps, especially when they had no pressing medical problem. For this reason, the physicians offered inducements: free transportation, free hot lunches, free medicine for any disease other than syphilis, and free burials. (The free burials were important to poor subjects, who often died without enough money for even a pauper's grave; but USPHS couldn't keep this promise itself after its budget was reduced and had to be rescued by the Milbank Memorial Fund.) In return for these "benefits," the physicians got not only the spinal taps but, later, autopsies to see what damage syphilis had or had not done.

There seems no doubt that the researchers also resorted to deception. Subjects were told that they had "bad blood" and that the spinal taps were "treatment" for it; moreover, the researchers sensationalized the effects of untreated "bad blood." USPHS sent the subjects the following letter, under the imposing letterhead "Macon County Health Department," with the subheading "Alabama State Board of Health and U.S. Public Health Service Cooperating with Tuskegee Institute" (all of which participated in the study):

> Dear Sir:
> Some time ago you were given a thorough examination and since that time we hope you have gotten a great deal of treatment for bad blood. You will now be given your last chance to get a second examination. This examination is a very special one and after it is finished you will be given a special treatment if it is believed you are in a condition to stand it.[32]

The "special treatment" mentioned was simply the spinal tap for neurosyphilis, a diagnostic test. The subjects were instructed to meet the public health nurse for transportation to "Tuskegee Institute Hospital for this free treatment." The letter closed, in capitals:

> REMEMBER THIS IS YOUR LAST CHANCE FOR SPECIAL FREE TREATMENT.
> BE SURE TO MEET THE NURSE.

To repeat, the researchers never treated the subjects for syphilis. In fact, during World War II, the researchers contacted the local draft board and prevented any eligible subject from being drafted—and hence from being treated for syphilis by the armed services. Although penicillin was developed around 1941–1943 and was widely available by 1946, the subjects in the Tuskegee study never received it, even during the 1960s or 1970s. However, as will be discussed below, it is not clear how much the subjects with late noninfectious syphilis were harmed by not getting penicillin.

The First Investigations   In 1966, Peter Buxtun, a recent college graduate, had just been hired by USPHS as a venereal disease investigator in San Francisco. After a few months, he learned of the Tuskegee study and began to question and criticize the USPHS officials who were still running it.[33] By this time, the physicians supervising the study and its data collection had been moved to the newly created Centers for Disease Control (CDC) in Atlanta. CDC officials were annoyed by Buxtun's questions about the morality of the study; later in 1966, having invited him to Atlanta for a conference on syphilis, they harangued him and tried to get him to be silent. He expected to be fired from USPHS; he was not, though, and he continued to press CDC for 2 more years.

By 1969, Buxtun's inquiries and protests led to a meeting of a small group of physicians at CDC to consider the Tuskegee study. The group consisted of William J. Brown (Director of Venereal Diseases at CDC), David Sencer (Director of CDC), Ira Meyers (Alabama's State Health Officer from 1951 to 1986), Sidney Olansky (a physician at Emory Hospital who was knowledgeable about the early years of the study and had been in charge of it in 1951), Lawton Smith (an ophthalmologist from the University of Miami), and Gene Stollerman (chairman of medicine at the University of Tennessee). In general, this group avoided Buxtun's questions about the morality of the study and focused on whether continuing the study would harm the subjects. Meyers said of the Tuskegee subjects, "I haven't seen this group, but I don't think they would submit to treatment" if they were told what was going on.[34] Smith (the ophthalmologist) pressed hardest for continuing the study; only Stollerman repeatedly opposed continuing it, on both moral and therapeutic grounds. At the end, the committee overrode Stollerman and voted to continue the study.

Also in 1969, Ira Meyers told the physicians in the Macon County Medical Society about the Tuskegee study. These physicians did not object to the study; in fact, they were given a list of all the subjects and agreed not to give antibiotics to any subject for any condition, if a subject came to one of their offices. It should be noted that although this medical society had been all white in the 1930s, during the 1960s its membership was almost entirely African-American.

In 1970, a monograph on syphilis was published, sponsored by the American Public Health Association, to give useful information to public health officers and venereal disease (VD) control officers. This monograph stated that treatment for late benign syphilis should consist of "6.0 to 9.0 million units of benzathine penicillin G given 3.0 million units at sessions seven days apart."[35] The first author listed on the monograph is William J. Brown, head of CDC's Tuskegee section from 1957 to 1971. Brown had been on the CDC panel in 1969 (when the monograph was probably written) and had argued for continuing the Tuskegee study, in which, of course, subjects with late benign syphilis received *no* penicillin.

The Story Breaks   In July of 1972, Peter Buxtun, who had then been criticizing the Tuskegee research for 6 years and was disappointed by CDC's refusal to stop it, mentioned the Tuskegee study to a friend who was a reporter for the Associated Press (AP) on the west coast. Another AP reporter—Jean Heller, on the east coast— was assigned to the story, and on the morning of July 26, 1972, her report appeared on front pages of newspapers nationwide.[36]

Heller's story described a medical study run by the federal government in Tuskegee, Alabama, in which poor, uneducated African-American men had been used as "guinea pigs." After noting the terrible effects of tertiary syphilis, the story said that in 1969 a CDC study of 276 of the untreated subjects had proved that at least 7 subjects died "as a direct result of syphilis."

Heller's story had an immediate effect. (It might have made even more of an impact, but it was competing with a political story which broke the same day—a report that the Democratic candidate for vice president, Thomas Eagleton, had received shock therapy for depression.) Some members of Congress were amazed to learn of the Tuskegee study, and Senator William Proxmire called it a "moral and ethical nightmare."

CDC, of course, responded. J. D. Millar, chief of Venereal Disease Control, said that the study "was never clandestine," pointing to 15 published articles in medical and scientific journals over a 30-year span. Millar also maintained that the subjects had been informed that they could get treatment for syphilis at any time. "Patients were not denied drugs," he said; "rather, they were not offered drugs." He also tried to emphasize that "the study began when attitudes were much different on treatment and experimentation."[37]

The public and the press, however, scorned Millar's explanations. One political cartoon, for instance, showed a frail African-American man being studied under a huge microscope by a white man in a white coat with a sign in the background: "This is a NO-TREATMENT study by your Public Heath Service."[38] Another cartoon showed ragged African-American men walking past tombstones; the caption read: "Secret Tuskegee Study—free autopsy, free burial, plus $100 bonus." Another showed a white physician standing near the body of an African-American man, partially covered by a sheet; the chart at the foot of the hospital bed on which the body lay read "Ignore this syphilis patient (experiment in progress)"; in the background, a skeptical nurse holding a syringe asked, "*Now* can we give him penicillin?"

CDC and USPHS had always feared a "public relations problem" if the Tuskegee study became generally known, and now they had one. So did the Macon County Medical Society: When its president told the *Montgomery Advertiser* that the members had voted to identify remaining subjects and give them "appropriate therapy," USPHS in Atlanta flatly contradicted him, retorting that the local physicians—African-American physicians—had accepted the Tuskegee study. The society then acknowledged that it had agreed to continuation of the study but had not agreed to withhold treatment from subjects who came to the offices of its members, whereupon USPHS documented the physicians' agreement to do exactly that.

The Aftermath   Almost immediately after Heller's story appeared, Congress commissioned a special panel to investigate the Tuskegee study and issue a report. (The report was supposed to be ready by December 31, 1972; as we will see, however, it was late.)

Also almost at once, senators Sparkman and Allen of Alabama (both Democrats) sponsored a federal bill to give each of the Tuskegee subjects $25,000 in compensation. The southern African-American electorate had been instrumental in electing these two senators and many southern members of Congress in the 1960s and 1970s, as well as presidents Kennedy and Johnson.

On November 16, 1972, Casper Weinberger, Secretary of Health, Education, and Welfare (HEW), officially terminated the Tuskegee study. At that time, CDC estimated that 28 of the original syphilitic group had died of syphilis during the study; after the study was ended, the remaining syphilitic subjects received penicillin.

In February and March 1973, Senator Edward Kennedy's Subcommittee on Health of the Committee on Labor and Public Welfare held hearings on the Tuskegee study. Two of the Tuskegee subjects, Charles Pollard and Lester Scott, testified; one of them appeared to have been blinded by late-stage syphilis. These two men revealed more about the study: Pollard said they had not been told that they had syphilis; both said they thought "bad blood" meant something like low energy. Kennedy strongly condemned the study and proposed new regulations for medical experimentation.

In April 1973, the investigatory panel that had been commissioned when the Tuskegee story broke finally issued its report, which did not prove to be very useful. Moreover, for some reason this panel had met behind closed doors, and thus reporters had not been able to cover it.[39]

On July 23, 1973, Fred Gray, representing some of the Tuskegee subjects, filed a class-action suit against the federal government. Gray, a former Alabama legislator (in 1970, he had become the first African-American Democrat elected in Alabama since Reconstruction), had been threatening to sue for compensation since Heller's story first broke, hoping for a settlement. He presented the suit as an issue of race, suing only the federal government and omitting the Tuskegee Institute, Rivers, the Tuskegee hospitals, and the Macon County Medical Society.

Eventually, the Justice Department decided that it couldn't win the suit in federal court, since the trial would have been held in nearby Montgomery, in the court of Frank Johnson, a liberal Alabama judge who had desegregated southern schools and upgraded mental institutions. Therefore, in December 1974 the government settled out of court.

According to the settlement, "living syphilitics" (subjects alive on July 23, 1973) received $37,500 each; "heirs of deceased syphilitics," $15,000 (since some children might have congenital syphilis); "living controls," $16,000; heirs of "deceased controls," $5,000. (Controls and their descendants were compensated because they had been prevented from getting antibiotics during the years of the study.) Also, the federal government agreed to provide free lifetime medical care for Tuskegee subjects, their wives, and their children. By September 1988, the government had paid $7.5 million for medical care for the Tuskegee subjects. At that time, 21 of the original syphilitic subjects were still alive—each of whom had had syphilis for at least 57 years.[40] In addition, 41 wives and 19 children had evidence of syphilis and were receiving free medical care.

By the time this settlement was reached, more than 18 months had passed since Jean Heller's first story, and the Tuskegee issue was no longer front-page news: Even the *New York Times* was giving it only an occasional short paragraph or two on inside pages. The issue was, after all, complicated; ethical standards had changed over the long course of the Tuskegee research; and, as noted above, the special panel commissioned to evaluate the study had met in secret. The public, therefore, had more or less forgotten about the Tuskegee study.

ETHICAL ISSUES: RACISM, INFORMED CONSENT, AND HARM TO SUBJECTS

Deception and Informed Consent

Two related ethical issues in the Tuskegee study are deception and informed consent. As has already been noted, the researchers undoubtedly deceived the subjects about "bad blood" and the spinal taps. Moreover, according to J. D. Williams, an African-American physician who was an intern at Tuskegee Institute Hospital when the study began (he was 73 when the story broke in 1972), the subjects did not know that they were part of a study, did not even know what syphilis was, and did not know that they weren't being treated with available drugs.[41] Assuming that such deception did take place, was it justified? What does it imply about informed consent?

The federal panel established in 1972 faulted the Tuskegee researchers for deceiving subjects and for failing to obtain subjects' informed consent. A counter-argument has been advanced by one apologist for the Tuskegee study: R. H. Kampmeier, an emeritus professor of medicine at Vanderbilt Medical School who worked as a syphilologist during the decades of the study.[42] Kampmeier considers it unfair to condemn a study undertaken in the 1930s on the basis of lack of informed consent—a legal notion which first appeared in court decisions in the 1960s. He argues that this amounts to judging earlier research by modern standards. He also describes such criticism as "tilting at windmills" because it would presumably apply to most of the great researchers of the past, who never bothered with consent: Does it really make sense to call someone like Pasteur unethical? Furthermore, Kampmeier cites a study by USPHS in 1943 involving use of penicillin with 35,000 syphilitics; this study is considered a landmark, but it did not obtain informed consent from its subjects. He notes, in addition, that during the early years of the Tuskegee study, it was accepted practice for physicians to walk into a patient's room and simply announce that they were taking out the patient's gallbladder.

The medical historian and physician Thomas Benedek also dismisses the issue of informed consent as "anachronistic" with regard to the Tuskegee study, noting that USPHS did not require informed consent until 1966.[43]

It is true that informed consent in medical experiments was mandated by court decisions during the late 1960s, and that before then it had not been a legal requirement. Still, the accepted presumption was always that physicians would neither harm patients nor allow harm to occur ("First, do no harm"), and this presumption would also seem applicable to physicians who were doing research with human subjects. Advocates of patients' rights argue that failure to adhere to this presumption—leading to situations like the "landmark" USPHS study of penicillin and syphilis—is what created the need for laws about informed consent in the first place.

Moreover, it can be argued that we need to distinguish between obtaining consent for procedures which might benefit subjects (*therapeutic* procedures) and *not* obtaining consent for procedures which might harm subjects (*experimental* procedures). On this argument, informed consent would always be required for experimental (potentially harmful) procedures and thus would represent a legitimate criticism of the Tuskegee study.

Finally, we can ask some rather simple questions. Granted that telling patients or subjects the truth was not legally required before 1960, and granted that this was not always a medical norm, was it really *not* wrong for the Tuskegee researchers to lie to their subjects, even in the 1930s? Did the researchers really believe they were doing no wrong?

Racism

Another issue in the Tuskegee study is racism. The study, of course, began long before the civil rights movement; it took place in the deep south—in Alabama—and all its subjects were African-American. Under such circumstances, was it only a coincidence that the subjects were deceived and left untreated? Would white subjects have been used in the same way?

In *Bad Blood*, James Jones sees the Tuskegee study as a result of pervasive racism in American medicine during the 1930s and earlier, and Kampmeier acknowledges that few whites of the time transcended this racism. It is important to realize exactly how bad the 1930s were for African-Americans: To take just one example, black students at Tuskegee Institute lived in fear of rural white toughs just outside the campus. In such a racial climate, it seems very probable that the researchers in the Tuskegee study would be willing to withhold the truth—and treatment—from African-American subjects.

Also, although studies in nature were still important in medicine of the early 1930s, there was no reason why a study in nature of syphilis should have used only African-American subjects. On the contrary: Some physicians believed then that syphilis ran a different course in different races, and this would imply the need for a parallel study of untreated white syphilitics. There was no parallel study of white subjects and it is hard to imagine that an analogous study of whites could have been undertaken or even contemplated.

The Tuskegee study continued for 40 years, during which the American racial environment changed significantly. In 1969, when CDC decided to continue the Tuskegee study, all of the following events had already taken place: the bus boycott in Montgomery led by Rosa Parks (1955); integration of Rich's department store in Atlanta by students (1960); the Freedom Riders (1961); integration of the University of Alabama in Tuscaloosa, despite Governor Wallace's posturing at the "schoolhouse door" (1963); discovery of the bodies of Cheney, Schwerner, and Goodman (1964); the Voting Rights Act (1965); the assassination of Martin Luther King, Jr. (1968); and riots in Watts and Washington, D.C. (1967 and 1968).

Another reason that the study of syphilis in blacks interested whites was that whites feared infection from blacks. Especially during the syphilophobia campaign, upper-class whites feared infection from black domestic servants.

Research Design

As has already been seen, the Tuskegee study was certainly not an example of good research design.

For instance, Kampmeier's justification of the Tuskegee research was based on a claim that untreated syphilitics fared no worse than syphilitics who were treated. A claim like this could be tested only through careful use of controls: That is, by comparing untreated subjects (an experimental group) with treated subjects (a control group). As noted earlier, the Tuskegee study originally started to follow 275 men with syphilis who had received a small number of arsphenamine injections and who might have served as a control group, but they were not reported on after 1936. Thus in the Tuskegee study the "controls" were actually the approximately 200 men who initially did *not* have syphilis at all. This means that the Tuskegee study could not compare treated and untreated syphilitics, and thus that it never learned—and never could have learned—anything about the effectiveness of treatment versus nontreatment.

It can be argued that, as a study in nature, the Tuskegee research was not supposed to learn anything about treatment versus nontreatment but was simply intended to discover what happens as untreated syphilis runs its course. Even on these terms, though, it is not clear how the study can be justified. In studies in nature, controls of some kind are still needed, so that the researchers can be reasonably sure that what they observe over time in, say, untreated syphilitics would not also be found in treated syphilitics or in nonsyphilitics. Since after 1936 the Tuskegee study had no control group of treated subjects, it could learn nothing about the course of untreated syphilis as opposed to treated syphilis. And although it did have a "control group" of sorts, of people without syphilis, its handling of these "controls" seems to have been so questionable that it could not even have learned anything useful about untreated syphilitics as opposed to nonsyphilitics.

To begin with, recordkeeping was poor, records were often lost, and—as was mentioned earlier—the names of the syphilitic subjects were often confused with the "controls." Furthermore, the researchers assumed (naively, given the high rate of syphilis in Macon County) that the "controls" would remain unaffected; as it happened, though, many "controls" eventually contracted syphilis and had to be switched to the "subject" group. (Note that "controls" who became subjects in the "study in nature" group were also given no treatment by the researchers.)

Even the handling of the syphilitic subjects themselves was careless enough to cast any findings into doubt. During the course of the research, many of the 399 syphilitic subjects, who were supposed to remain untreated, actually did get some treatment—neosalvarsan or, later, penicillin—outside the study or outside Macon County. James Lucas, a CDC physician, said later that "effective and undocumented treatment had been given to the vast majority of patients in the syphilitic group,"[44] and that the value of the study was thus undermined. The researchers could not be sure which subjects had received such treatment and therefore could not drop them from the "study in nature" group. As a result, no one could know whether what was observed really represented the consequences of untreated syphilis.

In short, even as a study in nature the Tuskegee study proved nothing. Before the study began, it was already known that morbidity and mortality were higher for syphilitics than for nonsyphilitics and (from Boeck and Bruusgaard's research) that not all people with late latent syphilis would die of syphilis; the Tuskegee research added nothing to this existing knowledge.

As Lucas remarked, the Tuskegee study was bad science. Anyone who wanted to argue that its subjects had been inadvertently sacrificed to science would have to acknowledge that the sacrifice was in vain: Nothing of scientific value was gained.

Media Coverage

In defending the Tuskegee study, Kampmeier criticized the news media: In October 1972, he first objected to the "great hue and cry" in the media a few months earlier, and second to the journalists' claim that "treatment was purposefully withheld to evaluate the course of untreated disease." He said about *Time* and *AMA News* (later *American Medical News*): "In complete disregard of their abysmal ignorance, members of the fourth estate bang out anything on their typewriters that will make headlines."[45] Neither of Kampmeier's objections seems well-founded. The answer to his second objection suggests that the media did a better job than he said, while the answer to his first objection suggests that the media did a worse job.

To begin with the second objection, Kampmeier attacked the media for reporting the damaging aspects of the study, such as the withholding of treatment; but withholding treatment was indeed, and precisely, the intention of the study. Here it seems undeniable that the media reported the situation accurately.

With regard to the first objection, Kampmeier's description of a "hue and cry" seems exaggerated. Actually, in terms of how much of a hue and cry journalists did raise in 1972, how much they *should* have raised, and how much they would raise today, the media seem to have botched the story. Coverage shrank within days—in newspapers, the story moved to back pages, where it was covered in only short paragraphs—yet the Tuskegee study surely deserved more attention than that. The issues were complicated and involved racism, at a time when the United States was undergoing racial turmoil; today, such a story might receive weeks of nationwide scrutiny in the national media.

The role of professional journals can also be questioned. Before Heller's story broke, the Tuskegee study had been reported routinely and repeatedly in medical journals: There were at least 17 articles between 1936 and 1972. In 1964, for instance, an article in *Archives of Internal Medicine* was titled, "The Tuskegee Study of Untreated Syphilis: The Thirtieth Year of Observation."[46] In other words, no attempt was made to conceal the study within the medical profession. Despite this, no professional publication or editor, and no physician, ever alerted the general media to the story.

Harm to Subjects

One of the most important ethical issues of the Tuskegee case has to do with whether the subjects were *harmed*. When we discuss whether, or how, the subjects of the Tuskegee study were harmed, it is important to be clear about counterfactual conditionals in philosophical discourse. A *counterfactual conditional* is a deceptively simple statement of the form "If *X* had not happened, then *Y* would not have happened," and it is *not* permissible in a logical argument.

For example, Kampmeier argued that if the Tuskegee study in nature had never been conducted at all, its subjects would still have received no treatment and therefore would have been no worse off. It is apparent why such a claim cannot be proved. In this case, an infinite number of other things might have happened if the Tuskegee study had not taken place. Some local organization might have provided neosalvarsan (as the Rosenwald Foundation had originally intended). Somebody like John Steinbeck might have written a novel about Macon County, arousing national concern, as *The Grapes of Wrath* did about migrant workers; then, the pressure of public opinion might have led to a federal program to provide neosalvarsan or, later, penicillin—ironically, such treatment might well have been provided through USPHS.

The problem of counterfactual conditionals cuts both ways, however: We cannot say that if the Tuskegee study had *not* been conducted, the subjects would have received treatment and therefore would have been better off. Again, many other things might have happened: The subjects might not have received treatment from another source (this was Kampmeier's supposition); they might have failed to benefit if they did receive treatment; they might have been killed or disabled in combat during World War II (recall that the researchers prevented the subjects from being drafted); and so on.

Are Spinal Taps Traumatic?   One issue of harm arises with regard to the spinal taps which many of the Tuskegee subjects were given. Some physicians regard spinal taps as an insignificant harm, justified by the need to prove that neurosyphilis is present or absent; some of them would argue, further, that lying about such an insignificant procedure is not an enormous concern. It is understandable that from the perspective of physicians who constantly see devastating diseases and injuries, a spinal tap is not tremendously significant; physicians and researchers who deal continually with life-threatening heart attacks, terminal cancer, kidney failure, and psychotic self-mutilation may feel that only laypeople, who lack this kind of experience, would protest vehemently about spinal taps.

Patient advocates, on the other hand, emphasize that most physicians and researchers have never undergone a spinal tap themselves: That is, professionals who describe a spinal tap as "insignificant" are thinking in terms of administering a tap rather than receiving one. A spinal tap is not simply a minor procedure like taking a blood sample. Some patients, though admittedly only a small minority, will experience bad side effects, such as being unable to stand for a week without a severe headache; 1 in 1 million will become paralyzed. In December 1988, a malpractice suit brought against Medical Center Hospital of Vermont on behalf of a 28-year-old woman who had gone into a coma after being incompetently "tapped" by a resident was settled out of court for $2.7 million.[47] "Tapping" someone involuntarily—i.e., without obtaining informed consent—is legally battery; and researchers who need healthy volunteers for spinal taps now offer as much as $500.

It is interesting to note, moreover, that paid volunteers may not be representative of the general population: Many people would not undergo a nontherapeutic tap for $5,000 or even $10,000, and some would not do it for any amount. There is no reason to believe that people would have been any more likely to consent to a nontherapeutic tap at the time of the Tuskegee study in the 1930s.

Fundamentally, defenders of the Tuskegee study say that the spinal taps were not traumatic and that lack of consent was therefore not a serious issue. Its critics say that such an attitude was at the heart of the problem. Today, patient advocates argue that physicians can become blind to the needs and rights of people outside medicine. Physicians who are also researchers may be especially likely to develop such a blind spot, since they have a conflict of interest—they are torn between serving science and preserving the rights of patients and subjects.

Withholding Treatment: Can "Studies in Nature" Injure Subjects?   A more general and more crucial ethical issue arises from the fact that the subjects in the Tuskegee study were not treated for syphilis: What harm, if any, resulted from nontreatment? This question might seem odd or even absurd; that is, it might seem obvious that since the subjects were left untreated, they must have been harmed. However, the issue may not be that simple, and according to some commentators—especially some physicians—there is no proof that the Tuskegee subjects were harmed by nontreatment.

At the outset of the study, when penicillin was not yet available, what was withheld from the subjects was heavy-metals treatment, particularly neosalvarsan. Neosalvarsan was expensive and cumbersome to administer; thus the subjects might not have received it even if they had not become part of a study based on nontreatment. (For one thing, as noted earlier, it required 20 to 40 injections over the course of 1 year; these cost $1 each, and during the Depression, few Alabama sharecroppers could afford them.) Moreover, Boeck and Bruusgaard's research showed that the benefits of heavy metals were controversial. Historian Benedek, for instance, has reviewed the medical evidence available in 1940 and concluded that in 1937 untreated syphilitics had actually lived longer and in better condition than those who were partially treated with heavy metals.[48]

But medical professor, Ben Friedman says, with regard to heavy metals:

> In the 1940s it was known that patients receiving as few as 20 injections of arsenicals rarely developed symptomatic aortic disease. Since we could not determine in advance which of the latent syphilitics would, after 20 or 30 years, develop symptomatic aortic disease, it was necessary to treat all of them. One cannot maintain that some small number of syphilitics deprived of treatment did not therefore suffer injury.[49]

Furthermore, as early as 1934 the major professional organization of physicians treating syphilis, the Cooperating Clinical Group, had demonstrated that use of heavy metals improved Bruusgaard's statistics and had therefore recommended neosalvarsan, mercury, and bismuth as therapy for all syphilitics.[50] Thus even if many patients might not be able to afford such therapy—and even though many might be expected to fail to complete the lengthy course of treatment—it would certainly seem that all patients should at least have been informed about the recommended procedure.

Later in the study, of course, penicillin became available. An early form of penicillin had been discovered by Alexander Fleming in 1929, though its value was not appreciated until it was tested in 1941; as a result of wartime production, penicillin became generally available by 1946.[51] The implications of this development with regard to harm in the Tuskegee study are disputed.

Kampmeier—who has argued in public what many physicians argue in private—believed for several reasons that withholding penicillin had not been harmful. First, he called latent syphilis a "chronic, granulomatous, self-limiting disease," which would imply (as Boeck and Bruusgaard thought possible) that it may not be devastating or fatal without treatment. Second (perhaps on the basis of later or better information), he held that according to "incontrovertible evidence," the late manifestations of latent syphilis have occurred within 20 years "in almost all instances": That is, with or without treatment. Third, he argued that definitive proof of the effectiveness of penicillin was not published until 1948—and this proof was only for primary syphilis, not for the secondary or tertiary phase. What his second and third arguments would imply is that, by the time penicillin became available as a proven therapy, the Tuskegee subjects (who originally had latent, or secondary, syphilis) could no longer have been helped by it; the damage of syphilis had already been done.[52]

Historian Benedek argues similarly with regard to aortic disease (which is more frequent among African-American than white syphilitics). According to Benedek, aortic disease occurs in only 10 percent of untreated syphilitics and begins 15 to 20 years after the initial infection—after which it does its permanent structural damage. He cites as an example 70 syphilitic subjects who were examined in 1948, when all of them had had syphilis for at least 18 years, and implies that penicillin would most likely have been ineffective for them, since it would not have reversed such damage. Benedek maintains that giving penicillin to latent syphilitics in the 1940s "might have exerted a definitely beneficial effect on the prognosis of only 12.5 percent of the subjects." He notes, paradoxically, that virtually all the syphilitic subjects of the Tuskegee study who were alive in 1973 had outlived the nonsyphilitic "controls." Benedek concludes:

> The Tuskegee study had been in progress for 12 years when the possibility of dramatic improvement of treatment appeared, for 16 years when new insights into the ethical implications of research began to be advocated, and was 39 years old when it abruptly became the subject of severe criticism for ethical deficiencies. . . . The righteousness of the ethical critics fails to take into account that in the context of the 1930s thoughtful physicians could detect no ethical dilemma in an investigation such as the Tuskegee study, and also refuses to accept the evidence that very little would have been accomplished therapeutically by initiating penicillin treatment in the 1950s.

Some defenders of the Tuskegee study have pointed to Erlich's experience in 1910, when the hoped-for "magic bullet" had turned out to be unreliable, sometimes simply missing its target and sometimes hitting the wrong target and killing the patient. In the early 1940s, who could be sure that penicillin might not be another disappointment? Benedek emphasizes that physicians in the 1940s did not know optimal dosages of penicillin and had no way to determine at that point whether or not penicillin would have any effect on long-term syphilis. (Kampmeier went further; in 1974, he said, dramatically, "Today—26 years later—we know no more about the effectiveness or ineffectiveness of penicillin in late latent syphilis than in 1948."[53]) These commentators are saying, in effect, that hindsight is always 20/20: At the time, the picture was less clear.

Most physicians disagree with Kampmeier's claims about penicillin. His argument that it was not proven effective until 1948 is especially weak. As Professor Friedman notes, "Penicillin replaced all the [heavy-metal treatments] and was available in adequate doses after 1946. . . . After Mohoney's studies in 1943 it became apparent that penicillin in adequate dosages was effective" for early syphilis. Also, the prophylactic effect of penicillin on latent syphilis was expected and had been proven: "The progressive decline in syphilitic heart disease since 1930 from the fourth highest cause of heart disease to almost total disappearance is strong indirect evidence that penicillin has a preventive effect." It can also be added that Benedek's estimate of how many subjects might have been helped by penicillin in the 1940s—12.5 percent—is hardly a negligible figure.

Practically speaking, though, it would be difficult to prove conclusively that syphilitics are harmed by not getting penicillin and thus to prove that the Tuskegee subjects were harmed. The reason why such proof is lacking is that since the introduction of penicillin, everyone with syphilis has been treated with it. To obtain proof *now* that withholding penicillin is harmful, it would be necessary to set up a study comparing an experimental group and a control group—that is, comparing treated and untreated syphilitics. In other words, to *prove* that the Tuskegee study was harmful or unethical, another harmful, unethical study would have to be done.

What can we conclude, then, about harm in this case? First, from a moral standpoint it may not be necessary to prove that the Tuskegee subjects were harmed by being left untreated (this point is discussed further below). In other words, the study cannot be excused simply by saying—as CDC tried to say—that it can't be proved to have harmed anyone. It may have been only a matter of luck for the researchers that the study caused no more harm than it did.

Second, a crucial point about harm is that when penicillin became available, *it should have been hypothesized that penicillin might help subjects with latent syphilis.* For all anyone knew at the time, penicillin could have prevented lethal aortic heart disease. At the very least, therefore, the originally untreated latent syphilitics should have been divided into two groups, one of which would receive penicillin. After penicillin became available—and everyone else with syphilis was getting it—continuing to withhold it from the Tuskegee subjects was tantamount to using them as involuntary, unknowing "controls" for the rest of the nation.

Effects on Subjects' Families   To critics of the Tuskegee study, one especially troubling aspect of the issue of harm is that no effort was made to survey syphilis in the subjects' families—their wives and children. Benedek read correspondence in the National Library of Medicine and discovered that "virtually all subjects were or had been married" and that the subjects had an average of 5.2 children. Keep in mind, moreover, that the researchers' disregard of families took place in a county where the rate of congenital syphilis was 62 percent.

When we consider the subjects' families, another disturbing issue is the fact that the 399 subjects were not told they had syphilis. Wouldn't the husbands in the study want to know that they had syphilis? Even if they were originally in the latent stage, wouldn't they need to know that they might become infectious again—that they might then infect their wives and thus give future children congenital syphilis? Did the researchers withhold the truth because they accepted the racist myth that African-American men couldn't refrain from sex?

Today, we know that late syphilis is almost never reinfectious; but when the Tuskegee researchers began their study, over 60 years ago, they did not know this. These researchers thus simply took a chance with the wives and children of their subjects. Either the researchers failed to consider possible harm to the subjects' families, or they decided that possible harm didn't matter compared with the goal of the study in nature.

Motives of Researchers

When the Tuskegee study was debated within USPHS and CDC, many physicians and administrators assumed that if no harm could be proved, nothing immoral had been done; this is also one basis of Kampmeier's argument. Focusing on consequences, however, is only one way of judging morality. Another way—and in this case perhaps a more appropriate way—is to focus on *motives* or *intentions*.

It is important to understand that in medical research, provable harm is a very self-serving standard. To see why this is so, consider that physicians and medical researchers seldom want to be held to the analogous standard of provable benefit: They typically argue that "benefit" needs to be no more than likely, "probable," or even "possible." This argument, moreover, is perfectly reasonable. Suppose, for instance, that no treatment were reimbursable unless its benefit to patients had been conclusively proved. Since it is estimated that as much as one-third of all medical practices are scientifically unproven, much of medicine would then have to be free. (Here is one example: Though the cost of hospital care is much higher in ICUs than in normal rooms, there is no proof that patients do better in ICUs.) But this reasonable argument about benefits would seem to apply equally to harm—and if it does, provable harm would not be a necessary or fair criterion.

As with benefit, then, a better criterion may be likely, probable, or possible harm. If we adopt such a standard, we do not ultimately need to prove that harm has been done; instead, we may consider motives or intentions in light of whether harm was likely. From this point of view, it should be emphasized that people do not exist to serve medical science. Human beings—of any race, rich or poor, sick or well, educated or uneducated—have a right to control their bodies and their medical treatment without risk of harm from researchers.

To argue that the Tuskegee researchers acted immorally in terms of motivation, then, we do not necessarily have to claim that they were motivated by racism or malice or even self-interest. They may have been motivated, primarily, simply to conduct a study in nature and thereby to learn something. The point is that, given a likelihood of harm, they should also have been motivated to protect their subjects. Since harm was possible, their motivations should have included an intention not to do harm. Instead, through systematic deceit and nontreatment, these researchers put their subjects at risk of harm, depriving them of their rights.

UPDATE: OTHER CONTROVERSIAL AMERICAN MEDICAL RESEARCH ON CAPTIVE POPULATIONS

IRBs

In 1972, the federal government required all institutions that conducted human medical experimentation and received federal funds to have Institutional Review Boards (IRBs). The original function of IRBs was to review proposals for medical research before these experiments were evaluated for funding; later on, IRB reviews were expanded to cover research on humans in the social sciences. Today, IRBs—which scrutinize written proposals—are the first line of defense against abuses in medical research.

Before the criticisms by Beecher and Pappworth in the 1960s and the revelation of the Tuskegee study in 1972, support for outside review of medical research (IRBs), or for peer review, was lukewarm. Afterward, however, medical research was forced to operate under quasi regulation in a multistage process. (As discussed in Chapter 9, after Gennarelli's animal studies were revealed, similar quasi regulation came to animal research.)

Later Analyses of Tuskegee

James Jones, the author of *Bad Blood*, later found many documents that had been filed by the Tuskegee researchers. *Bad Blood* was published in 1981, 9 years after Heller's first story and 49 years after the Tuskegee study had begun.

In the 1990s, the Tuskegee study attracted renewed interest. In 1992, Sidney Olansky, then age 78 and still practicing in Atlanta as a dermatologist, was interviewed on the television show *Prime Time Live*. Olansky had been in charge of the Tuskegee study in 1951 and had been at the CDC meeting which decided to continue the Tuskegee research in 1969. He supported Kampmeier's defense of the study and—like Kampmeier—did not believe that anyone could be proved to have been harmed by the study. In fact, like almost all the physicians who have ever been interviewed about the study, even in 1992 he did not believe that anything unethical was done. After the interview was broadcast, Olansky was upset by the reaction. "They made me look like a mad scientist and a bigot," he said.[54] Leaflets were distributed around his office building, urging his patients to "stop Olansky"; he received hate mail and a telephone call from a woman in California calling him a "murderer." Olansky's son David, also a physician (the two were in practice together), observed about his father, "These are very proud men. They know their intentions were good and they can't accept people questioning that. There's so much ego involved in medicine. They just can't admit that their methods, in retrospect, might have been wrong."[55]

Also in 1992, on a special *Nova* broadcast devoted to the Tuskegee study, some of the other Tuskegee physicians echoed Olansky's sentiments.[56] They did admit that nothing was learned from the study, but they refused to admit that they had done anything wrong. Among the people quoted by *Nova* in defense of the study were John Cutler, who had harangued Peter Buxtun at the CDC syphilis conference in 1966; and David Sencer, who had been a director of CDC and had convened the 1969 meeting.

During the early 1990s, *Miss Ever's Boys,* a play about the Tuskegee study written by the physician David Feldshuh, became popular around the country. Feldshuh's drama placed the study in its historical context and emphasized the deliberate omission of penicillin, the nontherapeutic spinal taps, and the benign deception. In 1992, *Miss Ever's Boys* was produced at the Alabama Shakespeare Festival in Montgomery and was given a special one-night performance in nearby Tuskegee, at which four survivors of the Tuskegee study were present. It was later made into a movie and shown on cable television.

Some months after Olansky had been interviewed on *Prime Time Live,* a replay was seen by the most famous of the Tuskegee survivors, Charles Pollard, who remarked: "I don't think I'd have anything to say to that man. I think I'd hit him in the face."

On May 11, 1997, President Clinton met four of the eight survivors to apologize for the Tuskegee Study on behalf of the federal government, saying that, "What the United States did was shameful, and I am sorry."[57]

At the time of the President's apology, the youngest survivor was 87 and the oldest (who did not have a birth record) was between 100 and 109.[58] The federal government has paid more than $10 million to members of the study and their heirs, who numbered more than 6,000 people, including 22 wives, 17 children, and two grandchildren, any of whom may have contracted syphilis as a direct result of the lack of treatment for syphilis of men in the study.[59] One of the most pervasive of the effects of the study was a lingering, widespread distrust by the black community of medical experiments.

Other Controversial American Experiments

In 1994, it was discovered that many physician-researchers had subjected over 16,000 American patients to radiation experiments from World War II to the mid-1970s.[60] At least 435 experiments were conducted by the Department of Energy or its predecessors in 21 states. Among the initial findings was the revelation that physicians working for the government had used many Americans as human guinea pigs in radiation experiments.

The purpose of these experiments was to study effects of exposure to radiation in order to determine safe levels of exposure for workers in programs such as the Manhattan Project (which developed the first atom bomb). In one experiment, about 130 male prisoners, most of whom were African-American, were paid $200 to undergo x-ray radiation of their testicles; afterwards, these men got vasectomies. In another, an indigent 36-year-old Texan who had injured a leg was given a shot of plutonium in the injured leg, which was then amputated.

Some terminally ill patients at Strong Memorial Hospital at the University of Rochester were injected with plutonium between 1945 and 1947 to study what kind of physical damage would occur to people in nuclear war.[61] In contradiction to testimony that all patients injected were terminally ill, documents later revealed that at least 11 patients were healthy. One of these was an 18-year-old boy. Eda Charlton, a woman who entered the hospital with a mild case of hepatitis, was secretly injected with plutonium-239 to study how the body eliminates radiation and was then followed for years so that the effects could be observed. (She died of a heart attack in 1938.) None of these patients or their families were ever told about what had been injected into them or why. Two were still alive in 1971 but all had died by 1995.

There were also studies of radioactive isotopes used in diagnosis and research. (The Veterans Administration was a pioneer in using such radioisotopes to diagnose thyroid disease, brain tumors, and leukemia.) In the late 1940s, at Vanderbilt University, 819 pregnant women were injected with radioactive iron as part of a nutritional study; a follow-up study in 1960 found that three of their children had died of rare forms of cancer.[62] In this research on the thyroid, no consent was obtained because researchers believed the dosage was so low that no harm could occur.

In 1995, the President's Committee on Human Radiation Experiments, formed to investigate these experiments, concluded that the government should apologize to all those who were involuntary subjects of the tests and should compensate people who may have been injured.[63]

In 1991 in Operation Desert Storm, military personnel were forced to take antibiological-warfare experimental vaccines. Federal law stated that soldiers could not refuse such vaccinations under operational conditions. Subsequently, many soldiers became sick. For years afterwards, the Pentagon and Department of Defense denied that their sickness was service-related. In a story broken nationally by the *Birmingham News* and pushed hard by it for years, the military's own records showed many causes of such sickness, especially of possible causes acting in combination. Bioethicist Arthur Caplan, a member of the Presidential Advisory Committee on Gulf War Illnesses, listed a minimum of the following possible causes of illness in these veterans: sand storms, biological weapons, oil fires, contaminated water, rare microorganisms, the above vaccines, chemical vapors from bombed Iraqi storage areas, unspent rocket fuel, and high levels of stress.[64] In all these events, there seems to be a repeated pattern of physicians and scientists working for the military or federal government who deliberately subjected vulnerable, captive populations to harm in the name of a vague, greater good.

Tuskegee and HIV Prevention in Africa

In 1994, a federally sponsored study—the 076 regimen—proved that giving the drug AZT (zidovudine) during pregnancy cut the risk of transmission of HIV from mother to child by two-thirds.[65] CDC, NIH, and WHO set out to export these dramatic results to prevent the 1,600 babies born with HIV every day worldwide.

In the fall of 1997, executive editor of the *New England Journal of Medicine*, Marcia Angell, claimed that American research in Africa to study AZT, in which pregnant, HIV-infected black women were given placebos, was like the Tuskegee study because researchers were permitting many babies in their care to be born with preventable HIV infection.[66]

The newly funded research in countries of Africa had subjects who were: (1) black, (2) female, (3) poor, (4) mostly illiterate, (5) victims of STD's, and (6) without other available treatment. In addition, studies in both cases were conducted by magisterial but distant governmental agencies, very much like the Tuskegee study, Dr. Angell charged, and therefore immoral.

Dr. Angell's comparison of these studies to the Tuskegee study sparked a firestorm of angry rebuttals, the heat of which was exacerbated when Public Citizen, a consumer rights organization founded by Ralph Nader, and specifically its Health Research Group (run by Sidney Wolfe, and Peter Lurie), joined in her charges.[67] All argued that AZT was a proven treatment for reducing transmission of HIV from mother to child, that it was being deliberately withheld from a control group, and that such withholding was immoral.

Researchers first defended themselves by arguing that, because of the lack of money, women in these countries would never have gotten AZT if the research had not been done. So the women were no worse off than they had been before.

Angell and others replied that it had long been established, for ethical reasons, that placebo-controlled studies could not be done on American women. Once AZT had been proven as an effective treatment for preventive transmission of the virus, it was the standard treatment for all pregnant, HIV+ women. In essence, they denied that a double standard should exist in medical research between developed and developing countries. "If it is unethical to do placebo-controlled trials in America, it should also be unethical to do them in third world countries," they said.[68] They charged that such a double standard violated the Nuremberg Code and Guideline 15 of the International Ethical Guidelines for Biomedical Research Involving Human Subjects, which prohibits a double standard between host country of researchers and country of subjects.

Apologists for the study, including officials in developing countries, replied that it was "ethical imperialism" to impose American ethical standards on African countries.[69] Moreover, they noted, many of the local officials were black and had lost children to HIV, so they were hardly like the white physicians of the Tuskegee study.[70]

The sponsoring agencies, which included those doing research funded by Belgium, Denmark, and France, replied that 300,000 children get infected every year with HIV by perinatal transmission, and that if they could prove—via a placebo-controlled trial—that a shorter regimen could reduce transmission by half, then they could save 150,000 thousand children a year. As such, if delays were caused by the skeptics' criticisms—in putting off proof for a year or more—then such delays might actually cost many children their lives.

Central to the defense of these studies by public health agencies were two more claims: A placebo-controlled trial of HIV transmission could be done faster and with fewer subjects than an AZT-controlled study, and that once good results were obtained, African and Asian governments would give all pregnant, HIV+ women the new, smaller dosage of AZT. Researchers also made procedural defenses, arguing that various review committees in both countries had approved the studies and that, unlike the Alabama men, the women themselves had given consent. (Subsequent interviews by the *New York Times* cast doubt on how much the women understood—a claim disputed by local health officials in Africa, who said the women really had understood.)

Angell and others argued that placebo-controlled studies were not necessary to prove such results, that retrospectively comparing dosages of AZT to other treatments or to each other could prove the same thing. More important, they strongly denied that, given the poverty of such countries, a proven, reduced dosage would later be given to all pregnant women in such countries. Even a cheap AZT regimen for $80, they pointed out, was 11 times what was normally spent on the average African's medical care.

Champions on both sides claimed that justice was on their side.[71] Hence this dispute was essentially one of philosophical medical ethics, not factual medicine. For researchers, the risk-benefit ratio had to be different for poor, illiterate women in backward countries who otherwise would not have gotten treatment. For critics, this was the same reasoning that led to the Tuskegee study and to the Nazi experiments: The thinking that deliberately allowing harm to occur to some vulnerable patients in medicine is justified to increase general knowledge to help a greater number of future patients, in example, "they're going to get it anyway, so we might as well study them to learn something."[72] As Angell criticized, "People can't be used as a means to a noble end."[73]

Philosophically, on one side there is Jeremy Bentham, utilitarianism, and public health ethics. On the other side is Immanuel Kant, his axiom that people can never be used as a "mere means," and his belief that ethical principles are not local but universal.

On February 18, 1998, CDC suspended the studies, announcing that the experimental, reduced-dosage treatment had been proven effective in reducing mother-to-child HIV transmission, that is, $80 worth of AZT in the last 4 weeks of pregnancy cut transmission in half.[74] Both sides claimed victory at this early cessation of the American-sponsored studies. Columnist Ellen Goodman noted that the Tuskegee study had not ended, but had been merely exported.[75] Meanwhile many thousands of subjects in third world countries continued to be subjects of HIV-vaccination studies, many of which were placebo-controlled.

The Krieger Lead Paint Study

On August 23, 2001, the federal Office of Protection from Research Risks began an investigation into a study of preventing retardation in children from lead paint that six of seven judges on Maryland's highest court had likened to the Tuskegee Study.[76] The new study, conducted in the mid-1990s by the Kennedy Krieger Institute, an affiliate of Johns Hopkins Medical School, recruited healthy children and their parents from 108 families to live in East Baltimore in houses with varying amounts of lead contamination.

East Baltimore is largely occupied by poor black families. Ingesting lead-based paint is a known cause of mental retardation in small children.

According to a spokesperson for the Kennedy Krieger Institute, the study was designed to find cheaper ways to reduce lead contamination so that landlords in poor areas there would not abandon their property.

One issue was whether, when they signed consent forms, the parents understood the nature of the study. "It can be argued that the researchers intended that the children be the canaries in the mines but never clearly told the parents," Judge Dale R. Cathell said in a scathing decision.[77]

Five days before, on August 18, 2001, the OPRR had halted all federally funded research at Hopkins after Ellen Roche had died in a study there of a drug to prevent asthma. Like Jesse Gelsinger, Ellen Roche was a healthy volunteer who died as a direct result of her decision to participate in medical research.

A Hopkins physician/administrator on television then denounced suspension of Hopkins's research monies, claiming Hopkins had only killed one person in medical research in many decades and that lives would be lost from such a suspension because of delayed cures. Normally, when a hospital kills someone, its spokesperson does not go on television to attack the messenger but says he is very sorry for the death. In this case, the denouncement motivated reporters to dig further, uncovering the Krieger case and interesting details about the workings of the IRB (see below).

According to the *Washington Post*:

> Maryland Court of Appeals Judge Dale R. Cathell, who wrote last week's scathing opinion, said the board instructed Kennedy Krieger researchers to write consent forms for study participants that skirted federal regulations requiring disclosure about risks.
>
> The Court of Appeals ruling ordered trials to be held in lawsuits filed against Kennedy Krieger by two women, Viola Hughes and Catina Higgins, whose children were involved in the study. Hughes's daughter now suffers from learning disabilities and cognitive impairments, both of which are often associated with lead poisoning, according to their attorney. Higgins says researchers withheld tests results that showed high levels of lead contamination from her. . . .
>
> Kennedy Krieger is a major institution in the study of lead paint abatement. Marc Farfel, who conducted the study, said today that it identified more effective ways to remove lead hazards and prompted legislation forcing landlords to remove those hazards.
>
> Farfel and Kennedy Krieger Chief Executive Gary W. Goldstein said they were concerned about the wording of Cathell's opinion and saw no parallels between their study and the Tuskegee experiments.[78]

The investigation by OPRR later revealed that the IRB at Johns Hopkins, which supposedly had reviewed and discussed the ethics of the Krieger study, had rarely met.

At least on the surface, the Krieger study did resemble the Tuskegee Study in that poor black people were deliberately recruited for a study where harm to them was foreseen. The harm was rationalized as going to occur anyway, like a study in nature, because such people would likely live in such housing if the study did not occur. Revelation of the Krieger study did not do much to further relations between Baltimore blacks and Hopkins, relations which had been historically frayed because of problems there in the 1960s from screening for sickle cell disease.

FURTHER READING

Thomas Benedek, "The 'Tuskegee Study' of Untreated Syphilis: Analysis of Moral Aspects versus Methodological Aspects," *Journal of Chronic Diseases*, vol. 31, no. 1, 1978.

Alexee Deep, "Placebo-Controlled Zidovudine Trials in the Developing World," *Princeton Journal of Bioethics*, vol. 1, no. 2, Fall, 1998, pp. 21–39.

James Jones, *Bad Blood*, Free Press, New York, 1981.

CHAPTER 12

Adult Heart Replacement

The First Heart Transplant and Artificial Heart

*T*his chapter focuses on two very famous cases of heart replacement in adults: surgeon Christiaan Barnard's first heart transplant into Louis Washkansky in 1967 in South Africa and surgeon William DeVries insertion of a Jarvik-7 artificial heart into Barney Clark in America in 1982. Although one case was 15 years after the other and on a different continent, were the ethical issues raised by the two cases remarkably the same.

THE FIRST HEART TRANSPLANT

Background on Transplants

Most early attempts at transplating organs, skin, limbs, or blood between humans ended in death because the immune system rejected the foreign bodies and created a lethal condition known as "graft-versus-host disease." As a result during the nineteenth century, England and several other countries banned blood transfusion.

In 1900, an Austrian physiologist, Karl Lansteiner, found that human red blood cells exist as distinct types. Lansteiner used letters of the alphabet arbitrarily to designate blood groups: A, B, AB, and O. Landsteiner's monumental discovery explained in part why most early transplants had failed and went unappreciated for 30 years, until he received the Nobel Prize in 1930.

The technological key to the first transplant was the heart–lung machine, developed between 1931 and 1953 by the surgeon John Gibbon and further improved in the early 1960s. Before the heart–lung machine was devised, the few operations that could be done at all had to be done in one minute, while the heart was stopped and the brain was without oxygenated blood. Early versions of heart–lung machines were problematic because blood clots formed on their surfaces (which were made of a synthetic substance, Mylar). In a later version, air bubbles supplied the blood with oxygen and were removed by greasy foam; but if the bubbles were not removed, or if the debubbling mixture returned to the blood, the patient would die. The slightest mishap with the heart–lung machine—an electrical failure, a leak, contamination—turned the machine into a killer.

The kidney has always been thought to be the easiest organ to transplant. Attempts to transplant it occurred from the 1930s to 1950s, based on innovations by Alex Carrel in 1902 in suturing blood vessels. These attempts failed because the immune system rejected the transplanted organ as a foreign substance.[1]

Using identical twins to avoid the problem of rejection, surgeons at Peter Brent Hospital in Cambridge, Massachusetts, transplanted the first kidney successfully in 1954. In 1959 Murray and colleagues at Brigham Hospital transplanted a kidney from a nonidentical twin to his brother, who had undergone total-body x-ray treatment. Such irradiation suppressed the immune system, allowing the organ to thrive.

But for most recipients, irradiation was fatal because in suppressing the immune system, it destroyed the body's ability to resist infections from viruses and bacteria.

In the 1960s, physicians began to learn how to selectively suppress the immune system by using irradiation, steroids, and Azathioprine (also called Imuran), which inhibits the functioning of T-cells or lymphocytes. Cambridge University's Roy Calne in 1962 used predisone and Imuran to achieve the first step toward successful transplantation.

An important figure on the path toward heart transplants was the surgeon Owen Wangansteen, under whom Christiaan Barnard would study. Wangansteen was the mentor of most American transplant surgeons, including three pioneers of modern heart surgery—Baylor's Michael DeBakey, Stanford's Norman Shumway, and UAB's John Kirklin.

As a medical student, DeBakey devised a booster pump that became the essence of the heart–lung machine and which made open-heart surgery possible in the 1960s. Shumway discovered that cardiac nerve connections, which are severed during transplantation but are too numerous and too fine to be reconnected didn't actually matter because the heart has an independent electrical ignition that triggers its beats and rate. He also discovered that it was better not to transplant a whole heart but instead to leave the upper walls (atrium or auricles) intact, thereby reducing operating time by half. Kirklin would later perfect cardiac surgery for congenital defects and pioneered the use of computers to aid heart surgery.

In 1967 Pittsburgh's Thomas Starzl transplanted a liver and Christiaan Barnard transplanted a heart.

THE OPERATION

Christiaan Barnard a young, 44-years-old surgeon, performed the first heart transplant on December 3, 1967. He grew up poor in South Africa but trained between 1955 and 1957 under famed Minnesota surgeon Owen Wangansteen in Minneapolis–St. Paul. Barnard also studied with Richmond, Virginia, surgeon David Hume between 1966 and early 1967 to learn about immunosuppressive drugs.

In 1967 Owen Wangansteen helped Barnard return to South Africa with a heart–lung machine. Did Wangansteen expect Barnard to then transplant a heart? Probably not. As Barnard says in his autobiography, Wangansteen treated him as a student, not as a colleague or trailblazer. Another transplant surgeon, Thomas

Starzl, says in his own memoirs that everyone expected Barnard to start doing kidney transplants rather than a heart transplant.[2] (Barnard did perform a kidney transplant in 1967 and wanted to do another, but then became intrigued by the possibility of a heart transplant.) On the other hand, the transplant surgeon Donald Kahn of Birmingham, Alabama, a friend of Barnard's, believes that Norman Shumway and others implicitly gave Barnard permission to attempt the first heart transplant.[3] Most probably, though, no one really thought that a heart transplant would be attempted until the problem of immune rejection had been solved.

This first heart transplant was not performed, as might have been expected, at a prestigious center of medical research, but at an obscure hospital in Cape Town, South Africa, called Groote Schuur—"big barn" in Afrikaans. Groote Schuur was associated with the University of Cape Town Medical School; set deep into the slope of a mountain above Cape Town, the hospital was a landmark visible from all over the city. It looked like a resort hotel, with even-spaced windows and double wings and an ancient forest on both sides. Ambulances brought patients from the city to either of two entrances—one for whites, one for nonwhites.

Barnard had quietly begun to assemble a team at Groote Schuur to perform the first human heart transplant. He did set up the best organ-transplant team outside the United States; even so, however, facilities at Groote Schuur were much more primitive than at American transplant centers. Other physicians at Groote Schuur were close-mouthed about Barnard's plans, and no American hospitals were informed.

Barnard had asked the cardiologists at Groote Schuur to refer to him a possible candidate for a heart transplant. He approached Velva Shrire (his superior, the chief cardiologist at Groote Schuur) and obtained permission for the transplant; Shrire also gave him the name of a patient—Louis Washkansky, 55 years old and dying. Louis Washkansky was white, a salesman with a fondness for playing cards, drinking, eating, smoking, and in general living life fully. As a young man, he had been athletic (a weightlifter and an amateur boxer); during World War II, he had served in the army. He was a big, intelligent man with a ferocious desire to live, exuberant, extroverted, and well-liked. He was married and was a macho type, pretending to his wife that everything was fine, snitching cigarettes, never slowing down, flirting with nurses.

Louis Washkansky was about as sick as a cardiac patient can be and still live. He had diabetes, coronary artery disease, and congestive heart failure; his flabby heart was so swollen that it extended across the entire inside of his large chest, from wall to wall. Washkansky had first been hospitalized in 1965: He felt an attack coming on, got to the hospital an hour later, and climbed the stairs to the cardiac unit—where his heart collapsed. He could not breathe at night and was kept breathing with drugs. In April 1966, he was diagnosed as in terminal cardiac failure and given only a month or two to live.

In October 1967, amazingly, he was still alive. He was deteriorating, though: He needed to take 15 pills a day; and at one point, in September 1967, he had developed so much edema (swelling from fluids) in his legs that drainage holes had to be opened. He then spent 5 days without sleep, sitting in a chair with water running down his legs into basins. His skin was almost black from lack of epidermal circulation. It was about at this point that he was referred to Christiaan Barnard.

When he was approached about the transplant, Louis Washkansky did not hesitate. He knew he was dying, and his life had been hellish for 2 years. Barnard said that he told his patient, "We can put a normal heart into you, after taking out your heart that's no longer good, and there's a chance you can get back to normal life"—and that Louis Washkansky replied, "So they told me. So I'm ready to go ahead."[4]

After obtaining this consent, Barnard waited 3 weeks for a donor. Meanwhile, the patient developed fulminant pulmonary edema—a sign of imminent death—and Barnard was afraid that his chance to perform the first heart transplant would pass. This had happened to other surgeons: Two patients of James Hardy in Mississippi, for instance, had died before donors could be found.

•

On the afternoon of December 2, 1967—a Saturday—25-year-old Denise Ann Darvall left her home, driving in a car with her brother, father, and mother. After parking the car, Denise and her mother walked a few blocks to a bakery, which was half a mile below Groote Schuur Hospital. A few minutes later, Ann Washkansky, Louis's wife, on the way up the mountain to visit him at the hospital, saw a crowd gathered at the scene of an automobile accident.

The accident had occurred without warning, when Denise Darvall and her mother left the bakery. A speeding car smashed into the mother, killing her instantly and throwing her against her daughter. Denise herself had been thrown through the air and killed on impact, but she was rushed up to Groote Schuur Hospital; though she was brain-dead, her heart was still healthy.

Shortly after Denise's arrival at the hospital, Barnard spoke to her shocked father, Edward Darvall. At a moment like this, everything depends on people's trust in the medical profession: Edward Darvall, who had just learned of the death of his wife and daughter, also had to accept Barnard's right to ask a very delicate, sensitive question. When Barnard approached Edward Darvall, he said, "We have a man in the hospital here, and we can save his life if you give us permission to use your daughter's heart. . . ." According to Barnard, Edward Darvall replied simply, "If you can't save my daughter, try and save this man."[5]

The operation took place during the early hours of December 3, 1967. As we've seen, Louis Washkansky had already been told about, and consented to, a possible transplant. Within 2 minutes of being informed that a donor had become available, he reaffirmed his consent. Blood typing was done (Denise Darvall was type O, a universal donor; Washkansky was type A). Calls went out to the transplant team; as the story is told, some of the team members arrived at the hospital in pajamas, and some were breathless because their car had broken down and they had run up the mountain to Groote Schuur.

As he was rolled into surgery, Louis Washkansky was still awake. For the first time, he felt "kind of shaky," like a person "going into the ring when you don't know who you're up against." He said that Barnard, as his surgeon, was his manager, but now he wanted to know what his opponent looked like. Barnard says that, though he told his patient nothing, he thought to himself, "I knew what [his opponent] looked like. He was the Skoppensboer—the wild Jack of Spades. He was death and against him I had only the King of Hearts."[6]

Denise Darvall was declared dead after her heart had actually stopped beating; surgeons then opened her body, preparing it for Barnard's excision of the heart. Meanwhile, in an adjacent room, in preparation of the excision of *his* heart, Washkansky was anesthetized, given drugs to produce paralysis and prevent spontaneous breathing, and placed on the heart–lung machine. The two operations that were about to take place had to be precisely coordinated.

At this point, everything almost failed. Washkansky's femoral artery, where a tube was attached, was so narrow from buildup of cholesterol that the machine couldn't force blood into his heart. The pressure on the tube climbed to 290, just below the point where the lines would blow, spilling gallons of blood over the room. Frantically, Barnard and other surgeons reattached the line directly to Washkansky's aorta, and gradually the pressure dropped.

Barnard then walked to the next room and excised Denise Darvall's heart, leaving part of the wall attached to it like the lid of a jack-o-lantern. He put her heart into a basin of chilled fluid and walked 31 steps back to Washkansky's operating room, where he gave it to a nurse to hold.

Then, Barnard cut out Washkansky's flabby heart. (As he peered down into Washkansky's huge, empty chest cavity and looked at the two hearts, he said, "This really is the point of no return."[7]) Next, he sewed Denise Darvall's heart (with the attached wall) into Louis Washkansky's chest, where it looked quite small.

The two operations had taken five hours, but cardiac surgeons regarded the surgery itself—the cutting out of the patient's own heart and the transplantation of the donated heart—as relatively simple. The interesting questions were, first, whether the transplanted heart would start beating in a foreign body; and if it did start beating, whether it would then be rejected.

The operation team therefore watched expectantly, hoping that the transplanted heart would simply start beating spontaneously as the patient's blood temperature rose to normal. This did not happen in Washkansky's case (though it would happen, later, with the second transplant patient); and reports differ about what took place next. According to United Press International (UPI), the transplanted heart began to beat after Barnard shocked it slightly, whereupon Barnard gasped, "Christ, it's going to work!"[8]—one surgeon at the operation described this effect as "like turning the ignition switch of a car."[9] But according to Barnard's own account, things were not so easy. A human heart does not always start beating when shocked; and Barnard says that although Louis Washkansky's new heart did start and continue to beat after the first shock, it then stopped. Moreover, at first the new heart didn't take over from the heart–lung machine. Thus it was only after another attempt that the new heart began to beat regularly, whereupon the patient was quickly weaned from the heart–lung machine, which was then turned off.[10]

The Postoperative Period

After working all night, the surgeons had finished the operation at 7 A.M. on December 3. An hour later, Louis Washkansky regained consciousness and tried to talk. Thirty-six hours later, a hungry Washkansky ate a soft-boiled egg and toast.

Louis Washkansky was encouraged to eat—to get protein into his system— but his recovery progressed slowly. He had five rough days immediately after surgery, when his urine output, enzymes, and heart rate were problematic. Also, worried about immunological rejection of the heart, Barnard's team flooded Washkansky with gamma ray radiation from a cobalt unit and administered both prednisone and Imuran (azathoprine), and the patient did not tolerate these treatments well. By day 5, he said, the constant tests were "killing me. I can't sleep. I can't do anything. They're at me all the time with pins and needles. . . . It's driving me crazy."[11]

On the sixth day, though, Louis Washkansky received steroids to prevent rejection of the heart; this began five very good, happy days when he laughed, visited with his family, and wanted to go home. At this time, Barnard told a press conference that if his patient's progress held, he would "have him home in three weeks."[12]

In retrospect, however, these five good days were the eye of the hurricane, merely a brief period before Louis Washkansky's body really began to reject his new heart. As this rejection process went on, he began to feel, as he said, "terrible": He suffered from constant pain in the shoulders; dark circles formed under his eyes; his heart and breathing rates climbed; on the thirteenth day, a shadow of unknown origin could be seen on his lung x-ray. Moreover, his personality changed: This vibrant, forceful man became sullen and irritable. In addition to the threat of rejection, there was also a danger of infection. Unfortunately, most posttransplant symptoms can indicate either rejection or infection, and treatment of one problem can exacerbate the other. It was therefore necessary to wait for a definitive diagnosis, even if the delay entailed a risk of death.

By the fourteenth day after the operation, Louis Washkansky felt that he was dying. He couldn't force himself to eat. He had lost bowel control. He had such severe pain in his chest that he preferred to lie in his own feces rather than try to move. Barnard said that he was "constrained" to insert a nasogastric tube in order to feed his patient, but Washkansky didn't want it. To Washkansky, it didn't look as though he would ever be normal again; he had lost his dignity and hence his will to live.

By day 15—December 18—there were spotty, mottled patches on Louis Washkansy's legs, indicating circulatory failure. He was breathing with difficulty, and x-rays showed that the patches on his lung had grown ominously larger. As Washkansky gasped desperately for each breath, Barnard decided that he should be placed on a respirator. Washkansky resisted this: He had been on the respirator when he first woke up after the operation, and he knew that reconnecting it would mean giving up speech; and in any case he continued to feel that he was near his end. Barnard disagreed; on December 18, he told Washkansky that there was "a chance" to be home by Christmas. Washkansky replied, "No, not now." His bed was in a sterile tent, and despite his extreme weakness, he grabbed the sides of the tent in an attempt to prevent Barnard from entering to reopen his tracheotomy hole.

As Barnard entered, Washkansky persisted in refusing, saying, "No, Doc."

Barnard replied, "Yes, Louis,"[13] and put him on the respirator. Washkansky would never speak again.

On December 19 or 20—day 16 or 17—Ann Washkansky called, telling Barnard that reporters were saying Louis was dying. Barnard lied to her and said that the reporters were lying. (Both Barnard and Washkansky saw Ann Washkansky as weak and unable to bear the truth.) New x-rays now showed that bilateral pneumonia, klebsiella, and pseudomonas had infiltrated Washkansky's lungs. Penicillin had been administered earlier, but though it had killed one organism, it had allowed others to grow. The anti-immune drugs given to suppress rejection had also allowed all these organisms to flourish.

On December 20—day 17—Ann Washkansky was allowed to see Louis, but she wasn't told it might be the last time. Barnard urged her to encourage her husband to keep fighting. Louis Washkansky, now on the respirator, couldn't speak, and his wife didn't understand why. She was told not to touch him because of germs. All Louis Washkansky himself could do at this last visit was, with enormous effort, open his eyes and move his arm a bit.

After his wife had left, the patient received 40 percent oxygen; then, as his breathing continued to worsen, this was increased to 100 percent. Between midnight of day 17 and 1 A.M. of day 18, the physicians gave him drugs to help his breathing, but it was too late: Germs had overrun his lungs. Louis Washkansky began to suffocate.

After 2 hours of Louis Washkansky's dying gasps, Denise Darvall's heart went into wild fibrillation from lack of oxygen and stopped beating. Even then, Barnard was not ready to give up; he rushed a team together to put Washkansky on a heart–lung machine. At this point, another physician challenged him, arguing passionately that it was "madness" to continue and that Washkansky was "clinically lost." Reluctantly, Barnard agreed. At 6:30 A.M. on December 21, after having lived 18 days with a transplanted heart, Louis Washkansky died.

The next morning, Barnard watched the postmortem, which showed that lobar pneumonia had destroyed the lungs; thus the heart–lung machine would ultimately have been useless. The heart itself and Barnard's surgery were perfect.

In 1968 Barnard became one of the most famous people in the world, gracing the cover of *Time*, appearing on major television shows, and meeting the President of the United States, Lyndon Johnson. In his second autobiography, he admits that fame went to his head, and he brags about how many beautiful women he bedded, including actress Gina Lollobrigida; he also admits there that all this ruined his first (and possibly his second) marriage.[14] His third marriage also ended in divorce. In 1984 he took $4 million for saying on film that a facial cream, Glygel, reverses aging in skin (it doesn't), for which famed dermatologist Norman Orentreich called him "a huckster." Barnard died of an asthma attack at age 78 on September 2, 2001, beside a swimming pool at a luxury hotel on Cyprus.

BARNEY CLARK'S ARTIFICIAL HEART

Background on Artificial Hearts

Left Ventricle Assist Devices (LVADs), which would become popular again in the 1990s, are called a halfway technology. Although not a cure, an LVAD was better than death, since it could keep a heart patient alive in a state of semisickness. Thus attempts continued to develop a true artificial heart.

The National Institutes of Health (NIH) committed $1.5 million for an artificial heart in 1964 and $8.5 million in 1967, hoping to test one by 1972. During the early 1970s, NIH became pessimistic about artificial hearts and switched most of its grants to LVADs; but in general between 1965 and 1982, NIH continued to support LVADs, mechanical assist devices, and artificial hearts, all together pouring $200 million into them.

Before Barney Clark's operation, Houston surgeon Denton Cooley had disastrously implanted a crude artificial heart inside Haskell Karp. Without permission, Cooley used a device developed by his fellow surgeon at Baylor College of Medicine, Michael DeBakey. Karp wasn't told that implantation of the device had killed a dozen experimental calves. Cooley also failed to get permission from Baylor's Institutional Review Board. DeBakey later forced Cooley's resignation from Baylor.[15]

Cooley defended himself by claiming *therapeutic privilege,* according to which a physician may lie for a patient's good in extreme situations. But the patient rights movement was already discrediting this notion by insisting on patient autonomy. Moreover, therapeutic privilege only covered everyday medicine, not experimental research.

BARNEY'S CLARK'S OPERATION

Barney Clark, the first patient to receive an artificial heart and live to talk about it, practiced dentistry in Utah for 30 years. A member of the Church of Latter Day Saints, he was also a heavy cigarette smoker.

In 1970, at age 49, he began to feel unwell. Seven years later, he retired as a dentist, and a year after that, the slightest exertion left him breathless. He was then diagnosed with emphysema, an incurable, obstructive lung disease, and cardiomyopathy, a disease where the muscles of the heart weaken and quit pumping blood. He then quit smoking, but it was too late.

Over the next 4 years, powerful drugs such as captopril and hydrazaline, which dilated his blood vessels, kept him alive, but by the end of November 1982, he was clearly dying. He had initially scoffed at the idea of receiving an artificial heart, but people sometimes change their minds when approaching death.

In Salt Lake City, physician Willem Kolff had been working on an artificial heart for 2 decades in a research lab funded by the University of Utah. Considered brilliant for inventing the first hemodialysis machine (see next chapter), Kolff paired with Robert Jarvik, an ambitious young medical student whom Kolff had helped get into Utah's medical school. Jarvik, after whom the first artificial heart was named, went to work in Kolff's lab after medical graduation, and never did an internship or residency, thus never being directly responsible for the care of sick patients.

The surgeon who would implant the Jarvik-7 was 36-year-old William DeVries, a 6 foot, 5 inch, blonde-haired Nordic man with a lean, tanned face. Because of his rugged good looks and macho daring in surgery, some American reporters lionized him as a medical John Wayne or Humphrey Bogart, a "man's man" in American surgery.

The Implant

In a biological heart, blood is pumped by the powerful lower part—the two ventricles. The device called the Jarvik-7 was in effect a replacement for the ventricles. It was made basically of molded polyurethane with two chambers of plastic and aluminum holding an inner diaphragm; the two chambers were separated by a wall of thin membrane through which blood could pass. The diaphragm in the Jarvik-7 was a substitute for the membrane and muscles of the ventricles. The source of power for this diaphragm was air from a compressor (the kind used by auto mechanics), brought up by 6-foot tubes inserted through the patient's stomach. The compressor itself weighed 375 pounds and was carried around on what physicians at Utah called a "grocery cart."

The Jarvik-7 worked as follows: The compressed air inflated the diaphragm, which compressed the right ventricle, which in turn pushed blood into the lungs for oxygenation and then back to the left ventricle; the left ventricle then pushed the oxygenated blood to the body. The Jarvik-7 also contained synthetic valves; these were the same commercial valves routinely implanted by heart surgeons, and as in a natural heart, there were four of them (analogous to mitral, tricuspid, etc.). The opening and closing of these valves against the walls of the Jarvik-7 produced clicks that were audible when an ear was pressed to the patient's chest.

•

DeVries had scheduled Barney Clark's surgery for December 2, 1982—almost 15 years to the day after Christiaan Barnard's first heart transplant. Meanwhile, Barney Clark—who already had chronic atrial fibrillation—began to experience ventricular tachycardia ("V-tach"), a potentially fatal condition. During the evening of December 1, according to DeVries, Clark's heart had weakened to a point where his life was in immediate danger,[16] and so the operation began that night at 11 P.M. rather than the next morning as planned. On his way to the operating room, Clark joked, "There would be a lot of long faces around here if I backed out now."[17]

As the surgery began, at DeVries's request, the sounds of Ravel's *Bolero* filled the operating room. Upon opening the chest, DeVries found a flabby, enlarged heart: It was twice the size of a normal heart and was merely quivering rather than contracting; one physician who was present described it as looking like "a soft, overripe zucchini squash."[18] DeVries first cut away the lower part of the heart, the two ventricles; then he stitched two Dacron cuffs to the intact upper part, the atria. He then had to connect to these Dacron cuffs—with Velcro fasteners—the two plastic ventricles of the Jarvik-7. However, the patient's atrial walls were paper-thin (this was an effect of the steroids Barney Clark had been taking), and when the Velcro fasteners were snapped, the pressure ripped the atrial stitches; the cuffs therefore had to be restitched into a new section of heart wall and the fasteners gently snapped into place.

The cuffs then held; but when the Jarvik-7 was turned on, it didn't work—it was not pumping blood out of its left ventricle. DeVries, increasingly frustrated, tried for 1 hour to get it to work correctly. He opened the ventricle by hand three times, each time running the risk of introducing air into the blood and causing a stroke. (Until the patient awakened, DeVries would not know if he had managed to avoid this.) At one point, DeVries reportedly exclaimed, "Please, please, please, work this time!"[19] Finally, he replaced the faulty ventricle altogether with parts from another Jarvik-7 and got the machine working, 2 hours after it was supposed to have started. Jarvik, who had scrubbed and entered the operating theater when his machine was implanted, helped DeVries to get it working; throughout this ordeal, he was very nervous.

The operation, having taken all night, concluded about 7:00 A.M. on December 2.

A few hours after the surgery, when the anesthesia wore off, DeVries watched anxiously as Barney Clark opened his eyes. If the patient had missed a bad stroke, he would be able to respond to requests to move his extremities; he was therefore asked (without explanation) to move each arm and his toes. He did so, and everyone felt relieved, though his surgeons would now watch to see if his immune system would rebel against the Jarvik-7.

Later that day, at a press conference, university physicians enthusiastically described the operation as a "dazzling technical achievement," something "as exciting and thrilling as has ever been accomplished in medicine"[20]; it would also be called "one of the most dramatic stories in medical history."[21]

•

People are often shocked when they visit an intensive care unit or see a patient after major heart surgery; certainly Una Loy Clark was when she saw her husband.[22] Barney Clark had a hole in his throat through which a breathing tube ran, a feeding tube running into his stomach, a bladder catheter, and of course the two hoses connecting the Jarvik-7 through his upper abdomen to the 375-pound air compressor at his bedside.

Like Louis Washkansky, Clark felt horrible after the operation. Also, though he had not suffered a massive stroke, he experienced what is called *intensive care psychosis* (or *acute brain syndrome*), which involves confusion, delirium, massive loss of memory, and periods of semiconsciousness. On December 4, more surgery was required to repair ruptured alveoli (air sacs in the lungs).

On December 6, he felt somewhat better and asked DeVries how he was doing. DeVries replied, "Just fine"; but seconds later, Barney Clark began to have seizures—involuntary shuddering from head to toe—perhaps caused by the dramatic increase in blood flow after implant of the Jarvik-7. A muscle tranquilizer (Valium) and an anticonvulsant (Dilantin) were injected. For the next several hours, the patient was unconscious and the seizures continued, though gradually the quivering became confined to his left leg and left arm. Throughout the next months, he would have continuing periods of confusion.

The following days were bad. DeVries later said that during this period, there were times when Barney Clark wanted to die and one time when he asked directly, "Why don't you just let me die?"[23] This reaction, however, is not uncommon after traumatic surgery, and it often passes. Still, Barney Clark was depressed by his lack of energy, his difficulty in breathing, and his stupor. Several times, he told a psychiatrist, "My mind is shot."

On December 14, things got worse when one of the $800 welded commercial valves inside the Jarvik-7 broke. The patient's blood pressure dropped dramatically, threatening his life, and DeVries had to operate again to replace the valve.

Nineteen days after implantation of the Jarvik-7, Barney Clark was doing much better, and DeVries said there was a good chance that he would eventually go home. Instead, complication after complication began to develop. Heparin was administered to prevent clots by keeping the blood thin, but this medication also caused severe bleeding (from normal sores and cuts that didn't clot and therefore didn't heal). On January 18, a persistent, severe nosebleed had to be surgically sealed.

More serious was the patient's underlying emphysema: It created pneumothorax (escape of air from the lungs into the chest cavity), requiring another operation to relieve pressure on Barney Clark's weak, smoke-damaged lungs. From January to March, Clark complained of conditions caused by this emphysema: He constantly complained that he was never able to get a good breath. In fact, he was suffocating—a situation unrelated to the Jarvik-7. On February 14, Barney Clark left the surgical ICU for a private room, but on February 15 he went back to the ICU because he needed a respirator; he spent the next 9 days in the ICU, presumably on the respirator.

On February 24, however, he was able to return to the private room, and his best week was at the end of February. On March 1, he made several videotaped interviews with DeVries. One of these was edited, and parts of it were released to the public on March 2; two others, in which Clark had nothing positive to say, were not released at all. According to the cardiologist Thomas Preston, the final short segment that was released "came from an extensive interview in which, encouraged by Dr. DeVries, Clark issued a semblance of a positive statement."[24] This clip showed the best moment to be found in the interviews: Although Barney Clark— tethered to a huge machine, in some pain, and apparently not fully conscious— did not look like a happy man, he claimed that he was glad to be alive and that he was not sorry he had undergone the operation. Moreover, it seemed possible that he might improve.

The next day, however—March 3—he developed severe nausea and vomiting; some vomit was aspirated, and this led to pneumonia. On March 21 he developed reduced renal function and a high fever. This was the beginning of the end.

On March 23, 1983, at 10:02 P.M., having lived 112 days with his artificial heart, Barney Clark died of multiple organ collapse. Large doses of antibiotics had killed most of the useful, benign bacteria in his colon; thus necrosis of the colon developed and produced toxins that entered his blood. This was accompanied by increasing expansion of his extremely fragile veins, to the point where they could no longer transmit blood. Degeneration of the colon and veins in turn led to the death of the kidneys, brain, and lungs, since little blood was reaching these organs, and the blood that did reach them was increasingly septic.

The Jarvik-7, of course, continued pumping. Una Loy Clark was asked if she wanted to be present when it was turned off; she said that her husband was already dead and left the room.[25] Someone (it was not revealed who) stopped the machine after a few hours. It had beaten 12,912,499 times.

The Aftermath

Following Barney Clark's death, public and professional reactions were mixed. Some people called the operation "one of the boldest human experiments ever attempted"; others concluded that it had failed to prove its worth, and that even if it had been worthwhile, it would represent one of the most expensive therapies in existence. The university's IRB and the FDA postponed any further implants until more data could be studied (though, as we will see, DeVries was allowed to perform three more implants). A few months later, predictably, Kolff defended the artificial heart: "A number of doctors were opposed to the artificial kidney and wrote articles against it. I decided not to respond at all. . . . I still have the same policy now [for] people [who] tell us that the artificial heart has no future. . . ." DeVries made a surprising comment: "After the first two days, 95 percent of the issues we were dealing with concerned ethics, moral value judgments, communications with the press—problems I had never thought about."[26]

A few weeks after Barney Clark died, the hospital corrected an "oversight": It revealed to irritated reporters that it had not informed them about another valve failure. Within days after Barney Clark's death, a valve had broken and killed Ted E. Baer, a 220-pound ram that had lived 297 days with an artificial heart—the world's record for survival by a mammal.[27] (Ted E. Baer was the model for "Flash" and his "Craig 2000" artificial heart on the television series *St. Elsewhere*.)

ETHICAL ISSUES

First-Time Surgery: Pressures to Be First

The surgeon who had trained the longest and seemed to be the most careful about insuring a good first result was Norman Shumway at Stanford in California (he did transplant the first heart in America shortly after Barnard jumped the gun). Some people claimed that Stanford's research ethics committee was too cautious and had stayed Shumway's hand, so Shumway had tacitly consented to Barnard's operation, but this is unclear. It is also true that perhaps a dozen heart surgeons around the world could have done what Barnard did.

So why do we give so much fame to the physician who goes first? Isn't it arbitrary to glorify who did the first heart transplant and ignore the great heart surgeons who laid the foundation and who could've done so themselves?

For example, Adrian Kantrowitz performed a heart transplant on a newborn very soon after Barnard's operation on Louis Washkansky. Kantrowitz needed an anencephalic infant as a heart donor for his patient and found one two days after Barnard's first; if it had taken him less time to find the donor, Kantrowitz would have been first and it would be his name that is famous today, even though the baby who received the heart died after only a few hours.

One factor in the issue of publicity and "being first" is, of course, the media. The media tend to feed the public's hunger for medical breakthroughs; and this tendency can lead to journalistic inaccuracy and sensationalism, and to medical haste and imprudence. (One Brazilian patient first learned of the possibility of a heart transplant when he woke up with another heart inside him.)

In the case of the first heart transplant, Barnard both wanted media attention and did not know how to handle it. He allowed the first conversation between Louis Washkansky and his son after the operation to be filmed by a television crew. Allowing reporters and cameras into Washkansky's hospital room, even in sterile gowns, can hardly have been best for the patient (it also seems inconsistent, since later the patient's wife was not allowed to touch him because of the danger of infection). Barnard seemed to relish publicity even while complaining about it. He held daily, candid briefings until doing so became overwhelming and the government information office took over. He favored American journalists and was criticized for taking payments from them for access to himself and Washkansky. (Barnard justified this by saying that the money would benefit his program and therefore future patients.)

Reporters understandably focused on the enormous symbolism of the fact that the operation had been done in the first place: a heart that once lived inside another human now pumped blood inside another human body. It is also true that the realities of Louis Washkansky's death were little understood. Reporters didn't seek out other surgeons and other surgeons didn't seek out reporters. Most reporters had too little medical background to understand what was occurring. The public was also more interested in a medical miracle than in clinical details of the patient's death.

Fifteen years later in the case of the first artificial heart, the media were much more critical, even hostile, with William DeVries and Robert Jarvik. Even before the initial surgery, reporters swarmed around the University of Utah Medical Center in Salt Lake City.

On the whole, journalists were unhappy with the conditions under which they were allowed to report the story. For one thing, the Clark family signed an exclusive contract with a magazine, and other reporters felt left out. Also, DeVries's attitude toward his patient was protective, and reporters resented this (as described in Chapter 6, the same kind of conflict had arisen when the first baby was born through in vitro fertilization). For their part, DeVries and the university officials said that they did not want a "media circus," although they themselves initially alerted the media about the operation

During the postsurgery period, the physician-administrator Chase Peterson, the university's vice president for health affairs, ran interference with the media and functioned as a public-relations professional. At one point, reporters exploded when Peterson said there would be no further briefings. The hospital later changed this policy, but reporters became angrier and angrier as weeks went by and the hospital kept trying to put the best spin on the facts about Clark's deteriorating condition.

In sum, with the first heart transplant, the media adored Christiaan Barnard and asked no tough questions. Fifteen years later, the media roasted the team of Utah physicians that performed the first artificial heart operation.

Quality of Life

One of the most important ethical issues in both cases concerned the resulting quality of life for the recipient. In both cases it was poor.

Both Barnard and DeVries correctly emphasized that for the first case, the question was not how long the patient could live, but whether. *That* a heart could be transplanted or *that* an artificial heart could run a human body was indeed a discovery and an achievement of fact to defy skeptics.

But then reflection set in. Did Washkansky have 17 days worth living? Did Clark have 112? Or was it merely what the *New York Times* said, that Clark got "112 days of dying"?[28]

Questions of quality of life really arose with the next recipients. Philip Blaiberg was the case Barnard wanted and exemplified the most basic standard of success for quality of life for all such operations: he could walk out of the hospital on his own power.

Following Barnard's success with Blaiberg, surgeons around the world went wild trying to transplant hearts. Magazines called 1968 the "year of the transplant." During 1968, 105 hearts were transplanted. After 1 year, of the 105 heart-transplant patients, 19 had died on the operating table, 24 had lived for 3 months, two had lived for 6 to 11 months, and one had lived for almost a year. Of 55 liver transplants in 1968 and early 1969 (15 months after Barnard's landmark operation), 50 patients failed to live as long as 6 months. Clearly, most of these early transplants were failures; the immune system was simply too powerful.

Most reporters also missed the fact in 1968 that 25 percent of transplant recipients became temporarily psychotic. Massive dosages of immunosuppressive drugs produced initial euphoria, followed by catatonia, severe depression, hysterical crying, and even permanent psychosis.

One of the great figures of medicine, Francis Moore, says that the year 1968 saw "epidemics" of chauvinism and of surgeons' egos: "It was the only example I know in the history of transplant medicine where everyone went nuts."[29] Nobel Prize winner (1954) Andre Courmand of Columbia University called Barnard's operation a stunt: "Merely demonstrating that it is technically feasible" to transplant a human heart, he said, was unethical.[30] Physician Norman Staub said Barnard's operation was "grandstanding."[31]

Many cardiac surgeons were critical of heart transplants, and they were not alone. Actually, in animals or humans, organ transplants were rarely successful for more than 1 month, let alone years; and to knowledgeable observers, the death rate in early heart transplants was appalling. As we've seen, 1968 had been called the "year of the transplant"; but the following years were by no means the "decade of the transplant"—they seem to have been the "decade of the high-tech last gasp."

In January 1969, the Montreal Heart Institute suspended heart transplants because of poor results, and this suspension provoked widespread discussion about whether a general moratorium should be called. For example, the surgeon Thomas Starzl (who specialized in liver transplants) and several other surgeons declared that they would observe a moratorium until more was learned; and three prominent cardiologists suggested a 3-month moratorium on heart transplants until further evaluation could be done.

For the rest of 1969, almost everyone cooled off on transplants; the number of transplants fell dramatically. In that year, Senator Walter Mondale of Minnesota suggested a presidential commission to evaluate transplants and related research. Many surgeons (not surprisingly) disliked the idea of a commission and said that surgeons should do the evaluating. The surgeon Walton Lillhei, for one, attacked "self-appointed critics" who "are better versed in the art of criticism than in the field under study . . . [and are] frustrated by their own inability to create." But the "self-appointed critics" were correct.

At the end of 1969 and the beginning of 1970, Massachusetts General Hospital, which is associated with Harvard Medical School and whose surgery department was chaired by Francis Moore, rejected a heart transplant program because of concerns about poor outcomes, costs, and poor quality of life for recipients.

Harvard's decision was significant and influential, and throughout 1970, most heart surgeons observed a moratorium on heart transplants. By tacit common consent, Norman Shumway, who had been the first American surgeon to transplant a heart, did not observe the moratorium. Using carefully selected patients, he studied who could benefit from such transplants. Most surgeons did observe the moratorium and heart transplant programs withered.

In the early 1980s, cyclosporin, a drug that selectively blocks immune rejection of foreign tissue, was discovered and revolutionized organ transplants. Thereafter, the number of organ transplants soared dramatically.

Today, 75 percent of heart transplant patients survive for at least 3 years, and more than 31,000 heart transplants have been performed in America. Dirk van Zyl, Barnard's sixth heart transplant patient, died in 1996 of diabetes unrelated to his transplant, the longest-living heart transplant recipient at 23 years. Sara Remington, the first infant in the world to receive a heart transplant in 1984 celebrated her tenth birthday in 1994.

Even today, life after a heart transplant is often not the miracle reported in popular media. Taking cyclosporin for life often causes cancer, and many recipients are in and out of hospitals for complications.

For recipients of the artificial heart after Barney Clark, quality of life was, quite frankly, terrible. The unfolding story of their misery continues the sad story of the artificial heart.

Because of concerns about Barney Clark's quality of life, Devries's referrals from physicians in Utah dropped to almost zero; claiming that he was unhappy with red tape, he moved in 1984 to Humana Hospital in Louisville, Kentucky, a for-profit center where he said he would be given a freer hand and (reportedly) three times his former salary.

As has been noted, after Barney Clark died the FDA allowed DeVries three more such operations. At Humana, on November 25, 1984, DeVries implanted a second Jarvik-7 into William Schroeder (nearly 2 years after Barney Clark's operation). "Bionic Bill" was 51; he was not only younger than Barney Clark but also much healthier (he had no emphysema), and he lived much longer, 21 months. However, he suffered a stroke only 19 days after his operation (probably from a clot formed where the Velcro connectors attached to what was left of his natural heart wall); thereafter he had a cascade of strokes, repeated bouts of endocarditis, and numerous other problems. Eventually he underwent a tracheotomy, a surgically created hole in the neck to the trachea, usually performed to insert a breathing tube. On August 6, 1986, he died of suffocation.

On February 17, 1985, Murray Haydon became DeVries's third recipient of a Jarvik-7. He started to suffocate on the seventeenth day after the implant, and he too had a tracheotomy. Murray Haydon soon became dependent on a breathing tube connected to a respirator, and he also experienced various infections; he lived for 10 months and 2 days. After he died (on December 19, 1986), an autopsy revealed that a hole from a catheter in part of his natural heart wall had not healed, and so blood had poured into his lungs.

The fate of the fourth recipient, Jack Burcham, helped the public to understand the realities of mechanical hearts. Going into surgery, Jack Burcham thought there was little risk; but he lived only 10 days (April 16 to 25, 1985) after a disastrous operation in which DeVries found that the Jarvik-7 wouldn't fit inside his chest. When Jack Burcham left the operating room, "his chest, draped with sterile dressing, . . . [was] only partly closed around the device."[32] The autopsy showed that large blood clots had clogged the valve openings in his artificial heart. Afterwards, DeVries admitted that the surgery had probably shortened the patient's life.[33]

Eventually, DeVries was forced out of the artificial-heart business. Referring physicians were afraid that he was more absorbed with the Jarvik-7 than with his patients; some patients were afraid that after what was supposed to be routine cardiac surgery, they might "wake up . . . with an artificial heart."[34]

Many physicians didn't refer patients to DeVries because they saw only miserable outcomes, grandstanding, and obliviousness to clinical realities; given DeVries's desire for success and his financial conflicts of interest, physicians simply didn't trust DeVries to do what was best for his patients. For some time, DeVries continued to claim that the Jarvik-7 could be successful, but he was a voice in the wilderness.

In regard to heart replacement in general, one sometimes wonders about the relationships between surgeon and patient after miserable results. Certainly, an ethics of care highlights the poignancy of such relationships. Does the patient blame the surgeon for failure? Does the research surgeon grow hardened? Surgeon P. M. Clark eloquently expresses such feelings:

> It is sometimes hard to meet the eyes of patients who have improved enough to have been moved to the regular postop floor and finally become alert enough to communicate their despair and disappointment. . . . Often, after entering the experience with great hope, patients for whom transplantation has been a series of setbacks clearly articulate their feelings of betrayal: "No one ever told me it could be like this."
>
> Certainly they were told that there would be no guarantees, and that it would be hard, and that there would be setbacks, but probably not how hard, or what some of the worst-case scenarios could be. When they were told, "You have to have a transplant or you're going to die," they were left a very slim margin for decision making. These people need to know not only what it will be like not to be dying any more, but what it may be like to not live so well.[35]

Continued Pressure to Be First: Hand Transplants

In 1998 a group of international doctors performed the first hand transplant in France. The hand donor was a 41-year-old man who died in a motorcycle accident, and the recipient was 48-year-old New Zealander Clint Hallam. A year later Louisville's Jewish Hospital performed the first hand transplant in the United

States on 38-year-old Matthew Scott who lost his hand in a firecracker accident. Before the first hand transplant, many doctors debated whether surgery of a nonvital organ such as the hand was ethical. Unlike heart and liver transplants, a hand transplant was unnecessary for survival, and the recipient still had to take antirejection drugs to suppress the immune system, which could increase the risk of infection, cancer, and even death.

Medical and Technical Problems

Is it ethical to try to achieve a "first" when the essential, underlying problem remains unsolved? Barnard technically transplanted one dog's head to another, but of course never began to connect the millions of nerves of the two dog's brains to the rest of their bodies.

In Barnard's case, before cyclosporin there was no way to selectively suppress the immune system's rejection of the foreign, transplanted heart. But the very drugs that suppressed the immune system also left the body open to infection from underlying disease or the incisions of the operation.

In 1953 Peter Medawar had discovered protein markers, or antigens, on the surface of cells and found that white blood cells (T-lymphocytes) recognize foreign antigens and then signal antibodies to attack. Highly specific antibodies develop against highly specific antigens. In 1968 Jean Dausset identified different kinds of white blood cells and suggested that they might be typed as Landsteiner had previously typed red blood cells. Dausset, who won a Nobel Prize in 1980 for his research, also advanced extremely important ideas about tissue typing and matching for transplants. Tissue typing has to do with antigens, which dictate the immune response (the term *tissue* is rather misleading here; *antigen typing* would be more accurate). There are many types of antigens, and so the process of typing them is long; but Dausset argued that they could be matched. He also argued that since the posttransplant immune response is controlled by antigens in cells of donor tissues, the closer the match between donor and recipient, the less the immune response would be. Further, he believed that specific donor antigens provoking rejection could be identified, and thus that an inappropriate donor could be screened out. It was soon verified that antigens can be typed and matched, and analysis of past operations indicated that this would significantly improve transplants.

With most new medical discoveries come new ethical issues, and tissue typing was no different. Surgeons hoarded possible donors and did not share them with other surgeons, who better tissue-matched a patient at another hospital. Everyone in the 1970s needed a system that matched donor organs and patients, but that system was not created in America until the 1980s, when the United Network for Organ Sharing (UNOS) was established.

The artificial heart presented medical problems similar to that of heart transplants before cyclosporin in that preventively treating one kind of problem worsened another. With transplants, surgeons fought infections with antibiotics and by holding off immunosuppressive drugs but thereby lessened chances of acceptance of the foreign organ. If they gave immunosuppressive drugs, infections flourished.

With artificial hearts, blood clots have always tended to form on joints and surfaces of mechanical surfaces. When such clots break free, they travel in the blood to the small vessels in the brain, lodge there, and cause brain damage (strokes). Blood-thinning medications, such as Heparin, are given to prevent or reduce clots, but when such medication was given to postoperation patients such as Barney Clark, they bled out of their sutures.

DeVries's results were castigated in three signed editorial reviews in the *Journal of the American Medical Association* in 1988. The general agreement was that:

> At the time of the device implantation or at autopsy, thrombi have frequently been identified as components of the mechanical heart. Prolonged, although temporary, use of prosthesis, similar to a permanent heart substitution, only provides time to increase the number of thromboembolic events and to allow further establishment of infection.[36]

In 2001, AbioMed of Massachusetts obtained permission to implant three of its totally implantable, titanium artificial hearts in patients at Jewish Hospital in Louisville (DeVries was not involved). (Two others were implanted at the Texas Heart Institute in Houston, and one each at UCLA Medical Center and Hahneman University Hospital in Philadelphia.) AbioMed's criteria of success were minimal: they wanted to prove, for dying patients with less than 30 days to live, that they could extend their life to 60 days.

Robert Tools received the first AbioMed and lived 151 days. Three other patients lived for 92, 78, and 32 days, and another died on the operating table. At this writing, a sixth was back in the hospital, and one, the biggest success, Tom Chriserson, was approaching one year. Blood clots forming on the device and causing strokes are still the major cause of death and problem to be overcome.

Two final problems with artificial hearts deserve mention. First, they are prone to causing infection, and DeVries's patients certainly suffered that problem. Second, once implanted, they must work perfectly, forever, with no margin of error, unlike dialysis machines or pacemakers, which can be erratic and not kill the patient. With failure of an artificial heart, loss of blood to the brain will kill the patient within 15 minutes.

Criteria of Success

Perhaps more than any other area of medicine, surgery escapes the scrutiny of ethics committees and federal agencies because it is difficult to monitor experiments in surgery (especially when there are no drugs or devices to prove effective or to regulate). So how should surgeons prove that their results are worthwhile? Merely that the patient lived?

This was certainly an important issue in the case of Barney Clark and one way to put this issue is to question whether implanting an artificial heart was therapy or research. In general, there are two ways in which a procedure that is not well established may be used ethically with a human patient. An *experimental* procedure (research) is permissible if the patient is dying (and has given informed consent); though such an experimental procedure should be based on good research design and supported by animal studies, no therapeutic benefit needs to be claimed. If the patient is not dying, however, the procedure must be *therapeutic* (therapy): That is, it must be expected to have a definite benefit for the patient. The difference between therapy and experimental procedures is important; although some researchers try to get around the entire issue by talking about "therapeutic research," this blurs a useful distinction.

Note that when the FDA gave DeVries permission to implant an artificial heart in a future patient, it *exempted* him from having to prove any therapeutic benefit. This implies that the surgery was experimental; and that also seems to have been Barney Clark's understanding.

In this regard, it is relevant to consider what, in general, makes any surgical intervention (such as the Jarvik-7) therapeutic. Outcomes of surgical interventions can be graphed in terms simply of how many patients live how long (see below). The two axes are time (*x*) and morbidity, or percent of patients alive (*y*). On such a graph, a surgical intervention can be represented by one line (call this line A) and a nonsurgical approach by a second line (B). Plotting begins, of course, at the left of the *x*-axis (time 0) and the top of the *y*-axis (100 percent of patients alive).

For patients with terminal cardiac disease, line B (no surgery) will slope downward steadily. Line A (surgery) will at first fall downward very sharply—more

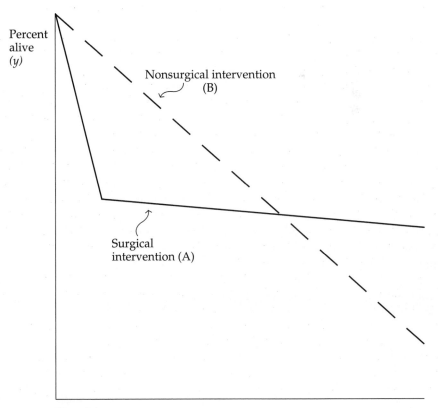

sharply than B—since the assault of the surgery itself will cause some patients to die immediately or very soon; thereafter, however, if the surgery is therapeutic, line A will slope much less steeply and may even level off, as the patients who survive surgery do better. Initially, then, line A will be behind line B, but later it will meet, cross, and move ahead of line B. With successful therapeutic surgery, in other words, although mortality will initially be higher than in a nonsurgical approach, it will later be significantly lower.

Surgeons routinely use a graph like this to assess probable outcomes. (Note also that such a graph could be helpful in illustrating and explaining anticipated benefits and problems to patients, and thus in obtaining their genuine informed consent.) In deciding to implant the Jarvik-7, though, DeVries did not use this kind of analysis, and many critics felt that he was irresponsible.

In fact, what chance did this particular procedure have with this particular heart- and lung-impaired patient? Although opinions differed, the predominant evaluation seemed to be that the chance was extremely slight and therefore that the implant was not therapeutic.

Costs

Two separate basic issues about costs arose in this case: the cost for the individual patient and the cost for society. In 2002 a heart transplant costs about $210,000, and bills for immunosuppression drugs (for the rest of the patient's life) are $15,000 a year. Eighty percent of commercial insurers and 97 percent of Blue Cross/Blue Shield plans cover heart transplants. Medicaid programs in 33 states and the District of Columbia also cover them.

In 1999 about 2200 hearts were transplanted in America, plus 4700 livers and over 12,000 kidneys. Remarkably, about 900 lung transplants were also done that year.

With regard to the individual patient, how much did this artificial heart cost, who would pay for it, and would it be cost-effective? Barney Clark's total bill was more than $250,000, and although the Clarks had contracted to pay for his treatment, they were released as the costs zoomed. Hospital administrators at the University of Utah had not initially expected this—according to Chase Peterson, they expected that the patient would die in a few days or be discharged in a few weeks—and later the hospital decided not to allow a second implant unless funding was provided in advance. The editor of *Journal of the American Medical Association* questioned the cost-effectiveness of the treatment: "How much is one more day of longer life worth? Is every life worth the same amount and if not, why not?"[37]

Artificial hearts also cost society dearly. NIH invested over $8 million in research leading up to the Utah project and over $200 million nationally in similar projects between 1964 and 1982. Was this the best way to spend limited funds? Should such expenditures be continued? Moreover, if the artificial heart was successful, could society afford to pay for it? The Office of Technology Assessment estimated that 60,000 Americans might use artificial hearts, at a cost to Medicare of $5.5 billion a year. If that happened, artificial hearts could easily become an exorbitant program.

Prevention or Expensive End-Stage Remedies?

Treating crises with expensive interventions only after an illness has become devastating does not save as many lives per dollar spent as a preventive approach. From the viewpoint of utilitarian ethics of public health, the millions spent on artificial hearts or heart transplants would be better spent on preventing people such as Louis Washkansky or Barney Clark from smoking in the first place. Glamorous high-tech operations are dramatic, but might not the money spent do more good for more people if spent in other ways?

The *Progressive* magazine complained at the time of the Clark case that a "medical establishment grown fat on chemicals and technological wizardry is not willing to empower people so they can prevent illness."[38] The *Progressive* argued that artificial hearts might benefit only the small number of cardiac patients who could afford them and hence were "qualitatively different from the basic advances in immunology which have saved million of lives, even among populations not directly treated."

Of course, almost everyone believes that an ounce of prevention is worth a pound of cure, but several arguments can be made to the above critics.

First, it is not always easy to establish that lives are saved by preventive measures. For example, if we cannot afford both artificial hearts and antismoking programs, we should go for the antismoking programs—assuming that those programs will save more lives than artificial hearts. But can we be sure of that assumption? Lives saved statistically are always mere claims, and because there are too many variables, it is difficult to be certain that such lives would not have been saved anyway.

Second, with regard to heart disease, heredity is believed to be the leading factor; thus, even if some lives are saved statistically by preventive measures, many people will develop heart disease anyway.

Third, it is necessary to take human nature into account, and it is only human nature for most of us to become more passionate about saving an identifiable life than about supporting distant preventive programs. Things are more real when the dying patient is right before you. An ethics of care certainly advocates giving the dying person before us a heart replacement.

Fourth, can't cardiac surgeons co-exist with utilitarians in public health? Can't we urge teenagers not to smoke, then try to help them when they fail? Is it really an either-or situation?

In reply, this issue is at least partly a matter of emotion versus reason, and in such a situation it is important not to abandon reason altogether. Even though prevention may be hard to document and partially unsuccessful, and even though human nature may insist on saving identifiable lives, we should not conclude that prevention should always be disregarded in favor of identified end-stage cures. This is especially so in discussing what is just to fund or priorities in national health policy.

For example, several states such as New York and Washington recently put very high state sales taxes on cigarettes, especially the kind of individual packs bought by teenagers from vending machines and from convenience stores. Such packs may cost over $7. Such a policy is a very tough judgment in public policy that society wants to discourage smoking in young people.

A similar judgment must occur about how far society wants to pay for heart transplants, liver transplants, and even lung transplants (for smokers?). Such issues will be discussed more in the next chapter in the context of allocation and distributive justice, where these issues are naturally discussed.

Patients: Informed Consent

The issue of patients' informed consent arises in allocating replacement organs because it is by no means certain that potential recipients understand what lies ahead. The media paint a sunny picture of organ transplants, typically citing only 1-year survival rates. Within medicine there has been a reconceptualization of transplants from "experimental" to "therapeutic"; and potential donors are urged to give a "gift of life." Thus there is a widespread perception among the public that a healthy transplanted organ will function for the recipient's lifetime. The reality is somewhat different.

Journalists have generally not understood, or have not reported, the long-term problems of transplants. If the recipient lives long enough, rejection of transplanted organs appears to be nearly universal. This is the familiar problem of rejection of foreign tissue by the immune system, and it does not seem to be solved by getting a closer match between donor and recipient. One-third to one-half of heart transplants are rejected after 5 years. Kidney transplants began in 1951 and today are closest to being truly therapeutic rather than experimental; but even so, over 50 percent of transplanted kidneys are rejected after 10 years.

To prevent rejection of a transplanted organ, continuous maintenance on cyclosporin is usually necessary. However, malignant lymphoma often develops in patients maintained on cyclosporin, and long-term exposure to cyclosporin often destroys the kidneys or liver and may produce brain damage. Cyclosporin also has lesser effects, such as excess facial hair in women patients. Moreover, the efficacy of cyclosporin appears to fade after several years.

In the 1990s, claims were being made for FK 506 as a "miraculous" antirejection drug (especially by the surgeon Thomas Starzl of Pittsburgh, who had by then retired); but there was less than full disclosure about its outcomes and about continuing problems associated with it. Fox and Swazey expressed concerns about the toxicity of FK 506, and in 1994 it played a role in the poignant case of 15-year-old Benny Agrelo of Coral Springs, Florida. Benny had been maintained on cyclosporin for 5 years after a primary liver transplant at the University of Pittsburgh; when that transplant failed, he received a second liver from the same team in 1992 and was then put on FK 506.

By the summer of 1994, FK 506 had made him unable to read for even 5 minutes without a blinding headache and was causing such severe pain in his joints that he was unable to play any sports; he decided that the drug was not worth it and that he wanted to stay home and die. His request was not honored: As he kicked and screamed, he was dragged from his home and returned to the hospital accompanied by two ambulances, five police cars, social workers, and his mother; before being strapped to a stretcher, he had managed to kick out a windowpane. Benny was held in the hospital for 5 days before a judge decided that he could not be forced to take FK 506. He died in August 1994.

Fox and Swazey's long study of organ replacement led them to some dismal conclusions. They argue that the reclassification of organ transplants as "therapeutic" was done not because of medical evidence but rather to make transplants eligible for reimbursement and to obtain publicity in order to increase the number of donors. They add:

> In the context of the growing organ shortage "crisis," the theme of organ transplantation as gift of life was framed and addressed primarily as a social policy problem of supply and demand. Exhortations to "make a miracle" happen through organ donation were accompanied by a structured forgetting of some of the darker emotional and existential implications of what it involved.[39]

There is evidence to bear out this conclusion, since several programs have a decade or more of experience and have performed hundreds of transplants. As Fox and Swazey—who were participant-observers for over 40 years—report, some patients and families never imagined that "it could be as bad as this."

Patients' informed consent, then, can be a serious issue with organ replacement. In the case of heart transplants, where the alternative is often certain death, the patient's awareness of probable long-term problems after a transplant is perhaps not a major ethical issue. However, in the case of kidney transplants, there is an ethical problem, since an alternative exists: Patients can be maintained indefinitely on dialysis.

How much does a candidate for transplantation understand about the experimental nature of an organ transplant? How much can such a candidate understand, given that these patients are seriously ill and often desperate? How is informed consent to be obtained in this situation?

Update: LVADs Extend Lives and Raise Questions

In 1998 the FDA allowed cardiac surgeons to insert left ventricle assist devices (LVADs) into patients as bridges to heart transplants. Being on the pump, which costs about $60,000, gave patients 408 days of life compared to 150 on drugs. The operation also costs about $100,000.

In a trial at 20 American cardiac transplantation centers, patients ineligible for a transplant and put on the HeartMate LVAD lived 250 days longer than those in a control group. Nearly a fourth of patients lived for 2 years (and, presumably, would have otherwise have died within a few months). The beauty of HeartMate is that, if the machine fails, the patient's original heart continues pumping, keeping him alive.

Although the FDA may approve the HeartMate for a limited class of patients, most insurance companies do not yet pay for it. At least a hundred thousand Americans a year could use a HeartMate. The worry is that use of LVADs will skyrocket if the government pays for them. In 1974 dialysis began with 600 patients, but after Medicare began paying for dialysis and kidney transplants, costs escalated to today's cost of $12 billion a year for 300,000 patients, roughly 5 percent of Medicare costs.

Conflicts of Interest

A significant issue in this case had to do with actual or potential conflicts of interest, and this in turn had to do with the profit motive. As we have seen, NIH was supplying public funding for the development of artificial hearts; nevertheless, private profitmaking became an important factor.

For one thing, Robert Jarvik was allowed to patent his machines. For another, the Jarvik-7 was made by a private corporation—Symbion, Inc.—which had been formed in 1976 by Willem Kolff and four others, including Jarvik and Jarvik's secretary. A for-profit hospital chain, Humana (which then owned 91 hospitals nationwide), was also involved. Moreover, DeVries had stock in Symbion; and though the University of Utah had forced him to divest himself of his holdings, Humana saw no conflict of interest.

Originally, Symbion simply owned prototypes of artificial hearts; its research and salaries were paid for by the University of Utah, and in return the university would receive 5 percent of sales of any Jarvik hearts and a small amount of stock. On this basis, Symbion limped along for 5 years; then, in late 1981, Kolff went public, looking for venture capitalists to underwrite its expansion. A struggle for power ensued between Jarvik and Kolff (Kolff later characterized this as a son rebelling against a father figure), and Jarvik and others squeezed Kolff out of management. Although Kolff retained some influence, Jarvik became the president of Symbion.

In 1982, Symbion needed more money, and Jarvik received $1 million each from Humana, Hospital Corporation of America, and American Hospital Supply. These companies were betting that artificial hearts would succeed and become profitable—in other words, they were betting that patients would soon have to buy a commodity which had already been financed by tax dollars. As one vice president said, Symbion's biggest advantage was that "it had the university as its research arm and its development arm subsidized by the government."

Humana, for its part, agreed to pay for 100 implants—if successful progress was made. Although these recipients would pay nothing, Humana of course expected a return on its investment: It wanted publicity, and as a major stockholder in Symbion, it wanted the Jarvik-7 to become routine.

When physicians become involved with high finance, competition increases and what is at stake becomes more than the patient's welfare. It seems clear that Jarvik and DeVries did have conflicts of interest; it also seems clear that such a situation undermines trust between physicians and patients. (Indeed, in a case like Barney Clark's, where "consent" may be mostly symbolic, trust becomes paramount and anything that undermines it is even worse than usual.) Furthermore, because of the involvement of Humana other financial issues seemed to mushroom. Could a for-profit hospital really afford major clinical research? If Humana was sponsoring such research just for publicity, would its commitment to research end if it found the publicity disappointing? And if its goal was publicity, would it really scrutinize research carefully? Some critics predicted that Humana's IRB would be largely a rubber stamp. "I'm not aware," said Arnold Relman, editor of *New England Journal of Medicine,* "that Humana has any experience in medical research. This makes a serious research problem into a public-relations commercial campaign."

Concerns about Donors: Criteria of Death

Although Barnard did not discuss this with Edward Darvall, he must have had some concern about whether Denise Darvall's "brain death" would be generally accepted as such. His criteria were certain to be scrutinized for any sign of conflict of interest or Frankensteinian overeagerness.

Louis Washkansky needed a heart in the best possible condition; and if Barnard had waited too long before excising the donor heart, he might have lost it. Barnard's brother Marius, who was also a surgeon on the transplant team, described a disagreement between them over when Denise Darvall's heart should be removed.[40] Marius Barnard wanted to remove it before it stopped beating (to ensure the best possible conditions for Washkansky); instead, Christiaan Barnard waited until the donor heart had stopped beating (which would have taken several minutes—a long time in heart surgery), and then waited another three minutes to be certain it wouldn't resume beating spontaneously. One ethical question here concerned who the patient was, Louis Washkansky or Denise Darvall. In this regard, did Marius Barnard have a conflict of interest? Did Christiaan Barnard have such a conflict? In such a conflict, whose interests should have come first?

A noteworthy point is why the donor's heart stopped at all, since Denise Darvall had a healthy heart. Actually, the surgeons had placed her on a respirator, and they had to cause her heart to stop by turning the respirator off; this damaged the heart slightly and was done only to deflect anticipated criticism. As the surgeon Thomas Starzl explained much later:

> [Standards of brain death] were not in effect during the first trials . . . and would not be until 1968. Rather than trying to maintain a strong heartbeat and good circulation in the cadaver donors, the legal requirement before the end of 1968 was the opposite. Because all such donors were incapable of breathing if the brain actually had been destroyed, they were supported by ventilators. The steps to donation began with disconnection of the ventilator, which the public called "pulling the plug." During the 5 to 10 minutes before the heart stopped and death was pronounced, the organs to be transplanted were variably damaged by oxygen starvation and the gradually failing and ultimately absent circulation.[41]

Because of ethical considerations, then, recipients like Louis Washkansky received damaged hearts that could have been supplied in better condition.

On the other hand, most transplant surgeons at the time realized that they had little choice in this matter. For one thing, moral caution coincided with their professional interests. Transplant surgery depended entirely on altruistic, voluntary donations, and any suspicious or doubtful procedures would sabotage donations. Even as late as 1985, a Gallup poll showed that 44 percent of Americans hadn't signed organ-donor cards because they feared being declared dead prematurely.

Another consideration at the time was that some influential conservative critics were claiming that a heart should be transplanted only when it had stopped beating. To these commentators, taking a beating heart from a body, even a brain-dead body, was ghoulish. In 1968, for example, one pioneering cardiac surgeon, Werner Forssmann, publicly criticized Barnard.[42] Forssmann had developed cardiac catheterization and had experimentally put tubes into his own heart nine times; in 1956, he had won the Nobel Prize for medicine. He was troubled by the "macabre scene" of two surgical teams at work in adjoining rooms, one team waiting, knives in hand, for a young donor to die; the other placing a patient on a heart-lung machine. (Partly because of such concerns, Japanese surgeons only recently began to perform heart transplants.)

In the United States today, by law in all states, the physicians who declare a potential organ donor brain-dead may not be members of the surgical transplant team; and several sets of criteria for brain death have been developed. The highly conservative Harvard criteria (which, however, do not require a heart to stop beating before removal) appeared the year after the first heart transplant, not by coincidence.

Criteria for death are discussed in Chapter 2; but it is worth noting here that although a person can be defined as dead when breathing and heartbeat have ceased, this is a fairly crude, undefinitive criterion. In the Washkansky case, for instance, Denise Darvall's heart could probably have been restarted easily with a small electric shock and (with supportive treatment) could have kept on beating in her brain-dead body; countless patients have been resuscitated in this way. Louis Washkansky himself could have been maintained for a while on a heart–lung machine; but of course he would have been dependent on it, and when it eventually became contaminated, sprang a leak, or broke down, he would have "died" again.

Non-Heart-Beating Organ Transplantation: "The Pittsburgh Protocol"

As this chapter has revealed, the issue of exactly how a patient, whose body is a potential source of organs, gets declared dead, has simmered in the background of organ transplantation for nearly half a century. Between 1954 and 1967, organs for transplantation either came from living, related donors (e.g., a kidney from one twin to another) or by patients who were dead ("cadavers"). Patients who were declared dead were so declared by cardiopulmonary criteria, that is, their hearts stopped beating and they stopped breathing. This criteria was not ideal because when tissue no longer receives blood, damage occurs very fast, and such damage often occurs while the heart is stopping.

With the Harvard definition of brain-death in 1967, declaration of death in cadavers switched to neocortical criteria, allowing retrieval of organs from cadavers who had their breathing and circulation maintained artificially by respirators. Because the organs procured from patients declared dead this way were not injured, and because all states passed neocortical brain-death laws, procurement of organs for transplantation switched almost entirely to use of the neocortical standard because now organs could be transplanted in better shape for the receiving patient.

In recent years, improvements in automobile safety have reduced the pool of such bodies while burgeoning numbers of transplant programs have learned to transplant sicker people. Supply has dropped while demand has soared.

The University of Pittsburgh Medical Center has perhaps the most aggressive and voluminous transplant program on the globe. In 1993, it developed a protocol to start obtaining organs from patients who were declared dead by the old cardiopulmonary criteria. The novel idea of the Pittsburgh protocol was to manage death in the small class of patients where the cause of death has not damaged the organ already and where the patient or the family has already signed a "do not re-suscitate" order. For example, a patient on a respirator is moved to the operating room where his respirator is removed, breathing stops, the surgical team waits two minutes for breathing to resume, the patient is declared dead, and then his organs are removed.

The official name of this protocol is the *non-heart-beating cadaver donors (NHBCD)*. This phrase is not felicitous, for it seems to be an oxymoron (can a cadaver be a "donor"?).

The Pittsburgh protocol declares death after two minutes during which no pulse is detected and while ventricular fibrillation, asystole, or electromechanical dissociation occurs. It also allowed drugs to be administered, such as vasodilators and anticoagulants, that were solely administered to maximize health of the organs to be transplanted. It declares that death occurs when there is *irreversible* loss of cardiac function, as opposed to the neocortical standard, which declares that death occurs when there is irreversible loss of all brain-activity, including brain stem activity.

A 1997 study requested of the prestigious Institute of Medicine (IOM) by the Secretary of Health and Human Services, Donna Shalala, distinguished between "controlled" and "uncontrolled" NHDBs. Before the Harvard, neocortical defini-tion of death was adopted, patients died in "uncontrolled" ways as their hearts stopped beating and injured their other organs. In the Pittsburgh protocol, the IOM said, "the (deaths of) donors are controlled because the timing and thus the process of donation are controlled through the timing of (withdrawal of) life sup-port."[43] These patients generally suffer from severe head-injuries or progressive neurological illness.

One aspect of the new protocol that some people have trouble accepting is that the judgment of irreversibility differs from the judgment about lack of neocortical activity. The only way to know if such changes truly are irreversible is to start cardiopulmonary resuscitation (CPR), but in the Pittsburgh protocol, of course, the *family and/or competent patient has already and explicitly declined CPR.*

This point cannot be stressed too much. Consent of the patient (or his family) distinguishes physician-assisted dying (ethical to some) from murder (ethical to none). If the family or patient had NOT given informed consent, then the staff might be charged with accelerating death to harvest organs.

Another point to stress here is that CPR on a dying or elderly patient is a bru-tal way to die and often involves breaking chest bones. It is a peculiar form of tor-ture practiced in our "advanced" and "modern" society. Fewer than 15 percent of hospital patients who receive CPR ever leave the hospital.[44]

Hence the essential idea of the Pittsburgh portocol: Because the family, the patient, and the physicians believe the patient is going to die soon, why not man-age the death to create life and good for others? So from a family's or dying pa-tient's point of view, something good may come out of a NHBCD, a gift of life to another person.

A 1993 conference explored the ethical issues of the Pittsburgh protocol, but did not achieve a consensus. Although all agreed that the *dead-donor rule* should continue, that is, that organs should only be taken from dead patients, they could not agree on whether families should be allowed to consent to organ procurement under the new protocol. "The Pittsburgh protocol gives an interpretation of irreversible that comes down to a low probability of auto-resuscitation and excludes the possibility of interventions that could restart the heart."[45]

Critics object on Kantian grounds that the patient is not being treated as "an end in himself." Alan Weisbard argued that the Pittsburgh protocol indirectly brings about the death of some people to benefit others.[46] Medical sociologist Renée Fox thinks it "morally offensive" to ask families, nurses, and residents to be involved in this effort, and criticizes the "macabre" public policy championing maximal organ transplantation.[47]

It is not clear that everyone understands what is going on here, because it would seem that Kantian ethics would allow patient/family decisions to donate based on autonomy. So long as a decision is informed and autonomous, why couldn't families of dying patients choose "no CPR" to help another person get an organ? Isn't that universalizable?

Other commentators accept the utilitarian justification for the Pittsburgh protocol but believe that is disastrous public policy because it undermines public trust in the system. In other words, people are too stupid to understand the protocol, they already don't trust the organ procurement system, and the new protocol will only make matters worse.

As discussed in Chapter 2 about Karen Quinlan's case, many in the public mistakenly believe that death is a uniform "metaphysical" event rather than a decision by physicians. Second, because there is the need to maximize donation of organs for transplants, there is great need to keep public trust. Given that the public has a mistaken belief, there is the problem that educating it about the realities of death conflicts with maintaining the present level of organ donation. In other words, the paradox is that the more we go into details about all of this, the more uneasy people may be about the whole situation.

In April 1997, the controversy made national news in the worst way when a bioethics professor in Cleveland went to a district attorney, charging that transplant surgeons at the famous Cleveland Clinic were about to violate the law. The headline of the *Cleveland Plain Dealer* was, "'Murder, She Said'" and a few days later, *60 Minutes* interviewed bioethics professor Mary Ellen Waithe and broke the story nationally. Many bioethicists criticized Professor Waithe's elevation of a dispute in public policy to charges of illegal activities with overtones of criminal mischief.

The *60 Minutes* story on the Cleveland Clinic revealed that the University of Wisconsin Medical Center had been using a NHBD controlled-death protocol to harvest organs for over 20 years. During this show, a particular point of contention was whether the administration of heparin and regitine accelerated the death of donors. Heparin, a blood thinner, prevents formation of clots, and regitine widens blood vessels, keeping organs perfused with blood.

The claim that administration of heparin and regitine hasten death is hotly denied by surgeons at centers using the new protocols. The Institute of Medicine study vindicated such surgeons, noting the NHBD protocols across the country were:

> divided evenly between allowing the use at some stage in the donation process of one or both of these agents and expressly prohibiting or not mentioning them.

In most cases, careful administration is appropriate. Nevertheless, because under certain circumstances in certain patients, there is a concern that these agents might be harmful, *this report recommends case-by-case decisions on the use of anticoagulants and vasodilators* and consideration of additional safeguards such as involvement of the patients' attending physician in prescribing decisions.[48]

The Institute of Medicine also recommended waiting five minutes, rather than two, before declaring death after life-support was removed.[49]

One final reflection concludes this discussion of the Pittsburgh protocol. It is not clear that most people will be able to understand the history and issues of this protocol (especially since few will have had a course in bioethics!), and there might be better ways to increase supply of organs. The Pittsburgh protocol at best is estimated to create 1,000 controlled NHBD deaths, but this is probably an inflated estimate (only 1 percent of cadaveric organ donors between 1993 and 1996 came from controlled NHBDs). Alternatively, allowing states to offer families a small reward to transfer organs from neocortically-dead patients, such as $1,000 toward funeral expenses, might go just as far to increase the supply of organs. Indeed, in 1997, Pennsylvania became the first state to authorize such payments, which are financed by hospitals, philanthropies, foundations, and private individuals.

FURTHER READING

Robert M. Arnold, Stuart Youngner, and Renie Shapiro, eds., *Procuring Organs for Transplants: The Debate over Non-Heart Beating Cadaver Protocols,* Baltimore, MD.: Johns Hopkins University Press, 1995.

Christiaan Barnard and Curtiss Bill Pepper, *One Life,* Macmillan, New York, 1969.

Renée Fox and Judith Swazey, *The Courage to Fail: A Social View of Organ Transplants and Dialysis,* 2d ed. rev., Chicago, IL, University of Chicago Press, 1978.

Institute of Medicine, *Non-Heart-Beating Organ Transplantation—Medical and Ethical Issues in Procurement,* Washington, D.C., National Academy Press, 1997.

Thomas Starzl, *The Puzzle People: Memoirs of a Transplant Surgeon,* Pittsburgh, PA, University of Pittsburgh Press, 1992.

CHAPTER 13

Allocation of Artificial and Transplantable Organsed

The God Committee

*L*ife-saving experimental treatments are sometimes scarce, and this brings us to the issue of allocating limited medical resources. Transplantable organs illustrate such scarcity; another example once was hemodialysis, which is in a sense an artificial kidney. Our case study in this chapter is a lay committee in Seattle in the 1960s, the Seattle Admissions and Policy Committee, dubbed the "God committee," that decided which patients in renal (kidney) failure would receive dialysis—and therefore which patients would live. The God committee also starts our discussion of how organs for transplant are distributed. The issues involved include not only selection of recipients by merit but also informed consent and certain aspects of organ donation.

BACKGROUND: ORGANS AS SCARCE RESOURCES

An Artificial Kidney: Hemodialysis

The kidneys remove toxins accumulated by normal cellular metabolism in the blood. When both kidneys completely fail, unless the cleansing function of the kidneys is somehow replaced, toxins will accumulate to a lethal level.

Hemodialysis (literally "tearing blood apart") can substitute for the kidneys: It removes blood from the body and sends it through cannulas (tubes) where a semipermeable membrane removes toxins by osmosis into a surrounding solution; then the cleansed blood returns to the body. Today, an adult in renal failure needs hemodialysis—or simply *dialysis*—for about 4 hours two or three times a week.

The physician Willem Kolff (whose work on artificial hearts is discussed in Chapter 12) invented the hemodialysis machine in the Netherlands in 1943. Kolff used a converted fuel pump from an automobile to force blood out of the body and to return it after cleansing. This early dialysis machine presented a daunting problem: Every time dialysis occurred, a new connection had to be made between the cannulas and the patient's arteries and veins. Because each artery or vein could be used only once, eventually all the available sites for connections would be exhausted.

In 1960, Belding Scribner in Seattle invented a permanent indwelling shunt making it unnecessary to reoperate in this way. He attached a piece of tubing permanently to one vein and one artery that allowed blood to flow continuously. The shunt contained connections for the cannulas of the dialysis machine and could be shut off between dialyses, like a spigot. For the first 3 weeks, Scribner did not realize that the combination of a workable dialysis machine and a permanent shunt meant that his 16 patients could be maintained indefinitely: He did not fully realize that he and Kolff had created an artificial kidney.[1]

Scribner's technological innovation meant that Kolff's dialysis machines could be used on the thousands of patients dying from renal failure. The Hartford foundation provided them about $250,000 a year for 16 patients on experimental, chronic dialysis. This breakthrough led to something wonderful: Thousands of patients who would once have died now could live. However, it also led to a potential tragedy: Some patients who could live would die if no way could be found to dialyze them and, this fact created a new ethical problem: selection of patients for dialysis.

The potential for tragedy and the accompanying ethical issues were not immediately obvious, because at first the procedure was only seen as experimental. Although both Kolff's dialysis machine and Scribner's shunt worked in the first few cases, no one knew if patients could survive for many years on chronic dialysis and return to normal life. When it gradually became clear that we had a long-term artificial kidney, the problem of selection arose.

Donated Organs: Supply and Demand

The ethical problem of allocating hemodialysis resembles the problem of allocating organs for transplantation. Why such problems arise with transplantable organs can be seen easily with a little background.

First, the base number of available organs for donation has not changed much over the past decades, despite numerous campaigns aimed at increasing it.[2] Second, while the supply drops, the demand for transplantable organs has steadily increased. Let's look at these two factors—supply and demand—in somewhat more detail.

With regard to *supply,* less than 20 percent of American adults sign forms agreeing to be organ donors. Various reasons explain this. For one thing, young adults notoriously do not think about death and thus do not sign donor cards. Other people resist the idea of "desecrating" a corpse by removing organs. In addition, members of groups who consider themselves victimized by American history or present American Society do not sign donor cards because they consider themselves more likely to be declared dead prematurely. Still another factor in reluctance to sign a donor card is concern about "brain death." (These last two factors were both illustrated in 1968, in the case of Bruce Tucker, who was African American. When Bruce Tucker's heart was transplanted after massive head trauma, Tucker's family sued because it had not consented, and also because Tucker had not been legally dead when his heart was removed.[3])

Of course, even in the absence of a donor card, organs may be donated by the family of a dead or dying patient. However, if the family refuses, American surgeons do not take organs and this practice lowers the number of organs donated, though it also reduces the number of lawsuits.

One factor that causes many families to hesitate is that the medical team working on behalf of a potential donor and the team working on behalf of a potential recipient may be at cross purposes. A treatment that might be indicated if the potential donor had a chance of surviving—or a treatment which might itself offer a very remote chance of survival—could be contraindicated in terms of preserving organs for donation. For example, victims of head trauma should, for their own well-being, be kept as dry (internally) as possible, whereas organ banks need well-hydrated donor organs.

Furthermore, suitable donors are mainly young, healthy adults with good organs; in practice, this almost always means young adults killed in motor vehicle crashes. Unsuitable donors who are older die in most other ways or have certain conditions when they die. For instance, the many Americans who are HIV-positive and the 1 million with hepatitis B or C can never donate organs.

Ironically, successful efforts to prevent motor vehicle accidents: restraints and seats for infants and children, helmets for motorcyclists, a legal drinking age of 21, lower speed limits, and laws and social pressure against drunk driving reduce the number of donatable organs. Safer vehicles with mandatory air bags also reduce the number of available organs. These measures especially reduce deaths among Americans under 40—the age group most likely to have donatable organs.

Another factor in increased demand for transplantable organs is improvements in transplant technology; another is that as more and more reimbursement becomes available, especially for elderly patients, more and more patients become potential transplant recipients.

Given the increasing need for donor organs, and their persistent scarcity, it is not surprising that in the United States over 4,000 patients die each year while waiting for a donor organ. This imbalance between supply and demand has naturally created pressure for change, but most of the proposed changes are controversial.[4]

For example, at least 14 European countries use *presumed consent*: A dead person is assumed to be a potential donor unless he or she has specified otherwise. However, presumed consent would probably not work well in the United States, where mistrust of the medical system is already a factor preventing donation—any attempt to establish the presumptive system here would only increase that mistrust. *Mandated choice* has been legislated in some states where all adults are required to volunteer or exclude themselves as organ donors at some appropriate time (in most cases, when they apply for or renew a driver's license).[5]

There have also been calls for replacing our traditional nonmarket system of organ allocation with a commercial system of selling and buying organs, but as will be discussed later, the ethical problems with any commercial system are enormous.

A development which many observers considered ominous was the Ayala case. Abe and Mary Ayala conceived a child for the acknowledged purpose of creating a bone marrow donor for their daughter Anissa; the baby, Marissa Ayala, was born on April 3, 1990, and the bone-marrow transplant took place on June 4, 1991. (In June 1992 Marissa was the flower girl at Anissa's wedding, at which time both sisters were well.) What Abe and Mary Ayala did was said to have already been done before and has been imitated since then in a few cases,[6] and it seemed only a step away from conceiving a child in order to obtain, say, a donor kidney.

Another development which many people found disturbing was the attempt to have severely brain-damaged babies declared brain-dead in order to use their organs for other infants.

Scarcity of human donor organs has also been a factor in attempts to perform xenografts—transplants from animals to human patients, as in the Baby Fae case and two cases in which baboon livers were transplanted by a team led by Thomas Starzl. It also explains the Pittsburgh protocol to use non-heart beating cadaver donors.

SEATTLE'S "GOD COMMITTEE"

When Belding Scribner developed his shunt, inpatient dialysis cost $20,000 a year.[7] Dialysis was then still considered experimental, and as with all experimental therapies, insurance companies refused to pay for it; thus Scribner's hospital— Swedish Hospital in Seattle—had to provide some treatment free. The first dozen or so patients constantly felt in danger of losing their treatment.

Because the cost of dialysis was so high, Swedish Hospital soon told Scribner that it could not take any more dialysis patients (the hospital also noted a shortage of beds). By then, though, Scribner and others had a year's experience with managing problems of caring for dialysis patients, and they decided that dialysis could be done as an outpatient procedure. Swedish Hospital agreed to oversee an outpatient program, and in 1962, it began long-term, or *chronic,* outpatient dialysis.

The outpatient dialysis center created at Swedish Hospital in 1962 could serve 17 patients, but many more were eligible; from the beginning, then, there was an ethical problem—in the words of the title of a seminal article, "Who Shall Live When Not All Can Live?"[8] An advance in treatment had thus created a specific problem of distribution.

Instead of leaving the problem of distribution to be dealt with by individual physicians for individual patients, Swedish Hospital and King County Medical Society took an unusual step of forming an Admissions and Policy Committee in 1961 to make crucial decisions about selection. Remarkably, this committee consisted of laypeople; although there was a surgeon on the committee, and although physicians on an advisory committee screened applicants for medical suitability. The intent was to take the burden of decision off physicians, since a physician would naturally want his or her own patients to be accepted.[9] The committee, was supposed to represent the community, and had seven members: a minister, a lawyer, a housewife, a labor leader, a state government official, a banker, and the surgeon. Two physicians familiar with dialysis served as advisers. The committee worked anonymously.

The committee first limited candidates simply to residents of the state of Washington who were under age 45; candidates also had to be able to afford dialysis, which generally meant that a candidate's insurer had to agree to pay for it. Almost immediately, however, too many patients applied and additional criteria became necessary. The committee then began to consider whether a candidate was employed, was a parent of dependent children, was educated, was motivated, had a history of achievements, and had any potential to help others. Eventually, the committee also asked for and considered analyses of a candidate's ability to tolerate anxiety and to manage his or her medical care independently; it also considered whether or not a candidate was likely to use his or her symptoms to get attention. In its deliberations, the committee would evaluate the personality and personal merit of the candidate, the strengths and weaknesses of the candidate's family, and the family's emotional support for a patient on chronic dialysis. By its own rule, the dialysis committee did not meet candidates personally.

It should be noted that this committee struggled with issues of distribution in the era before bioethics. At the time, no philosophers were writing about ethical issues of allocating artificial or natural organs; indeed, no philosophers were writing about bioethics at all.[10] Nevertheless, Scribner, who had evidently been involved in establishing the committee, wrote in 1972, "As I recall that period, all of us who were involved felt that we had found a fairly reasonable and simple solution to an impossibly difficult problem by letting a committee of responsible members of the community choose which patients [would receive treatment]."[11]

In May of 1962 (at about the time when Seattle built its Space Needle), Belding Scribner went with one of his patients to Atlantic City, where a convention of newspaper publishers and editors was being held. Scribner hoped to obtain public support for more dialysis machines; but he also described the selection committee to reporters,[12] and it was his account of the committee—rather than his appeal for more dialysis—that made the front page of the *New York Times* the next day.[13]

Life assigned its first woman reporter, Shana Alexander, to cover the story of the committee; she spent 3 months interviewing people in Seattle, and her report appeared in November 1962.[14] She coined the term *God committee:* to describe the committee playing a godlike role in deciding who would live and who would die. She also described in detail the committee's criteria, which came to be called the *social worth standard* and which were seen as implying that some candidates were more worthy than others.

According to Alexander, in response to criticisms that they were "playing God," some committee members argued that if they didn't do the choosing, someone else would (an argument which recalls the existentialist philosopher Jean Paul Sartre, who held that "Not to choose is still a choice"). Other members had pointed out that dialysis was an experimental treatment: "We are picking guinea pigs for experimental purposes," two members said—"not denying life to others."[15] But as dialysis became increasingly safe, this justification would become untenable.

In the spring of 1963, the front page of the *Seattle Times* showed nine of the center's dialysis patients with the heading, "Will These People Have to Die?"[16] As a result, the Boeing Corporation and the U.S. Public Health Service offered temporary financing. The next year, Scribner gave the Presidential Address to the American Society for Artificial Internal Organs, entitled "Ethical Problems of Dialysis Selection."[17] In 1965, Edwin Newman narrated an NBC documentary on the Seattle committee, *Who Shall Live?* That year, Congress had added to social security two national medical programs—Medicare for the elderly and Medicaid for the indigent—but dialysis was not yet covered under either of them. On the documentary,

Congressman Melvin Laird (later secretary of defense) asked why, if the United States could have a space program, it couldn't have a dialysis program to save lives;[18] the powerful Congressman John Fogarty demanded that the AMA take a stand about federal support for production of thousands of dialysis machines. National interest grew about the story, and indirectly, about bioethics.

•

The media shaped all these events. Shana Alexander said that when Scribner went to Atlantic City, he had been angling to get the magazine with the largest circulation of its time to bring this story to the nation; and the medical sociologist Judith Swazey agrees that Scribner set out deliberately to get publicity.[19] Undeniably, he did get publicity; but the story he wanted to get across seems to have been simply the need for more dialysis machines, and the story he got amounted to an exposé of the selection committee.

Thirty years later, Scribner said that he had been "totally naive" about the kind of national publicity which developed; he also said that he had taken "a lot of flak" about the committee's existence, especially from an early article in *UCLA Law Review*.[20] He claimed then that he had had nothing to do with the committee, which had been created and supervised by the King County Medical Association (here, though, he is not entirely convincing); he also said that he "hated the goddamn committee" and did everything possible to circumvent it when he had a dying patient who wasn't selected. Scribner also claimed that Alexander had not interviewed a single patient[21]—a claim she flatly denied, to his face.[22]

With regard to the story in the *Seattle Times,* this report could not have been written without the cooperation of nephrologists (kidney specialists) at Swedish Hospital and at the University of Washington. As always, medicine thought of local and national media largely in terms of public relations,[23] and these physicians were using the *Seattle Times* to seek funds. Their success may have set the pattern of using the media when emergency financing is needed for patients with organ failure, i.e., the rule of rescue.

During the late 1970s—when widespread questioning of authority became part of the American culture—the media became less willing to participate in this kind of rescue. Reporters would begin to insist that if physicians wanted to use the media to rescue patients, it would have to be a two-way street. With the Barney Clark case in 1982, the media had grown independent, and physicians who tried to use journalism for their own ends often found that they had a tiger by the tail.

ETHICAL ISSUES: FROM SOCIAL WORTH
TO THE MEDICAL COMMONS

The Public Arena

For reasons that were mixed and complex, Belding Scribner did something that went against a medical practice going back decades or even centuries: He made public a moral dilemma that hitherto had been discussed only among physicians. Bringing this issue to the public's attention was controversial within medicine.[24] As would also be true in the case of Karen Quinlan, many physicians felt that such ethical issues should be handled only within the profession.

By letting this genie out of its bottle, Scribner began to educate the American public about the many ethical problems in medicine. Different moral opinions among physicians now began to be expressed publicly by scholars. In retrospect, this process was perhaps inevitable: Since ethical issues in medicine affect so many people so intensely, probably they were bound to reach the public sooner or later.

Selecting Recipients

Ethical problems of selecting patients remain the same whether the resource to be distributed is a donor organ or dialysis. In this section, we'll consider four specific major issues having to do with selection: social worth, systems of distribution of donor organs, retransplants, and the rule of rescue.

Social Worth   As we have seen, the Seattle dialysis committee took social worth into account—though the committee itself did not use this term. Medical sociologists Renée Fox and Judith Swazey (who spent 30 years studying the American experience with artificial kidneys and transplantation)[25] reviewed the minutes of the committee's meetings and described its social worth criteria as follows:

> Within these very general criteria, the specific, often unarticulated indicators that were used reflected the middle-class American value system shared by the selection panel. A person "worthy" of having his life saved by a scarce, expensive treatment like chronic dialysis was one judged to have qualities such as decency and responsibility. Any history of social deviance, such as a prison record, any suggestion that a person's married life was not intact and scandal-free, were strong contraindications to selection. The preferred candidate was a person who had demonstrated achievement through hard work and success at this job, who went to church, joined groups, and was actively involved in community affairs.[26]

Some critics have argued that social worth should never be used as a criterion, because any such standard implies that some people are worth more than others and is therefore inherently unjust. Immanuel Kant, for instance, would oppose any social worth standard; his ethical philosophy would seem to entail impartial, random selection by lot, say, or by drawing straws. Two severe critics of the Seattle committee—a psychiatrist and a lawyer—remarked:

> The magazines paint a disturbing picture of the bourgeoisie sparing the bourgeoisie, of the Seattle committee measuring persons in accordance with its own middle-class suburban value system: scouts, Sunday school, Red Cross. This rules out creative conformists, who rub the bourgeoisie the wrong way but who historically have contributed so much to the making of America. The Pacific Northwest is no place for a Henry David Thoreau with bad kidneys.[27]

George Annas, both a lawyer and a bioethicist, criticized the Seattle Committee for preferring housewives over prostitutes, working men over playboys, and scientists over poets.[28]

On the other hand, in 1969 the philosopher Nicholas Rescher argued, in a classic article, that the Seattle committee had been just in using criteria which included social worth.[29] Rescher favored considering life expectancy, number of dependents, potential for future contributions to society, and past achievements. (Less controversially, he also supported screening candidates for medical problems that were likely to make them do poorly on dialysis, since otherwise dialysis machines would be wasted.) He suggested that such a selection system might be based on points, with ties broken by a lottery.

Annas also argued that some criteria of social worth can be just at some stage of the selection process, though he says that justice requires these criteria to be consciously formulated and made public. That is, if one rule is going to be "always prefer housewives to prostitutes," this should be explicitly defended. Private rules allow discrimination based on race, sex, class, or wealth.

In fairness to the committee, we should note that dialysis at home soon became an official goal because six patients could be supported at home at the same cost as a single patient in the hospital. That being the case, at least two aspects of social worth loomed large: the psychological support of the patient's family and the patient's own attitude or capability.

A passive, uncooperative patient can usually be handled adequately in a hospital setting, but not necessarily at home. Fox and Swazey, for instance, devote an entire chapter to the case, around 1969, of a Native American patient named Ernie Crowfeather. Ernie Crowfeather—a criminal, though a charmer—received dialysis for 30 months but refused to comply with the medical regimen, hated his quality of life, drank, imposed his childlike needs on the staff, and finally turned down further therapy and died.[30] In selecting Ernie Crowfeather, the committee had apparently made an exception to its standards regarding patients' attitudes and capability; if so, the point is this: Was use of dialysis for this patient worthwhile, when it might have saved the lives of two or three others?

The issue of social worth has also emerged with regard to liver transplants, though in this context social worth can be particularly hard to disentangle from medical criteria. The liver is by far the most expensive organ to transplant: The surgery calls for a highly skilled team and takes a long time. A significant fact is that the most common cause of liver destruction, or end-stage liver disease (ESLD), is alcoholism; when alcohol is a factor, the condition is actually called *alcohol-related end-stage liver disease* (ARESLD). In the 1990s, a controversy arose about whether patients with ARESLD and patients who were nondrinkers should be equally eligible for liver transplants. This is partly a medical issue, of course, since it can be analyzed in terms of which patients will probably benefit from such a transplant; but there is also an element of social worth. Is a nondrinker more deserving of a donor liver? Can someone with ARESLD be held blameworthy for the loss of his or her liver and thus undeserving of a new one? Would a drinker keep on drinking, thereby destroying the new liver; or would drinkers be transformed by receiving the gift of life?

In the case of liver transplants (as in certain other medical situations), there is also another issue: Can candidates be excluded on the ground that they have voluntarily risked their health?[31] With ARESLD specifically, this question is complicated by disagreement over whether alcoholism is a disease (and thus involuntary) or a self-inflicted voluntary behavioral pattern. The disease model of alcoholism has prevailed for some time, but it has recently been attacked by the philosopher Herbert Fingarette.[32]

In 1992 two teams of clinical medical ethicists conflicted over this point. In Chicago, the physicians Alvin Moss and Mark Seigler argued that since ARESLD usually causes liver failure, since there is a dire shortage of livers for transplant, and since recidivism is likely among alcoholics, patients who develop liver failure "through no fault of their own" (that is, nondrinkers) should get livers before patients with ARESLD—whose condition "results from failure to obtain treatment for alcoholism."[33] Two medical ethicists at the University of Michigan with doctorates in philosophy, Carl Cohen and Martin Benjamin, found that argument defective: Cohen and Benjamin maintained that alcoholics should not be blamed for drinking and do in fact have satisfactory rates of survival after a liver transplant.[34]

Distribution Systems and Waiting Lists   A second issue in the selection of recipients is systems of distribution and how candidates are listed in such systems.

In the 1970s, no real system existed for distributing donated organs, and organs that became available in one medical center or one region of the country were not always shared with other centers nationwide. Some states even resisted the idea of allowing their donor organs to be used elsewhere and if a nearby state had a big transplant program, did not pursue organ donors aggressively.

By 1987, the National Transplantation Act (1984) and the federal Task Force on Organ Transplantation (1986) had created the United Network for Organ Sharing (UNOS). UNOS alleviated some regional competition. It also established a standardized system for deciding which patient will get the next available organ; before UNOS, lack of standardization had made this decision a significant ethical problem.

However, UNOS deals only with candidates who are already in the system. Thus how and when applicants get onto waiting lists for donor organs remains a pressing issue. Imagine that you are going to die if you don't get an organ, but you know that 100 other patients want the same organ for the same reason. Suppose you hear that someone in, say, Pittsburgh or Houston has received an organ because he or she knew the right surgeon and therefore got onto the right list. It's one thing to feel unlucky because you're in a life-threatening condition, but quite another to feel that you are going to die because someone else managed to get into line in front of you.

An especially vexing problem is the practice of *multiple listing*.[35] Some patients get themselves appointments with surgeons at more than one transplant center and have themselves worked up at each; but only people who can take time off from work, can afford to travel, and have generous medical plans can arrange for multiple listings in this way. For a patient who needs a kidney, being on several lists may not be necessary; for a patient who needs a heart or a liver, though, a multiple listing may be a matter of life and death. One criterion for receiving a heart or liver is locality: A candidate must be within the area of the transplant center. A patient who registers at half a dozen such centers (say, in southern California) can significantly increase the chance of being selected.

Multiple listing is generally permitted, but in July 1990, New York became the first state to ban it (New York is still the only state with such a ban). In 1992, some patients who were then multiple-listed argued in a hearing before UNOS that forbidding the practice denied them autonomy. They maintained that they had a right as individuals to choose their own physicians; that is, a ban on multiple listing would curtail their liberty right to contract for medical care.[36]

There are two powerful arguments against multiple listing. First, a primary attribute of a just medical system is equality of access, and the use of wealth to bump the line violates this norm. Second, multiple listing compromises the entire UNOS system because some people are getting listed above others arbitrarily. UNOS should be impartial not only in dealing with candidates who are already listed but also in the actual process of deciding who gets listed.

A similar problem surfaced in the early 1990s, when it was revealed that candidates for neonatal heart transplants were being identified prenatally and then being placed on waiting lists immediately, while they were still fetuses.[37] Because time accumulated on a waiting list gives a candidate extra points, such a practice would offer a significant advantage. In this case, prenatal listing was made possible by the ability to diagnose hypoplastic left heart syndrome (HLHS) in utero; but such early diagnosis is not uniformly distributed in the United States, and early listing of babies diagnosed in utero seemed unfair to babies who were not diagnosed until birth. Moreover, fetuses with HLHS remain relatively safe while they are in the womb, whereas at birth HLHS babies are almost always at great risk and are in NICUs. For these reasons, UNOS changed its policy in June 1992 and put fetuses on a separate list from babies. UNOS also decided to allocate a heart to a fetus only when no baby could use it.

Retransplants   A third issue in selecting recipients is raised by retransplantation. Since transplanted kidneys and hearts are often rejected, a retransplant is often necessary. In such a situation, the question arises whether a patient who needs a second (or third) transplant and a patient who is waiting for a first transplant should be treated equally, or whether either one should take priority over the other. This is a complex matter.

In the UNOS system, patients waiting for retransplants are treated the same way as first-time patients. This may not lead to the best possible outcomes. Consider the following statistics for heart transplants and retransplants from October 1, 1987, to December 31, 1991 [38]:

	Recipients	*One-year survival (%)*
First transplant	4,830	81.6
Retransplant	86	56.7

These figures indicate that retransplant patients fare much worse than first-transplant (or *primary-transplant*) patients; the reason is simply that retransplant patients tend to be sicker. If this were the only consideration, UNOS should probably give first-time patients priority over retransplant patients: That would maximize survival per heart and on utilitarian grounds would seem to be the only ethical policy.

However, statistics like these are not the only consideration. One other consideration, for instance, is that it is precisely the sickest patients who are most urgently in need—patients who are less sick may be able to wait a while.

There is also the human factor. Whatever might be argued about hypothetical or statistical cases, a transplant team in real life develops a bond with a patient and thus finds it extremely difficult not to use an available organ for retransplant to save that patient. This is understandable: The medical team has worked very hard—often over many months—to save the patient's life, and when an organ is rejected, the team members do not want to be forced by some system of regulations to stand back and watch the patient die while an available organ goes to someone else. In fact, medical staffs see this as patient abandonment; physicians emphasize their emotional attachment to such patients and insist that they cannot ethically abandon them. More simply, a retransplant patient is personally *known* to the surgeon and the transplant team, whereas a new patient is only an abstraction.

It is true that medical ethics cannot ignore human emotions or the intimate relationship between patients and physicians. On the other hand, it is reasonable to ask why identified patients should take priority over new patients: A new patient may be just as much in need, just as likely to benefit, and just as meritorious. It can also be argued that "patients who are better at forming relationships with transplant teams"[39] will be favored if the medical teams are allowed to exercise their own judgment. We might feel that if one patient has already received a donor heart, it is time for someone else to get a chance; why should a first-time candidate die so that a retransplant patient can have a second (or third!) donor heart? Kant would certainly favor universalizing the rule, "Each patient gets one organ before anyone gets two."

Some critics argue that transplant centers are biased in favor of retransplants not only for emotional reasons but also because they are evaluated in terms of posttransplant survival rates—the centers are not required to report how many patients die on their waiting lists. In addition, their medical criteria may be contradictory: In selecting candidates, these centers first maximize the chances of survival by emphasizing blood and tissue compatibility; but then, by favoring retransplant patients over first-time candidates, they fail to maximize survival.

This whole issue is highly controversial within transplant medicine. The case of Ronnie DeSillers, who received three liver transplants (at a total cost of over $1 million), caused very bitter feelings among physicians in Miami and among patients on waiting lists for liver transplants. In 1998, Danny Canal of Wheaton, MD received *three* quadruple organ transplants (the first due to multiple-listing). Perhaps one reason why such enormous resources were devoted to him was that he was an identified person who had a relationship with a medical team. Should such identified relationships be allowed to determine who will receive a treatment? It is perhaps because of this question that the issue is defined as a matter of justice.

The Rule of Rescue   A fourth problem in selecting recipients is a social problem known as the *rule of rescue*. The rule of rescue, named by the bioethicist Albert Jonsen,[40] refers to the strong social tendency to help an identified individual—in this context, a patient—rather than unidentified, anonymous, or statistical people who are equally deserving and equally endangered. Countless examples of the rule of rescue can be cited. If the story of a small child trapped in a deep well is followed closely on television, hundreds or thousands of people will probably send tens of thousands of dollars in contributions for the rescue effort; meanwhile, though, the story of another, equally deserving person in danger does not receive television coverage—and this second person is not rescued and therefore dies. Larry McAfee, discussed in Chapter 3, benefited from the rule of rescue when his private medical insurance ran out: He gained the attention of the media and thereby received special public funding in Georgia.

In the context of organ replacement, the rule of rescue has been used for nearly three decades to save a few children in organ failure. In 1982, hospital administrator Charles Fiske, successfully manipulated the media to obtain a liver donor for his daughter Jamie. When transplant teams favor identified candidates for retransplants over new candidates for primary transplants it is also an instance of the rule of rescue. Another instance was of course, the *Seattle Times* story "Will These People Have to Die?" in 1963, which was instrumental in getting support for nine dialysis patients.

The rule of rescue can obviously be used very successfully, but it involves serious ethical problems. To begin with, if one life is worth the same as another, the rule of rescue seems irrational and unfair.

Also, the criteria that drive the rule of rescue often seem irrelevant, trivial, or muddleheaded. Who gets to live shouldn't be decided by who gets on television. Who gets to live shouldn't be decided by who has been admitted to a hospital or has gotten into the system. Who gets to live shouldn't be decided by who is most photogenic. Who gets to live shouldn't be decided by who is cutest or most appealing.

Furthermore, the rule of rescue can mean that journalistic gatekeepers in effect are making decisions about who lives and dies. As newspaper and television editors quickly found out, the rule of rescue replaces a God committee with an assignment editor.

Finally, the greatest problem with the rule of rescue is that for every identifiable person who is saved, there will be any number of anonymous patients who are lost.[41]

Although originating in bioethics, the rule of rescue really exemplifies a much larger clash between kinds of ethical theories. On one side are *partialist theories* that favor special regard to identified people such as patients in the hospital, members of one's family, or members of one's country. The so-called "ethics of care" illustrates such a theory.

On the other side are *impartial theories,* such as Kantian ethics or utilitarianism, that regard each person as having the same moral worth regardless of his geographical location or other nonmorally relevant criteria. It is precisely the partiality of the rule of rescue towards an identified person that impartial theories despise, for such partiality seems to disvalue the worth of all the anonymous people who do not receive the medical resource.

This clash looms throughout medicine. Admission to the hospital may illustrate the rule of rescue when a powerful physician decides to admit a patient without medical insurance and to care for him. Obviously, the hospital cannot do so for everyone or it will be sought out by other patients without insurance and go bankrupt. Such an admission may give the patient hundreds of thousands of dollars worth of treatment that she would otherwise not get. Such an admission can also make the physician feel like a hero, even if it does not solve the greater structural injustices in the American system of medical finance (see the last chapter).

UPDATE

Seattle's God committee went on selecting and rejecting dialysis patients for nearly a decade. By 1971, however, many stories had dramatized the plight of patients in renal failure; and in that year Shep Glazer, the president of the American Association of Kidney Patients, testified dramatically before Congress. As the story goes (although it may be exaggerated), Glazer dialyzed himself before the House Ways and Means Committee, disconnected a tube from the machine, let his blood flow onto the floor, and said, "If you don't fund more machines, you'll have this blood on your hands."[42]

In 1972, Congress legislated a "right to medical care," of sorts, for Americans: It was limited to just one organ, the kidney. This was the End-Stage Renal Disease (ESRD) program, whereby the federal government would pay for a dialysis machine for any American who needed one. Faced with the ethical problem of which patients should be funded and how to select such patients, Congress took what was then the easy way out—it simply funded all patients.

Congress had passed ESRD as an amendment to the 1972 Social Security Act in a session lasting only 30 minutes. The impetus came from a coalition of kidney patients, lobbyists for some physicians, concerns over high rates of kidney failure in people of color, and concerns that too much money was being spent on space and the war in Vietnam and too little on dying people who might be saved. Impetus also came from a national media focus on desperate kidney patients, which might be traced back to the efforts of Belding Scribner.

By making dialysis available to all patients, ESRDA ended the problem of allocating it and thus ended the need for the God committee.

In retrospect, ESRDA was hastily conceived, and it set an unfortunate precedent—other groups, such as hemophiliacs, soon pressed for similar coverage. Sooner or later, of course, someone would have to pay the piper.

Advocates of funding for dialysis had predicted that costs would come down as more machines were produced. Senator Vance Hartke of Indiana, who was once considered a contender for the presidency, predicted that although ESRDA would cost $100 million the first year, its cost would drop sharply thereafter because of increased efficiencies in production; and Willem Kolff had said that a dialysis machine could be mass-produced for a unit cost of $200.

These predictions turned out to be wrong, because of the cost-plus reimbursement scheme that American medicine funded in the 1960s and 1970s. Under cost-plus reimbursement, physicians and hospitals were allowed to buy as many dialysis machines as they wanted (or anything else) and pass the cost "plus" a percentage of profit on to "third-party payers"—that is, to ordinary people who pay premiums for medical insurance and who have FICA taxes withheld. One effect of cost-plus reimbursement was that hospitals not only had no incentive to buy inexpensive dialysis machines but actually had an incentive to buy ever more expensive machines. The larger the cost, the greater their net profit (as a percentage of cost).

Thus it is no surprise that by 1991, instead of costing a few hundred million dollars or less, ESRDA was costing $4 billion a year for 150,000 Americans.[43] This yearly figure was at least 20 times higher than Hartke's prediction, and possibly 100 times higher, since Hartke had expected the cost to fall.

Cost-plus funding was replaced in 1983 by reimbursement by diagnostically related groups (DRGs); but until then, all possible candidates for dialysis received it, no matter how hopeless their other medical problems might be. Reports were circulating that blind patients with cancer and Alzheimer's disease were being dialyzed in intensive care units, and that nephrologists in centers with many patients were making hundreds of thousands of dollars a year. Anticipating unlimited profits during the 1980s, hundreds of dialysis clinics sprang up, some run by hospitals, some by for-profit companies.

Under ESRDA, Congress also reimbursed kidney transplants, which were not too expensive in the 1970s. After the development of cyclosporin, the number of successful renal transplants jumped from 3,730 in 1975 to over 9,000 in 1986. In addition to the question whether every dying kidney patient should receive dialysis, this development raised a new question: Should every dying kidney patient have a kidney transplant? Again, the basic problem seemed to be that, for this particular organ, everything was covered by federal funds—a situation that existed for no other organ or disease.

Update: UNOS and the Rule of Rescue

As we have seen, utilitarianism clashes with the ethics of care over retransplants and the same clash is writ large in America's national system of allocating organs for transplant.

A utilitarian wanting to maximize human life in the lifeboat selects the strongest rowers, tosses the weak, sick, and elderly overboard, and eats the dog on the long row to Africa. Similarly, a utilitarian wanting the maximal years per organ only allocates organs to first-timers (unless the organ will be wasted if it doesn't go for a retransplant). But the impartiality of utilitarianism makes it oblivious to, and even scorn, the partiality in the ethics of care. For impartial ethical theories such as utilitarianism or Kantian ethics, one human life is as valuable as another, regardless of whether that life is my father, my neighbor, my patient, or my fellow citizen.

Piggybacking this logic on some facts leads to a surprising conclusion about the way organs are allocated in America: giving organs first to the sickest patients does not maximize the most years per life per organ. Why? Because some patients are too near death to ever have a realistic chance of life with the new organ. If they die, the organ has been wasted.

Therefore, the best way to get the most organs per life is to give the organ to moderately sick people or even relatively healthy people just experiencing heart or liver failure. In that way, the most people live the longest with the given supply of organs.

Congress, many surgeons, and the families of many patients reject such an impartial system. As their loved one grows closer to death, they grasp for a solution. Even if it wastes an organ, they feel that after waiting for years on the list for an organ, they deserve a chance.

So strong is this feeling that in the fall of 2002, Congress *mandated* that the United Network for Organ Sharing (UNOS) allocate organs on the basis of "sickest first." Howard Eisen, head of Temple University Hospital's heart transplant program, disapproves, "What you're doing is giving hearts to people who will do less well with them. People are waiting longer, so they get sicker, and end up getting two operations when they would otherwise need one."[44]

FURTHER READING

Renée Fox and Judith Swazey, *The Courage to Fail: A Social View of Organ Transplants and Dialysis*, 2d ed. rev., University of Chicago Press, IL, 1978.

Renée Fox and Judith Swazey, *Spare Parts: Organ Replacement in American Society*, Oxford University Press, New York, 1992.

Thomas Starzl, *The Puzzle People: Memoirs of a Transplant Surgeon*, University of Pittsburgh Press, PA, 1992.

CHAPTER 14

Infants and Medical Research

Baby Fae and Baby Theresa

*T*his chapter discusses two major cases. In the first case, which took place in 1984, a baboon's heart was transplanted into an infant called Baby Fae. The second case, which took place in 1992, involved an anencephalic infant known as Baby Theresa whose parents wanted to donate her heart to another baby.

The Case of Baby Fae

BACKGROUND: XENOGRAFTS

Transplantation of an organ from one species to another is called a *xenograft*. Before the Baby Fae case, attempts to transplant animal organs to human patients had been rare, and those that were undertaken did not promise much.

In 1964, James Hardy implanted a chimpanzee heart into a 68-year-old man who lived 90 minutes.[1] In 1977, Christiaan Barnard piggybacked a baboon heart next to the heart of a 25-year-old Italian woman, who lived 300 minutes; later he used the same technique to implant a chimpanzee heart in a 59-year-old man who lived less than four days. During the 1960s, Thomas Starzl and Keith Reemtsma performed six transplants each with simian kidneys and had somewhat better luck, but they eventually abandoned these projects.[2]

BABY FAE: THE IMPLANT AND THE OUTCOME

The infant who came to be known as Baby Fae was born at Barstow Memorial Hospital in Barstow, California (a small desert town), probably on October 14, 1984. She was three weeks premature and weighed five pounds. Noticing her pallor, the pediatrician transferred her on October 15 to Loma Linda Hospital, a Seventh-Day Adventist facility near Riverside, California, about 60 miles from Los Angeles. Physicians at Loma Linda confirmed that she had hypoplastic left heart syndrome (HLHS). In HLHS, which affects 1 in 10,000 babies, the normally powerful left side of the heart and the aorta are underdeveloped and are too weak to pump blood. HLHS is almost always fatal within 2 weeks.

Because Loma Linda agreed to protect the privacy of Baby Fae and her family, their identity has never been revealed; and much of the information reported about them is uncertain or conflicting, as are some of the dates in the case (even the date of Fae's birth has been variously reported as October 12 and October 14). Evidently, Baby Fae's mother was 23 years old, a Roman Catholic, unmarried, unemployed, and with no medical insurance; Fae's father was a 35-year-old laborer. The parents had lived together for 5 years and already had a son (then $2^{1}/_{2}$), but they had never married, and at the time of Fae's death, they had separated or were about to separate. Two other people who were figures in the case were Fae's maternal grandmother and a 28-year-old man—a mechanic—who was often called the mother's boyfriend but may more accurately have been described as a family friend. This friend seems to have accompanied Fae's mother when the infant was transferred to Loma Linda.

At Loma Linda, Fae's mother was told that the infant had HLHS and would soon die; the baby was kept overnight in the hospital and then released to her. She had Fae baptized and took the child to a nearby motel, where they were joined by the grandmother, to wait for death.

•

On October 16, however, Baby Fae's mother received a call from Leonard Bailey, the 41-year-old chief of pediatric surgery at Loma Linda who had been aggressively pursuing animal-to-human heart transplants. Bailey had been away at a convention when Baby Fae first came to the hospital and when options were discussed with her mother, but now he wanted to discuss a xenograft—a transplant of a baboon heart. For the previous 14 months, Loma Linda's Institutional Review Board (IRB) had been considering the possibility of xenografts by Bailey, and it had recently granted him permission for five operations. His call surprised the family. Bailey said, "I think they were awestruck that their child might still have the possibility to live."[3] At this point, Fae's father joined (or perhaps had already joined) her mother and grandmother.

On October 19, at 11:30 P.M., Baby Fae was readmitted to Loma Linda and placed on a respirator, and her parents began to talk with Bailey. The surgeon seems to have discussed the operation for several hours with Fae's mother, father, and grandmother (and perhaps also the friend) during the early morning of October 20. Fae's mother and possibly some of the others also watched a slide show about the operation. Both parents then signed a consent form which had been reviewed in great detail by the IRB; they later signed a second form, but reports differ as to whether the second form was signed 6 hours, 18 hours, or 2 days after the first. At 6 A.M., antigen-typing tests began, to find the best match for Fae among potential baboon donors; these tests would take six days.

On October 26, as the immunologist Sandra Nehlsen-Cannarella waited for the results of the final tissue-typing tests, Baby Fae's heart was said to have started dying and her lungs to have started swelling with fluid. (The baby has been variously described as 12 days old, 2 weeks old, and "around" 2 weeks old on that day.) Whether Fae was actually dying at this point is important: According to the hospital's spokesperson, a baboon heart was used because there was no time to find a compatible human heart; but Bailey made little effort to find a human heart donor (though, as we will see, a possible human donor was available). In any event, the results of the matching tests were returned at 6 A.M., and the transplant surgery began at 7:30 A.M. The donor was a female baboon named Goobers, about 7 to 10 months old, purchased from the Foundation for Biomedical Research outside San Antonio, Texas. (This is an organization which has enormous animal colonies, including 2,500 baboons, and supplies many medical centers with primates for research.)

According to what was by then standard procedure, Baby Fae was placed on a heart–lung machine that gradually lowered her blood temperature to 68 degrees. Meanwhile, Goobers was waiting in the basement, three floors below Bailey's operating room, where Loma Linda kept primates in its animal quarters. Goobers was then sedated, and in 15 minutes Bailey excised her walnut-sized heart. He put the heart in saline ice-slush in a Tupperware container, which was in turn put into a picnic cooler. (This sounds rather informal but was standard for organ transplants nationwide.) Back in the operating room, Bailey removed Fae's defective heart and replaced it with Goobers's healthy one. Over the next 4 hours, he connected the transplanted heart and transplanted arteries. Then the heart-lung machine raised Fae's temperature to 98 degrees, and Goobers's heart began to beat spontaneously inside Fae.

On October 29, Baby Fae was weaned from her respirator. On November 5, in an exclusive interview with *American Medical News,* Bailey predicted that Goobers's heart would grow as Fae grew, and that Fae might live to celebrate her twentieth birthday.

On November 10—two weeks after the surgery—Baby Fae showed the first signs of rejection of the donor heart. By November 12, she was deteriorating and was put back on the respirator.

On November 12, 13, and 14, David Hinshaw, the former dean of Loma Linda Medical School, in his capacity as the hospital's medical spokesperson, held three press conferences. Hinshaw said that after an episode of rejection on November 12, Fae was "showing steady improvement"; on the fourteenth, he said that the "signs of rejection" were "reversing very definitely."

On November 15, at 7 P.M., Baby Fae developed a heart blockage and renal failure; her physicians started closed-heart massage and dialysis. At 9 P.M. (or perhaps 11 P.M., according to *Newsweek),* Fae died. It had been 21 days (or 20 days, according to the *New York Times*) since her transplant surgery.

ETHICAL ISSUES: FROM ANIMAL RIGHTS TO INFORMED CONSENT

Animal Donors and Animal Rights

Bailey's operation on Baby Fae generated intense ethical controversy about the use of Goobers. "This is medical sensationalism at the expense of Baby Fae, her family, and the baboon," said Lucy Shelton of People for the Ethical Treatment of Animals (PETA).[4] Animal-rights activists protested outside Loma Linda Hospital, claiming that using Goobers's heart was unethical because Fae's life was not intrinsically worth more than Goobers's. The philosopher Tom Regan condemned the operation and said that it had "two victims," Baby Fae and Goobers.

Regan's general philosophical view (discussed in Chapter 10) is that beings who "have a life" also have a right to life, and he held that Goobers had a biographical life of sorts in that it mattered to her whether she would live or have her heart cut out: "Like us, Goobers was somebody, a distinct individual." He also argued from the premise that all primates have equal moral value, concluding that Goobers did not exist as Fae's resource:

> Those people who seized [Goobers's] heart, even if they were motivated by their concern for Baby Fae, grievously violated Goobers's right to be treated with respect. That she could do nothing to protest, and that many of us failed to recognize the transplant for the injustice that it was, does not diminish the wrong, a wrong settled before Baby Fae's sad death.[5]

Regan also argued that even if human beings had obtained benefits in the past from using animals, such use was still wrong. In a possible—but if so, incorrect—reference to the Tuskegee study, he said:

> In the 1930s, we intentionally gave syphilis to prisoners to trace the disease. Suppose others benefited. It was still wrong. We recognize that there can be ill-gotten gains in the exploitation of human beings, but we are blind to the fact that this is exactly what we're doing with animals. We are morally inconsistent.[6]

Other animal-rights philosophers emphasized that the difference between Baby Fae and Goobers, considering how young both were and what their individual potential might be, was not as great as the difference between Baby Fae and an anencephalic baby.[7] Anencephalic babies almost certainly have no cognitive ability or potential cognitive ability, whereas a young baboon has already developed as much cognition and affect as a human newborn. Some philosophers contemplated the large breeding facility from which Goobers had been bought and offered the image of a similar facility supplying severely retarded humans as organ donors and research subjects. If this image is repugnant, they asked, why do we tolerate such a facility for primates—since primates are more like us than severely retarded humans are?

Needless to say, Bailey's views were diametrically opposed to all this. Bailey said that the ethical sensitivity of the animal lovers picketing his campus was "born of a luxurious society" and implied that only in California would surgeons have to confront issues of animal rights: "People in southern California have it so good that they can afford to worry about this type of issue."[8] Moreover, he held, "When it gets down to a human living or dying, there shouldn't be any question" of using an animal to save that human.

The director of Loma Linda's Center for Christian Bioethics argued similarly:

> On an ethical scale, we will always place human beings ahead of subhumans, especially in a situation where people can be genuinely saved by animals. That is the story of mankind from the very beginning. Animals, for example, have always been used for food and clothing.[9]

Predictably, Baby Fae's mother was unsympathetic to animal-rights activists: "They don't know what they're talking about," she said.[10]

This issue will probably not go away soon. There are always reports of imminent breakthroughs in research on the human immune system or animal genetics that would make xenografts feasible. Moreover, the persistent shortage of human donor organs makes xenografts seem necessary: Since patients die every day waiting for human donors, the ability to use animal donors successfully could save many human lives.

Therapy or Research?

One of the most important criticisms of Bailey's surgery had to do with whether it was therapeutic or experimental. This issue can be put more bluntly: Was Baby Fae a patient, or was she only a research subject—a victim?

A therapeutic procedure must offer a patient a reasonable chance; a procedure which offers little or no real chance is experimental. This medical distinction between therapy and experimentation can also be expressed in moral terms: In Kantian ethics, it is the difference between treating people as "ends in themselves" and using them as "mere means" to some other goal. In an essay in *Time,* Charles Krauthammer wrote:

> Civilization hangs on the Kantian principle that human beings are to be treated as ends and not means. So much depends on that principle because there is no crime that cannot be, that has not been, committed in the name of the future against those who inhabit the present. Medical experimentation, which invokes the claims of the future, necessarily turns people into means.[11]

Was Bailey's best scenario really possible? Was there any genuine probability that Fae could live to adulthood—to age 20, as he predicted—with a baboon heart? At one point, Bailey phrased his claim somewhat differently, saying that Fae had a chance to "celebrate more than one birthday with her new heart."[12] Was even this more modest scenario possible?

Bailey claimed passionately that the operation was therapeutic:

> I have always believed it would work, or I would not have attempted it. . . . There was always therapeutic intent. My dilemma has been educating the university and the medical profession.[13]

This commentary was made 9 days after the operation, when Baby Fae was still alive and seemed to be doing well; and Bailey actually implied then that xenografts might be preferable to human transplants.

Bailey's immunologist, Sandra Nehlsen-Cannarella, also felt that the operation was intended to be therapeutic; she argued that Baby Fae could have accepted the heart if a good enough match was found with compatible lymphocytes. Nehlsen-Cannarella tested for compatibility, using Baby Fae's reaction to her own blood and tissue as the control: She tested Baby Fae's mother and some other relatives (finding a weak immune reaction), some lab workers (strong reaction), herself (strong reaction), three baboons (strong reaction), and three additional baboons (surprisingly, a weak reaction); she found a "very, very weak" reaction with one more baboon—Goobers.[14] From these tests, she concluded that she was not confronted with across-the-board rejection of xenografts.

There is considerable similarity between human blood and the blood of other primates (in fact, this is evidence of common ancestry); thus we might expect to find some close matches between humans and primates. Moreover, some humans react strongly against other humans: One-third of humans have a "preformed antibody" against tissue from other humans and 70 percent of humans have a preformed antibody against baboon tissue, but 70 percent is not 100 percent. Baby Fae was among the other 30 percent, and Bailey gave this considerable weight: He claimed that ignorance about human-baboon matching explained Hardy's earlier failures in xenografting.

The medical profession strongly opposed Bailey. It rejected his claim of therapeutic benefit; saying that therapeutic intent did not create therapeutic *probability*. Almost any operation has some possibility of being therapeutic, and in this sense all surgeons could say they intend their operations to be therapeutic—but that would make the concept of therapeutic surgery meaningless.

The medical profession also opposed Bailey over tissue typing. In 1970, Paul Teraski had discovered that although tissue typing can improve transplantation within families, it cannot improve transplants outside families. Thomas Starzl wrote in 1992 that whereas transplant surgeons initially resisted Teraski's findings—in the early 1970s—they gradually came to accept the limitations his results suggested:

> Twenty years later the only controversy is whether matching under all circumstances means enough to be given any consideration in the distribution of cadaver kidneys. By exposing the truth, Teraski had made it clear that the field of clinical transplantation could advance significantly only by the development of better drugs and other treatment strategies, not by vainly hoping that the solution would be through tissue matching.[15]

Most transplant surgeons agreed.

The surgeon John Najarian at the University of Minnesota—the foremost American expert on pediatric transplants—said at the time of the Baby Fae case: "There has never been a successful cross-species transplant. To try it now is merely to prolong the dying process."[16] He also said that Fae's death on November 15 was "reasonably close to what could be expected," because 3 weeks was about how long it usually takes for rejection to do its damage. The physician Kenneth Stoller maintained that Bailey had performed, over 7 years, "about 160 cross-species transplants, mostly on sheep and goats, none of whom survived more than 6 months."[17]

In November 1984, in a review of xenografts, the editor of *Journal of Heart Transplantation* concluded:

> These clinical attempts demonstrated that primate hearts could be acutely tolerated by the human body, at least for a few days, but no evidence was found to suggest that these grafts could be accepted for prolonged periods of time with the available methods of immunosuppression. . . . Using presently available means

of immunosuppression and immunomanipulation, there is no evidence that a vital organ can be transplanted from one species to another and result in prolonged survival of the recipient. . . .

From the experimental data and past clinical attempts, there is nothing to indicate that primate hearts will be tolerated by a human infant for months or years using today's means to induce and control tolerance. The Loma Linda surgical team has not informed the medical community, as yet, of any new evidence that might suggest the contrary.[18]

The case against Baby Fae's transplant as therapy may be summed up as follows:

- *First.* As noted above, it had been known since the mid-1970s that (with the exception of family members) better antigen matches (tissue typing) between donor and recipient would not improve transplants.
- *Second.* Even the best of matches would still require long-term maintenance on cyclosporin. Bailey claimed that infants can be given larger dosages of cyclosporin than adults;[19] but cyclosporin eventually produces toxic side effects or loses its efficacy. The autopsy on Baby Fae (which was not released until some months after her death) indicated that her kidneys may have been poisoned by cyclosporin.
- *Third.* Bailey also argued that since an infant's immune system is not fully developed, babies might tolerate organ transplants better before their immune systems develop. But this is not certain; and even if it were true, any initial success would be expected to be followed by failure as the baby's immune system developed and rejected the xenograft.
- *Fourth.* Only one real heart xenograft had been tried previously, and this had a disastrous result.
- *Fifth.* Loma Linda was a small medical institution (it had only 5,000 students); in their zeal to perform a xenograft, the staff may have been blinded to their own limitations.
- *Sixth.* Bailey himself was a relative amateur: He had never performed a human heart transplant, and he had never published any articles on his animal-to-animal xenografts.

Taking all this into account, Baby Fae probably had no chance of surviving for even 1 year, let alone reaching her twentieth birthday; thus the surgery was not therapeutic but experimental. *Nature* concluded that "the serious difficulty over [Bailey's] operation . . . is that it may have catered to the researchers' needs first and to the patient's only second."[20] In his essay in *Time,* Krauthammer said that Baby Fae had lived and died in the realm of experimentation:

Only the bravery was missing: no one would admit the violation. Bravery was instead fatuously ascribed to Baby Fae, a creature as incapable of bravery as she was of circulating her own blood. Whether this case was an advance in medical science awaits the examination of the record by the scientific community. That it was an adventure in medical ethics is already clear.[21]

Furthermore, even as an experiment, the surgery on Baby Fae was dubious. AMA and medical journals criticized Bailey and held that xenografts should be undertaken only as part of a systematic research program with controls in randomized clinical trials.[22]

Was Alternative Treatment Possible?   One obvious alternative to a xenograft for Baby Fae was a human donor heart. Should Bailey have sought a human heart for Fae?

As we have seen, Loma Linda claimed that the xenograft was necessary because Baby Fae was at the point of death and no human heart was available. Bailey argued that it would be impossible to find a heart because the donor would have to be under 7 weeks old, and criteria for neonatal brain death were problematical ("You can have a flat EEG on a newborn, and yet the baby will survive").[23] Most neonatal transplants come from anencephalic babies; and Bailey maintained that most parents of such infants would refuse to accept the fact that their baby was brain-dead, and in any case would not agree to donate the baby's organs. He described the baboon heart as Baby Fae's "only chance to live".

An associate surgeon at Loma Linda defended Bailey:

> It would have to be the sort of case where an infant fell out of a crib and was declared brain dead but the heart was okay. Then all these tests would have to be done to insure a proper matching. With Baby Fae, we had five days to do those tests, getting the best possible [animal] donor. With a human heart, we might not have been able to keep the recipient alive.[24]

However, Paul Teraski, director of the Southern California Regional Organ Procurement Agency, said that an infant heart had indeed been potentially available on the day of Baby Fae's xenograft. Teraski added, "I think that they [the Loma Linda team] did not make any effort to get a human infant heart because they were set on doing a baboon."[25] (It is worth noting that in his memoirs, the surgeon Thomas Starzl describes Teraski as a "symbol of integrity" in the transplant community.[26])

Since Bailey had been preparing for a xenograft on a human patient—in preparation, he had performed more than 150 transplants on animals—it is hard to believe that he wasn't looking for a first case. In fact, Bailey himself admitted:

> We were not searching for a human heart. We were out to enter the whole new area of transplanting tissue-matched baboon hearts into newborns who are supported with antisuppressive drugs. I suppose that we could have used a human heart that was outsized and that was not tissue-matched, and that would have pacified some people, but it would have been very poor science. On the other hand, I suppose my belief that there are no newborn hearts available for transplantation was more opinion than data or science, but it is scientific to acknowledge that the whole area of determining brain death of newborns is very problematical.[27]

Also, the available heart may have been too big or had preformed antibodies against other human tissue, and thus would not have worked.

There was another possible alternative. The pediatric surgeon William I. Norwood had developed surgery for HLHS that was less radical than a heart transplant—it attempted to repair the left ventricle—and had performed his operation many times at Children's Hospitals in Philadelphia and Boston, with a success rate of 40 percent. Bailey claimed that children did not do well enough after the Norwood procedure to justify this operation for Baby Fae, but given his extensive efforts to develop xenografts, was he an impartial judge?

Informed Consent

In a case like Baby Fae's, involving an infant, the issue of informed consent has two aspects. First, since informed consent can obviously never be obtained from infants themselves, is it ethical to subject an infant to an experimental procedure? Second, when parents consent to such a procedure for an infant, is their consent genuinely informed?

For many critics, what was objectionable about Bailey's surgery was not that it was risky or experimental—after all, surgery can discover what is possible or impossible only by trying. What was objectionable was, rather, that Bailey used a baby, who could not consent. In the decades since the earlier attempts at xenografts, the only new developments had been cyclosporin and better tissue matching, and these critics argued that both could have been used with a xenograft in a consenting adult.

Bailey argued that he had chosen an infant not to circumvent consent but for medical reasons: He said that immunorejection of a xenograft might be less in an infant whose immune system was not yet fully developed, and that infants can be given larger dosages of cyclosporin than adults.[28] As we have seen, this defense did not seem convincing in terms of establishing Fae's surgery as therapy, and for the same reasons it does not seem to justify his choice of an infant rather than an adult. Even if Fae survived for a while, he would have had to anticipate that she would reject the xenograft when her immune system did develop; moreover, cyclosporin evidently poisoned her kidneys. In other words, Bailey could not really justify using a baby—an unconsenting subject—on the grounds that the risk would be lower.

In addition to the specific questions about whether using Fae made sense medically or ethically, a more general question is whether parents should ever volunteer children as research subjects. The conservative theologian Paul Ramsey has argued that it always wrong for parents to volunteer their children as subjects of nontherapeutic research:

> If today we mean to give such weight to the research imperative, . . . then we should not seek to give a principled justification of what we are doing with children. It is better to leave the research imperative in incorrigible conflict with the principle that protects the individual human person from being used for research purposes without either his expressed or correctly construed consent. Some sorts of human experimentation should, in this alternative, be acknowledged to be "borderline situations" in which moral agents are under the necessity of doing wrong for the sake of the public good. Either way they do wrong. It is immoral not to do the research. It is also immoral to use children who cannot themselves consent and who ought not to be presumed to consent to research unrelated to their treatment. On this supposition research medicine, like politics, is a realm in which men have to "sin bravely."[29]

On the other hand, a Catholic theologian, Richard McCormick, holds that parents can volunteer children for low-risk nontherapeutic research.[30] McCormick's argument is based on the Roman Catholic tradition of applying natural law to ethics; according to McCormick, adults should volunteer for low-risk, nontherapeutic research for the general good, and therefore infants should also be volunteered. That is, adults should choose for a child not as the child would actually choose in adulthood, but as the child ought to choose in adulthood.

Interestingly, neither Ramsey nor McCormick uses the utilitarian justification—the greatest good for the greatest number. To many people, though, utilitarianism offers the most natural justification: Since HLHS is a congenital defect of babies, how can treatment of HLHS be advanced unless some babies with the condition are used as subjects of research?

•

With regard to the second aspect of informed consent in the Baby Fae case—the *parents'* consent—some critics asked whether that consent had indeed been informed.

Many people wondered, for instance, whether Fae's parents fully understood the alternatives in her case. Had Bailey carefully described the Norwood procedure to the parents? Were they aware of the Norwood procedure, and did they realize that it might be used to keep Fae alive until a human donor heart was found? Were they informed that a human donor was available on the day of Fae's surgery?

Another consideration here is that Fae's mother had no medical insurance. The xenograft was offered free, whereas Fae's family would have had to find the money for the Norwood procedure or a human transplant—or, very probably, would have been unable to find the money.

Furthermore, were the parents really informed about the probable outcome of the xenograft? That is, did they understand the experimental nature of the surgery? Loma Linda had decided to follow the normal procedure of IRB review in Baby Fae's case (although as a religious, privately funded institution it was exempt from NIH rules); still, no matter how good the resulting consent form may have been, it is doubtful that Baby Fae's family entirely grasped the situation: Almost all other surgeons were skeptical about the baby's chance of survival to adulthood.

William DeVries's implant of an artificial heart was described as having demonstrated only the "clinical feasibility" of the device—not its "clinical usefulness." Did Baby Fae's parents understand that Bailey's xenograft might be of this nature, a demonstration of feasibility rather than usefulness?

The law professor Alexander Capron summed up the issue of whether Fae's family had given truly informed consent:

> Doubts linger, not only about the adequacy of the information supplied to Baby Fae's parents but about whether their personal difficulties made it possible for them to choose freely, and whether the realization that their child was dying may have left them with the erroneous conclusion that consenting to the transplant was the only "right" thing to do.[31]

An old saying among physicians may sum up this situation: "Beware the surgeon with one case."

In fact, lack of informed consent had also been a problem with xenografts on adults. The law professor George Annas emphasized that in previous attempts to implant animal hearts in humans, consent was minimal and the patients (or subjects) were similar to Baby Fae in being vulnerable and poor. In 1963, Keith Reemtsma at Columbia University had implanted chimpanzee kidneys in a 43-year-old African American man who was dying of glomerulonephritis. In 1964, James Hardy at the University of Mississippi had implanted a chimpanzee heart into a poor deaf-mute who was dying, was brought to the hospital unconscious, never consented to the operation, and survived for only 2 hours. These operations were experimental, not therapeutic, and were characterized by exploitation and lack of consent. Annas saw Baby Fae's case as a continuation of such practices. Calling Bailey the champion of this "anything goes" school of experimentation, Annas concluded:

> This inadequately reviewed, inappropriately consented to, premature experiment on an impoverished, terminally ill newborn was unjustified. It differs from the xenograft experiments of the early 1960s only in the fact that there was prior review of the proposal by an IRB. But this distinction did not protect Baby Fae. She remained unprotected from ruthless experimentation in which her only role was that of victim.[32]

Costs and Resources

One ethical issue in the Baby Fae case was rarely if ever mentioned: money. That is not unusual; there is a conspiracy of silence in medicine about money and therapeutic treatment. Money was a significant issue here, however, and it merits discussion.

For one thing, as noted above, money was almost certainly a factor affecting the parents' informed consent. Baby Fae's mother was poor, and she had no medical insurance. Fae's family could not have paid for a human heart transplant, which might have cost $100,000; nor could they have paid for the Norwood procedure, which would have cost nearly as much, plus travel expenses and lodging in Philadelphia, where Norwood practiced. This helps explain why Loma Linda did not seek a human donor heart for Fae and why it did not pursue the Norwood procedure. But because of its interest in xenografts, Loma Linda provided the transplant of Goobers's heart free. Bailey and Loma Linda contended that, medically, the xenograft was Fae's only chance; that was probably not true, but the xenograft was undoubtedly her only chance financially.

There was also a broader financial issue. As with artificial hearts, many critics questioned whether so much money should be spent on a single case when the same amount of money could have done so much good for so many others. Although Loma Linda never revealed the cost of Fae's surgery and the associated treatment, it was probably at least $500,000. Would it make sense to perform, say, 500 to 1,000 such operations a year, at cost of maybe $1 billion, while thousands of babies are born deformed because their mothers could not afford prenatal tests like amniocentesis and sonograms?

The Media

Some issues in the Baby Fae case had to do with the media.

For one thing, although the case drew an enormous amount of attention in the media, Fae's family shunned publicity. As we have seen, the family's identity was never published, and certain details that might have identified them were withheld or unclear, including the date of Fae's birth. Also, Loma Linda and Bailey seemed to withhold more than just identifying details. Their account of events leading up to the surgery was confusing; hospital spokespersons gave occasional misstatements of fact; and Loma Linda refused to release a copy of the consent form which Fae's parents had signed. Some journalists complained about secrecy and invoked the public's right to know.

This situation formed an interesting contrast to the case of Barney Clark's artificial heart 2 years earlier at the University of Utah. Just as many reporters came to Loma Linda as to Utah (more than 300), but they got much less information. For instance, William DeVries, the surgeon in the Clark case, had held daily press briefings; Bailey held fewer press conferences. Reporters accused Loma Linda of ineptitude in handling their requests and said that certain aspects of the case begged for clarification. Loma Linda may have decided that it could learn a lesson from the Clark case—that it was better to give scant information than to try to satisfy the unending demands of reporters.

If Bailey and Loma Linda were accused of reticence, though, they were also accused of publicity-seeking, self-promotion, grandstanding, and adventurism. Bailey was also described as practicing *celebrity surgery*.[33] The surgeon Keith Reemtsma, for one, said that he himself would give no news conferences at all until his patient had been permanently discharged from the hospital and until he had prepared and submitted a scientific paper. Reemtsma argued:

> Science and news are, in a sense, asymmetrical and sometimes antagonistic. News emphasizes uniqueness, the immediacy, the human interest in a case such as [Baby Fae's]. Science emphasizes verification, controls, comparisons, and patterns.[34]

The bioethicist Alex Capron argued similarly: "There was a time when the public learned of biomedical developments after they had been reviewed by, and generally reported to, the researchers' scientific and medical peers"—a procedure that protected everyone's dignity and also meant that the public would learn only of genuine advances "rather than merely being titillated by bizarre cases of as yet unproven import."[35]

For its part, the press had also learned a lesson from the Clark case. When it came to the coverage of Baby Fae's story, perhaps never before had such accurate, detailed criticism from medical professionals been presented to the American public. Journalists were careful to include commentary about Bailey's claims from other surgeons and cardiologists, and (as the quotation above from Reemtsma suggests) many of these were highly critical of Bailey. Some of the people in medicine whose observations and analyses were reported saw Fae's surgery as a stunt which could only be damaging to medicine and Bailey himself as a maverick, as lacking good judgment, or even as incompetent.

UPDATE

Bailey attempted no more xenografts. Because of the pressing need for organs, however, there have been some attempts by others.

On June 29, 1992, Thomas Starzl's team at the University of Pittsburgh transplanted a baboon liver into a 35-year-old man with hepatitis B. About 30 percent of patients waiting for a human donor liver—many of them under age 45—die before getting one; also, hepatitis B will attack any human liver. However, hepatitis B does not attack baboon livers, and Starzl hoped that the immunosuppressor FK 506 and four other drugs would allow the xenograft to "take." The patient lived about 70 days. After his death, it was revealed that he had HIV infection; but according to the autopsy, this infection had not contributed to his death. The autopsy said that an "antirejection drug . . . hastened an infection that killed him." (Probably, the drug was FK 506.)

In October of 1992, a woman patient at Cedars Sinai Medical Center in Los Angeles received a pig liver as a "bridge" while she waited for a human liver, but she died 32 hours later.

On January 11, 1993, another man with hepatitis B received a baboon liver at the University of Pittsburgh; this patient was 62 years old and near death when the surgery took place. He died on February 6, 1993, never having regained full consciousness. The cause of death was an infection triggered by stitches in the abdominal cavity that either had been incorrectly sewn or had "fallen out of place."[36] After the experience, the surgeon, John Fung (who had by then replaced Starzl after Starzl's retirement), described himself as "somewhat emotionally drained."

Since 1905, various baboon organs have been transplanted to humans in 33 operations. So far, none have been successful.

•

Various studies have reported success in transferring human genes into pigs and thereby breaking down one barrier to using pigs as a source of organs[37]—organs of transgenic pigs may "take" better in human recipients. However, xenografts may continue to prove easier in theory than in practice. Even when initial immunorejection can be suppressed by drugs such as cyclosporin, a more lethal "hyperacute" or "complement" rejection occurs in almost all xenografts (it also occurs in about one-third of human kidney transplants). In addition, transfer of genes into organs for xenografts may also introduce dangerous viruses into not only the rescued human patient, but into the entire human species. (SARS probably came from a non-human animal.)

The Case of Baby Theresa

BACKGROUND: ANENCEPHALY AND ORGAN DONATION

Anencephaly is a congenital neurological disorder characterized by absence of the cerebrum and cerebellum, as well as the top of the skull, resulting in exposure of the brain stem.[38] In the words of the Medical Task Force on Anencephaly, "Anencephaly does not mean the complete absence of the head or brain."[39]

Because there is a brain stem, an electroencephalogram (EEG) can be taken, and autonomic functions such as breathing and heartbeat may be present. Anencephalics thus do not meet the Harvard criteria of brain death or the criteria of the Uniform Brain Death Act (UBDA)—standards which are sometimes called *whole-brain* criteria.

Anencephaly is perhaps the most serious of all birth defects, because the baby essentially lacks the higher brain necessary for personhood. Anencephalics are said to be born dying with no hope of growth into childhood or adulthood. Because the open skull is vulnerable to infection, most anencephalics die within one week,[40] though in rare cases some have lived for a year.

Anencephaly occurs in a 1 in 500 pregnancies. Sonogram or maternal serum alpha-fetoprotein testing identifies most cases prenatally, and then 95 percent are aborted. Of the remainder carried to term, about 55 percent are stillborn.

The organs of anencephalics could be transferred to other babies born with congenital defects. When the recipient is an infant, a donor organ must also be very small. The possibility of using anencephalics as organ donors has existed for two decades. In 1967, a few days after Christiaan Barnard transplanted a heart into Louis Washkansky, Adrian Kantrowitz transplanted a heart from an anencephalic baby into another infant, who died 6 hours later.[41] Indeed, Kantrowitz had almost performed a similar operation 18 months earlier, but he was required to wait for the anencephalic donor's heart to stop beating (so that the donor would be legally dead) and then restart it—which proved not to be possible.

Supply of infantile organs for transplant is restricted. Few infants are involved in accidents that leave them brain-dead but with healthy organs. Babies who die as a result of abuse or from sudden infant death syndrome often have damaged organs that are unsuitable for transplantation.

In the United States, 2,000 babies a year need organ transplants; including 600 with HLHS (like Baby Fae), 500 with liver failure, and 500 with kidney failure. About 300 anencephalic babies are born alive each year.

The Ontario Protocol

In 1987, a conference of surgeons and medical ethicists in London, Ontario, drew up guidelines for using anencephalics as organ donors. In these, an anencephalic could become a donor only after being pronounced dead by the classical criteria of brain death. Also the potential donor could not live more than 1 week; this standard was meant to ensure that the donor was truly "born dying." At birth, an anencephalic was to be put on a respirator to preserve the organs, then taken off every 6 hours to see if it could breathe on its own. If a baby failed to breathe for 3 minutes, it could be declared brain-dead by three physicians independent of the transplant team.

The respirator is necessary in this protocol because the normal course of anencephaly is for the heart gradually to stop beating: This diminishes the blood flow, so that the organs become anoxic and start to deteriorate; by the time the brain stem is dead, the heart and kidneys are no longer useful for transplantation. Thus the Ontario protocol can lead to a dilemma, since providing intensive support to maintain the brain stem may mean that a potential donor will not meet criteria of brain death.

The leading authority on anencephaly, the pediatric neurologist Allan Shewmon at UCLA, severely criticized the Ontario Protocol. Shewmon held that anencephalic babies should not be used as donors at all because there was no consensus in neurology on determining brain death in such infants for purposes of donation.[42] The Ontario protocol was not applied to an actual case until February 1988.

•

One of the people involved in the events leading to Baby Theresa's case was Baby Fae's surgeon Leonard Bailey. After his xenogafts failed, Bailey tried to use anencephalic babies as donors, and he had been involved in the Ontario Protocol. Bailey and Loma Linda Hospital—both well known because of the Baby Fae case—tried to use the media to help them become a national surgical center for treating HLHS babies through organ transplants from anencephalics.

In October 1987, a Canadian couple, Karen and Fred Schouten, learned after 8 months of pregnancy that their fetus, named Gabriel, was anencephalic. They decided to bring it to term and to donate its organs. When the baby girl's heart began to fail she, was ventilated and UNOS was alerted. No potential recipients were found in Canada or in the northeastern United States.

Meanwhile, at Loma Linda Hospital, Bailey was working with another couple, Alice and Gordon Holc (by chance, also Canadian), whose 8-month fetus had HLHS and who needed a heart transplant. Publicity had caused them to come to Loma Linda. The Schoutens and Gabriel were flown to Loma Linda. There, the Holcs' baby, Paul, was prematurely delivered by cesarean section to take advantage of the available donor heart. Three hours later, Schouten's heart was excised and transplanted into Paul Holc's chest. The surgery took 6 hours.

This was the first time a transplant from an anencephalic baby to another infant resulted in a baby who could grow up and lead a normal life. In gratitude to the Schoutens and to Leonard Bailey, the Holcs named their baby Paul Gabriel Bailey Holc. Gabriel Schouten's mother later said that she felt very good about her decision and how it had benefited Paul Holc: "Paul is very special to me because he has a part of our baby inside him. One day maybe I'll see him. I hope he comes to me when he's 30 years old and says, 'Hi. Guess what? I made it.'"[43]

•

Bailey had not applied the Ontario protocol in the Schouten-Holc case (perhaps because he was waiting for it to gain consensus). The first case in which the Ontario protocol was followed was that of Michael and Brenda Winners and their anencephalic baby, at Loma Linda in February 1988. The Winners case resulted in a sad anticlimax: No recipients were found at all. This was the first of 12 unsuccessful attempts by Bailey and Loma Linda to transplant organs from anencephalic babies to other babies.[44] Of these 12 potential donors, 10 lived beyond the 1-week limit, one could not be matched to a recipient, and in the remaining case the physicians decided against a transplant. In 1988, Bailey and his department of surgery announced that they had suspended his transplant program to reassess the situation.

There was a de facto moratorium on transplants from anencephalics until the issue was raised again, in the spring of 1992, by the case of Baby Theresa.

BABY THERESA:
THE PATIENT AND THE LEGAL CONTROVERSY

In 1991, in Fort Lauderdale, Florida, Laura Campo and Justin Pearson—who were not married—conceived a child. Laura Campo had no medical insurance for prenatal care and did not see a physician until her twenty-fourth week of pregnancy. During her eighth month of pregnancy, she learned that the fetus was anencephalic. Because this diagnosis was made so late in the pregnancy, no abortion could be performed; Laura Campo would say later that if she had known the diagnosis earlier, she would have aborted the fetus.

After hearing a talk show about organ donation from anencephalics, Laura Campo decided to bring the fetus to term to serve as a source of organs. This decision entailed a cesarean delivery: Since an anencephalic is likely to have a swollen head, vaginal delivery may kill it, and so a cesarean is performed to keep the organs healthy for transplantation—and also to give the infant a chance in case of misdiagnosis.

The baby, a girl, was born on March 21, 1992, and named Theresa Ann Campo Pearson. Some of the physicians expected her to die within minutes, but she did not. Pictures of Theresa showed a beautiful baby wearing a pink knitted cap that covered the top half of her head. Underneath the cap was no skin, no skull, and no cerebrum. The physicians and Theresa's parents said that when the cap was removed, they could actually look down directly on the brain stem.

Before her organs could be donated, Baby Theresa had to be declared brain-dead. But Florida used the strict Harvard standard of brain death, and Theresa did not meet that standard. (As we have seen, most anencephalic babies do not.) The neonatologist Brian Udell said that unless the baby was declared brain-dead, he would not remove the organs.

Laura Campo and Justin Pearson then asked Judge Estella Moriarty of the circuit court to rule Theresa brain-dead so that the baby could be an organ donor. However, because Theresa had some very minimal brain activity and did not meet the Harvard criteria, Judge Moriarty ruled otherwise on March 28: "[I am] unable to authorize someone to take your baby's life, however short—however unsatisfactory—to save another child. Death is a fact, not an opinion."[45]

The couple appealed to Florida's District Court of Appeals, which immediately delivered an emergency opinion, affirming Judge Moriarty's decision. The appeals court had also been asked to certify the case as one of "great public importance"—a certification which is necessary for an appeal to Florida's supreme court. The appellate court declined to do this.

Amidst a great deal of national publicity, the parents then appealed to the Florida Supreme Court to issue an emergency ruling. The supreme court replied that without certification of the case by the lower court as of great public importance, it lacked constitutional authority to make an emergency ruling.

On March 29, Theresa began to experience organ failure, in spite of support from a respirator. At this point, the neonatologist said, "We had to tell the parents [that] all they were doing was prolonging the baby's death."[46] The respirator was then removed. Theresa died on March 30 at 3:45 P.M. By that time, her organs were useless for transplantation.

•

On the day of their baby's death, Laura Campo and Justin Pearson appeared on the *Donahue Show* to plead for a change in Florida's laws regarding brain death. Laura Campo seemed very upset and depressed, and it was questionable whether she should have been allowed to undergo the strain of being on the show. A calm, eloquent surgeon joined them and discussed the need for donor organs.

On September 1, the Florida Supreme Court heard arguments in the case of Baby Theresa. On November 12, 1992, it issued a ruling that anencephalic newborns are not considered dead for purposes of organ donation.[47]

ETHICAL ISSUES: FROM INFANTS TO CONGENITAL BRAIN DEATH

Infants as Donors

The case of Baby Theresa raised basic questions about infants as donors. Should any baby be used for the good of another baby? If so, what are the criteria? What are the social consequences?

One argument against using infants as organ donors is their vulnerability. In general, the more vulnerable patients are, the less defensible it is to do something to them without their consent, and babies are the most vulnerable of all. Babies cannot consent; nor can their consent be inferred.

Indeed, when an infant's organ is used as a transplant, who is giving what as a "gift"? Terms like *donation* and *gift of life* seem inappropriate. Since no baby ever consents to donate his or her organs, a baby cannot really be described as providing a "gift." More accurate terms are: "organ salvage," "organ transfer," "organ recovery," and "organ reassignment." In brief, when infants' organs are used as transplants, *donor* and *donation* are euphemisms.

Anencephalics as Donors: Brain Death and Other Issues

One vital question in the debate over anencephalics as donors has to do with brain death. Some critics have argued that there are no good criteria for brain death in infants, and whether or not this is true in general, brain death in anencephalic infants is indeed unclear.

Anencephaly is a medical term describing a range of gross congenital brain deficits, all of which entail no chance of normal brain function but some of which do not entail immediate brain death.[48] The fact that some babies do not die within the first week—and thus could not be donors under the Ontario guidelines—illustrates this problem. Actually, some kinds of anencephaly are something like persistent vegetative state (PVS); therefore, some anencephalic infants could survive indefinitely with supportive care. One critic has said, "I have an uneasy feeling that what lurks behind the anencephalic issue is the vegetative state issue."[49]

Some commentators have suggested creating a new category of legal brain death, or an exemption from the usual legal criteria of brain death, to allow for transfers of organs from anencephalic babies. Such a special category or exemption is needed for organ donation because anencephalic infants are neither dead nor necessarily about to die immediately, and simply allowing them to die naturally could destroy their organs. The parents of Baby Theresa hoped that her case would help create pressure for such an exemption in Florida. Disability advocates opposed changing the Florida law, however: "Treating anencephalics as dead equates them with 'nonpersons,' presenting a 'slippery slope' problem with regard to all other persons who lack cognition for whatever reason."[50]

Two physicians considered a proposal to adopt a system used in Germany, where anencephalics are considered "brain-absent" and therefore brain-dead. They rejected this proposal for the United States, though—and the idea of a special exemption. They argued as follows:

> Not only are the brains of such infants not completely absent, but there is also a remarkable heterogeneity of morphologic and functional features in the infants considered anencephalic. . . . The causes of the neural-tube defects, including anencephaly, are complex and multiple—a fact that confounds the issue and supports the concept that the condition is quite variable. It is worrisome, but not surprising, that the diagnosis of anencephaly is occasionally made in error. Indeed, too many errors have been made for the diagnosis to be considered reliable as a legal definition of death. We conclude that anencephalic infants are not brainabsent and that the condition is sufficiently variable that the establishment of a special category is not justified.[51]

This analysis notes another problem with anencephalics as donors: The diagnosis of anencephaly, even as a range, is often problematic. As discussed in the case of Baby Jane Doe, diagnosing brain size or brain function at birth is uncertain. Some people fear that overzealous physicians and parents, wanting to bring some good out of a tragedy, might declare a baby anencephalic when in fact the baby had some lesser defect—say, a gross congenital malformation of the brain such as microcephaly. There are anecdotal reports in the popular media of retarded children, allegedly diagnosed at first as anencephalic, who are now functioning well.

Still another problem: If borderline anencephalics can become a source of organs, there might be a tendency to use infants with closely related disorders such as atelencephaly (incomplete development of the brain) and lissencephaly (unusually small brain parts). Some say that "'the slippery slope is real,' because some physicians have proposed transplants from infants with defects less severe than anencephaly."[52] Judge Moriarty wrote in her medical review, "There has been a tendency by some parties and amici to confuse lethal anencephaly with these less serious conditions, even to the point of describing children as 'anencephalic' who have abnormal but otherwise intact skulls and who are several years of age."[53]

Much of this debate has to do with personhood. In the context of anencephaly and organ donation, the question may boil down simply to this: How fast do we want to change our standards of personhood to create more organs for transplantation?

•

An issue closely related to anencephalics as donors is anencephalics as *patients*. If organ donation becomes a possibility, who is the patient?

Some critics have asked whether less was being done for anencephalic babies when these babies were seen as potential organ donors. Alex Capron described the situation as follows: "By far the most fundamental problem . . . was trying to sustain an anencephalic's liver, heart, and kidneys without temporarily giving life to its brain stem, the one organ that needed to die for transplant to begin."[54]

According to the Ontario protocol, a potential anencephalic donor is to be maintained on a respirator (this keeps the organs suitable for donation) but periodically removed from the respirator to see if independent breathing will occur (so that brain death can be declared if such breathing does not occur): Would this removal be in the best interest of the anencephalic infant? Is the anencephalic infant really being seen as a patient?

A counterargument here is that with anencephaly, birth is not morally relevant. That is, most fetuses diagnosed as anencephalic are aborted, so the actual birth of an anencephalic does not make a moral difference. If abortion is appropriate in anencephaly, why should it be considered immoral to do less to prolong the life of an anencephalic who is a potential organ donor? Since anencephalics almost always die a few days after birth (and since similar but less severe conditions are only infrequently misdiagnosed as anencephaly), why not allow physicians to kill anencephalics painlessly and transplant their organs at the optimal time? Some critics would consider this line of reasoning to be a *conceptual* slippery slope and hence, a person to reject the conclusion.

Another question has to do with the anencephalic *fetus*—specifically, the idea of keeping such a fetus alive to be used later as a source of organs. There seems to be a real distinction between keeping a fetus alive for this purpose and simply using the organs of a baby who has accidentally become brain-dead or who has unexpectedly been born anencephalic, and some critics would see a line here that should not be crossed.

There is also a *statistical* issue. As noted earlier, most anencephalics will be identified in utero and almost all of these will be aborted. Of the approximately 650 anencephalics brought to term each year in the United States, between 55 and 66 percent will be stillborn. Of the approximately 300 anencephalics who are born alive and survive immediately after birth, about half will be possible donors of hearts, kidneys, and livers; the others will be unacceptable for various reasons, including organ malformation, low birthweight, and withholding of consent by the family. The number of possible donors would be further reduced after blood and tissue typing. Taking all this into account, one study estimates that only about 30 recipients a year would benefit from using anencephalics as sources of organs.[55]

Given that serious problems exist about using anencephalics as organ sources, is this figure—30 babies a year—large enough? Would it justify changing our criteria of brain death? Would it justify the costs involved? In the Holc case, the surgery alone cost $140,000; in addition, there were costs of flying everyone to Loma Linda and, for the Schoutens and the Ontario hospital, the cost of keeping Gabriel Schouten alive for a week. Consider that thousands of pregnant women in the United States get no prenatal care and that as a result, many babies are born with preventable defects. Isn't the system biased in favor of dramatic surgical cases and against these anonymous women and their children? Is this justifiable?

UPDATE

Paul Holc turned 13 years old on November 21, 1998, his last public event. Eddie Anguiano, aka Baby Moses, also turned 10 about this time. At this time, Loma Linda surgeons had transplanted hearts into 195 babies under 6 months of age and into 82 babies over 6 months, and 205 of these 277 babies are still alive.[56]

Today—and after a great deal of professional discussion—there is general agreement that anencephalic babies are poor candidates for organ donation after brain death, and that not enough babies would be benefited by transplantation to justify changing legal standards of brain death specifically for anencephalics. There is also general agreement that Bailey's program was premature, and that Bailey was a maverick.

Conjoined Twins

On any given month, two desperately ill infants will be treated in any major children's hospital and no one will take notice. Spectacular surgery may occur, and teams may spend weeks nurturing each child back to health, but the public is indifferent.

Now make one change and have the two infants enter the hospital as conjoined twins, connected either at the head, sternum, or more globally. For some reason, now everyone takes notice. Why is that?

It may be in part a modern version of a freak show, the kind of thing that once accompanied traveling circuses, where people paid to see animals and humans with various kinds of congenital abnormalities. It may be in part a kind of grandstanding by the hospital and surgical team, saying, "Hey. We can do this and nobody else can. We're the top dog!" More charitably, it may be just another version of the Rule of Rescue: we can separate these two conjoined babies, give them separate lives, and feel good about doing so.

Certainly this situation has played out several times in North America and England over the last decades. In 1993, Laura and Ken Lakeberg of Minnesota had conjoined twins, surgeons at Loyola Hospital in Chicago said the twins could not be safely separated, but surgeons at Children's Hospital of Philadelphia (CHOP) said they could do it if Loyola couldn't, and they did. When Americans sent thousands of dollars for care of the children, the father scandalously spent it on cocaine.

Children can live and grow into late adulthood and stay conjoined. Eng and Chang lived into their 70s, married separate women, and fathered many normal children. Long-term studies of twins separated do not show as glowing results as might be expected.

In September 2002, the United Kingdom went hysterical when two conjoined twins were flown in from Malta (the Maltese government had previously contracted with the U.K. for the care of several such severe cases). The facts were that both children would die unless they were separated; if separated, the strongest would probably live.

The extraordinary aspects of this case were, first, that the parents refused the operation, wanting both to die, seemingly because they thought the kids would be regarded in Malta as freaks (regardless of the outcome). Second, British religious and ethical leaders decried "killing Mary to save Jodie" as "murder" and as "something that can't be permitted." A long, agonizing battle ensued in the courts and press, resulting in a decision to proceed with the operation, with the justices declaring it to be "one of the most difficult decisions we've ever made."

All of which showed a society at an immature level of dealing with such problems, analogous to Americans' immaturity in not allowing respirators and feeding tubes to be withdrawn in the 1970s and 1980s. In such cases in America, there would *never* be an issue of ever letting both die for fear of being charged with euthanasia.

A different criticism, much more cogent, was that surgeons and parents were prejudiced against life as a conjoined adult, thinking that quality of life was so low for both people that likelihood of death for one during surgery to "free" the other was preferable.[57] This, of course, is a much more subtle issue and one that is harder to evaluate. It might even be true that a conjoined child, faced with possibly killing his connected twin, might prefer to stay conjoined. Indeed, some adults living as conjoined twins (conjoined at the head, neck, or sternum) made exactly this criticism, but they were mostly ignored by medicine and society.

In August 2002, after staying at the hospital for two months, two 1-year old Guatemalan twins joined at the head ("craniopagus twins") were separated by UCLA surgeons in a 22-hour operation. The story received saturation coverage nationwide, illustrating again the Rule of Rescue.

FURTHER READING

George Annas, "Baby Fae: The 'Anything Goes' School of Human Experimentation," *Hastings Center Report*, vol. 15, no. 1, February 1985, pp. 15–17.

Denise Breo, "Interview with 'Baby Fae's' Surgeon," *American Medical News*, November 16, 1984.

Charles Krauthammer, "The Using of Baby Fae," *Time*, December 3, 1984.

Thomasine Kushner and Raymond Belotti, "Baby Fae: A Beastly Business," *Journal of Medical Ethics*, vol. 11, 1985.

Judith Mistichelli, "Scope Note 5: Baby Fae—Ethical Issues Surround Cross-Species Organ Transplantation," National Reference Center for Bioethics Literature at the Kennedy Institute of Ethics, Georgetown University, Washington, D.C., January 1985.

PART FOUR

Classic Cases about Individual Rights and the Public Good

CHAPTER 15

Involuntary Psychiatric Commitment

Joyce Brown

*I*n many large cities across the United States, daily life involves seeing homeless people. Panhandlers and derelicts, many of whom are mentally ill, roam the streets. In 1983 New York City, where the case of Joyce Brown look place, had 10,000 visibly homeless people; although the city made shelters available at night, homeless people often refused to use them. The problem of what to do with homeless people had become both a national and a local controversy.

BACKGROUND: INSANITY AND IDEOLOGY

A Brief Historical Overview

Ideas about insanity have varied greatly during different periods of human history.

Scholars have speculated that early humans believed in prehistory that the voices characteristically heard by schizophrenics came from gods or spirits. One scholar even suggested that the first human being to have an identifiable thought experienced it as an internal voice and was terrified by it, and that the human brain evolved as bicameral in order to control such "voices."[1] If so, the voices in schizophrenia might be a throwback to an earlier stage of humanity.

The ancient Greeks generally believed that mental illness was caused when angry gods took people's minds away, but, Hippocrates and his followers held that mental disorders, like physical disorders, had natural causes; and Plato thought of insanity as an imbalance where one part of the mind dominates the others.[2]

The Middle Ages abandoned the naturalistic approach substituting instead demonic possession, so exorcists were hired to drive out demons. Insane people were sometimes confined on a ship ("ship of fools") which sailed from port to port, taking on food and water but never allowing its human cargo to disembark.

During the fifteenth century, belief intensified in demonic possession and witch hunts began. Persecution of witchcraft did not end until the eighteenth century, and throughout this period many mentally ill people were treated as witches. However, one historically famous institution for mental patients, Bethlehem Royal Hospital in London, was established in the sixteenth century; actually, it had been founded much earlier as a religious organization and had housed a few mental patients then. Bethlehem Hospital—whose name is the origin of the term *bedlam*—had more patients than it could handle, though, and simply released many of them to wander as beggars.

Serious concern for the mentally ill developed in the eighteenth century, as fervor against witchcraft diminished and the concept of natural causes of disease took held. An important figure was the French physician Philippe Pinel (1745–1826), who became head of the Bicêtre Hospital for the Insane in Paris. Patients at Bicêtre had been kept chained, but Pinel insisted on unchaining many of them, with dramatically therapeutic results.

In the nineteenth century, approaches to mental illness were mixed. Some Philadelphians, for example, paid admission to mental hospitals, where they gawked at mental patients in chains and prided themselves on their own normality. More enlightened treatment was provided by the Society of Friends, who saw God (not Satan) in the insane. Early in the century, Quaker institutions practiced "moral treatment," allowing patients to roam the grounds freely and work in gardens. This moral treatment also included trying to create a homelike atmosphere for patients while isolating them from the conditions that were thought to have brought on their insanity, such as marital and financial problems.

In the twentieth century, treatments based on modern psychiatry have been developed; there has also been a new emphasis on patients' rights, and on the molecular-biological-chemical causes of insanity.

Patients' Rights

The twentieth-century approach to patients' rights initially came about as an alternative to imprisonment in jail and commitment in a mental institution. Early in the twentieth century, it was accepted that the insane needed "therapeutic justice" rather than criminal justice. Since insanity was not a crime, no legal proceedings were required to commit a person thought to be insane to an institution. It was simply assumed that the committing psychiatrists would always act in the patient's best interests. Later in the century, this assumption would be challenged and intensely debated.

In the 1960s and 1970s, views clashed about mental patients, dramatized in movies such as *King of Hearts* (1966) and the Oscar-winning *One Flew Over the Cuckoo's Nest* (1975). Lawyers who defended patients' autonomy argued that psychiatric diagnoses were subjective, that large public mental institutions were coercive, and that checks and balances were needed. These lawyers led the patient-rights movement to batter down the locked doors of psychiatric wards.

On the other side, many psychiatrists argued that psychiatry was benevolent, that the insane needed treatment, and that apathy was dangerous. They emphasized that some forms of insanity have a biochemical basis—which could be identified and treated.

Opposed to them was the existentialist psychiatrist R. D. Laing, who saw insane behavior as an inner, mental defense against a brutal, manipulative, terrifying world. In Laing's view, the young woman in the book *Sybil* (which was published in the 1960s and also became a film) would have developed her multiple personalities to distance her original "self" from the torture inflicted by her vicious mother. Similarly, Joyce Brown—the allegedly deranged street woman whose case is the subject of this chapter—might have muttered to herself and yelled obscenities at others as a defense against wrongs inflicted on her (this interpretation may be supported by the fact that her muttering and shouting seemed to increase when rough-looking men appeared).

Another important dissident psychiatrist, Thomas Szasz, led a revolt within the profession. Szasz saw no problem with patients who voluntarily sought help; he held that the proper role of psychiatrists was to help patients who had already identified themselves as troubled. He objected most to forcing help on people—such as Joyce Brown—who did not see themselves as mentally ill and who resisted intervention. For Szasz, involuntary commitment rarely benefits patients and is carried out chiefly to rid society of people who act strangely.

Szasz's basic position was this: A physical disease, such as AIDS or cancer, has a physical cause. Some mental illnesses also have a physical cause in the brain, and these mental illnesses are real. But other "mental illnesses" have no physical cause; they result merely from problems in living. A "mental illness" with no physical cause, Szasz held, is a "myth," not a disease. A disease is caused by something physical (a microbe, a lesion); so if a condition is not physical, it is not a disease at all.

Szasz concluded that nonbiological psychiatry could not be objective, or value-free; he held that it was "much more intimately related to problems of ethics than is medicine in general."[3] Consider that interpersonal relations—relationships between wife and husband, between the individual and the community, among colleagues, among neighbors—inevitably involve stress, conflict of interests, and strain. Much of this disharmony has to do with incompatible values, and to pretend that psychiatrists can offer value-free approaches is ludicrous: "Much of psychotherapy revolves around nothing other than the elucidation and weighing of goals and values—many of which may be mutually contradictory—and the means whereby they might best be harmonized, realized, or relinquished."[4]

Who, Szasz asked, can correctly define norms of "correct" and "psychotic" behavior? He was especially opposed to the classification of personality disorders as mental illness. (As discussed in the Baby M case—Mary Beth Whitehead was said to have a personality disorder. This kind of diagnosis aroused Szasz's suspicions, particularly because it seemed to be made for purposes other than helping the person who was supposed to have the disorder.) According to Szasz, psychiatry generally presumes that love, continued life, stable marriage, kindness, and meekness indicate mental health; and that hatred, homicide, suicide, repeated divorce, chronic hostility, and vengefulness indicate mental illness. These presumptions are evaluative, not factual.

A study by D. Rosenhan, "On Being Sane in Insane Places," was also significant in the patients-rights movement. In this study, several sociologists, psychiatrists, and others voluntarily entered mental hospitals, saying that they were "hearing voices"—a differential diagnosis of schizophrenia.[5] Once committed, they acted normally and no longer mentioned voices; however, they had been labeled "schizophrenic" in their medical charts, and the staff continued to treat them as schizophrenic. Ironically, although the staff did not see through the sham, the genuine patients did.

Deinstitutionalization

Deinstitutionalization of mental patients in the United States began in the 1970s. In 1972, in *Wyatt* v. *Stickney*, a federal judge in Alabama, Frank Johnson, ruled that a committed mental patient must either receive treatment or be released. Johnson's decision specified the institutional conditions necessary to ensure minimal treatment: at least 2 psychiatrists, 12 registered nurses, and 10 aides for every 250 patients. This standard is indeed minimal, but most states had been failing to meet it for years. Johnson also required state mental institutions to provide individualized treatment plans, to allow patients to refuse invasive treatments such as electroconvulsive therapy (ECT) and psychosurgery, and to establish the least restrictive conditions necessary for treatment.

Johnson's ruling was the precursor of a decision by the United States Supreme Court in 1975, in *O'Connor* v. *Donaldson*.[6] In 1943, at age 34, Kenneth Donaldson got into a fight with coworkers over politics and was knocked out; his parents, considering him crazy, petitioned a Florida judge to commit him to a mental institution. He was committed, was given 11 weeks of electroshock treatment, and was then released. In 1956, while he was visiting his parents in Florida, his father asked for a sanity hearing, saying that Kenneth Donaldson had a persecution complex; the son was then committed to Florida State Mental Hospital, where he was held for 15 years. Throughout those 15 years, he petitioned the courts many times, asking for a hearing; meanwhile, he rarely saw a physician and never received treatment. In the institution, he was presumed insane and—like Rosenhan's impostors—could not prove otherwise. Finally, in 1971, when his case was about to be heard, he was released.

A lawyer then helped him bring suit for damages against the superintendent of the institution, J. B. O'Connor, and the case eventually reached the Supreme Court. The Supreme Court decided for Kenneth Donaldson, ruling that he should not have been held against his will, even if he was mentally ill, unless he had been dangerous to himself or others and had no means of existing outside the institution. It also upheld a lower court's awards of $38,500 in compensatory damages and $10,000 in punitive damages.

More generally, the *O'Connor* decision established two conditions as necessary for involuntary commitment:

1. Suffering from mental illness (being "insane").
2. Being dangerous to others *or* being dangerous to oneself.

Note that *both* conditions—(1) insanity and (2) danger to oneself or others—had to be met for involuntary commitment. *Dangerousness* was subsequently interpreted as imminent risk to life (or threats of such risk) or imminent risk of bodily harm; *imminent* meant within days or hours. The arbiters were two psychiatrists. Evidence of dangerousness to oneself would consist of:

(a) Threats of suicide.

(b) Gross neglect of basic needs.

Dangerousness to oneself was eventually stretched to include gross *incapacity* to take care of basic needs.

With these legal changes, the courts moved rapidly from a medical model of civil commitment, which had been used in the early 1960s, to a patient-rights model in the 1970s. An important factor in this change was that a third requirement for commitment was added to the two *O'Connor* conditions:

3. Provision of the least restrictive environment by the institution.

Conditions 1 (mental illness) and 2 (dangerousness) applied in all states, since the Supreme Court had established them; two-thirds of the states also applied condition 3 (least restrictive environment).[7]

O'Conner v. *Donaldson* used the "clear and convincing" standard of evidence for the kind of laws states can pass and still be legal under the U.S. Constitution. *O'Conner* v. *Donaldson* said this standard was met by laws that specified the two necessary conditions of mental illness and dangerousness. Of interest, the dangerousness must be caused by the mental illness, and if a patient exhibited a different kind of dangerousness not caused by his mental illness, that would not be grounds for commitment.

These legal developments entailed the release of many mental patients from large state institutions, because such institutions often could not provide individualized treatment (as required by *Wyatt*) and were not the least restrictive environment: Arrangements such as halfway houses were less restrictive.

Other factors also contributed to deinstitutionalization. For one thing, new psychotropic medications allowed much more outpatient treatment. Also, the Kennedy administration had advocated small, community-integrated facilities rather than large, impersonal state institutions: In the words of President Kennedy, "Reliance on the cold mercy of custodial isolation will be supplanted by the open warmth of community concern."[8] Other factors included tight budgets, psychiatrists who sought lighter workloads, and a general distrust of authority in the early 1970s.

All these factors combined to empty American mental institutions. In most states during the early 1970s, 50 percent of the patients in state institutions were released; in some other states, 75 percent were released. In 1955, nearly 560,000 patients had lived in state mental institutions; in 1988, there were only 130,000. Nearly 500,000 mental patients were deinstitutionalized over the course of 30 years. All levels of government saved money, the American Civil Liberties Union was appeased, and mental patients flooded into communities.

However, the warmth of community concern envisioned by John Kennedy did not appear. Communities opposed halfway houses in their midst, and few such facilities were created. Mental patients living in the community lived more often on warm-air grates than in group homes, which were scarce and—where they existed at all—understaffed. Bag ladies were seen on more city streets. Charities set up soup kitchens for hungry street people. Soup kitchens and food banks were a sign that deinstitutionalization was not working; but in the 1980s, Reaganites hailed them as proof that government intervention was unneeded.

In short, deinstitutionalization failed. It failed because government funds were never allocated for community homes; because communities themselves rejected such homes; because mental health services were fragmented between county, state, and federal agencies; because housing was scarce; and because the legal pendulum had swung toward autonomy for mental patients.

During the 1970s, many people struggled to make deinstitutionalization work, but the system was not a system, and it was not too long before psychiatry—among other groups and many individuals—revolted. A number of prominent psychiatrists chastised liberals who resisted committing schizophrenics. One former director at the National Institutes of Mental Health (NIMH), who had been a leader of the deinstitutionalization movement, questioned the ethics of mental health administrators and accused them of allowing a new form of profitable segregation: "poor blacks working with other poor blacks while white mental health professionals worked with their own kind."[9] In 1976, a famous psychiatrist reviewed deinstitutionalization and concluded that it was a failure, that some involuntary confinement was needed to help the mentally ill, and that civil liberties lawyers were often enemies of the insane.[10]

THE CASE OF JOYCE BROWN

Project Help

By the 1980s, both mental health professionals and the general public in New York wanted something done about the situation there. Pedestrians found themselves having to step around or over derelicts sleeping on the street; people entering offices, stores, concert halls, and even their own homes had to step over derelicts huddled in doorways. Homeless panhandlers seemed to be almost everywhere. Subway cars were taken over by the homeless, who slept in them all day—many homeless people stay awake all night and sleep during the day, when life is somewhat less dangerous. During the winter, some of the homeless who preferred the streets to the city shelters died of exposure. (Reluctance to go to a shelter in New York City is not entirely unreasonable: Most of the inmates in these shelters are men who use crack cocaine.)

Many of these homeless people were—or certainly seemed to be—insane; and in 1983, the administration of Mayor Ed Koch started Project Help to evaluate homeless mentally ill people for possible psychiatric treatment. The city runs 11 acute-care hospitals with some psychiatric units; but since these municipal hospitals could provide only short-term care, the Koch administration also negotiated for some of the scarce beds in New York State mental hospitals for long-term care of extremely dysfunctional homeless people.

Originally, Project Help was a voluntary program: That is, except for people considered dangerous to themselves or others, the project intervened only with mentally ill people who wanted to be helped. On this basis, however, most of the people it tried to help resisted its efforts. City administrators were thus confronted with a difficult issue. Could insane homeless people just be left to "die with their rights on"? Or could these people be forcibly picked up for psychiatric evaluation in a hospital? Forcible evaluation, possibly leading to involuntary commitment, might seem to violate these people's freedom; but surely it might also help them, and didn't they desperately need help?

In October of 1987, this reasoning led Project Help to broaden its standards for involuntary commitment beyond the legal requirements of mental illness and dangerousness. It added two new criteria: self-neglect and a need to be treated.

The first person picked up by Project Help under its new criteria was a 40-year-old African American woman calling herself Billie Boggs. She had been deliberately chosen as a test case; Mayor Koch, who had seen her and spoken with her on the street, was personally involved in that decision. At about the same time, almost 100 other homeless people were also evaluated under the new criteria, and 38 of them were brought to Bellevue Hospital's inpatient psychiatric unit; none of them made a legal issue of it. The case of Billie Boggs, however, did become a legal issue and would soon attract national attention as a symbol of the conflict over whether or not to impose involuntary treatment on homeless people who are mentally ill.

Billie Boggs = Joyce Brown

Billie Boggs's real name was Joyce Brown (Bill Boggs was actually the name of a man who was prominent on local television). For 1½ years, Joyce Brown had been sleeping at night on an air grate outside a Swensen's ice cream parlor on Second Avenue and 65th Street, on the upper east side of Manhattan (ironically, in a neighborhood with the highest per capita wealth in the United States). During the day, she panhandled on the street. At a nearby delicatessen, she would buy chicken cutlets, ice cream, cigarettes, and toilet paper.

Joyce Brown had become a familiar figure in the neighborhood, and to many people her physical appearance suggested mental illness. Her teeth were very unclean; her matted, tangled hair was pushed underneath a bulky white knit cap. All winter, she went without gloves; the only clothing she had seemed to be a striped blouse, beige pants, and a green sweater, though she kept sheets and blankets nearby and slept under them when she went to her air vent at night.

Joyce Brown's behavior also seemed to suggest derangement. She had a glazed look, muttered as she panhandled, and often carried on a dialogue with herself. She sometimes sang "How Much Is That Doggie in the Window?" Once, when a resident of the block gave her some money, she tossed it back, while screaming angrily at an invisible man. One neighbor described her in a letter to the *New York Times* as "full of rage." She seemed to dislike men especially and would curse at any she encountered on her side of the street, although she liked babies in strollers. She sometimes defecated and urinated in the gutter. On bitterly cold nights, people in the neighborhood sometimes tried to have the police pick her up, but she always resisted.

For some time, psychiatrists working in Project Help had been observing Joyce Brown on the street, and on this basis they had judged her insane. On October 28, 1987, she was forcibly removed from the street by Project Help and brought to the emergency room of Bellevue Hospital. She identified herself at Bellevue as Billie Boggs and also as "Ann Smith" (another alias she sometimes used) and said that she had lived on the street for 5 years and had no parents or other relatives. In the emergency room, she was injected with 5 mg of Haldol, an antipsychotic drug; and 2 mg of Ativan, a fast-acting short-term tranquilizer. She was then taken to a new, 28-bed, locked psychiatric unit on the nineteenth floor.

The Legal Conflicts

After Joyce Brown was evaluated at Bellevue, Mayor Koch was informed that she was neither sufficiently insane nor sufficiently dangerous for involuntary commitment; he replied, "You're loony yourself." Here, Koch said, was a woman whom compassionate people should help, but who could not be helped because of legalistic quibbles. He also believed (and this belief was probably shared by most New Yorkers and visitors to the city) that the civil liberties of homeless mentally ill people were being overemphasized, to the detriment of quality of life in the city's public places. He and Project Help, therefore, decided to pursue her commitment on the basis of their new additional criteria. Bellevue, although it did not consider her dangerous enough for commitment, had diagnosed her as schizophrenic and in need of treatment—and need for treatment was one of Project Help's new standards.

In any event, once a person is brought to a psychiatric facility by the police or emergency-room personnel, release is unlikely in practice until a commitment hearing before a judge has been held and concluded. (For commitment hearings, hospitals usually have a designated room in the psychiatric unit.) Moreover, the law in New York State is that, without a hearing, involuntary injections are allowed only in emergency rooms; and in the psychiatric unit at Bellevue, Joyce Brown exercised her right to refuse further drugs. Therefore, she could be given no drugs in the psychiatric ward until a separate hearing was held on involuntary drug treatment.

•

Joyce Brown's commitment hearing began on November 5, 8 days after her arrival at Bellevue, and it would take 3 days. Judge Robert Lippman of the state supreme court, presided. Lippman was then 51 years old, and lived on the upper east side; appropriately enough, he had worked for 17 years as a Legal Aid lawyer in the Bronx.

And he was known in the legal community as an advocate for the poor and homeless. Joyce Brown had called the American Civil Liberties Union (ACLU) from Bellevue and asked for their help; she had received a team of ACLU lawyers, on the condition that she would waive confidentiality and agree to publicity for her own sake and that of other homeless people. New York City's attorney opposed Joyce's ACLU lawyers.

Both the mayor's office and ACLU treated the hearing as a test, and Judge Lippman apparently also saw it in those terms. Such hearings are almost always closed to the public, but because this case had the potential to set a precedent— and because of the publicity it had already generated—Lippman allowed the press to attend. However, only the testimony of witnesses who consented could be reported by the press.

On November 2, a few days before the commitment hearing, a sketch of "Billie Boggs" had appeared on a television news show, and three women recognized her as their sister. As the commitment hearing began on November 5, these three women were present. Outside the hearing room, they identified her to reporters as Joyce Brown. They had been searching for Joyce Brown for 1½ years. The three sisters were all married, had all worked for years, and were all living in what they described as comfortable homes.

As the hearing proceeded, Joyce Brown's sisters gave the press many details. They said that she had never married and had no children, and they described her background.[11] Their family was from Elizabeth, New Jersey, and their father was a Methodist minister; as children, all the girls had gone to church every Sunday. Joyce was said to have been a "bright, attractive, and happy-go-lucky child." Joyce Brown graduated from both high school and business school and had then had several jobs at Bell Laboratories. During these years, her sisters said, she had been a "big, healthy girl" who wore nice clothes and jewelry and "always drove around in a new Cadillac."

In her twenties, however, according to her sisters, Joyce Brown became increasingly dependent on heroin and, later, cocaine; it can be noted that this is the age at which the first signs of schizophrenia often appear. She worked for 10 years as a secretary for the New Jersey Human Rights Commission; but in 1982, she was arrested by the Newark police, charged with assault, and found guilty of harassment. At about this time, her conduct deteriorated: She became belligerent and less able to support herself; her mental health and her job performance plummeted. In 1985, at age 38, she was fired because of absenteeism and her use of heroin and cocaine. She had been living with her sisters and their parents in turn, but now she left her family and went to a shelter in Newark, where she was expelled for assaulting others there.

Her sisters admitted that they then tricked her into a voluntary commitment in the psychiatric ward of East Orange General Hospital in New Jersey. There she was diagnosed as psychotic and given antipsychotic drugs, though she resisted these injections. She was held for 2 weeks, during which—again because of assaults on others—she was put in restraints in an isolation room. After these 2 weeks, she was released.

She then fled New Jersey and began to live on the streets of New York, on the upper east side, under various aliases. She avoided shelters for the homeless, considering them dangerous for unattached women. For some time, she did not contact her sisters, fearing that they would have her committed again. But her sisters said that in July 1986 they received an abusive telephone call from her in Manhattan, and that they then spent much of the next year looking for her along Manhattan streets.

The sisters emphasized, "Behind every homeless person there is a family that just wants to find them and help them."

•

When Joyce Brown herself testified at her commitment hearing, she appeared to be intelligent and articulate. She called herself a "professional street person" and was able to answer a number of probing questions.

Why had she torn up paper money? She said that she needed $7 a day and had torn up only additional money that was forced on her. "If money is given to me and I don't want it, of course I am going to destroy it," she said; she explained that she might be robbed if she did not. "I've heard people say: 'Take it. It will make me feel good.' But I say: 'I don't want it. I don't need it.' Is it my job to make them feel good by taking their money?"[12]

Why did she defecate on herself? "I never did," she replied; though she added that she had used the streets because no local restaurant would let her use its restroom. "I offered to buy something and they still refused."

Why had she used aliases such as "Billie Boggs"? "To prevent my sisters from finding me."

The attorney for the city argued that Joyce Brown had to be committed because she was endangering herself through self-neglect. Four psychiatrists testified for the city that she suffered from chronic schizophrenia, that she was clearly psychotic and should be treated in an institution, and that she would deteriorate if she was left on the streets. One of the psychiatrists for the city, Luis Marcos, was a vice president of its public hospital system and an advocate of the new criteria adopted by Project Help; he was therefore challenged about his ability to give unbiased testimony. He said in reply, "This is not political psychiatry"; he also stated that Joyce Brown's self-neglect was so severe that she had to be helped against her will. He noted that schizophrenia was consistent with being bright and having periods of rationality.

ACLU, on the other side, asked for an injunction to free Joyce Brown. Three psychiatrists testified for ACLU that she was not psychotic, not dangerous, not unreasonable in her answers, and not incapable of caring for herself on the streets. One of these three, Robert E. Gould of New York Medical College, testified that she was living on the street by choice.

One of Joyce Brown's sisters started to testify but was not allowed to continue after the ACLU attorneys objected. She had begun to describe how her sister's condition had deteriorated over the years, and the objection was sustained on the ground that this evidence was not relevant to Joyce Brown's present competence. (The sisters saw this as a ruling that the testimony of family members was irrelevant, and they resented it.)

By the third day of the commitment hearing, Joyce Brown appeared self-confident. She spoke slowly, deliberately, and with assurance and even smiled a few times at the judge. She told him that passersby on her street chatted with her every day: "They tell me about movies, they tell me about restaurants. They are executives, lawyers, doctors. They are established in their fields. If I asked for large amounts of money, they would give it to me."

In his summation, one of the ACLU attorneys said that the city had not proved that Joyce was dangerous to herself or others: "The only evidence the city had is that she goes to the bathroom in the streets. I see that in New York City every day, because there's a lack of public restroom facilities." The attorney for the city said in her summation: "Decency and the law and common sense do not require us to wait until something happens to her. It is our duty to act before it is too late."[13]

On November 12, Judge Lippman ordered Joyce Brown freed. He had found her "rational, logical, and coherent" throughout her testimony;[14] he said that she "displayed a sense of humor, pride, a fierce independence of spirit, [and] quick mental reflexes"; and he noted that she met none of the conditions set forth in *O'Connor* v. *Donaldson*. He stressed that even if all the psychiatrists had diagnosed her as psychotic, the city had still not met the requirement of dangerousness to others or oneself. "I am aware that her mode of existence does not conform to conventional standards, that it is an offense to aesthetic sense," he commented. Nevertheless, "she copes, she is fit, she survives." Moreover, "she refuses to be housed in a shelter. That may reveal more about conditions in shelters than about Joyce Brown's mental state. It might, in fact, prove she's quite sane."

Judge Lippman also complained: "There must be some civilized alternatives other than involuntary hospitalization or the street." He did not invalidate Project Help itself, and even praised it as a step in the right direction. Forced to decide for one side or the other, however, he ruled that the City had not proved Joyce Brown incompetent.

•

After the hearing, Joyce Brown's sisters talked again to reporters. They called Lippman's decision "racist" and "sexist." They argued that if his own wife or mother were sleeping on the streets, "he would not stand for it." They also insisted that Joyce Brown needed treatment. As the psychiatrist Robert Gould left the hearing with Joyce Brown's sisters and reporters, he challenged the sisters: "Can't you understand that a lot of people are frightened that the Mayor has unilaterally decided to change the statute and pick up your sister?" One sister replied, "The Mayor is absolutely right. I have lived with her. You have not lived with her." Gould replied, "Is it possible that your sister doesn't want to live with you because you are so angry?" [15]

At this time, the sisters revealed that after Joyce Brown was hospitalized for schizophrenia in East Orange, they had gotten her declared mentally disabled and she had accordingly received $500 a month in social security disability payments, which they had been holding for her. Joyce Brown had persisted in refusing the money, though, saying that she rejected the "lie" that she was mentally disabled.

At the same time, Joyce Brown and her ACLU lawyers held a press conference, at which she said, "I didn't want to play the game before, but now I am . . . . I am going to get an apartment, . . . go back to work, and get my life together." She criticized the city for spending $600 a day on her care: "I could be living at Trump Tower." [16]

One question that had been raised was why she had appeared so rational at the hearing; in response, the psychiatrists at Bellevue had acknowledged that she had seemed sane but had claimed that she improved rapidly in the hospital. Joyce Brown dismissed their claim, saying—as she had been saying all along—that she had never been crazy in the first place. She objected to being taken into Bellevue like "cattle" and said that, given her options, living on the street was a rational choice. (Her sisters dismissed this argument: "You might be able to survive one winter," one of them said, "or even two. But you can't survive that way forever.")

Mayor Koch blasted Judge Lippman's decision: "If anything happens to that woman, God forbid, the blood of that woman is on that judge's hands." Reminded by a reporter that Lippman had found Joyce Brown lucid, Koch replied, "This woman is at risk. When she lay on the ground in the rain, in the snow, uncovered— was that lucid?" [17] When asked if Joyce's commitment was "political psychiatry," Koch asked, "Who would claim that?" When told that it had been Joyce Brown herself, he replied, "That alone proves she's crazy." [18]

The city and Koch appealed to a five-member New York State Appellate Court, and one of its members stayed Judge Lippman's order of release pending its own hearing. This higher court agreed to hold its hearing extraordinarily soon—within 2 weeks—but until then, Joyce Brown would have to remain at Bellevue. She was reportedly bitter but accepted the decision.

During the weeks before the hearing on their appeal, city officials sought and obtained an order to see if Joyce Brown had lupus cerebritis, a genetically caused, incurable degenerative brain syndrome. After negotiations, she allowed a blood sample to be taken. On December 12, the result was found to be negative; this embarrassed the psychiatrist who had made the provisional diagnosis—he seemed to have been grasping at a straw.

At the appellate hearing, ACLU argued that Joyce Brown would not return to the streets but would live in a supportive residence for the homeless. The city argued that where she would live was irrelevant: "She was not hospitalized because she was living on the streets [but because] 3 psychiatrists said she needed medical and psychiatric help." According to the city, she was schizophrenic and should remain under psychiatric care for her own good (though the city did not argue that she was dangerous to herself or others), and her decision not to return to the street did not affect this situation; the case was not about homelessness but about mental illness. It was pointed out that in New York, the homeless tended to be poor, African American, or Hispanic; in contrast, Project Help was aimed at mentally disturbed people on the streets, who—according to the city—were typically white, middle-class people with chronic undifferentiated schizophrenia. (It was also said that many of these people were not New Yorkers.)

In short, the city attorneys told the justices that the city could help Joyce and should be allowed to do so; and having won 11 previous challenges to its various commitment programs over the last decade (including Project Help under the original criteria), it hoped to win this one too.

Joyce Brown's attorneys replied that she did not want help, did not need help, and was entitled to live as she pleased. (She herself did not testify before the appeals court.) While awaiting the decision, she told reporters that she was ready to return to work. "Tomorrow I could sit at a typewriter and take shorthand," she said. "I am not insane. I am homeless." She also said that she had known before the test for lupus that she did not have it and was not in poor health, claiming, "You have to be in good physical shape to survive on the street."

•

The city won on appeal. On December 19, the appellate court held (3–2, with the two dissenting justices disagreeing vigorously) that Judge Lippman had ruled incorrectly that the city had not provided enough evidence for commitment, and that Lippman had placed too much emphasis on Joyce Brown's testimony instead of the testimony of the psychiatrists who believed she would harm herself. Surprisingly, the majority noted that a very high standard of proof was required in this case—"clear and convincing evidence" rather than the weaker "preponderance of evidence"—and that the city had met the higher standard.

In an unusual move, the appellate court reviewed detailed testimony in the case, especially that of a social worker who said she had observed "fecal matter" on the sheets in which "Miss Boggs" wrapped herself. The appellate court also reviewed the testimony of one psychiatrist who said that Joyce Brown had told him she often defecated and urinated on herself. In addition, the court found that "the evidence presented in this case clearly and convincingly demonstrated Ms. Boggs's past history of assaultive and aggressive behavior."[19] The majority justices gave little weight to Joyce Brown's lucidity during her commitment hearing, attributing it to "a week of hospital treatment."

The two dissenting justices argued that the city's case could be "narrowed to one claim," which was that "she is dangerous to herself" because "she is likely to provoke others to do injury to her." They considered that commitment to prevent such possible harm was an "extreme remedy" and "somewhat offensive." They were dismayed that their colleagues had dismissed Lippman's assessment of Joyce Brown's lucidity in court: " . . . If the court's [Lippman's] judgment of her mental condition is to be completely ignored, then what was the purpose of the hearing in the first place?" Finally, they stressed that in Joyce Brown's six previous hospitalizations,[20] disinterested psychiatrists had unanimously concluded that she was not dangerous to herself.

After the decision of the appellate court, Mayor Koch said, "Up until this moment, the only treatment has been care, loving, a safe environment. Now we will seek to treat her medically." However, to medicate Joyce Brown against her will, under New York State law, the city still had to get a court order.

One month later, on January 19, 1988, a state judge ruled that she could not be given drugs against her will. Bellevue Hospital promptly released her, saying that if she could not be treated with drugs, there was no further point in holding her.

ACLU then appealed the earlier appellate decision on commitment to New York's supreme court, the Court of Appeals, which declined to hear the case because it presented "no novel, constitutional or substantial case for this court to review," and because the case was moot after Joyce Brown's release from Bellevue.

All together, Joyce Brown had been held for 84 days. One member of the city council noted that the city had spent more than $42,000 for her stay at Bellevue and suggested that in this case "the mayor's ego got in the way of what was right." After her release, Joyce Brown held forth:

> I was incarcerated against my will. . . . [I was] a political prisoner. The only thing wrong with me was that I was homeless, not insane. You just can't go around picking everyone up and automatically label them schizophrenic. I'm angry at Mayor Koch, the city and Bellevue. They held me down and injected me. . . . They took my blood against my will. . . .
>
> I need a place to live; I don't need an institution. . . .
>
> People are treated differently just because of your economic status, [because of] what you look like and where you live. . . .
>
> I was mistreated, mentally abused, and I will never, ever, forget this.[21]

The Aftermath

Joyce Brown was released to live in a hotel for women run by a nonprofit agency. She received several job offers and worked temporarily as a secretary in the ACLU office. Interviewed there, she said that after leaving Bellevue, "I was supposed to have deteriorated within 3 or 4 days," and then noted with a smile that 3 weeks had passed and, "I'm fine. I'm working."

In fact, in early 1988 Joyce Brown became something of a celebrity. She received half a dozen movie and book offers. On February 15, she dined at Windows on the World, a restaurant atop the World Trade Center, where the waiters congratulated her. She shopped at Bloomingdale's, Saks Fifth Avenue, and Lord and Taylor; these shopping sprees were paid for by two television shows—*The Donahue Show* and *60 Minutes*—which were broadcasting discussions of her case. She seemed to flourish with attention.

Joyce Brown herself appeared on *The Donahue Show*. During this show, a hostile immigrant said that he had found a job and bought a house "in just 25 years," and he wondered why she couldn't do the same. He said, "You're an intelligent woman. How come you're homeless? I'm sure you can find a job." She replied, "Right now I'm trying to get a job. Mr. Donahue, do you need any help around here?" (The audience laughed heartily.)

Joyce Brown also lectured to students at two law schools—Cardozo and Harvard. The title of her speech was "The Homeless Crisis: A Street View." At the time, she said, "It looks like I have been appointed the homeless spokesperson."

Then things began to go worse for her. She had eventually decided to accept the disability benefits which her sisters had been accumulating for her, but her sisters now resisted; they said they would release the money to her when the ACLU lawyers stopped "manipulating her" for political purposes.

Her roommate at the hotel said that Joyce Brown had "a lot of anger inside" and frequently talked to herself. One day, while walking to work, she was heard muttering racial slurs and obscenities. She dismissed these incidents as misinterpretations of her habit of singing popular songs to herself.

On March 21, 1988, Joyce Brown was seen begging on a street in the Times Square area and shouting obscenities at passersby. When asked how she was doing, she insisted, "I'm not insane."[22]

On May 10, she collapsed on the street and was admitted to a hospital for dangerously high blood pressure; she had always refused medication for hypertension.

On September 6, she was charged with having been in possession of a small amount of heroin ($40 worth) and two hypodermic needles in a Harlem housing project shortly after her release from Bellevue.[23] This incident in particular made many people who had sided with Koch, including the essayist Charles Krauthammer, feel vindicated.[24] On December 27, 1988, she pleaded guilty to disorderly conduct and was conditionally discharged.

•

By July of the next year—1989—Joyce Brown was living in a supervised residence for formerly homeless women, in Manhattan.

During that month, Project Help announced that it had picked up and helped 466 homeless mentally ill people since adopting its new criteria in 1987. It estimated that 800 to 1,000 such people were still out on the city streets.

When New York City officials planned Project Help, they assumed that people such as Joyce Brown would stay for a few weeks in psychiatric hospitals and would then be moved into community facilities, where they could live under supervised conditions. As the people picked up by Project Help were actually evaluated, however, they turned out to be far sicker than had been expected. Thus many more permanent places were needed in psychiatric hospitals than had been planned for.

ETHICAL ISSUES: FROM CRITERIA OF BENEFIT TO IDEOLOGY

Criteria for Commitment: Applying the *O'Connor* Standards

One issue in the Joyce Brown case was the *O'Connor* standards for involuntary commitment. The five appellate justices had to decide whether or not Joyce Brown could be committed under the *O'Connor* criteria, but because the legal issue was obviously in her favor, they would in effect be deciding whether or not those standards were morally sufficient. In other words, Joyce Brown clearly could not be committed under the existing legal criteria established by *O'Connor,* and so the justices had to decide whether those criteria should be changed or radically reinterpreted for reasons of compassion.

In its argument to this appellate court, New York City used a moral argument: that the traditional legal standard allowed too much risk of harm. The city maintained that personal liberty had been valued too highly and could result in ultimate harm to the mentally ill.

The city's argument hung on two points. The first of these was that homeless mentally ill people will eventually come to harm if they are simply left alone. In Joyce Brown's case, if she stayed on the street, hurling insults at people and sleeping unguarded, she would eventually be attacked.

The second point was independent of the first; it appealed simply to humanitarian considerations. Here, the city argued that governments have an ancient right—or duty—known as *parens patria* ("parent of the country"). *Parens patria* originated in English common law, under which the king or queen had a royal prerogative to act as guardian for incompetents. In modern law, state attorney generals exercise the same right in bringing antitrust suits on behalf of citizens. On this basis, the city held that it had a responsibility to protect people, like Joyce Brown, who were deteriorating, and that it would be degrading and unmerciful to let them continue to live without help. To say that society cannot help them because helping them would violate their rights was to value their personal liberty over their sanity, their health, and their survival. The city noted that while this appeal was taking place, three homeless men had been found frozen to death in Central Park.

Of course, not everyone agreed with these two points, or with the city's case as a whole. Some people, including Joyce Brown herself and Judge Lippman, considered the first point an especially poor argument: After all, she had already lived 11½ years on the street and seemed to have come to no harm.

However, Charles Krauthammer, a well-known writer who wrote for *Time* and *New Republic,* supported the city. He argued that Joyce Brown should be committed not because she was dangerous but because she was helpless.[25] For every insane person committed who protested, he emphasized, hundreds did not protest and appeared to like warm beds and regular meals. Still, it must be noted that Joyce Brown herself said she wasn't helpless and indeed didn't appear to be.

Motives for Commitment

In the controversy over Joyce Brown, motives for commitment became an issue. Were those who argued for commitment—and even some of those who argued against it—genuinely motivated by altruism, or did they have ulterior, nonaltruistic motives? In this regard, the general question of public altruism arose, along with various arguments about nonaltruistic motivation.

Altruism and Its Limits   Altruism as such is a persistent ethical problem of civilized life. How much should any individual do for strangers who appear to be in need? In face-to-face meetings with apparently needy strangers, few of us are completely indifferent, but most of us experience doubts and self-conflicts about what to do.

Charles Krauthammer argued that the ethical response to people like Joyce Brown should be based on societal rather than individual responsibility. The Joyce Browns of a community need facilities and staff to care for them, he held, and to implement this kind of solution he urged higher taxes. Krauthammer said, "To expect saintliness of the ordinary citizen is bad social policy," but "society must not leave the ordinary citizen with no alternative between ignoring the homeless and playing Mother Teresa. A civilized society ought to offer its people some communal act that lies somewhere in between, such as contributing to the public treasury to build an asylum system to care for these people."

There are, however, arguments against Krauthammer's position. One counterargument is theoretical: Individuals do have a moral duty to be altruistic but are only too ready to abandon their duty and let society take over. Three authors argued along these lines in a legal journal:

> Most of us profess to believe that there is an individual moral duty to take care of a senile parent, a paranoid wife, or a disturbed child. Most of us also resent the bother such care creates. By allowing society to perform this duty, masked in medical terminology, but frequently amounting in fact to what one court has described as "warehousing," we can avoid facing painful issues.[26]

There is also a practical argument against Krauthammer's position: Societal altruism may be lacking or grossly inadequate. In a case like Joyce Brown's, it can be argued that no real treatment exists and commitment is no more than getting the insane off the streets.

Nonaltruistic Motives   In the case of Joyce Brown, almost everyone on both sides claimed to be motivated by altruism—to have her own best interests in mind—and almost everyone was accused of having hidden, nonaltruistic motives.

Mayor Koch and New York City, for example, were accused of wanting Joyce Brown committed simply because she was a public nuisance. Her sisters were accused of wanting her committed because she was a family nuisance. Both Judge Lippman, who decided in her favor, and the appellate justices who decided against her were accused of racism: Lippman, it was said, considered it not inappropriate for a black woman to live in filth on the street; the appellate justices were said to be presuming that a black woman was probably incompetent. ACLU was accused of manipulating Joyce Brown to further its own agenda. Some psychiatrists were accused of being the city's rubber stamp and of using "treatment" for purposes of restraint or even punishment; psychiatrists on the other side were accused of patient abandonment.

The truth is probably that many people involved in the case, as participants or commentators, had mixed motives. This is neither surprising nor particularly sinister: Most of us have mixed motives most of the time.

With regard to Mayor Koch, the columnist A. M. Rosenthal (a former editor of the *New York Times*) said that he himself saw Joyce Brown almost every day from his Second Avenue apartment and believed that Koch was trying to get therapy for her, not rounding up a political dissident.[27] To Rosenthal, it seemed that the city had wanted to be compassionate and gotten its hands slapped for trying: Thus the case symbolized a situation where the law seemed helpless. Some people argued that her commitment was arbitrary because of the original psychiatric evaluation "on the street," but Rosenthal held that it was not; an arbitrary commitment would have been based only on secondhand evidence such as the possibly biased reports of her neighbors, but Joyce Brown had been given a hearing at Bellevue and had been represented by attorneys. The Project Help program, Rosenthal concluded, "is an attempt to help, not a program of incarceration."

The motives of Joyce Brown's affluent neighbors also came in for considerable scrutiny. ACLU, noting that Joyce Brown did not want to leave the street and had never been proved dangerous, argued that her presence embarrassed the rich people in her neighborhood. New York City has thousands of people like Joyce Brown, so why, then, was there no similar outcry about all the others? Why did no one write letters to the *New York Times* about the Joyce Browns in the Bronx?

Norman Siegel, executive director of ACLU, extended this argument to Koch and the city as well: "In sweeping up the homeless, the Mayor is attempting to place these people out of sight and out of mind and hide the crisis from the public consciousness." Siegel claimed that Project Help targeted areas seen by tourists and inhabited by the rich.

As noted earlier, quality of life in public places was a consideration for Koch and the city. However, the consideration they emphasized was treatment; and the city's mental health commissioner maintained that patients had been picked up in affluent areas simply because homeless people gravitated to such areas, which were safer and offered better opportunities for begging.

Paternalism, Autonomy, and Diminished Competence

Paternalism in medicine is treatment of adult patients as incompetents who do not know their own best interests, and an important set of issues in Joyce Brown's case had to do with paternalism versus patients' autonomy.

Many philosophers, physicians, and legal scholars have discussed the conditions under which paternalism might be justified. One condition is temporary incompetence, followed by a return of competence; in this situation, paternalism would be justified if the patient himself or herself later agreed with it. (A suicidal patient, for example, may later be glad to be alive.) In Joyce Brown's case, the city might have argued impressively for paternalism if its psychiatrists had brought forth at least one patient who had been forced to undergo psychiatric treatment and was now sane and grateful. No such patient testified for the city, however.

Questions about patients' competence are important in any discussion of paternalism. In this regard, one question has to do with the basic concept of competence. The American legal system tends to treat mental patients as if they were either totally competent and autonomous, or totally dysfunctional and subject to mandatory treatment. Many observers think this is a false dichotomy which can be harmful to patients. Competence, on this argument, is not an either-or matter but a matter of degrees; and over the last decade, American bioethics has increasingly seen competence in this way.

Another question has to do with what constitutes proof of incompetence. This issue is not necessarily clear-cut: The psychiatrist Virginia Abernethy argues, for instance, that "disorientation, mental illness, irrationality, [and] commitment to a mental institution are not conclusive proof of incompetence."[28]

Abernethy describes the case of "Ms. A," a highly intelligent, very independent woman who lived alone in a large house with six cats, in an unheated garbage-strewn room. After a fire in her house (which had apparently started when she burned some debris to keep warm), Ms. A was hospitalized but found competent and released. As winter came, a concerned social worker investigated; he found her with her feet black, ulcerated, and bleeding. When he tried to get her to go with him to a hospital, she chased him away with a shotgun. The police later came and forcibly hospitalized her. At the hospital, her feet were diagnosed as gangrenous, and surgeons wanted to amputate; when she refused, psychiatrists began to evaluate her.

It turned out that Ms. A's feet had blackened once before, a few years earlier, and she had recovered. She now hoped for another recovery, but the psychiatrists interpreted this as psychotic denial and tried to get her to say that she wanted to live, so that they could amputate. She refused, avoiding their questions. Ms. A was faced with a dilemma: Either she had to let the surgeons amputate (a drastic operation which she did not want), or she had to let the psychiatrists conclude that she was in denial and therefore psychotic. It might seem unfair to present a patient with such a choice—a choice between two highly undesirable outcomes—and it might also seem that in such a situation trying to avoid the choice would be reasonable. However, according to Abernethy, "Her rejection of the two-choice model became the grounds, finally, for concluding that Ms. A was not competent to refuse amputation."

Abernethy analyzed the psychodynamics of this process as follows. First, a false aura of medical emergency "pervaded the psychiatric consultations and judicial process." Second, "Ms. A herself was quick to anger and regarded most interactions with medical personnel as adversarial." Third, Ms. A's anger created anger in those evaluating her competence: "Professionals who think of themselves as altruistic, or at least benevolently motivated, may be particularly sensitive to hostility because they feel deserving of gratitude." Abernethy says that psychiatrists are outcome-oriented and cannot tolerate a patient's self-destructiveness, even in the name of autonomy and even when self-destruction results from an underlying disease that they ultimately cannot stop. Abernethy notes, moreover, that "hope (disbelieving the physicians' pessimistic prognosis) is not a criterion of psychotic denial."

In some ways, Joyce Brown was similar to Ms. A. Like Ms. A, Joyce Brown did not accept her diagnosis (schizophrenia) or her prognosis (that she would come to harm if left alone); she hoped that she was sane and could take care of herself. Also like Ms. A, Joyce Brown saw psychiatrists as enemies who wanted to treat her against her will. Both women were acknowledged to be generally competent, but both were evaluated as having a *focal incompetence,* a specific incompetence to make decisions about their own treatment. Abernethy notes, "The criterion of a focal delusion is dangerously liable to error because a patient can easily be seen as delusional in an emotionally charged interchange, when in other circumstances he addresses the same issue appropriately."

Actually, the concept of focal incompetence—particularly in psychiatric commitment—is a two-edged sword: If an incompetent patient cannot *refuse* treatment, how can such a patient *consent* to treatment? In the majority of cases, consent of incompetents is allowed for psychiatric admission and rarely challenged; this is hardly logical. Abernethy sums it up: With regard to commitment, "Competence is presumed and does not have to be proved. Incompetence has to be proved."

Homelessness and Commitment

What was the real issue in the Joyce Brown case—insanity or homelessness?

City officials claimed that Joyce Brown's insanity was the true issue and her homelessness merely a side issue. Her ACLU lawyers disagreed: "The Joyce Brown story has captured the issue of the homeless that a lot of people have been trying to deal with for years."[29] The real problem, ACLU implied, was how to get homeless people off the streets, not how to treat the mentally ill; city officials didn't seem worried about schizophrenics who camped out in bad neighborhoods. ACLU suggested reinstituting public baths (which had been widely available in the city during the depression and earlier) and using condemned housing as temporary shelters. Incarcerating the homeless for their own good was a cheap solution; building homes for street people was much more expensive.

No one could deny that the housing situation in New York City was bad: Affordable housing was rare. On a talk show about this issue in 1988, for example, one man said he had been working 15 months in Manhattan as a home health aide. He made $4.50 an hour and brought home $130 a week. Just to rent a room—with no stove, no sink, and no refrigerator, and not in pricey Manhattan, but along a noisy elevated train line in an outer borough—would cost him 2 weeks' pay in security ($250) at the outset, and then 1 week's take-home pay ($130) in rent each month. (Today, the same room would cost at least $300 to $400 a month, and might be much farther away.)

On one talk show, a member of the audience said to Joyce Brown, "But a woman of your obvious intelligence, why would she be happy to spend the rest of her life on the street?" Joyce Brown replied, evidently referring to such housing problems:

> I didn't say I was going to spend the rest of my life on the street. I'm not a career homeless person, I have skills, I'm very intelligent, I am employable, but at that particular time that was my choice. I had a limited choice and that's what I chose to do.[30]

The problem of creating permanent housing for the city's homeless had frustrated many good minds. The city maintained over 1,000 families in squalid welfare hotels at exorbitant rates, using funding from the Emergency Assistance for Families act and the primary nationwide welfare program, Aid to Families with Dependent Children. The city would have preferred to use these funds to rent permanent housing for such families (in fact, it would later pressure the Clinton administration to allow this by threatening to block health care reform). Critics feared, however, that providing rented housing would encourage more people to depend on government handouts; they also pointed out that the city was one of the most expensive places in the United States in which to subsidize public housing. On the other hand, government subsidizes everyone who owns a home or condominium, since the interest on a mortgage is deductible for federal and state income taxes; and it can be argued that the poor and homeless not only deserve similar subsidization but also need it far more.

Moreover, it seemed in Joyce Brown's case that the dangers the city envisioned for her—and used as one basis for committing her—may have had more to do with homelessness than with schizophrenia or incipient schizophrenia. A lone woman sleeping unprotected on a sidewalk is indeed in danger, but that has little to do with mental illness. In other words, although the city insisted that the case was about mental illness, the dangers it emphasized seemed to come from life on the street.

The crucial point here may be this: The city would not have tried to commit Joyce Brown if she had not been homeless, since Project Help was aimed at *homeless* mentally ill people. Was that reasonable? What does homelessness have to do with committing the insane?

In this regard, we might argue as follows. Presumably, anyone—homeless or not—should be committed if the legal criteria for commitment are met: insanity, dangerousness, and (in some states) a least restrictive environment for treatment. Presumably, also, no one—homeless or not—should be committed if these criteria for commitment are not met. Project Help's intention was to broaden or loosen those criteria by applying different standards, but *only* for homeless people. Was that justifiable? Shouldn't the same standards apply for everyone? Isn't that what we mean by "equal justice for all"?

Two final points should be made here. First, some people simply tried to infer insanity from homelessness, arguing as follows: It is dangerous to sleep on the streets of Manhattan. No one but an insane person would sleep there. Therefore, those who sleep on the street are insane. This, of course, begs the question of mental illness.

Second, some people argued that homeless people, regardless of sanity or insanity, should be taken to shelters or otherwise incarcerated for their own safety. In 1972, the United States Supreme Court overturned a vagrancy law in Jacksonville, Florida, under which vagrants had been jailed without hearings or due process. No such law existed in New York; nevertheless, one Queens Democrat said during the Joyce Brown case that homeless people refusing to go to shelters should be "accommodated overnight in a cell" for their own protection.[31] To many critics, such remarks suggested that programs like Project Help entailed a real danger of abuse: that they might sooner or later be extended in ways which would represent a wide threat.

Psychiatry and Commitment

A potential for psychiatric abuse was also seen in the Joyce Brown case. Shortly after Joyce Brown was picked up, one of her ACLU lawyers (Robert Levy) and the psychiatrist Robert Gould discussed this in the *New York Times*.[32] They emphasized several possible abuses: involuntary roundups, handcuffing, forcible injections of medication, and confinement in locked wards. Joyce Brown herself had been given medication and kept in a locked ward against her will; and Levy and Gould said that she had been examined at least five times previously and had been found "not to require involuntary hospitalization." Indeed, nearly half of the 215 people brought to emergency rooms by Project Help were found "not to require involuntary hospitalization." Gould and Levy argued that to allow "preventive detention based solely on nebulous predictions of future self-destructive behavior" would invite abuse. They raised the specter of "totalitarian regimes" that would use psychiatry for political control.

When confronted with arguments like this, Mayor Koch replied, "This is not political psychiatry! This is not Russia! We're trying to help this woman!" The director of the psychiatric unit at Bellevue, David Nardacci, a 32-year-old psychiatrist, said that he had chosen to be a physician, not a lawyer; and as a physician, he was more concerned with helping people such as Joyce Brown than tiptoeing around legal pitfalls.

The issue of broadening criteria for commitment is again relevant here. How broadly should standards of commitment sweep? If we want to argue that these standards should be broadened enough to allow us to treat the Joyce Browns, aren't we thereby allowing psychiatric abuses to develop? How many people might be forced into mental hospitals by uncaring or even malevolent relatives? (Isn't this what Barbra Streisand portrayed in *Nuts)?* How many psychiatrists might use medication, time-out rooms, restraints, and continued commitment not as treatment but as punishment for patients who thwart their will?

•

A related issue concerns the limitations and potential contributions of psychiatry. When people like Koch argue in terms of helping the mentally ill, it is fair to ask how much psychiatry can be expected to help. Part of the debate about Joyce Brown's case concerned the ability of psychiatry to help schizophrenics.

Judge Lippman, for example, noted that he could place little faith in psychiatry because the four city psychiatrists and the three ACLU psychiatrists who had testified, although equally qualified, had disagreed dramatically. Lippman concluded, "It is evident that psychiatry is not a science amenable to the exactness of mathematics or the predictability of physical laws."

Most psychiatrists, of course, would object strongly to this evaluation of their profession; and many psychiatrists argue for involuntary commitment of schizophrenics. They point to schizophrenics who were dysfunctional but who gained years of ability (or at least minimal functioning) after being made to take medication.

They say that such patients stabilize and become free from delusions and that many patients, if they take their medication regularly (an important condition!), can even return to life outside institutions. The psychiatrist Paul Chodoff defended limited involuntary commitment as follows:

> Is freedom defined only by absence of external constraints? Internal physiological or psychological processes can contribute to a throttling of the spirit that is as painful as any applied from the outside. The "wild" manic individual without his lithium, the panicky hallucinator with his injection of fluphenazine hydrochloride and the understanding support of a concerned staff, the sodden alcoholic—are they free? Sometimes, as Woody Guthrie said, "Freedom means no place to go."[33]

In fact, people suffering from paranoid schizophrenia can make amazing improvement as a result of treatment. One patient, for instance, believed that the grounds crew mowing the lawns were communicating with themselves in secret "motor language" about his faults. After weeks of medication, he began to doubt bizarre beliefs like this one. After more weeks on medication, he really wasn't sure. Still later, he admitted that the belief was probably false. Finally, after more medication, he concluded one day, "How did I ever think that?"[34] Chemicals can change even our deepest thoughts (witness Prozac), and such change may be beneficial. Since some schizophrenia might be either caused by, or manifested in, chemical disturbances of the brain, this finding is not surprising.

One editor of *U.S. News and World Report* defended psychiatric treatment for Joyce Brown by arguing that she had lost the "rational freedom of choice offered by medicine that can alleviate mental anguish and paranoia."[35]

Suffering and Commitment: Benefit and Harm

One columnist argued that the ethical questions in this case boiled down not to whether people like Joyce Brown were likely to harm themselves, but to whether they were suffering. Another columnist agreed, saying that Joyce Brown should be taken off the streets before she died there "with her rights on."[36] These writers thought that it should be enough to convince a judge that a mentally ill person was in distress and that treatment would help.

But was the matter really so straightforward? To say that commitment is justified to end suffering assumes first that a person is really suffering, and second that involuntary psychiatric commitment can ease his or her suffering. This is a somewhat narrower issue than the general issue (discussed previously) of the uses and limitations of psychiatry.

Consider the first assumption, that the person is suffering. When someone such as Joyce Brown protests that she does not need or want help, it can be asked—as Thomas Szasz asked—who can determine that she is "suffering" enough to be locked inside a psychiatric ward? Who bears the onus of proof, patient or psychiatrist?

With regard to the second assumption, that involuntary commitment can help, consider the nature of involuntary commitment. What Joyce Brown feared most was another commitment to an inpatient unit like the one at East Orange Hospital.

Would she really be helped by involuntary psychiatry, involuntary medication, and involuntary therapy—in a locked unit within a large public institution?

Joyce Brown's court-appointed psychiatrist (who of all the psychiatrists involved in the case was the most likely to be impartial) had found that she suffered from serious mental illness and would benefit from medication—but that she would suffer more from forced treatment than from the mental illness itself. In such a situation, for one thing, Joyce Brown might harm herself while trying to resist the administration of antipsychotic medications and tranquilizers. Also, commitment might destroy her fierce independence; and if it did not—if she continued to resist—she might end up with a lobotomy, like McMurphy in *One Flew Over the Cuckoo's Nest.* Moreover, the long-term side effects of antipsychotics and tranquilizers can be as bad as the original disorder: Antipsychotic drugs such as neuroleptics administered over years create tardive dyskinesia in 10 to 25 percent of patients; this condition impairs voluntary movement, is untreatable, and persists in two-thirds of the affected patients when the medication is stopped.

It can also be argued that the potential benefits of involuntary treatment cannot be defined objectively. Most psychiatrists, of course, tend to think that people such as Joyce Brown benefit from living on medication and thereby losing their inner voices and delusions. But aren't benefit and harm, above the level of basic needs, defined by each person's own self-concept and life plans?

> When faced with an obviously aberrant person, we know, or we think we know, that he would be "happier" if he were as we are. We believe that no one would want to be misfit in society. From the very best of motives, then, we wish to fix him. It is difficult to deal with this feeling since it rests on the unverifiable assumption that the aberrant person, if he saw himself as we see him, would choose to be different than he is. But since he cannot be as we, and we cannot be as he, there is simply no way to judge the predicate for the assertion.[37]

Isn't it a rather shaky application of paternalism to say that Joyce Brown had to be treated so that she could obtain someone else's idea of a benefit? Psychiatrists imply that mentally ill patients suffer internal pain; but if that is so, why don't all patients want to get rid of it? Isn't it illogical—isn't it begging the question—for psychiatrists to explain that patients don't want to get rid of this pain "because they're crazy"?

UPDATE

Recently, the term *homeless* has been attacked by a new wave of critics as inappropriate for the wandering mentally ill; instead, these critics emphasize substance abuse. They have challenged ACLU's view that people such as Joyce Brown were primarily victims of a greedy or indifferent society which failed to provide affordable housing; they say there is evidence that as many as 85 percent of panhandlers are alcoholics, substance abusers, or mentally ill—and that all of these need treatment.[38] These new critics advocate mandatory treatment and police intervention to prevent panhandling, or begging. They also urge people not to give money to beggars, saying that those who do give money are "enablers of addiction."

There also seems to be a greater tendency to see mentally ill derelicts as dangerous. This trend had already begun a few years before Joyce Brown's case, when Juan Gonzalez, a homeless man suffering from symptoms like hers, went berserk on the Staten Island Ferry and killed two people with a sword. As a result, there was considerable public pressure for incarceration of mentally ill people who were "potentially dangerous"; and the concept of "potential danger" is now often used to justify temporarily holding someone for a cool-down observational period. (Actually, Gonzalez had been picked up for just such an observational period; but although he was diagnosed as a paranoid schizophrenic, he had not been considered imminently dangerous to others and had thus been discharged.)

In 1991, Keven McKiever, a homeless man who had gone to Bellevue Hospital seeking care and was turned away, stabbed Alexis Walsh, a former Radio City Rockette, to death. In 1993, Christopher Battiste, a homeless mentally ill drug abuser, allegedly murdered an elderly woman in the Bronx on a Sunday morning as she came home from church.

The most prominent of these cases in the 1990s was that of Larry Hogue, a homeless, mentally ill African American who was a veteran of the war in Vietnam. Larry Hogue sometimes lived peacefully on a street corner on the upper west side of Manhattan; but when he took illegal drugs, this "wild man of 96th Street" (as he was called on *60 Minutes*), became hostile and violent. A state judge ruled that he could be involuntarily committed against his will for detoxification, but that he would have to be released "as soon as he decides to seek outpatient care."[39] In 1994, shortly before he was due to be released from Creedmore Hospital, he escaped, committed a robbery for small change, and was soon picked up. He has since been returned to Creedmore.

The courts and the general public have come to expect psychiatrists to be able to predict dangerousness among the mentally ill, but it is debatable whether they actually can. In general, to assess the potential for violent behavior, emergency-room psychiatrists simply ask patients about their own tendencies toward violence and their own past acts of violence.[40] This is hardly a sophisticated predictive tool, though in practice it seems to work better than anything else.

There has been at least one significant legal development with regard to *O'Connor* v. *Donaldson*. In some states, the *O'Connor* criteria have been interpreted to mean that a person must commit an *overt act* in order to warrant a hearing for involuntary commitment. This interpretation is controversial and has in general been opposed by relatives, who can often perceive a pattern of threats and hostility and do not want to wait until someone is injured or killed before a commitment hearing can take place. At present, courts and legislatures are struggling with the implications of this "overt act" requirement.

•

The sheltered, or supervised, group home remains an elusive ideal. Whether we are discussing severely physically disabled people, welfare reform, or the mentally ill homeless, the best living facility for many people is a supervised group home. Living in such a home is much better than being warehoused in a large institution or—obviously—than being left to fend for oneself on the cold hard streets. Supervised group homes, especially if they are located in safe neighborhoods, are often a perfect compromise between institutionalization and independence.

The problem, then, is not with group homes as a concept but rather with the practical matter of getting group homes for those who need them. Funding has been one difficulty. In New York, for example, places in group homes are very scarce; in fact, the shortage of such beds has created a crisis in the city since 1988. In those homes that did exist, budgets were cut, so that some staff members had to be fired and some patients released. The funds saved were used by legislators for other projects; and now no one seems to know how to get the funding back. Meanwhile, deinstitutionalization has continued. In 1993, in New York, 2,400 new group home beds had been planned in preparation for the release of 1,000 more inmates from large institutions in 1994, but the number of new beds was later cut to 800. When New York State's highest court ruled in February 1993 that New York City must provide housing for homeless mentally ill patients discharged from city hospitals, the city said it would cost $300 million to do so and disputed the ruling.[41]

In 1999, two schizophrenic men not taking their prescribed medications pushed innocent people in front of oncoming subway trains in New York City, killing a young woman named Kendra Webdale and leaving the other without legs. Both had a history of violence. In previous years, similar events had occurred:

> Reuben Harris, who suffered from paranoid schizophrenia and had 12 hospitalizations and a history of violent behavior, pushed Song Sin to her death in the same manner in 1995. Jaheem Grayton, who also had a history of violence and severe mental illness pushed Naeeham Lee to her death after struggling to steal her earrings in 1996. Mary Ventura pushed Catherine Costello into the path of a subway train in 1985, 3 weeks after being discharged from a psychiatric hospital.[42]

These cases and others resulted in passage in 1999 of *Kendra's law* in New York, where a psychiatrist or relative can force hospitalization for a mentally ill person who has been hospitalized within the last 3 years, who has a history of violence, and who will not take his medication.[43] Forty states have now implemented such Assisted Outpatient Treatment (AOT) programs, in which outpatients can be forced to take their medications by court order and under supervision while still essentially remaining outpatients.

A White House conference on mental health, convened by Tipper Gore in 1999, caused brief interest in expanding medical insurance to cover mental illness, but critics complained it would make premiums soar for everyone. Critics also said it would create more workers without medical insurance because rising costs would force more employers to drop coverage. The only solution, such critics said, was a national system not based on if or where one worked.

Homelessness remained a major problem in 2002, with many homeless people plagued by drug problems, mental illness, or extreme poverty (or often, all three).

Many cities emulated New York City Mayor Rudolph Giuliani, who in the mid-1990s forced homeless people off the streets and into many city-funded shelters. Cities such as Sacramento, California, Seattle, and Atlanta simply forced homeless people to move out and closed shelters.

Attitudes also changed. Urban revitalization made new couples in old neighborhoods intolerant of homeless beggars. In 1986, six million Americans formed a 4,000-mile human chain from coast-to-coast to raise money to feed and help the homeless, but in 2002, the prevalent attitude had become that homelessness was a problem of mentally ill substance abusers who were losers under the capitalist system. No one denied that lack of affordable housing caused homelessness, but few citizens felt government should raise taxes to build such housing.

When some cities tried to build group homes for the homeless or mentally ill, fights ensued. Residents on Earle Street in one of the oldest neighborhoods in Greenville, South Carolina, sued in 1994 when charities tried to open a sixth group home there. All around the country, certain neighborhoods of each city became categorized as an area for group homes, where too many were built, thus making any other neighborhood passionately resist having even one such home, lest others follow.

•

Unconfirmed reports have indicated that Joyce Brown was in and out of psychiatric hospitals in the 5 years from 1989 to 1994, and it would seem that her primary problem was drugs rather than schizophrenia. As of this writing, she was living in an apartment on her own, drug-free. The problem of both Joyce and Larry Hogue appeared to be schizoid tendencies exacerbated by illegal drugs.

FURTHER READING

Alice Baum and Donald Burnes, *A Nation in Denial: The Truth about Homelessness,* Westview, Boulder, CO, 1993.

Paul Chodoff, "The Case for Involuntary Hospitalization of the Mentally Ill," *American Journal of Psychiatry,* vol. 133, no. 5, May 1976.

Saul Feldman, "Out of the Hospitals, onto the Streets: The Overselling of Benevolence," *Hastings Center Report,* vol. 13, no. 3, June 1983.

Charles Krauthammer, "How to Save the Homeless Mentally Ill," *New Republic,* February 8, 1988.

J. Livermore, C. Malmquist, and P. Meehl, "On the Justification for Civil Commitment," *University of Pennsylvania Law Review,* vol. 117, November 1968.

CHAPTER 16

Ethical Issues and Genetic Disease

Nancy Wexler

*T*his chapter takes up ethical issues in presymptomatic testing for genetic diseases focusing on the case of Nancy Wexler, who helped develop a test for Huntington's disease (HD), a fatal neurological genetic disorder. Tests for hereditary forms of breast cancer are also discussed, as well as the death of Jesse Gelsinger.

BACKGROUND: GENETICS AND EUGENICS

DNA, Genes, and Genetic Disorders

In 1953, in *Nature,* James Watson and Francis Crick published their description of the double-helix structure of deoxyribonucleic acid (DNA), the nucleic acid responsible for transmitting hereditary characteristics.[1] This description included the basic mechanism for copying genetic material from one cell to another and, in reproduction, from one generation to another. Their discovery moved the study of genetics from observational inference to molecular biology.

The basic unit of life is the cell. The basic unit of heredity is the *gene,* which consists of DNA, though not all DNA takes the form of genes. Genes are carried on chromosomes; a *chromosome*—which consists of DNA and other material—is a macromolecule composed of repeating nucleotides. Normally, the nucleus of each human cell contains 46 chromosomes. The germ, or sex, cells, however, have 23 chromosomes each; thus the union of sperm and egg provides the 46 (23 + 23) chromosomes for every new human being, and genes are inherited in pairs consisting of one gene from the father and one from the mother.

As a result of the work of Watson, Crick, and others, we know that each of the 46 chromosomes contains an enormously complicated strand of interwoven DNA: This is the famous double helix. Each strand is composed of combinations of four chemical (nucleotide) bases in approximately 3 billion pairs (in each pair, one bit is on each side of the helix); thus the total number of pairs is about 138 billion.

The pattern of the four nucleotide bases in the 46 double helices is a person's genetic code. Scientists believe that about 30,000 to 40,000 sequences of these pairs of bases are genes, with the number of genes varying from chromosome to chromosome.

The Human Genome Project began in October 1993 and finished early in 2003.

If we think of the 46 strands of human DNA (each with its 3 billion base pairs) as, say, North America, the Human Genome Project provides a map of the territory and its major highways; on this map, the 30,000 to 40,000 genes are the towns and cities. The largest gene, comparable in size to Los Angeles, is the gene for muscular dystrophy, composed of 2 million base pairs. The genes for globulin and insulin are like towns, with only about 1,000 base pairs each. At the beginning of the Project, scientists already knew the location of a few cities, but many of the towns remained to be found. Even today, we do not know the functions of over 50 percent of genes.

•

Genetic diseases are inherited disorders. It is possible that most of us actually have genes for inherited disorders but are *heterozygous* for these disorders: That is, we have a dissimilar pair of genes for an inherited disease or trait. If a gene is *dominant*, it will be expressed, or shown, in a heterozygote; if it is *recessive*, it will *not* be expressed in a heterozygote. However, even though heterozygotes may not show a trait themselves, they are *carriers* who can pass the gene for the disorder along to their offspring. If two parents who are heterozygous for a disorder both pass on the gene for the disorder to an offspring, that person will be *homozygous* for the disorder—will have an identical pair of genes. A disease or trait will always be expressed in a homozygote.

As many as 15 million Americans may have moderate to severe genetic disease.[2] According to a definitive list compiled by V. A. McKusick (and updated online daily), there are over 10,000 diseases with an established gene locus.[3] This is a large figure; in fact, every family may include someone who is a potential victim of genetic disease or is susceptible to a disorder that may be linked to genetic causes, such as alcoholism, cancer, or coronary artery disease. Genetic diseases are estimated to account for over one-third of acute-care hospitalization of children under 18.

Several single disease-causing genes have already been discovered, and physicians are attempting gene therapy to treat some of these diseases. The Jesse Gelsinger case, discussed at the end of this chapter, was one such attempt. Francis Collins, who became head of the Human Genome Project in 1993, predicted that:

> The Human Genome Project will change the face of medicine. It's very possible that in the future a physician will give an 18-year old patient a physical exam that includes a test of his or her DNA for hundreds of diseases with known genetic components. Family histories are useful, but genetic exams will give the doctor a much more precise tool to assess risks and give advice. The physician will be able to tell the patient whether the risk is high, low, or average for a given condition and to make life-style recommendations based upon known risks. There will be personalized schemes for a new kind of preventive medicine and I think it will prove very appealing.[4]

The Eugenics Movement

Before genetics became a science, a number of ill-founded popular ideas about heredity were influential in the nineteenth and early twentieth centuries. One notorious example is *phrenology*, a pseudoscience based on the idea that the size and shape of the head determined intelligence and character. (Vestiges of phrenology may still be found among novelists who write as if character can be inferred from a person's face. George Eliot lampooned this notion in *Middlemarch:* "So much subtler is a human mind than the outside tissues, which make a sort of blazonry or clock-face for it.") What passed as "science" then was based on more or less crackpot versions of Charles Darwin's theory of evolution by natural selection, particularly his concept of "survival of the fittest." What Darwin meant by *fittest* was simply "best adapted"—he was referring to the "fit" between an organism and its environment—but many people misunderstood this to apply to one's social position.

One prominent misinterpretation was *social Darwinism,* which saw Darwin's theory in terms of group competition in human societies. Social Darwinists were elitists: They held, for one thing, that social advantages implied biological superiority, and that therefore the upper classes would prevail in this competition. They were also racists: They claimed that the fittest races would prevail in the struggle for existence; and they predicted that blacks, whom they saw as biologically unfit to compete with whites, would not survive into the twentieth century. Social Darwinism can most charitably be described as unsophisticated. It was not based on any real understanding of evolution, and it failed to take account of the vast numbers of organisms involved in the attempt to survive, the enormous length of time over which evolution works, or the role of adaptive mutations.

Eugenics—another of these popular pseudosciences—flourished from about 1905 to 1935. This was a movement to improve humanity by improving hereditary characteristics, a goal it intended to accomplish through selective breeding. Its ideas came from various sources, including social Darwinism and Malthusian theory, though some of these were dubious to begin with and others were misapplied. The term *eugenics* was coined in the late 1880s by Francis Galton. Galton was Charles Darwin's cousin, and his particular misinterpretation of Darwin's theory took the form of claiming that famous people were the most "fit," a notion which famous people naturally liked.[5]

During the 1880s, chromosomes were first discovered in cell nuclei; around 1900, it was hypothesized that chromosomes carried genes, Gregor Mendel's laws of inheritance were rediscovered, and William Bateson coined the term *genetics* for this new field of study. At the same time, Karl Pearson, Charles Davenport, and others popularized some crude notions of genetics: This was the origin of the eugenics movement, which was to become hugely influential.

Eugenic organizations were formed worldwide, especially in Germany, Austria, Scandinavia, Italy, Japan, and South America; but as historian of science Daniel Kevles writes, "the center of this trend was the American eugenics movement. Its headquarters was at Cold Spring Harbor on Long Island, New York, and its leader was Charles Davenport."[6] This point bears emphasizing: Although many people identify modern eugenics with Nazi Germany, it was actually in the United States—with its heterogeneous population—that eugenics was most widely championed. Politicians, popular media, and even many scientists espoused eugenics, advocated "eugenic marriages" and sterilization of the unfit, and declared that the American "breeding stock" was declining through interbreeding with unfit races.

In the United States at the beginning of the twentieth century, a few prominent families—largely of English, Swiss, German, and Dutch ancestry—had enormous wealth and power; they controlled many newspapers, magazines, and even universities, and thus they exerted a great deal of control over the ideas of the time. These families, on the whole, were greatly concerned about breeding, and they were afraid that the purity of Americans with backgrounds like their own would be contaminated if their children interbred with the Irish, Italians, Turks, Jews, Asians, African Americans, or anybody else whose origin was different.

Wealthy and powerful families were concerned not only with preserving the purity of their own stock but also with controlling the growth of groups from other backgrounds. They were appalled by the many progeny of Irish, Italian, and Greek immigrants and saw Malthusian doom approaching. (Because predominantly Catholic ethnic groups tended to have more children, anti-Catholic sentiment grew.) The upper classes also agreed, almost unanimously, that the "unfit" had no right to bear children. A prominent New York urologist, William Robinson, proclaimed:

> It is the acme of stupidity to talk in such cases of individual liberty, of the rights of the individual. Such individuals have no rights. They have no right in the first instance to be born, but having been born, they have no right to propagate their kind.[7]

It is worth noting that even on their own terms and in the context of their own time, these ideas made little sense. The combination of social Darwinism and eugenics is almost immediately self-contradictory: If the white race and the upper class were destined to emerge triumphant, why worry about excessive breeding among "lower" races and classes? If the lower races and classes were so unfit that they were destined to die out, why try to prevent them from breeding?

Probably, eugenics seemed plausible, and became so influential, mainly because it was part of a general climate of bigotry. The newspaper magnate William Hearst and Theodore Roosevelt, for instance, thundered against "yellow niggers" who were invading the United States from Asia. When Henry Ford ran for president in the 1920s, he said he would rid the country of the "Jew bankers," whom he accused of having forced the United States into World War I; later, he would accuse them of causing the Depression.[8]

•

During its height, from about the turn of the century to the early 1930s, the eugenics movement had a significant effect on legislation in the United States.

One effect was mandatory sterilization. The forced sterilization of 225,000 people, mainly "mental defectives," in Nazi Germany is of course notorious; but it is less well known that although the Nazis were more systematic, secretive, and biased by racism, the United States also practiced large-scale involuntary sterilization.[9] In 1907, Indiana became the first state to require sterilization of the retarded and criminally insane; it was soon followed by 30 other states. In each of these states, a board of experts ultimately decided who would be sterilized.

The number of mandatory sterilizations reached a peak during the 1930s. Most people who are aware of these sterilization programs at all believe that they took place mostly in the deep south or Appalachia, but in fact the leading state was California, where sterilizations accounted for nearly one-third of the national total;

Virginia was second and Indiana third.[10] All together, by 1941 over 36,000 Americans had been involuntarily sterilized, often for a vague condition described as "feeblemindedness" or because they had been born into large families on welfare. Some of these sterilization laws were not reversed until the 1960s.

Besides mandatory sterilization, the most important legacy of the American eugenics movement was the Immigration Restriction Act of 1924. This act, hailed by eugenicists as their greatest triumph, stemmed from the assumption that Asians, Africans, the Greeks, the Irish, and eastern and southern Europeans such as the Poles and Italians were "inferior" peoples; whereas the English, Dutch, Scotch, Scandinavians, and Germans, and possibly the French (if they were not Catholic) represented "superior stock." The act was enthusiastically signed by President Calvin Coolidge, who as vice president had declared, "America must be kept American. Biological laws show . . . that Nordics deteriorate when mixed with other races."[11] Interestingly, the term *melting pot*—which today is considered laudatory—was first used, pejoratively, by those lobbying for the Immigration Restriction Act.

This immigration act established quotas according to country of origin; although these quotas were based on how many people from a given country were already in the United States, in effect they made it very difficult for people from "inferior" countries to be admitted. The Statue of Liberty is often seen as a historic symbol of freedom, but after 1924, thousands of the world's "huddled masses" had only a glimpse of it before being turned away and sent back home.

The influence of eugenics also extended to the courts, and in 1927 it was reflected in a famous decision by the United States Supreme Court, *Buck* v. *Bell*.

Carrie Buck was a supposedly retarded young woman whose mother, Emma Buck, was also supposedly retarded; according to a crude IQ test, Carrie Buck's mental age was 9 years and Emma Buck's was 8 years. Carrie Buck had been committed to a state mental institution in Virginia at age 17 and had been pregnant at the time she was committed; she gave birth to a daughter, Vivian, inside the institution. Then as now, institutionalized women often became pregnant by guards or visiting relatives, and the institution's director (who was the "Bell" in the case) wondered if Carrie Buck could be sterilized so that she would not have another child.

Virginia officials asked Harry Laughlin, an influential geneticist who worked at Cold Spring Harbor, to determine whether Carrie Buck's retardation was hereditary. Laughlin did not see Carrie Buck; he relied simply on the reported mental ages of Carrie and her mother, and on the report of a social worker who said that Carrie had a strange "look" about her. On this basis, Laughlin declared that Carrie Buck "lived a life of immorality and prostitution," and that she and her mother belonged to the "shiftless, ignorant, worthless class of anti-social whites of the South."[12]

The Supreme Court, by a vote of 8 to 1, upheld the legality of sterilizing Carrie Buck and handed down an order for her sterilization. Justice Oliver Wendell Holmes wrote the opinion in *Buck* v. *Bell*, saying, "Three generations of imbeciles are enough,"[13] and concluding, "The principle that sustains compulsory vaccination is broad enough to cover cutting the Fallopian tubes."[14] Holmes noted that science should guide public policy and emphasized that what the public good would gain in "sound genetics" would outweigh individual rights of the retarded to procreate. Such was the ethos of America in the 1920s.

•

"Sound genetics," however, is more complicated than Holmes or his contemporaries realized. At the time, some crucial information about genetics was lacking or poorly understood, and this led to several incorrect assumptions.

One area of ignorance was recessive inheritance. If a trait is recessive, it will be expressed only in a homozygote—a person who has received an identical pair of genes for the disorder. The existence of recessive genes explains why normal people can produce impaired children: Two unaffected carriers can each pass a gene for a recessive trait to a child, who will then be homozygous for the trait. Recessive inheritance also explains why genetically impaired people can produce normal children: If a defect is recessive, and an affected person mates with someone who is not a carrier, their child will not have the defect. Such instances must have been observed often (and also apparent instances—Carrie Buck's daughter Vivian was considered bright by her teachers and was doing well in school before she died at age 8 of an intestinal disorder), but their significance was not appreciated.

A second area of ignorance was the complexity of inheritance. In 1927, eugenicists and others assumed, mistakenly, that each trait was inherited through a single gene (a person with 378 traits, in their view, must have 378 separate genes). Thus they thought that there was a specific, inheritable gene for retardation; and Charles Davenport held, around 1930, that prostitution was caused by a gene for "innate eroticism."[15]

A third area of ignorance had to do with mutations and chromosomal breakage. Because the eugenicists and their contemporaries did not know about these aspects of genetics, they believed—again mistakenly—that retardation could be eliminated from the gene pool if all retarded people could be prevented from reproducing.

A fourth area of ignorance had to do with determining exactly which traits are inherited. Almost nothing was known about what is and is not inherited, and this too led to mistaken ideas; Davenport, for example, believed that poverty and criminality were hereditary. Actually, it is often difficult to distinguish inherited from acquired traits even today: Nature is not easily separable from nurture. Psychologists continue to debate whether intelligence is determined primarily by hereditary or environmental factors; and as recently as the 1980s, the Harvard psychologist Richard Herrnstein argued that criminality ran in certain families and suggested a genetic link.[16] However, retardation is now known to be caused by many factors and combinations of factors, including nonhereditary causes such as alcohol abuse during pregnancy.

A fifth area of ignorance was population genetics. The eugenicists hoped to perfect humanity through selective breeding, but population genetics have since shown that a regression to the mean will occur. *Regression to the mean* is the inherent tendency in stable populations to return to an average value over time; in population genetics, this tells us that the underlying causes creating a mean value in a population will eventually normalize any deviant values. (This applies, among other things, to baseball statistics, the stock market, lucky streaks, height in a family of many children, and efforts to improve humanity through human cloning.)

Finally, the eugenicists and their contemporaries did not realize how many generations are needed to eliminate a defect. Because they did not understand the difference between carrying an unexpressed gene and actually having a trait, they could not calculate that reducing the frequency of a defect from 1 in 100 to 1 in 1,000 might take 22 generations and that reducing it to 1 in 1 million might take hundreds of generations.

After about 1935, the eugenics movement declined in the United States. Many geneticists had supported the movement in its early years, but after the Depression, most abandoned it. This was partly because of its zealous emphasis on human perfectibility, partly because of its racism, and partly because its assumptions were being contradicted by the emerging facts of genetics.

By 1935, the geneticist Hermann J. Muller said that eugenics was "hopelessly perverted," a cult for "advocates for race and class prejudice, defenders of vested interests of church and State, Fascists, Hitlerites, and reactionaries generally."[17] Another leading geneticist, J. B. S. Haldane, said at the time of the sterilization programs that "many of the deeds done in America in the name of eugenics are about as much justified by science as were the proceedings of the Inquisition by the Gospels."[18] Advances in population genetics prompted Haldane to remark, "An ounce of algebra is worth a ton of verbal argument."[19]

The eugenicists' ideas about race were also being discredited—for example, they linked false assumptions that race represented a biological subspecies and that it determined behavior. To the eugenicists, designations such as *Irish, Italian, Polish, African American, Jewish,* and *Arab* were biological types; but to more advanced thinkers, such terms were political, religious, or ethnic generalizations.

In 1935—attacking the Nazis' eugenics program, which was based on, and designed to promote, "Aryan" racial superiority—Julian Huxley and A. C. Haddon maintained that race is not a uniform, biological type but a mixture of many peoples. They argued that "the word race should be banished, and the descriptive and noncommittal term ethnic groups should be substituted."[20] They denied the notion that any groups (such as blacks, Poles, or the Irish) were naturally promiscuous; they also denied that members of any such group naturally liked certain kinds of food or drink. In particular, they attacked the idea of promiscuity as a genetic trait; in general, they attacked the crude belief that genes influenced any highly specific human behaviors—a belief for which there was no evidence—and the hasty generalization that all people from a certain area (such as Ireland or Africa) had the same genes.

Eugenics, then, was being seen as bad science. One measure of how bad it was could be found in eugenicists' own debates over how to analyze World War I. Some of them said the war was dysgenic, because the best male stock went off and died; others said it was eugenic, because the remaining men had their choice of the best women; but those who considered it dysgenic said that the women would marry inferior men, to avoid being spinsters, and would therefore produce less perfect offspring. The decline and fall of eugenics can be discerned in this kind of nonsense. Much of the eugenicists' theorizing reflected male fantasies and biases (not many eugenicists were women); and all of it reflected complacency, since advocates of eugenics uniformly saw themselves as part of the "fittest" breeding stock.

In 1997, Sweden was forced to face a painful legacy when it was revealed that up to 60,000 Swedes were sterilized between 1935 and 1976—most of them under pressure to do so from local physicians and authorities—because of "inferior" phenotypes for bad eyesight, mental retardation, or "undesirable" racial characteristics.[21] What especially alarmed people was that Sweden's laws allowing sterilization weren't overturned until 1976.

However, although the idea of improving humanity by improving heredity—"positive eugenics"—was generally abandoned, a very different form—"negative eugenics"—trying to eliminate genetic diseases and disorders—appeared in the 1960s with prenatal testing and genetic screening. However, "eugenics" is now such a loaded term that it has little vaue in such contexts.

Genetic Screening

In the early 1960s, prenatal predictive tests made it possible to identify phenylketonuria (PKU) in fetuses. PKU is a recessive genetic disease in which there is an excess of the amino acid phenylalanine. If PKU is not diagnosed until after birth, when its symptoms appear, this excess will always cause retardation. However, retardation can be prevented and development will be normal if PKU is identified before birth, so that the infant can be put on a special diet as soon as it is born. The prenatal test for PKU is cheap and easy.

It was the development of the PKU test that led many well-intentioned people to advocate negative eugenics. If PKU, a genetic disorder, could be prevented by prenatal screening, what better justification could there be for making such screening mandatory? Most states accepted this reasoning and eventually required screening for PKU.

Subsequent studies showed that the PKU test was often unreliable and that if PKU was misdiagnosed in normal babies, they could be harmed by the special diet that was prescribed for it. Nevertheless, PKU screening did save thousands of correctly diagnosed children from retardation, because it targeted a specific deficit for which there was a known remedy.

If all genetic screening were this specific, and if all of the conditions it identified were so effectively treatable, such screening would be routine today. However, not all screening is so clear-cut.

Genetic screening actually forms a sort of spectrum. PKU testing—which can identify a specific, treatable condition—is near the successful end of this spectrum. An example of the opposite end of the spectrum is testing for an extra Y chromosome. In 1965, a team headed by Patricia Jacobs found that some male inmates of penal and mental institutions had an extra Y chromosome and suggested that this caused a condition characterized by antisocial behavior: It was called the *XYY syndrome.* Some newborns were then tested for *XYY* and later followed to see if their behavior was antisocial. Most scientists were opposed to *XYY* testing. They argued that *XYY* might not even be a syndrome; that even if it was, no treatment existed; and that testing positive could become a self-fulfilling prophecy: Parents and others might expect an *XYY* child to be antisocial, and this expectation could in itself cause the child to develop antisocial behavior.

Other forms of genetic screening have fallen at various points along the spectrum. These include screening for Tay Sachs disease, sickle-cell disease, Down syndrome, certain susceptibilities, and cystic fibrosis.

Screening for *Tay Sachs* disease—a rare, lethal condition found in Jews of eastern European descent—became possible in the 1960s and eventually became a major success. As with PKU, the gene for Tay Sachs disease could be identified in a fetus by a simple, cheap test; moreover, this test for Tay Sachs was highly reliable. Unlike PKU, however, Tay Sachs disease is not treatable. Thus if the fetal test was positive, the fetus would be electively aborted; if parents would not consider abortion, the Tay Sachs test was not given. Adults can also be screened for Tay Sachs; in this case, intervention would take the form of counseling two carriers not to have children together.

Initially, screening for Tay Sachs was only partially successful, because some parents were opposed to abortion and some people were afraid that they would be stigmatized if they were identified as carriers. But in the early 1970s, Jews themselves started encouraging such screening, in a program which had been given 14 months of careful preparation; this effort was centered in Brooklyn and included the matchmakers who arrange marriages in Orthodox Jewish communities. Since then, over 1 million young adults have been screened and over 2,400 pregnancies involving a risk of Tay Sachs disease have been identified and, presumably, ended.[22]

By contrast, screening for sickle-cell disease has been unsuccessful until recently. *Sickle-cell disease*, which affects mostly black people, takes its name from sickle-shaped cells (erythrocytes) in the blood; it causes acute abdominal pain, joint pain, and ulceration of the lower extremities. Its clinical course is variable (unlike that of PKU or Tay Sachs disease), and—importantly—some people with sickle-cell disease lead nearly normal lives.

Screening for sickle-cell disease is possible in both fetuses and adults, but when screening programs began, authorities failed to consider the possible consequences of identification. As with Tay Sachs, there is no cure for sickle-cell disease; thus if a fetus tested positive, the only intervention was elective abortion. However, since the condition might not actually be serious in any individual, abortion was controversial. In 1999, embryos were successfully tested for sickle-cell during IVF, resulting in only healthy babies.

With regard to screening adults, people confused carriers of the sickle-cell gene (heterozygotes) with those who actually had the disease (homozygotes). Because of this, some carriers were treated as if they had the disease itself: Some were denied medical insurance or even fired from their jobs. Some jurisdictions made screening for sickle-cell disease mandatory, making things worse.

Protests from the African American community finally defeated the early sickle-cell screening programs, and state laws mandating such programs faded into limbo. Sickle-cell testing of fetuses is now recognized as a paradigm of how not to set up a screening program.

In the early 1970s, it became possible to screen for *Down syndrome,* which is a chromosomal aberration. Screening for Down syndrome is done by amniocentesis and has been very successful. Such screening was initially opposed by critics who said its use would lead parents only to create perfect babies through repetitive tests and abortions. Today, pregnant women over age 35 or 40 are routinely tested; in fact, an obstetrician's failure to suggest such a test for a patient over about 35 may be grounds for a malpractice suit.

Some genes appear to be linked to certain diseases, such as cancer or coronary artery disease; and *susceptibility screening* for cholesterol, lipids, and HLA-antigens was developed in the 1970s. This can make early intervention possible; for instance, early identification and treatment of hypercholesterolemia may prevent a later heart attack. However, there is some potential for abuse in susceptibility screening: Employers might try to lower medical costs by screening job applicants and discriminating against people who test positive.

Screening for *cystic fibrosis* (CF) began in the 1990s. CF produces thick, excessive mucus in the bronchi; a person with CF must be continually thumped on the back to loosen these secretions and held upside down to drain them. Eventually, CF is fatal: It destroys the lungs, causing suffocation, usually by early adulthood, though the symptoms may not appear until the teenage years. One in 22 white people carries the gene for CF; since this gene is recessive, a child of two heterozygotes has a 25 percent risk of CF. Screening for CF can be done with fetuses (by amniocentesis) or children, but it is controversial. It is accurate and useful only if there is a family history of CF, but 80 percent of children with CF are born to families with no history of the disease. Also:

> Molecular biology has revealed that CF is not caused by a single type of mutation. Although one mutation is associated with 70 percent of all cases, and two others with 25 to 20 percent, more than 360 mutations have been linked to CF so far.[23]

The pediatrician and bioethicist Norman Fost has described CF screening in the general population as "metastasizing, despite the lack of evidence that it works."[24] A better strategy is pre-implantation diagnosis of CF embryos.

More recently, *ultrasound* and *maternal alpha fetoprotein testing* have become the most important methods of genetic screening in the world.[25] These techniques are used to screen for physical deformities and neural-tube defects; the intervention is abortion, which is usually noncontroversial, since these are gross defects. Ultrasound and maternal alpha fetoprotein screening are at the successful end of the spectrum, though it should be noted that they are generally possible only when they are covered by health insurance. In India and China, ultrasound is also used by the rich to ensure that first-born babies are male.

NANCY WEXLER AND THE TEST FOR HD

Nancy Wexler, who is a clinical psychologist, was born in 1945 in Washington, D.C., and graduated from Radcliffe College in 1967. In 1967–1968 she spent a postgraduate year in Jamaica; at this time, she and her parents and sister learned that a mysterious disease in her mother's family was Huntington's disease (HD), a devastating and fatal neurological disorder for which there is no cure and no treatment.

Nancy Wexler's mother, Leonore Sabin Wexler, had suddenly begun to experience strange symptoms at age 58. Over the next decade, Nancy Wexler, her sister Alice, and their father—Milton Wexler, a psychoanalyst—watched as Leonore Wexler deteriorated: She became emaciated and catatonic and finally died in 1978. What happened to Leonore Wexler had also happened to the folksinger Woody

Guthrie (1912–1967), who was the father of Arlo Guthrie and was portrayed briefly in the film *Alice's Restaurant.*

The gene for HD is dominant, and thus Nancy and Alice Wexler, and Arlo Guthrie, each had a 50 percent risk of HD. Since HD does not typically appear until its victim is in the thirties, forties, or fifties, this means there is a 50 percent chance that someone such as Nancy Wexler is carrying a genetic time bomb.

Huntington's Disease

HD is a severe, progressive neurological disease in which neurons in the caudate nuclei region of the brain are rapidly shed. The average age of onset is 36. Thereafter, HD progresses through four stages of roughly 5 years each.

In the first stage of HD, there are initially small losses of muscular coordination; then there are changes in personality, making the victim angry, hostile, and depressed. In the second stage, speech becomes slurred, facial expressions become grotesquely distorted, there is constant muscular jerkiness, the fists clench and unclench, the limbs flail involuntarily, and the victim frequently staggers and falls. In Nancy Wexler's words: "Gradually, the entire body is encompassed by adventitious movements. The trunk is writhing and the face is twisting."[26] During this second stage, the victim is likely to lose his or her job. In the third stage, the victim is incontinent, experiences severe mental deterioration, and becomes dependent on others, at home or in an institution. In the fourth and final stage, the victim stares blankly ahead and remains motionless.

Nancy Wexler has described this progression as follows:

> The gene is so sly, so sinister. It's like there's an orchestra playing, and there are these [wrong] notes. At first they're very soft, but they keep getting louder and louder. Finally, they're all there is.[27]

Some genetic diseases, such as Down syndrome, are apparent at birth; but HD, as noted above, typically appears during the thirties to fifties. Because its onset is so late, people with HD usually have children before learning that they are affected. Although the age of onset varies, HD will be completely "penetrant" if one lives long enough.

HD arrived in America in 1625, around the time of the *Mayflower;* it was brought by three affected men from the small English village of Bures. Their descendants include the physician George Huntington of Long Island, who first described the disease in 1872.[28] Originally, HD was called *Huntington's chorea* (from the Greek *choreia,* "dance") because of the victims' jerking and twisting.

In the past, victims of HD have been treated badly. During the era of witch-hunting, for example, because their distorted movements were said to resemble Jesus's writhing on the cross, they were believed to be worshipers of Satan (a strange inference) who were being tortured by God. Seven female descendants of the original three Englishmen were thought to be witches, and one was executed at Groton, Connecticut, in 1692. Some of the Salem witches also probably had HD.

At present, about 30,000 Americans have HD, and more than 150,000 Americans with an afflicted parent are at risk of HD. Almost all those affected are white, except for one large African American family around Baltimore.

People at risk of HD live with a genetic sword of Damocles over their heads, constantly wondering if each stutter, spill, or stumble is a sign of the disease. Nancy Wexler once said that for her, not a day went by without some thought of HD: "You become aware of all kinds of things you never noticed before—little muscle jerks in bed, or clumsiness. I remember dropping a carton of eggs and thinking, 'Oh, no! Is this the beginning?'"[29]

Finding a Genetic Marker for HD

Nancy Wexler entered a doctoral program in clinical psychology at the University of Michigan in 1968; she wrote her dissertation on HD and its effects and received her doctorate in 1974. In 1968, her father started the Hereditary Disease Foundation in Los Angeles, and she became its president in 1983. In 1976, she was executive director of the Congressional Commission for the Control of HD and Its Consequences. Throughout the late 1970s, Nancy Wexler

> . . . found out everything she could. She studied genetics. She organized patients' groups. She helped start a brain collection program so that the brains of HD victims would be available for research. She lobbied Capitol Hill for research funds. She convinced a wide variety of scientists such as molecular biologist David Housman of the Massachusetts Institute of Technology to study HD. Soon she was a driving force in the HD community.[30]

There are two kinds of presymptomatic genetic testing. First, there are *linkage tests*—tests for "markers" rather than for actual genes. A marker is linked to a gene and is usually inherited with that gene because marker and gene are close together in the DNA sequence.[31] Linkage tests require family histories and blood samples from family members.

Second, there are tests for the genes themselves—that is, for the actual sequence of DNA which constitutes a disease-causing gene (if there is such a single gene). Tests of this second kind are the ultimate genetic tests, because they detect the actual presence of a disease-causing gene. A test for a gene requires only a blood sample from the individual at risk.

The first goal of Wexler's Hereditary Disease Foundation was to find a cure. To do so it needed a marker for HD to use in a linkage test. The foundation believed that this could be done by finding a large number of people in a single family tree where HD had been inherited, taking blood from each member, and carrying out a genetic analysis; then, geneticists would examine tiny portions of the genetic map to see if some bit of DNA was to be found only in victims of HD. As early as 1977, Nancy Wexler had already lobbied Congress and obtained some funding. However, during the late 1970s:

> . . . there was considerable skepticism within the biomedical community as to whether this approach—called *genetic linkage analysis*—could possibly yield the desired information. "People thought it would take a hugely long time—maybe 50 to 75 years—to find a gene marker [for HD]," Wexler recalled.[32]

In 1972, a Venezuelan physician had discovered a large number of carriers descended from a common ancestor with HD named Maria Concepcion. All of them lived in and around the village of San Luis on Lake Maracaibo in Venezuela. In 1981, Nancy Wexler led an expedition there (the first of a number of annual trips). Her sister Alice, who had earned a Ph.D. in history, researched ancient records to determine where the gene had originally come from. Possibly, the source was a European sailor who jumped ship there in the early 1800s.

Nancy Wexler played a key role at this point. The subjects were reluctant to allow skin biopsies or give blood samples until, through an interpreter, she explained that she too was at risk of *el mal* ("bad thing" or "disease") and had herself undergone these procedures.

The next step was getting the blood samples and skin biopsies back to the United States. This was not easy, since the samples had to reach the American researchers within 48 hours, and San Luis is far away from any city. Recordkeeping was also difficult: Nancy Wexler's family tree of the 3,000 descendants was 100 feet long.

Next, of course, came the crucial part: actually finding a marker for HD, which would entail finding the general location of the gene. In 1979, the Hereditary Disease Foundation had held a workshop on using recombinant DNA, which had recently been developed, to find a genetic marker linked to HD. David Housman and James Gusella, a graduate student of Housman, were able to use these new techniques to look for a marker in the genetic karyotypes (these are somewhat analogous to blueprints) of the Venezuelan families.

Some predicted that finding a marker would take 5 to 10 years. Someone needed to find the general location of the genetic base pairs for HD—a sequence of perhaps only a few thousand—within the millions of base pairs of one chromosome. In August 1983 David Housman of MIT found a marker (G8) for HD on the far tip of the short arm of chromosome 4.

The next step was to identify the HD gene itself. The discovery of the G8 marker meant that the search for the gene could be restricted to the tip of chromosome 4, that is, to less than 0.03 percent of the human DNA. Even so, Gusella said in 1983, "We're still three to five years away from finding the gene—unless there's another lucky break."[33] In 1984, Nancy Wexler helped start the HD Collaborative Research Group to find the HD gene.

By the fall of 1987, though the gene itself had not been discovered, James Gusella was able to develop a linkage test for HD, using the G8 marker.

The HD linkage test (as is always true of such tests) could not be performed simply by drawing blood from an individual. It required blood samples from other family members because it depended on knowledge of grandparents' and parents' genes. Not only was blood from other family members needed to prove the existence of a case of HD, a family history was also needed. As a result of this and problems of recombination, the HD linkage test was often not 100 percent accurate. It might be 97 percent or only 75 percent predictive, depending on what was known.

Still, the linkage test represented a significant advance. Gusella and the geneticist Michael Connealy received primary credit for discovering the marker and developing the linkage test; Nancy Wexler was also listed as a principal codiscoverer.[34]

Marjorie Guthrie, Woody Guthrie's widow, who created an organization for HD descendants, also played an indirect role.

The Aftermath

As will be discussed under "Ethical Issues," the personal decision whether or not to take the HD linkage test was by no means easy: There were problems with both knowing and not knowing the answer.

In 1986, while the linkage test was being developed but before it was available, Nancy Wexler (who had become an associate professor of clinical neuropsychology at the College of Physicians and Surgeons of Columbia University in 1985) said that she herself would take it: "My feeling was that the advantages of knowing, even if the answer was yes, outweighed the disadvantages."[35] However, she later reconsidered that decision.

In May 1987, when the linkage test was first becoming available, Diane Sawyer (DS) interviewed Nancy Wexler (NW) and Alice Wexler (AW) for *60 Minutes.*

DS: Did you think you'd get the test if they ever had one?
NW: I was positive I would. Unquestionably. It never occurred to me that I wouldn't.
DS: And all of a sudden when you have the option, you're not so sure.
NW: I wasn't so sure. Exactly. I even said to people, "When the test is actually here, a lot of people are going to change their minds." It never occurred to me I would be one of them. That wasn't in the book.
AW: I would like to know I don't have it, but I absolutely don't want to know if I do have it.
NW: This is absolutely the hardest choice I've ever made in my life.[36]

Nancy Wexler now thought that people who took the test to end uncertainty would be fooling themselves: If the result was positive, she said, the question wouldn't be, "What if?" but "When?" For herself, she said there could be many bad outcomes: "If I found out that I was free of the disease, but Alice wasn't, I'd die." There would also be the worst possibility of all: Both she and her sister could test positive.

Alice Wexler said that she had tried to imagine the "unimaginable"—testing positive—but admitted that she had not really succeeded. She could not imagine sitting at her own desk and knowing that she had this lethal gene at work in her:

> If you have the certainty that you have the gene, and if you have the certainty that you're going to die this absolutely miserable death over many years, I'm not sure it's possible to keep on living, to use the knowledge constructively. I'm sure I wouldn't. I think I would be devastated by it.

Diane Sawyer then asked, "So some hope is better than possible bad news?" Alice replied, "Hope is better than despair."

Milton Wexler did not want either of his daughters to take the test; he said that a positive test would represent a "potential for madness" and might destroy the three of them.

At the end of the interview, Diane Sawyer asked Nancy Wexler, "Will you take the test?" and "Is there a right answer?" Nancy Wexler answered, "I think for each person there's a right choice."

•

In 1987, three medical centers in the United States offered the linkage test for HD. Surveys had predicted that between 60 percent and 80 percent of those at risk of HD would take the test; but of 1,500 people at risk in New England, only 32 signed up for preliminary genetic counseling and only 18 actually took the test.

In 1989, Nancy Wexler said that she had not taken the test. She said that she now felt happy, that knowing she was negative wouldn't make her very much happier, and that knowing she was positive would make her very unhappy.[37] (Since then, she has not discussed whether or not she has taken a test.)

At that time, Arlo Guthrie (who was then about 40) had also decided not to take the test. He was living with his wife and their four children in western Massachusetts and felt he had "escaped the trauma" that killed his father. Did he regret having children without knowing his status? No, he said: "Life is more important than learning about diseases. . . . I could've said I don't want to 'inflict pain and suffering,' . . . [but] life is wonderful! There's a lot to live for."[38]

Nancy Wexler agreed. To people who wanted to be tested so that they could decide, say, whether to go to law school, she said: "Go to law school! Develop your mind! What are you going to do if you're positive? Spend the rest of your life waiting to be a patient?"

Finding the Gene for HD

In 1983, when James Gusella created the linkage test for HD, he predicted that finding the gene itself would take 3 to 5 years, even though the effort could be concentrated on a small area on the upper tip of chromosome 4. As it happened, he had actually underestimated. Over the next 10 years, many false trails were followed and there were many tantalizing reports that researchers were on the edge of this discovery. Meanwhile, other researchers discovered the genes for other single-gene diseases: muscular dystrophy, cystic fibrosis, neurofibromatosis, colon cancer, ataxia, and sickle-cell anemia.

In March of 1993, a very large international team of six genetic laboratories announced that the exact molecular location of the HD gene had finally been found.[39] This discovery made possible a genetic test for HD, which began to be offered in 1994. The discovery also explained why the search had been so difficult and had taken a decade: The tip of chromosome 4 is very densely packed with genes and rife with "recombination," a situation in which genetic material may be passed on in unconventional ways.

Nancy Wexler heard the news of the discovery of the HD gene as she was just about to walk out the door on her way to another expedition to South America. "I felt like I walked into a brick wall," she said. "I was stunned. I was ecstatic. I was wandering around like a zombie after that."[40]

Nancy Wexler's View Today

During the 1990s, Nancy Wexler emerged as a champion for the choice "not to know now." She emphasized that, with diseases such as HD, "it's not whether you know, but when," since those with the gene will eventually experience symptoms. Comparing getting a genetic test to taking a test for cancer, she emphasized that a "DNA biopsy" may produce knowledge that is "toxic" to people unready for bad news, so counseling before testing to ensure informed consent is crucial.

Nancy and Alice also railed against a "macho attitude" among physicians and the media that portrays "those who took the test as somehow stronger, braver, more optimistic, more 'normal'" than people who choose not to know.[41] Both sisters emphasized that choosing to take the HD test would affect any at-risk person's life forever: "Once you have the information, you cannot give it back."[42] In a talk she gave around the world, Nancy closed by quoting Oedipus Rex: "It is but sorrow to be wise when wisdom profits not."

HEREDITARY BREAST CANCER

Breast cancer kills 50,000 American women each year, and it is estimated that 1 in 10 women alive today will develop breast cancer by age 80. During the last 20 years the number of women with age-specific breast cancer has risen 25 percent, and this figure is expected to rise due to the large number of women born just after World War II who are now in their forties.

In 1990, Mary Claire-King proved that one form of breast cancer was inherited on chromosome 17 and linked to a single gene, although she could not isolate the gene. After 4 years of intense competition from genetics labs around the world (similar to the race to discover the HD gene), the first gene for breast cancer, BRCA1, was discovered in 1994 by a team led by Mark Skolnick at the University of Utah. The gene was exceptionally long, consisting of more than 100,000 base pairs of DNA (about 10 times larger than the average gene). About a year later, a second gene, BRCA2, was discovered.

At first it was thought that these genes would only have limited use in presymptomatic tests because they seemed to only reliably cause breast cancer in women with familial histories of this disease, about 5 to 10 percent of breast cancer cases. Women with the BRCA1 gene and family history had an 80 to 85 percent chance of developing breast cancer. Because the vast majority of the breast cancer seemed not directly related to family history ("sporadic"), the discovery of this gene seemed to have only limited medical interest.

However, it was soon discovered that both genes play a role in causing hereditary ovarian cancer (a very deadly cancer) that comes before age 50, and probably play a role in the ordinary "sporadic" cancers in women with breast cancer with no family history of the disease. BRCA2 was also thought to play a role in causing pancreatic, prostate, and colon cancer, as well as other kinds of cancerous tumors. In a 1996 study widely reported in the media, one study discovered that BRCA1 in American Jewish women of Ashkenazic origin (90 percent of American Jews), caused more than 25 percent of breast cancers that occurred before the age of 40.

According to the popular "two hit theory," the presence of one of these genes is a necessary but not sufficient cause of developing cancer; the second "hit" comes from 15 to 20 years of environmental carcinogens such as cigarette smoking or exposure to chemical carcinogens.

Calling these genes "breast cancer genes" is misleading. They do not seem to be this so much as *cancer restraining genes:* When something goes wrong in them, cancer may develop. Such "tumor suppressing" or *inhibitor* genes regulate cell growth, but if one is defective (mutated) or if a defect is inherited, the neoplastic cell growth occurs that is the hallmark of cancerous tumors. For example, in the study of Ashkenazic Jews above, a deletion (i.e., mutation) of genetic material called the 185 de1AG deletion is linked to breast cancer.

Presymptomatic tests for breast cancer raise similar, but different, issues than testing for HD. No treatment exists for HD, whereas a controversial "treatment" exists for those with BRCA1 or BRCA2: prophylactic, radical mastectomy and oophrectomy (removal of ovaries). Many women who are diagnosed with breast cancer desire to cut everything out, and thus, they hope, maximize their chances of a long life. This desire prompted women in the 1960s to favor radical mastectomies over modified ones or lumpectomies, until it was proven that, for many women, lumpectomies offered just as long life as radical mastectomies. Will a positive test for one of these breast cancer genes prompt thousands of women to immediately have their breasts and ovaries removed?

Even doing so does not guarantee that all risk of breast cancer can be removed: It is almost impossible to guarantee that all breast tissue has been removed, and any tissue left behind retains the possibility (governed by the BRCA genes) to cause breast cancer. A statistical study in 1998 projected that prophylactic mastectomy gives 3 to 5 additional years of life in women with BRCA1 and BRCA2 mutations.[43]

Joseph D. Schulman, director of the Genetics and I.V.F. Institute in Fairfax, Virginia, and his wife, Dixie, of Ashkenazic Jewish origin, decided to offer the test in 1996 to any Jewish woman who wanted it for $295.[44] His decision to do so was condemned by many, but not all, in medical genetics. When asked whether it wasn't irrational to encourage mastectomies in women testing positive, Dr. Schulman replied, "There isn't a single rational person who believes that." Eighteen Jewish women took the test and two had the mutated BRCA1 gene: Dixie Schulman and her mother.

ETHICAL ISSUES

The Case for Knowledge

To begin with, some people at risk wanted to know because they felt that, for them, the relief of testing negative would outweigh the possibility of testing positive; also, some people felt that nothing is worse than uncertainty. In 1992, a Canadian study followed up 135 patients who had undergone linkage testing for HD.[45] It found that 1 year later, those who had tested negative felt much better off and, surprisingly, even those who had tested positive felt considerably better as a result of knowing for sure what would happen. The leader of this study reported that the patients who were positive for HD felt that knowledge "gave them control over their lives" and made them "live more in the present than in the future."[46]

In an editorial accompanying this study, Catherine Hayes, the president of HD Society of America, described how she heard of the test:

> For the first 33 years of my life, I lived at risk for HD. . . . One day in 1983, I heard on the radio that a genetic marker, a segment of DNA believed to be close to the gene for HD, had been discovered. It was clear to me that within a few years a presymptomatic test would be available. I had to stop the car because I was crying. I knew that I would take the test. Knowing, whatever the outcome, would be better than waiting and wondering day after day.[47]

In Hayes's case, the result was negative: "When I learned the results I cried and laughed," she wrote. "It took months for the news to sink in. I am still adjusting."

Another major argument for knowledge has to do with childbearing. If people at risk of a genetic disorder like HD do not know whether they are positive or negative, their decisions about childbearing may be misguided. People who would test negative and thus might safely have a child may feel that they are forced to remain childless; at the same time, people who would test positive may have children. Being born with HD is a fate that we would not wish on our worst enemy, let alone our own child.

Other arguments for knowledge have to do with the existing family of a person at risk. Consider the following example. A man who was at risk for HD but had decided not to take the test discussed his reasons before a large medical class. His reasons were greeted with respect; but as the class ended and the students started to file out, a woman cried out from the back of the room, "What about me and the kids?" It was the man's wife.[48]

This man's wife wanted to be able to plan for the future. If her husband was positive, she would sooner or later have to take care of him. She might also have been thinking, realistically enough, of money: If her husband was positive, he would need medical care and eventually custodial care, and they would have to start saving up for that or, if possible, arrange for life or health insurance. When HD strikes, moreover, the family will suffer emotionally; they might want to try to prepare themselves for this. Perhaps most important, they might try to make the most of whatever time remained before onset.

So, some of those at risk might want to be tested for the sake of their families; Nancy Wexler's decision not to take the HD linkage test, for instance, might have been more complicated if she had a husband or children.

There may be medical reasons for taking the test. For example, in one family involved in BRCA1 linkage study, one of two sisters was worried abut developing breast cancer and had planned to have her breasts removed as a preventive measure; she turned out to be negative and quickly canceled this plan. The other sister did not think she was at risk and had refused mammograms; she was shocked to find out that she had the BRCA1 marker. A thorough examination of her breasts found nothing, but a reexamination found a minuscule node, and one day later a biopsy determined that cancer had already begun; a radical mastectomy was performed. Without the linkage test, this woman might not have discovered her cancer until many years later.

Obviously, presymptomatic testing for breast cancer can allow some intervention at a very early state when necessary and allay the fears of women who are "certain" they have BRCA1 mutation but actually do not. In the families in this study, all the women greatly appreciated the fact that what had seemed to be a mysterious, random turn of fate had become testable and predictable. Although the women who tested positive did not like the news, and although some who tested negative felt guilty, most thought it was better to have a way to know.

The Case for *Not* Knowing

As we have seen, many people at risk of genetic disorders do not want to be tested themselves. Some general arguments against testing have also been advanced. What is the case for *not* knowing? We should note that there is some opposition, from very diverse sources, to the entire concept of genetic testing. Some people feel, for instance, that geneticists should not give such information to couples because of opposition to abortion.

The epidemiologist Abby Lippman is concerned that there will be social pressure on women to undergo genetic testing during pregnancy: "In today's Western world, biomedical and political systems largely define health and disease, as well as normality and abnormality."[49] According to the sociologist Dorothy Nelkin, information developed by the Human Genome Project could lead people to believe that differences in children's learning in schools are genetic rather than social or cultural.[50]

Harm to the Person at Risk   In general, many people at risk decide against knowing because they feel that the devastation of testing positive outweighs the possibility of testing negative; others feel that uncertainty (or "hope," as Alice Wexler put it) is preferable to knowing the worst. This, of course, is an individual, subjective evaluation.

With regard to HD testing, there have been concerns about possible harm to those at risk. One such consideration, for example, was raised by Nancy Wexler, who thought that people who tested positive might adopt a "sick identity."[51] That is, the knowledge that they had the gene would dominate their life and thoughts, rendering them incapable of pursuing their former goals. The knowledge can be "toxic," Nancy says.

The greatest harm to those at risk may come from discrimination by others. In one case, an at-risk patient for HD was a candidate for an organ transplant and one physician wanted to do the test so as to not "waste" an organ on someone testing positive.

Medical Insurance Discrimination   An important issue in genetic testing is confidentiality, or privacy. As the power of government has grown, the right to privacy has seemed increasingly important—especially in recent years, as information and surveillance have been computerized. One presidential commission on bioethics recommended that results of genetic tests should be held confidential.

The greatest form of discrimination comes from possible loss of medical insurance as a result of testing. Several national companies (such as Medical

Information Bureau of Boston) inform insurance companies about applicants who are risks[52]; thus there is considerable concern that insurers will raise premiums for families at risk or simply refuse to cover such families—in fact, for bioethicists, this is the major issue. In the United States, the logic here is indeed alarming: Genetics allows precise calculations of risks in family trees; an insurance company functions on the basis of such calculations; such a company exists to make money; the most profitable procedure for an insurer is to sell policies only to people with the best genetic health and either deny it to others or charge them a fortune for it. A related concern is that employers, to reduce their cost of insuring workers, will discriminate against people who represent genetic risks.

Not every country is subject to this logic, of course: Some health systems work on the basis of sharing risk, and in such a system everyone pays premiums to help cover the costs for those who become sick. Where a risk-sharing system exists—as in England, Canada, Australia, and the state of Hawaii—insurers and employers have no motive to learn the results of genetic tests; but in the United States, there is a powerful incentive to have this information. Patients testing positive for a genetic disorder like HD can then be excluded from the insurers's risk pool, and from the employer's personnel.

In the case of HD, any child of a person with this disease has a 50 percent risk; though risk—or probability—varies depending on the specific genetic disorder, there is always some incentive for insurers and employers to discriminate. Thus when parents give an insurer genetic information about themselves, they are giving information that may also affect the availability and cost of medical insurance for their children. When a child tests positive for a genetic disorder and the parents file for insurance, they may not realize what they are revealing about themselves.

It is therefore crucial to control the distribution of test results: that is, to decide who should and should not receive them. Many large institutions, such as the military, universities, and large companies, "self-insure" themselves and pass their losses along to employees through increased premiums. Moreover, some employers may not keep test results confidential, especially if key employees are involved; consequently, a positive result may keep an executive off the fast track. Violation of confidentiality might also keep a physician out of a medical group, a student out of a university or graduate school, and so on. According to one respected geneticist:

> [One day] it might be common for a physician to give patients a battery of DNA probe tests as part of an intake procedure. Such a panel of tests would likely include susceptibility markers. . . . Predictive testing would almost certainly appeal to the physician charged with performing the intake screens on prospective applicants to an HMO or to General Motors for that matter— . . . and thereby enable the employer to take appropriate "remedial" measures—such as not employing them [job applicants] in the first place.[53]

Congress has never passed the Human Genome Privacy bill, to ban insurers from access (even paid access) to genetic tests. This is a forward-looking bill which would cover testing to prevent the birth of children with genetic diseases. A task force of the Human Genome Project has recommended that:

all individual risk information be excluded from decisions about who gets insured, what they get insured for, and how much they get charged. We see no other practical, sustainable plan for health care coverage than community rating.[54]

Financial issues were also associated with BRCA1 linkage testing. For example, when one woman who tested positive decided to have a preventive radical mastectomy, her insurer thought she was being irrational and wouldn't pay for the surgery. She didn't want to tell the insurance company the real reason for her decision, because she was afraid the company would cancel her policy or raise her premiums, and perhaps even do the same for the rest of the family.

It is fair to point out that insurance companies want genetic information in order to keep people who test positive from buying the best medical insurance and running up enormous costs for the insurer to cover—and that the Human Genome Project reveals some of the gaps in our national medical nonsystem. However, it is also fair to observe that in the face of genetic advances, insurance companies might find a role to play other than the bad guy. For example, they might encourage individuals who test positive for genetic diseases to insure themselves for future care through monthly premiums.

What Are People Testing For?   A second consideration about harm to people at risk is that self-knowledge is seldom perfect. Many people simply cannot predict how they will react to testing positive—what they will feel or do if they learn the worst. Since HD, for example, cannot be cured or ameliorated, a positive test will tell someone like Nancy Wexler that she is certainly going to die an early, terrible death. We might argue that not everyone can deal with such knowledge, and that it is inhumane to give people such a diagnosis when no real treatment is possible; some critics have argued that people at risk of HD should not be burdened with more truth than they can carry.[55]

In this regard, in 1986, when scientists at a conference in Salt Lake City were debating whether the linkage test should be made available, Nancy Wexler said, "We have to understand that the day you tell someone he has this gene, his life and view of himself change forever. We're worried about the potential for suicide"[56] In medical genetics, it is usually assumed that suicide after a positive test would be a bad thing, that such suicide should be prevented at all costs, and that people who say they might commit suicide should not be tested.

Concerns about suicide are not groundless. Over 25 percent of the victims of HD attempt suicide and 10 percent actually carry it out[57]; and given the nature of HD, these figures are understandable. As Nancy Wexler points out, during the first stage of HD victims do not lose memory and can recognize relatives: "HD patients know their family and they know what's happening to them until the end. So in a way, it's worse than Alzheimer's."[58] A victim may become frustrated and enraged at being unable to do something as simple as tie a shoelace; later, the victim may feel ashamed and become depressed. People who are concerned about suicide often focus on the consequences of testing teenagers—a population which is already highly suicidal. Youngsters who are merely at risk of HD already agonize about going to college and spending their parents' money, and those who learned for certain that they had HD might be even more vulnerable. Nancy Wexler does not think the possibility of suicide should weigh against testing: "Suicide is not un-reasonable. It's not so awful that we can't discuss it or consider it."[59] She observed, "For some of my friends who have HD, knowing that they can commit suicide gives them a certain sense of control. They want to feel that if it gets too bad, they can have a way out. They can do something."

All this raises the question of whether people at risk who agree to a test really understand what they are doing. One HD counselor said, for instance, "When people say they want this test to find out if they have the gene so they can make de-cisions, they really want to find out that they don't have it. The trouble is that fifty percent of them do. And there's no way to prepare them."[60] Nancy Wexler agreed with this.

There is some evidence for this second argument. In the first pilot study of the linkage test for HD, although most people at risk (63–79 percent) originally said they would take the test, some changed their minds later.[61] It was found that some of these people had expected to test negative and had intended to take the test to confirm this expectation. Since in fact they had a 50 percent chance of testing pos-itive, this expectation indicated that they were in denial and were unprepared for a positive result; when they were given counseling which broke through their de-nial, they decided not to take the test. In this same study, it was reported of those who took the test, "Participants found to be probable gene carriers reported being surprised or shocked by the test result"[62]; they said they had not really expected to have the lethal gene. That too is a significant finding.

Not Testing as a Family Issue   In the case for not knowing—as in the case for knowing—another kind of consideration may be the family of the person at risk. In more ways than one, the results of testing for a genetic disorder like HD affect the entire family.

With regard to the person at risk, although other family members may want to know, it is also possible that they may not want to know: that the family may pre-fer uncertainty to despair. Also, it is important to keep in mind that in testing for something like HD, there is no such thing as testing only a fetus, say, or testing only a parent or only a child: A positive fetus reveals a positive parent; a positive par-ent reveals that any children are at risk; a positive child reveals a positive parent.

Some women at risk for breast cancer do not want to know, but it is difficult for them to not know. As with HD, testing one family member had inevitable impli-cations for others. Among the women of these extended families, confidentiality was very difficult to maintain. It was hard for any woman to hold out against the rest of her family and not discover her BRCA1 status: For example, once results are known for a grandmother and her granddaughter, the result for the intervening generation (the woman who is grandmother's daughter and the granddaughter's mother) may also be known. Or vice versa: In testing a middle-aged woman for the BRCA1 marker, one is also telling her mother and her daughter about their likelihood of having BRCA1. As with HD, then, each individual needs to realize that her decision to be tested has consequences for other people.

With regard to knowing versus not knowing, it is interesting to note that in the BRCA1 linkage study, girls under 18 years of age were not tested; it was felt that such a test might be overwhelming for them. A registry was proposed for results of BRCA1 linkage test, so that family members could provide information for their children without learning the results themselves.

One legal issue in this area is the family versus the individual's right to decline testing. Courts have ruled that, even in a life-and-death situation, relatives cannot be compelled to be tested for compatibility as possible bone-marrow or organ donors; such legal precedents suggest that the courts will not force relatives to participate in genetic tests.

Another, subtler issue was suggested earlier with regard to HD: Testing one member of a family has implications for other members. Any number of questions can arise as a result.

If a person has been tested early in life, could hiding the results from a spouse later be grounds for legal annulment? Does a prospective spouse have a right to know about the risk of a disorder like HD? Or does marrying "for better or worse" cover such questions?

Can one parent have a child tested in order to find out if the other parent is affected?

Suppose that a parent tests positive and refuses to tell his or her child. Suppose that a genetic counselor is aware of this. As the child approaches childbearing age, what should the counselor do? A counselor in such a situation might, of course, simply recommend general genetic tests, but suppose the child refuses. Would the child agree to testing if he or she knew that a parent was positive? If so, should the counselor violate the parent's confidentiality? To many people, the good of preventing another child with, say, HD outweighs the harm of violating privacy, especially where this is a strong sense that the affected parent had an obligation to reveal his or her disease to the family.

Catherine Hayes believes that:

> First and foremost, genetic testing must be viewed as a family issue, not an individual one. The person who enrolls in a testing program should be strongly encouraged to involve other family members, within reason. Testing one member of a family will affect other members. Persons who refuse to involve their families may not have considered fully the consequences for other members or for themselves.[63]

It is sometimes difficult to test just one member of a family:

> A case in point involves a pair of identical twins, only one of whom wanted to be tested. She swore that she would never reveal the results to anyone else in her family, in particular to her twin. Once she was informed of the results—that there was a high probability that she would have HD—the information spread quickly throughout the entire family. This meant that the twin who did not want to know her genetic status was now faced with the unwelcome knowledge that she too would probably have the disease.[64]

Hayes herself had five brothers and eight nieces and nephews. Though she herself tested negative, one of her brothers already has symptoms of HD and another has tested positive; both already have some children.

Actually, the family can be a very complex factor in the question of testing. Hayes notes, "Many medical professionals have difficulty viewing genetic issues in a family context. . . . Most researchers cannot possibly know what it is like to grow up in a family haunted by a genetic disease. . . . "Some family issues will reappear when we discuss confidentiality.

Counseling   Many people will not fully understand all the above implications of presymptomatic testing for genetically based diseases such as HD and breast cancer. As such, many ethicists and geneticists believe that it is crucial that individuals at risk get good counseling before they take a test, the results of which can never be "given back."

A presidential commission on bioethics emphasized that counseling should be guaranteed: "A full range of prescreening and follow-up services . . . should be available before a program is introduced."[65] Note, though, that the recommendation here is for making counseling *available* rather than *mandatory;* it can also be noted that counseling is not always even made available, especially to people who are not covered by health insurance. Others disagree, such as Joseph Schulman, who is offering the test for BRCA1 mutations *without* counseling. At the Salt Lake City conference in 1986, one scientist argued against paternalism: "I think we can trust people to make these decisions. I'm not so convinced we researchers should be dictating how the technology gets used."[66]

Many people who are not absolutely opposed to testing as such—and even some people who are generally in favor of testing—argue that it should not be offered without counseling. This may seem paternalistic; but it is true that some of those who test positive will wish they hadn't taken the test and some may develop emotional problems, and that counseling can be helpful in such situations. As a matter of public policy, should people, through their private physicians, simply be allowed to "buy" their own test results, or should counseling be required?

Counseling is important to prepare even those who test negative. One man in his late thirties had lived his life convinced he had inherited the HD gene from an affected parent. He lived life on the edge, pursuing risky activities such as sky diving and mountaineering, having only short-term relationships with women, and running up enormous debts. Because he "knew" he would have HD by 50, it made no sense to have a pension, marry, have kids, or worry about a long-term career. When he tested negative, he said, "My life fell apart. I lost my creative terror. I didn't know what to do."[67]

Embryonic and Fetal Testing   In vitro fertilization, or IVF, has had interesting implications for genetic testing. In IVF, several eggs are removed from the ovary, then fertilized with sperm in a petri dish; one or more (usually more) of the resulting embryos are then implanted in the womb. Since each embryo has its own genetic "DNA map," this map can be inspected for genetic defects before implantation, at the point when the embryo consists of eight cells: One cell can be removed and its DNA can be replicated for genetic testing. (It is believed that removal of this single cell does not change the embryo.) Any embryo in which a defect is found need not be implanted.

It should be noted that this kind of single-cell testing of embryos is possible only with IVF—and, in this regard, that IVF is expensive (costing about $8,000 per attempt), that it is typically not covered by insurance, and that it is successful in only about 14 percent of cases.

There are, moreover, issues about genetic testing of embryos, and also about genetic testing of fetuses. Consider fetal testing for CF, for instance. One woman who had two children with CF underwent amniocentesis and was relieved to discover that her third child was not at risk; she said, "I couldn't bear bringing another child into the world with cystic fibrosis,"[68] and in this she is probably typical of parents. On the other hand, drug treatments now allow about half of children with CF to live to age 30 (earlier, they rarely survived into their twenties),[69] and such improvements in life expectancy may continue. One New York physician who specializes in treating CF says that offering such a prenatal test is like telling people with CF, "It would have been better for all of us if you had not been born."[70] A similar argument is often made by some organizations of parents of children with Down syndrome and spina bifida.

A conceptual slippery-slope argument is sometimes made here. If embryonic or fetal screening is used to select against, say, Down syndrome or Tay Sachs disease, won't this create a slippery slope, eventually allowing parents to select against shortness, homosexuality, one sex or the other, or even unfashionable cosmetic traits? The bioethicist Arthur Caplan has predicted:

> I think the stance that we deal only with clear-cut disorders [in testing embryos] will last about five minutes. Once you can do that testing, the interest [of parents] will swamp my objections. The ability to choose the traits of your child will roar through with a whoosh.[71]

In one alleged case, a deaf couple wanted to screen prenatally for deafness in order to select *for* a deaf child.[72]

There have also been some financial arguments about embryonic and fetal genetic screening; in fact, opponents of a single-payer system of health insurance use such an argument. Caplan is concerned that a single-payer system might "unjustly" influence decisions about procreating by establishing criteria for what kind of procreation is appropriate and inappropriate: "You can have a kid like that [with a genetic disease] if you want, but we're not paying." Paul Billings, a medical geneticist who is an activist against discrimination, thinks this could lead to a resurgence of eugenics: "Whether you want to dress it up in economic incentives, if you have to sell your house and go broke to have a child of a certain type, that's eugenics."[73]

Resisting Genetic Reductionism   Most people now accept some form of *genetic determinism,* the idea that the characteristics of a human are totally caused by his genes ("it's all in the genes"). The successes of the Human Genome Project have predictably fueled this attitude, which is called *genetic reductionism.*

There is an ancient debate in biology going back to Aristotle about how much of human reproduction is determined by something fixed and formal and how much of reproduction is fluid. Aristotle incorrectly thought that only males contributed the formal cause in their semen, and that such semen acted on mostly passive matter. *Preformationism,* the idea that the development of the embryo is merely the unfolding of something present from the start in the seed, was found in human embryology even before Aristotle (e.g., in the Hippocratic corpus).[74] Preformationism dominated the medieval period, holding that humans were formed immediately at conception, such that embryogenesis was merely the expansion of a very small human (called a "homunculus"). According to this view, male ejaculation passed on a very small human; so Dalenpatius (1699) claimed to see homunculi in human sperm.[75]

Genes are best understood not just as simple mechanisms that cause traits in humans, but as functions whose expression in individuals is mediated by what happens in the environment. The "expression" of a gene is not contained in itself, but is determined by how the genes of a particular individual interact with many other things.

The author of the scientific section of the National Bioethics Advisory Commission's *Report* on human cloning put it this way:

> Indeed, the great lesson of modern molecular genetics is the profound complexity of both gene-gene interactions and gene-environment interactions in the determination of whether a specific trait or characteristic is expressed. . . . Recent scientific findings have revealed that a "one-gene-one-disease" approach is far too simplistic. Even in the relatively small list of genes currently associated with a specific disease, knowing the complete DNA sequence of the gene does not allow a scientist to predict if a given person will get the disease.[76]

We know that the environment plays a key and complex role in the formation of individuals during childhood. Not only do the expressions of genes in creating a phenotype depend on the child's early environment, but also (and what is not so readily appreciated) even the expression of genes in embryonic development depend to an unknown degree on the uterine environment. Much of the expression of genes in the phenotype is not caused by preformed, fixed templates (genes) that shape the passive matter of the embryo, but rather, the phenotype is caused by genes acting more like variables that can respond over a continuous range, depending on what happens around them.

To oversimplify, we know that there are some, rare, powerful genetic traits such that if an individual has gene X, the trait is always eventually expressed. The gene for Huntington's disease is like this, being fully penetrant if one lives long enough. Other diseases and traits need a gene from both parents for the disease or condition to be expressed, e.g., cystic fibrosis or blue eyes.

Importantly to us, we do not know how much or how little the uterine environment influences genetic regulation (as opposed to genetic structure) of embryonic development in the first 100 days of human life. We postulate that many traits or characteristics of adults may require a certain set of genes from one parent mixed with another parent, and with this mixture developing in the right kind of environment. That is another kind of genetic causation. Again, we don't know all of what happens here. We know that the presence or absence of certain proteins or amino acids influences development of the brain. For example, in PKU babies, the presence of excess phenylaline leads to an excess of phenylpyruvic acid that impairs development of the brain and results in mental retardation. But there may be all kinds of other causes of brain development and formation of personality of which we are now ignorant.

Once a fetus has gestated and become a baby, a tremendous amount of shaping of later traits occurs within the first two years of life. Genes have shaped some ranges of response here, but what happens now depends on parents, nutrition, and all the other factors in a child's world.

Finally, for diseases such as breast cancer, it may take from 15 to 30 years of the right environmental interactions with a genetic predisposition to cause the cancer. Even then, it may take many different factors coming together in just the right way to produce the disease. Such complexity makes it difficult to predict who will get a specific cancer, and also, to know how to prevent and treat such cancers.

One example of this complexity is seen in the naive early reports of discoveries of genetic causes of alcoholism, schizophrenia, and manic depression—reports that turned out to be premature. The implication seemed to be that psychiatric disorders would not be caused by single genes but by from three to five genes acting together, possibly (though not necessarily) in conjunction with environmental cofactors.

Ecogenetics studies such environmental-gene interactions. A paradigm here is the gene for xeroderma pigmentosum, a fatal disease which produces hypersensitivity to ultraviolet light, thereby causing melanoma. Another example is a particular gene on chromosome 15 that turns compounds in cigarette smoke into carcinogens. Another gene may turn charred meat into carcinogens but remain harmless if the person never eats such meat.

Ecogenetics may lead us to rethink some common assumptions about causes of disease. For example, two popular theories about cancer are that people cause themselves to develop it by exposing themselves to carcinogens (as by smoking and ingesting certain foods), and that it is caused by environmental carcinogens (such as toxic chemical emissions). Although these theories undoubtedly represent part of the truth, they do not explain why some people who are exposed to carcinogens remain free of cancer, or why some people who are *not* exposed develop cancer anyway. Ecogenetics is starting to provide an explanation: Researchers are beginning to find that some people have genes which detoxify carcinogens rapidly, whereas other people do not.

Such findings may seem to imply only that some people who are exposed to carcinogens can do very little to prevent cancer, but actually the implications are much more hopeful. Ecogenetics suggests that presymptomatic testing may give some people a small "window" of real preventive control, if they can be tested, informed, and advised soon enough. Genetic conditions predisposing people to cancer may be detectable before exposure to carcinogens such as cigarette smoke, asbestos, and industrial chemicals; and if so, what was once a matter of "fate" can become controllable through public health measures and individual motivation. People who are genetically less able to detoxify the effects of secondhand cigarette smoke, for instance, may choose environments where their exposure is minimal. The complex truths of ecogenetics all counter the simplistic myths of genetic reductionism.

In sum, the common view that it's "all in the genes" is false and it's false in more complicated ways than initially appear. All of which makes presymptomatic testing, embryonic testing, and genetic therapy much more complicated than they seem at first.

Gene Therapy

Gene therapy has become an issue in the 1990s. There are two kinds of gene therapy, though these are frequently confused. *Somatic therapy,* the less controversial kind, involves the somatic cells—that is, differentiated cells other than the sex (germ) cells. Somatic therapy attempts to treat a particular individual by altering disease-causing genetic material while leaving the patient otherwise the same; it is much like ordinary medical treatment. *Gametic* or *germ-line therapy,* in contrast, alters the hereditary genetic material of an individual and thus affects only future generations, not the patient himself or herself: The patient's descendants will inherit altered genetic material. Both germ-line therapy and somatic therapy are sometimes called "genetic engineering," a term so drastically misleading that it should be discarded.

After 20 years of debate over the ethics of such intervention, and many years of genetic testing on animals, somatic gene therapy was first attempted on September 14, 1990, on a 4-year-old girl with adenosine adaminase deficiency (ADA), a fatal disease resulting from lack of an enzyme; scientists at NIH attempted to insert the genes causing this enzyme into the girl. There were no controls. To date, the results of this experiment are controversial and uncertain, partly because the course of ADA varies in individuals and is uncertain.

On April 20, 1993, researchers inserted a deadened cold virus into the nose of a 23-year-old man with cystic fibrosis. The much-ballyhooed "genetic engineering" and "tampering with nature" came down practically to a patient using a nose inhaler the same way that millions do for the common cold.

This was a prototype for a study of somatic gene therapy in CF: The virus contained a healthy copy of the genetic material the patient lacked, and it was hoped that this somatic therapy would block the production of excess mucus. For the 30,000 Americans with CF, and the many heterozygotes who were silent carriers, this was the first real frontier of the new age of gene therapy.

At the end of 1998, predictions about quick successes from somatic gene therapy look like similar, false predictions made previously about quick discoveries of genes for HD and breast cancer. Thousands of patients have participated in many different attempts to create the first, successful case of somatic gene therapy, but not one true, universally accepted success has been achieved. Part of the problem is that viruses are unstable platforms for introducing new genetic material into the body.

Update: Testing for Breast Cancer

In 2002, a clinical trial proved that women with a BRAC1 or BRAC2 mutation undergoing prophylactic bilateral mastectomy have a "statistically significant" lower risk of breast cancer after 5 years. Both BRAC1 and BRAC2 are autosomal, dominant genes. The science of presymptomatic testing is complex. Many mutations of BRAC1 and BRAC2 carry varying degrees of risk, which must be interpreted and conveyed correctly to patients. In 2002, CHEK2 was discovered, another gene that, if mutation occurs, can cause breast cancer. With each of these genes, the same gene or same mutation may act differently in different families or in twins with different lifestyles. Even more important, either BRAC1 or BRAC2 may play a role in prostate, colon, ovarian, pancreatic or gallbladder cancers, as well as malignant melanoma, so knowing one has these genes might be important in preventing other cancers.

Presymptomatic testing remains controversial. In 2002, Myriad Genetics of Salt Lake City expanded its sales force from 85 to 600 agents to market BRAC analysis directly to doctors and their patients. The tests, which cost between $750 and $2,750 would only benefit the 5–10 percent of people with breast cancers linked to these genes. In some ways, marketing such tests is a win-win situation for Myriad. For the people who test positive, they get their money's worth and advance news. For the people who test negative, they get relief and will not complain about the money spent. The problem comes when thousands of people seek relief who are really not at risk: they will waste their money in getting a negative result. But it would be patronizing to say they can't spend their money as they choose, even irrationally.

If a woman has BRAC1, benefits of knowing early are that taking birth control pills reduces risk of ovarian cancer by 60 percent and taking the drug tamoxifen reduces risk of breast cancer by nearly half. Also, and more radically, prophylactic bilateral mastectomy increases longevity somewhat. About 2 percent of breast cancer is in men, and these same benefits apply to men.

Jesse Gelsinger's Death: Changes in Gene Therapy

In the fall of 1999, the death of Jesse Gelsinger stunned the medical research world and set back gene therapy for years. As reporters and congressmen investigated the death, problems emerged that changed the way regulators thought about funding genetic research on patients. In this sense, news of Jesse Gelsinger's death was like news of the Tuskegee syphilis study or Gennarelli's head-injury research on baboons in that the case revealed a pattern of problems over a long time that had to be remedied.

During the summer of 1999 in Tuscon, Arizona, 17-year-old Jesse Gelsinger heard about an experiment in gene therapy at the University of Pennsylvania for his inherited disorder, ornithine transcarbamylase deficiency (OTC).

OTC is a genetic disease where the liver fails to properly cleanse the blood of ammonia, a chemical produced in normal metabolism, resulting in toxic levels of ammonia. Many OTC newborns die around birth and half don't make it to age 5.

A regimen of drugs and diet originated by Penn researcher Mark Batshaw enabled Jesse to live to be a teenager. But without a cure, he would eventually die young of his disease.

The son of a handyman, Jesse worked as clerk in a grocery store and rode a motorcycle on weekends, as did his father, Paul. A friend said Jesse "wanted to prove he was a man as much as anything."[77] Penn researchers claim Jesse was informed that the experiment wouldn't help him, but that it might lead to a cure for OTC babies. His father testified at a later congressional hearing that Jesse's motives had been pure: "He was going to help save lives."

Jesse's death was unusual because he entered the study, in the parlance of the research, as a "healthy research volunteer." In the cold language of the lawsuit that followed, he entered as a young man in his prime and was rendered dead.

But why weren't studies done on dying OTC patients, as is usually done with potentially lethal, risky experiments? First, researcher James Wilson denied that the experiment could have been expected to kill Jesse. Second, OTC babies are essentially born dying; most babies die within days. It would be hard to prove that any genetic therapy did any good. Third, as emphasized by Penn's own bioethicist Arthur Caplan, parents of OTC babies are so desperate that they would consent to almost any study.

So researchers now made the fateful decision to seek adults with OTC whose livers were still functioning well and to inject an adenovirus into them that contained copies of the gene lacking in OTC patients. Adenoviruses are quite common in life, causing common colds. They easily infect human cells, and because the cell is the basic unit of the body, these viruses are a potential device or vector for transmitting new or better genes to patients with genetic diseases.

The fateful decision was backed by Penn's IRB and its media-connected bioethics department. It was also backed by the NIH committee with some oversight of gene therapy research, the RAC (Recombinant DNA Advisory Committee), whose power, however, had been significantly diminished before Jesse's death.

One of the main problems of all gene therapy is successful delivery of the new genes to a patient with defective or missing genes. If successful, the same virus that helped Jesse might also be the vector for any number of genetic diseases, especially those affecting the liver.

What actually happened to Jesse is quite grim. The definitive news account of Jesse's death was co-written by Rick Weiss, medical science writer for the *Washington Post*. The dramatic lead for this article began:

> Four days after scientists infused trillions of genetically engineered viruses into Jesse Gelsinger's liver as part of a novel gene therapy experiment, the 18-year old lay dying in a hospital bed at the University of Pennsylvania. His liver had failed, and the teenager's blood was thickening like jelly and clogging key vessels while his kidneys, brain, and other organs shut down.[78]

According to the factual summary of the case, drawn from medical reports in the wrongful death lawsuit, when the physicians injected Jesse with the virus, "he suffered a chain reaction including jaundice, a blood-clotting disorder, kidney failure and brain death" in quick, irreversible succession over 4 days. The legal charges brought were:

1. Wrongful death by negligent and reckless conduct
2. Strict products liability for a device causing death
3. Intentional assault and battery from lack of informed consent
4. Intentional infliction of emotional distress
5. Fraudulent misrepresentation of the study and the past efficacy of its vector/virus
6. Punitive damages due to actions that were "intentional wanton, willful and outrageous"
7. Fraudulent reporting to the Federal Drug Administration (FDA)[79]

Many of these legal charges grew out of ethical issues raised by the case. Chief among these were that:

1. *Harmful vector.* Researchers knew (or should have known) that the adenovirus used to transfer the genes was more toxic than normal vectors used in gene transfer because the virus had injured other adults with OTC. Researchers continued to deliver greater and greater concentrations of the virus despite the fact that ammonia was reaching more and more dangerous levels in Jesse's system, just as in a previous adult patient where the virus had caused severe damage to the liver.

2. *Lack of informed consent.* The Gelsingers were not told that other adults given the experimental virus had not done well and that animals given the virus had died (this information was omitted from the final consent form, even though the RAC had required it).

3. *Financial conflict of interest.* James Wilson, the University of Pennsylvania, and even the Penn bioethics department, each had a conflict of interest in the case because each received money through Wilson's academic center, the Institute for Human Gene Therapy, which in turn received money from Wilson's commercial bioetech company, Genovo, for commercial rights to patent and use Wilson's adenovirus, should it prove therapeutic for patients such as Jesse.

4. *Lack of reporting of adverse incidents to the NIH.* The National Institutes of Health and the Federal Drug Administration are charged by Congress with monitoring medical research, and researchers are supposed to promptly report to the NIH and FDA any serious downturn in an experimental subject's condition. Researchers at Penn failed to report very serious problems about the experimental virus.

5. *Inappropriate solicitation of patients.* Solicitation was made through newsletters and websites devoted to particular diseases, rather than through the filter of referral by a knowledgeable physician.

Jesse Gelsinger's death created a spotlight on medical research as reporters and congressional hearings dug into why he had died. What they found disturbed the public. First, investigations found that only 39 of nearly 700 adverse incidents had been reported to the NIH. What this means is that medical researchers were willfully avoiding scrutiny by the NIH and the press for their experiments in gene therapy. Because they hoped to gain money and fame from being the first to cure a genetic disease, they were also not privately sharing news of these adverse effects on patients. So no central clearinghouse existed for researchers to know how bad things had become. As a result of Jesse's death and investigations, much stricter reporting of these events is now required.

A second result of news of Jesse's death is changes in the way medical researchers are allowed to benefit financially by for-profit research on patients. Biogen, Inc., paid Wilson's Genovo $37 million in the 4 years preceding Jesse's death for rights to market genetic therapies to cure lung and liver diseases. Genovo shared that money with Wilson's Institute for Human Gene Therapy at Penn. Genovo also had a similar financial deal with Genzyme, a biotech company hoping to find cures for various diseases affecting how the liver functions.

Wilson denies that desires for profit played any role in his decisions about the virus or Jesse's case; instead he claims his main desire was to be first to cure a genetic disease.[80] Nevertheless, after the publicity and news of the death of Ellen Roche at Johns Hopkins, another healthy adult "rendered dead" by medical research on a potentially profitable drug to treat asthma, most research universities created special conflict-of-interest committees to monitor and regulate such conflicts among researchers. (Whether this is creating the simulacrum of solving the problem or really solving it remains to be seen.)

A third result of the case was that researchers in gene therapy stepped back and reassessed their field at an Asimolar-like conference that was at the site of the original Asimolar conference in 1975, where similar researchers created a voluntary ban on genetically modified organisms until they were proved safe. As a result of the conference in 2000, researchers concluded that adenoviruses should only be used as a last resort (to prevent death or a liver transplant) and not on healthy volunteers. They decided that they needed to curtail some of their current research until it could be proved safe. Harvard's hospital had stopped several studies on gene therapy for cystic fibrosis.

On-site investigation of Wilson's research by the FDA revealed a pattern of failure to obtain informed consent and the alarming fact that Jesse's liver was already beginning to fail when he was injected with a toxic virus that challenged the capacity of his liver. As a result of these transgressions and others aforementioned, the NIH on January 22, 2000, suspended all medical research at Penn until it was satisfied that Penn's researchers were able and willing to comply with federal law and regulations about research.

After stern rebukes from the U.S. Senate and especially physician Senator Bill Frist of Tennessee, the NIH and FDA vowed to better monitor medical research in the United States. As a result of closer scrutiny, several medical universities were cited for violations and, like Penn, had all their medical research temporarily suspended until they proved they were in compliance. These institutions included the University of Colorado Medical Center, the University of North Carolina, Johns Hopkins, and the University of Alabama at Birmingham.

An interesting sidebar in this story was the fact that famous bioethicist Arthur Caplan was named in the lawsuit over wrongful death and lack of informed consent. Caplan was quoted as having said to reporters that, "Not only is it sad that Jesse Gelsinger died, there was never a chance that anybody would benefit from these treatments. They are safety studies. They are not therapeutic in goal. If I gave it to you, we would try to see if you died, too, and if you did OK." . . . In regard to Wilson's adenovirus for delivering gene therapy, the suit claims Caplan told reporters, "If you cured anybody, you'd publish it in a religious journal. It would be a miracle. All you're doing is you're saying, I've got this vector. I want to see if it can deliver the gene where I want it to go without killing or hurting or having any side effects." In essence, the claim in the suit was that the Gelsinger family was not given the opportunity to understand the experiment in direct, simple language.

The Gelsinger family eventually settled out of court with Penn for an undisclosed sum. Penn regained its right to do medical research, although Wilson's gene therapy protocols were not resumed. The reason Jesse died was never completely clear because it was later found that the virus used on him differed from the originally engineered virus.[81] Did a mistake occur? Did the virus change? No one knows for sure.

Finally, the FDA and NIH became more vigilant. A new national oversight board was created to toughen up regulations about medical research, and a proposal was debated for regional, centralized IRBs rather than local and institutional ones.

The Carr Case

Carol Carr, 63, shot and killed two of her three sons inflicted with HD on June 8, 2002. Michael Randy Scott, 42, and Andy Byron Scott, 41, had been bedridden for 4 months at Sunbridge Care and Rehabilitation Center. Carr, whose husband died of HD in 1995, has another son, James, who recently had begun to exhibit symptoms of HD. Husband Hoyt Scott's mother seems to be the originator of the illness in the family; Hoyt's sister died from HD, and his brother committed suicide when he learned he was infected.

Carol cared for Hoyt as his stages of HD advanced over 2 decades until his death. Around the same time as Hoyt's death, the family learned that Michael and Andy were infected, and Carol took on the daunting task of caring for them.

Carol has been charged with two counts of murder, and, at this point, the verdict is quite unclear and controversial. Her defense team is trying to claim the incident was a "mercy killing," but Georgia law does not protect mercy killings. James and several other groups, such as HDSA, have rallied to support Carol and now several funds have been set up to pay for her defense and family expenses.

Carr's defense attorney, Virgil Brown, told reporters outside the courtroom, "Those boys were dead long before that day. For all practical purposes, only the disease died that day." He went on to say, "I see no evidence of malice aforethought. I see only love."

When Carr took the stand, she reportedly said, "I know what happened but I don't remember. I don't doubt I did it."

There have been other cases like the Carrs, where family members have killed others to protect them from a fatal, debilitating disease, but not quite as well publicized.

The media coverage of the Carr case has been intense and unrelenting. It has made James and Carol Carr famous and unintentional crusaders for the cause of Huntington's disease and mercy killings.[82]

FURTHER READING

G. Annas and S. Elias, eds., *Gene Mapping: Using Law and Ethics as Guides,* Oxford University Press, New York, 1992.

Catherine Hayes, "Genetic Testing for HD—A Family Issue," *New England Journal of Medicine,* vol. 327, no. 20, 1993.

"The Human Genome Project: Where Will the Map Lead Us?" *Bioethics*, vol. 5, no. 3 (special issue), July 1991.

Daniel Kevles, *In the Name of Eugenics: Genetics and the Uses of Human Heredity*, Knopf, New York, 1985.

LeRoy Walters and Julie Polmm, *The Ethics of Human Gene Therapy*, Oxford University Press, New York, 1997.

Alice Wexler, *Mapping Fate: A Memoir of Family, Risk, and Genetic Research*, Random House, New York, 1995.

CHAPTER 17

Preventing the Global Spread of AIDS

This chapter discusses debates, almost always ideological, about how to stop the spread of HIV infections around the world. HIV (*human immunodeficiency virus*) is the virus that invades the immune system to cause AIDS—*acquired immunodeficiency syndrome.* In contrast to versions of this chapter in earlier editions, this chapter emphasizes prevention of AIDS as a worldwide problem and as a challenge for international bioethics.

As background, this chapter discusses reactions in similar epidemics in past centuries, the history of the public's understanding and misunderstanding of AIDS, the transmission and clinical course of AIDS (including treatments), scandals over HIV infecting the blood supply, and the symbolic death of Kimberly Bergalis. It also discusses homosexuality as a moral issue and methods in public health of preventing spread of disease such as contact tracing, mandatory screening, and programs that exchange needles.

BACKGROUND: EPIDEMICS, PLAGUES, AND AIDS

Throughout human history, epidemics have terrified humans; one of the deadliest was the bacterial disease during the Middle Ages known as *the black death* and more generally, as *the plague.*

It had two forms: *bubonic plague,* the most common and classic, characterized by inflamed swellings of the lymphatic glands in the groin and armpits; it was carried by fleas which in turn were spread by rats and other small mammals to humans. So bites of fleas actually transmitted plague to humans. A virulent complication of untreated bubonic plague, *pneumonic plague,* involves the lungs and may be easily transmitted when one person coughs on another.

Both types of plague broke out many times before the great outbreak of 1348 in Europe, and both continued afterwards there until 1900. Plague still kills humans in remote parts of Asia, Africa, and South America. When plague occurred in 1994 in the city of Surat in India, thousands fled. In the 1990s in the American southwest, small mammals were found to be carrying plague and again in 2002 in Colorado at the Donner Pass.

Bubonic plague is now known to be caused by the bacillus *Yersinia pestis*, and today it is treatable in its early stages with antibiotics. However, its specific causative agents remained unknown for nearly 500 years, in part because the virulent, respiratory mode of infection of pneumonic plague made discovery of its true cause more difficult. All this made physicians reluctant to come near or study its victims, and during plague, many physicians either left cities for the countryside or gave up their profession.[1]

Untreated bubonic plague killed 50 percent of its victims and pneumonic plague killed all its victims. Daniel Defoe (1660–1731) tells us that during epidemics of plague in London: "It is scarce credible what dreadful cases happened in particular families every day. People in the rage of distemper, or in the torment of their swellings, which was indeed intolerable, running out of their own government, raving and distracted, and oftentimes laying violent hands upon themselves, throwing themselves out of their windows, shooting themselves."[2]

In the fourteenth century, astrologers claimed that plague resulted from the conjunction of Saturn, Mars, and Jupiter, while others said it resulted from sulfurous fumes released by earthquakes. The most popular theory was that plague resulted from supernatural causes, either as the work of Satan or as God's punishment of humans for sin.

During medieval epidemics, people marched from city to city across Europe, and once even the Pope crawled on his stomach through mud to beg for forgiveness for the sins that were bringing on plague. In so marching, unfortunately, they spread infected fleas: "Organized groups of 200 to 300 . . . marched from city to city, stripped to the waist, scourging themselves with leather whips tipped with iron spikes until they bled. While they cried aloud to Christ and the Virgin for pity, . . . the watching townspeople sobbed in sympathy."[3]

The fear and ignorance of the times required identifiable evil people to be punished, and Orthodox Jews, with their distinctive dress, fit the bill. They were accused of poisoning wells and spreading plague. When atonement processions reached cities, especially in Germany, they often attacked the Jewish quarter and burned Jews alive who were trapped inside. (When plague followed, Jews were blamed, not the procession.)

Leprosy, cholera, and syphilis also terrified people. Leprosy, or Hansen's disease, creates lesions on the skin and is usually, and slowly, fatal. People get infected through exposure over many months through the skin or mucosa, but this was learned only in the twentieth century. Before then, lepers were banished from society, forced to live in lepers' colonies in isolated places, and had to ring cowbells as they walked to warn people.

Great epidemics of cholera from infected supplies of water also created fear and loathing of innocent victims. During the American epidemic of 1813, Americans blamed those who fell ill as deserving it, especially wanton prostitutes, drunk Irish, lazy blacks, and in general, the dirty poor who lived along creeks where sanitation was poor. Ministers praised God for cholera for "cleansing the filth from society," just as some would later say that AIDS came from God to rid society of gays and intravenous drug users.

In 1854, physician John Snow made the insightful observation that cholera only broke out in the district that received water from the Broad Street pump; he then confirmed that cholera was spread in infected water and could be prevented with clean water. His ideas were slow to be accepted, and many Americans died in the third great cholera epidemic of 1862. Not until acceptance of the germ theory of disease at the turn of the century did authorities in public health stem the tide against recurrent epidemics of cholera.

Victims of syphilis were also blamed for their disease. As discussed in Chapter 11, authorities could not decide if their enemy was sin or spirochetes, and they often fought each other over the appropriate enemy rather than the disease itself.

A Brief History of AIDS

The first proven case of HIV was from a blood sample collected in 1959 from a man in Kinshasa, Democratic Republic of Congo. Genetic analysis of his blood suggests that HIV-1 may have stemmed from a single virus that existed in the late 1940s or early 1950s.

Researcher Beatrice Hahn and others at UAB proved in 1999 by DNA sequencing that the virus spread to humans from chimpanzees (*Pan troglodytes troglodytes*) in the west-central region of Africa; hunters were exposed to the blood of these primates through catching, killing, and cutting up these animals for bushmeat.[4]

Around 1978, gay men in the U.S. and Sweden, and heterosexuals in Tanzania and Haiti began to show signs of (what would later be called) AIDS. Between 1979 and 1981, Kaposi's sarcoma and Pneumocystis carinii pneumonia (PCP), rare diseases that usually indicate AIDS, unexpectedly showed up in gay males in Los Angeles and New York.

In June of 1981, the Centers for Disease Control (CDC) announced the discovery of a mysterious "gay-related infectious disease" (GRID) that had killed three gay men; only a month later, 108 cases of GRID were reported and 46 gay men were dead.

Three months after the first report of GRID in the summer of 1981, CDC announced that babies of drug-dependent women in New York City also had the disease; "GRID" was changed to *acquired immune deficiency syndrome* or *AIDS*.

In 1982, when physicians in New York and California had already seen hundreds of cases of AIDS, the incubation of AIDS and its causative agent were unknown. CDC guessed that incubation could be many years and that many thousands of people could be infected. At that time in 1982, no one who had been diagnosed with AIDS had lived more than 2 years, so the disease frightened everyone.

As early as 1982, CDC warned that donated blood could carry the agent causing AIDS. Blood then could have been screened for hepatitis, thereby indirectly screening for HIV, but this was deemed too expensive and, unfortunately, not done.

In 1983, Luc Montagnier and the Institut Pasteur (France) discovered that a virus, HIV, caused AIDS. Today his discovery is called HIV-1. In 1986, a second form, HIV-2, was also discovered in west Africa, where it may have been infecting Africans for decades. HIV-2 seems to develop more slowly and to be milder than HIV-1 (the United States has reported few cases of HIV-2).[5]

In 1984, the FDA approved the ELISA test for antibodies to HIV. Hence a means existed for determining whether donated blood or blood inside a person carried HIV.

Despite many rumors to the contrary, HIV is transmitted in only three ways: through blood, through semen, or to babies during birth or breast-feeding. Sharing needles to inject drugs transmits HIV because withdrawing blood from a user's vein to mix with a drug in the syringe also mixes the user's blood with blood left over in the syringe from a previous user. (This is why cleaning out the syringe with bleach reduces the spread of HIV. Together, using fresh needles and syringes really prevents spread of HIV this way.)

The website of the Centers for Disease Control gives a great deal more information on the transmission and treatment of AIDS. It also describes risks of many different kinds of behavior.[6]

Without treatment, HIV causes a progressive weakening of the immune system, resulting in the body's inability to ward off normal infections. Cells called T4 lymphocytes (or simply T4 cells) indicate the health of the immune system: the lower the number of cells, the worse the immune system is doing. When the count of T4 cells drops below 200, a person with AIDS usually gets *opportunistic infections* such as Kaposi's sarcoma, PCP, a fungal infection called oral thrush, or cervical cancer.

Possible use of the ELISA test in 1984 to screen donated blood caused controversy. Some vocal gay men argued that their donations of blood should not be "quarantined" and that HIV had not really been proven to cause AIDS. Blood banks worried that their income might drop if blood were screened (although they do not technically charge for blood, such banks make money classifying, transferring, and storing blood).

In May 1984, Stanford University started screening blood for HIV. Two months later, defending a decision not to screen, Health and Human Services Secretary Margaret Heckler said, "I want to assure the American people that the blood supply is 100 percent safe . . ."[7] Joseph Bove, MD, who chaired the FDA's committee overseeing the safety of the nation's blood, said the "overreacting press" was causing hysteria about blood.[8] When CDC counted 73 cases of deaths from AIDS caused by transfusion in March of 1984, Bove dismissed this danger: "More people are killed by bee stings."[9] Six months later, 269 people had died of AIDS from tainted blood.

In so assuring Americans, Bove and Heckler either lied, were incompetent, or were guilty of both. In March of 1985, most American blood banks began using the ELISA test to screen blood, a full year after they should have, and several years after blood could have been screened for hepatitis. Because of this lag, thousands of Americans and most hemophiliacs became infected with HIV. One of them was a teenager, Ryan White, who died at age 18 in 1990.

Also in 1985, a woman who was a prostitute and intravenous drug user tested positive for HIV. Now the disease seemed to be no longer just a gay disease.

In 1986, an organization called ACT-UP was founded to help people with AIDS. A year later, its demonstrations forced the FDA to shorten by two years its process for approving new drugs against AIDS. In 1987, AZT (zidovudine) became the first anti-HIV drug approved by the FDA. The recommended dose was one 100 mg capsule every 4 hours.

In 1996, protease inhibitors allowed people to live with AIDS and go back to work. Protease inhibitors block the protease enzyme, which is needed to create new, mature particles of HIV. These drugs in combination with AZT can cost

$10,000 a year and have some severe complications. Because they require an obsessive attention to daily regimens, few people who use them work regular jobs. In sum, they are by no means a cure for AIDS.

AIDS and Ideology

Throughout the last two decades, ideology has shaped how people react to HIV and AIDS. The following social history illustrates some of those battles, which provide background for understanding how the worldwide spread of AIDS might be prevented, the "case" of this chapter.

By the end of 1981, CDC realized that gay men were being killed by a new kind of infectious disease whose nature and transmission were unknown. CDC postulated that sex among gay men might spread the disease, especially sex with anonymous partners in bathhouses in cities such as New York and San Francisco. CDC called upon federal and state governments to fund studies, but nothing was done, perhaps because of prejudice towards gay men, but probably because no one was really prepared for a totally new, deadly epidemic to appear among humans (at the time, medical experts incorrectly believed that all known lethal infectious diseases had been discovered).

Also in 1981, gay men had recently begun to win some freedom from social prejudice: psychiatrists had removed homosexuality from their list of psychiatric illnesses. Resistance against oppressive police roundups began in June 1969 at a bar called the Stonewall Inn in Greenwich Village in New York City. Such resistance to harassment fostered a new pride in being gay and gay men to "come out" of the "closet" (of shame and secrecy in which they had been hiding about their sexual identity). In North America and Europe during the 1970s and 1980s, a new freedom among gay men and lesbians had also accompanied new freedoms among heterosexuals, caused in part by availability of birth control but also by more permissive attitudes towards both nonmarital sex and illegal drugs

But much hatred remained in the populace toward gay men and especially toward sexuality among gay males. As such, gay men reacted angrily when the Reverend Jerry Falwell, who founded Moral Majority, a religious political organization, blamed gays themselves for AIDS. In 1982, the Secretary of Moral Majority, Greg Dixon, wrote, "If homosexuals are not stopped, they will in time infect the entire nation, and America will be destroyed—as entire civilizations have fallen in the past."[10] (In 2001 when the World Trade Center was destroyed, evangelists Falwell and Pat Robertson blamed gays and atheists for the event, saying it was God's punishment on America.[11])

The head of the Southern Baptist Conference said that God had created AIDS to "indicate his displeasure with the homosexual lifestyle."[12] Monsignor Edward Clark of St. John's University in Queens, New York, claimed that, "If gay men would stop promiscuous sodomy, the AIDS virus would disappear from America."[13] Politician and media commentator Patrick Buchanan decried, "The poor homosexuals—they have declared war on nature and now nature is exacting an awful retribution."[14]

Reverend Falwell advocated shutting down bathhouses where gay men engaged in anonymous sex. Owners of such bathhouses countered with ads in gay newspapers extolling freedom and lambasting Falwell as a bigot. When gay activist Larry Kramer suggested that shutting down bathhouses might just save lives of gay men, he too was ridiculed as a bigot.

Between 1983 and 1987, conservative politicians and clergy engaged in a highly political war of words about AIDS. French philosopher Michael Foucault asserted that HIV did not cause AIDS and that HIV was not spread sexually. Foucault patronized bathhouses in the 1970s and died of AIDS in 1984, becoming one of the few philosophers in history to have his views empirically refuted by his own death.

In the *New York Review of Books*, contributing editor Jonathan Lieberson, also a graduate student in philosophy at Columbia University, wrote a long article in 1986 claiming that irrationality about AIDS was running wild, that only 10 percent of HIV-infected people would get AIDS, and that contact tracing should never be used to track down sex partners of HIV-infected men, even to save lives, because the newly won freedom of gay men and their sex lives was too important to sacrifice.[15] (Lieberson died of AIDS around 1989.)

As we have seen, it was in the midst of this passionate controversy that authorities weighed whether to test America's blood, first for hepatitis, and later with the new ELISA test. Each time, those against testing won the first rounds.

Between 1981 and 1986, gay men hoped that sex did not spread HIV, that HIV did not causes AIDS, and that most people infected with HIV would not get AIDS. That changed in 1986, when researchers announced that statistical projections indicated that almost everyone infected with HIV would get AIDS.

The Kimberly Bergalis Case

In December 1987, 21-year-old Kimberly Bergalis, a junior at the University of Florida in Gainesville, had two molars extracted by dentist David Acer, a dentist in Jensen Beach, Florida, who was a "preferred provider" on her family's CIGNA dental plan.

Fifteen months later, she developed a sore throat, ulcerated tonsils, and a fungal infection of the mouth, oral thrush—common first symptoms of HIV infection. After graduating in 1990, Kimberly tested positive for HIV, and CDC began to search for the source of her infection.

A typical sorority girl who during her college years had only two boyfriends, Kimberly passionately claimed she was a virgin and could not have obtained HIV sexually; nor had she received any blood transfusions. During the summer, her family and she learned—by watching television—that the CDC had concluded that her dentist could have infected her.

A young white male in his early thirties, Dr. David Acer was gay and had sexual relations with 100 to 150 men over the previous decade. In September 1987, he developed Kaposi's sarcoma. In July 1989, he sold his practice; in this process, his dental tools and records of patients were sold or destroyed. In September 1990, he died of AIDS.

In a letter to newspapers, published coincidentally on the day of his death, Dr. Acer explained that when he had tested positive for HIV, he had contacted the American Dental Association and asked it if he should continue to practice

dentistry. The ADA told him he could do so as long as he practiced safe procedures, which he averred that he had done. Nevertheless, when his former patients
tested themselves for HIV, six tested positive.

During this case, supporters and attackers of Dr. Acer and Kimberly Bergalis
tried to manipulate and interpret the facts to their liking. Gay supporters of
Dr. Acer claimed that Kimberly Bergalis was no virgin, and the same critics said
the same about the other five infected patients (although this became increasingly
hard to justify, since one patient was an older matron). Attackers of Acer said he
had deliberately infected his patients so that others would die of AIDS with him.

A new technique used by CDC solved one mystery in this case. By using DNA
sequencing, CDC revealed that Acer was the real source of infection in all six patients because the virus in his body matched that in his six patients.

All the families felt betrayed by the health professions. The dying of Kimberly
Bergalis was very public and painful. In 1991 and after she had lost her hair and
weighed only 70 pounds, she was barely able to travel to Washington to testify before Congress. There she advocated making it a federal felony for HIV-positive
health professionals to interact with patients without revealing their HIV infection.
The law never passed and Kimberly died in December 1991 at age 23.

The media and Congress at that time pushed hard for mandatory testing for
HIV of all health professionals and revelation of all HIV+ results to patients. Both
the American Medical Association and the American Dental Association issued
new guidelines that HIV+ practitioners should either inform their patients or not
perform any invasive procedures. These guidelines have never been enforced, in
part because the AMA and ADA do not have legal powers to enforce them. According to the CDC, no other Americans have been infected by health professionals infected with HIV other than the six patients of Dr. Acer.

Exactly how or why Dr. Acer infected his patients remains somewhat of a mystery. Certainly this question raises the most passion on all sides. The dental drill bit
or a suctioning tube could have been improperly sterilized, but dentists do not normally use such equipment on themselves. A very popular view is that the dentist deliberately infected normal, heterosexual people so that Americans would no longer
see AIDS as a disease of gay men. This view charges Dr. Acer with the murder of six
of his patients. What actually happened will probably never be known for sure.

THREE ETHICAL ISSUES IN STOPPING THE SPREAD OF AIDS

Homosexuality

Some people believe that teaching gay men how to practice safe sex condones sex
between men. Although similar objections can be made to teaching any kind of
safe sex, many people feel passionately that sex between men should not be tolerated by society or education.

Homosexuality has existed for thousands of years. In ancient Greece, bisexu-
ality among men was popular, and leading Greek men such as Socrates preferred
male lovers. Also Roman emperor Hadrian was gay, as well as King Frederick
the Great of Prussia, playwright Tennessee Williams, and novelist Gore Vidal.

Surprisingly, before the twelfth century, Christianity tolerated homosexuality more than in later centuries.

In 1991, cancer researcher Simon LeVay published a paper in *Science* asserting that a specific region of the X chromosome in 40 pairs of gay men was associated with their sexual preference for men. The media dubbed this "the gay gene."

Although some skeptics see homosexuality as a choice, virtually every gay man and lesbian as teenagers report fighting against their inclination because of the norm of heterosexuality in advertising and general culture. Because the culture is heterosexual and teenagers want to fit in, most gay and lesbian teenagers resist being attracted to members of the same sex and date heterosexually. Only after a long time do most gay men and lesbians accept their sexual orientation. As such, it appears to be more of a discovery than a choice.

Many people harbor the false belief that state or federal laws protect sexual orientation. That is false. Only if Congress, a state, a city, or a county passed such a law would it be illegal to evict or fire someone because of his or her homosexuality. As it is now, except for San Francisco and two cities in Colorado, it is legal to do so almost everywhere.

Indeed, in *Bowers* v. *Hardwick,* the U. S. Supreme Court in 1988 allowed Georgia to keep a law making forms of anal and oral intercourse illegal between members of the same sex. Ironically, a footnote to the decision did not allow the state to criminalize the same behavior among heterosexuals. Obviously, this decision violates Mill's harm principle (it also cries out for an explanation of why such sexual behavior between members of the same sex is sodomy, a crime, but not when between members of different sexes).

All of which is to say that worldviews that consider homosexuality an immoral choice or evil lifestyle will be seen by gay activists and champions of education as part of the problem of spreading AIDS because of homophobia. On the other hand, moralistic views will see tolerance of homosexuality as part of the cause of the spread of AIDS.

Needle Exchange Programs

Needle exchange programs (NEPs) prevent the spread of HIV by giving drug users a clean needle and syringe each time they inject drugs, eliminating the need to share a possibly contaminated syringe. One study in New Haven, Connecticut, achieved a 33 percent reduction in HIV transmission by giving out clean needles to at-risk persons. A 1992 study by the CDC of 23 NEPs seemed to show no increase in drug usage by giving out clean needles.

But do such NEPs encourage nonusers to try hard drugs? If there were no dangers of disease from using such drugs, might not more people use them? If they were legal and risk-free, wouldn't many more people try hard drugs, and hence, many more people become addicted?

In public health, we know about *the exposure rate*. What that means is that, in most populations, a small percentage of people will always become addicted after exposure to an addictive drug, be that drug alcohol or heroin. If the same, say, 2 percent of people always become addicted, and if the numerical percentage stays roughly constant, it matters a lot whether the population exposed is 20 thousand people or 20 million.

One justification of Prohibition was to keep the population low that was exposed to alcohol. Similarly, keeping cocaine and heroin illegal keeps low the number of people exposed to these drugs.

Finally, NEPs may inadvertently increase the population exposed to hard drugs by making it safer to try them. Defenders of NEPs claim this is not so, but critics dispute this claim.

HIV Exceptionalism

In the first decade of AIDS, authorities in public health bowed to pressure from AIDS activists and did not pursue contact tracing the way they had with other sexually transmissible diseases (STDs). Because of prejudice against gay men, it was feared that tracing the exposure to HIV might lead to some men losing their medical insurance or jobs. Besides, until 1986 when AZT arrived, authorities could offer no treatment, so the benefits of identification to identified men were scant.

Today, with AZT and protease inhibitors, early notification can save lives by helping those infected get prompt treatment. Also, if a person who has been identified as HIV+ knowingly practices unsafe sex, he can be charged with a crime. In 1997, Nushawn Williams knew he was HIV+ and infected 28 teenage girls; he went to jail for doing so. In this case, contact tracing prevented even more girls from becoming infected.

HIV exceptionalism is now generally regarded in public health as a mistake. It succumbed to too much pressure from gay activists, costing some of them their lives by not pursuing contact tracing.

STOPPING THE WORLDWIDE SPREAD OF HIV: FIVE VIEWS

In the first edition of this book in 1990, it seemed shocking that by 1987, 60,000 Americans had died of AIDS, more people than had died in Vietnam, and researchers then guessed that 10 million people could be infected worldwide. A few years later in 1992, gay rights activist Larry Kramer wrote:

> When I first became aware of this disease, there were only 43 cases in the United States; now there are 12 million people infected with AIDS around the world; within the next eight years, this figure could rise to 40 million. From 43 [people] to 40 million should be enough not only to cause some level of panic, but also to make everyone ask: how is this plague spreading so quickly? Indeed, 1 million new people worldwide were infected with the AIDS virus last year alone.[16]

Now 2 decades of AIDS have given us even more perspective, and also more shocking numbers, both for America and for the world. By 2001, AIDS had killed nearly a half a million Americans, including 200,000 white males, 200,000 black or Hispanic males, and 70,000 females. Worldwide by 2001, the virus had killed 20 million people and had infected another 40 million.

How to prevent the spread of AIDS is an urgent question. Answers affect millions, perhaps billions, of people who are at risk of HIV infection. More lives could be saved by stopping the spread of AIDS than by all of modern medicine's surgery, drugs, and high-tech interventions.

If moral actions create the greatest good for the greatest number of humans, then stopping deaths from AIDS is the greatest problem today of medical ethics. In the next 10 years, if past trends continue unchanged, the 40 million people now infected with HIV may pass it to another 40, 50, or 60 million.

In the countries of China, Russia, Ethiopia, Nigeria, and India—the five countries with the greatest concentrations of HIV infection—the number of people infected by 2010 could easily be 75 million. South Africa in 2002 has 5 million HIV+, mostly adults. Eastern Europe and Central Asia (the Ukraine, Kazakhstan, etc.) also have a million infected, due to large numbers of people using intravenous drugs.

Part of the controversy about reducing the spread of HIV is a moral one. Do we attack the behavior or the microbe in trying to stop the spread? Do we use nonmoralistic education or moralistic condemnation? Is money spent on education in developing countries helpful or wasted? Are cheap anti-AIDS drugs worthwhile when the numbers infected keep doubling and when many lack clean water? Would it be more efficient to instigate medical triage and ignore those dying in whole countries to concentrate resources where they might save the most lives? These are the questions for the rest of this chapter.

The following section sketches five views of how to stop AIDS from spreading further around the world. This section also features some exchanges between proponents of the different views.

The Educational Approach

In 2002, the Global HIV Prevention Working Group, funded by the Gates and Kaiser Foundations, praised Thailand as a model of how to reduce the spread of HIV. This country instituted a national campaign for 100 percent use of condoms, used advertising on television and community leaders to educate teenagers and drug users about the prevention of HIV, allowed free access to testing and counseling, and protected those infected with HIV against discrimination. These efforts reduced new infections by 89 percent in Thailand.

Similar efforts worked in Uganda when led by President Yoweri Museveni, and featured testimonials on radio and television by famous Ugandans diagnosed with HIV. During the 1990s, the rate of HIV infection dropped by half in rural areas and dropped by two-thirds in urban, pregnant women.

Efforts in education about AIDS focus on producing safe supplies of blood, educating injectors of drugs who use needles and syringes, offering small dosages of AZT to pregnant, HIV+ mothers to prevent transmission of HIV to their babies, and implementing programs promoting exchange of clean needles. They also work to improve the empowerment of women in countries where they are abused and treated like chattel.

Such programs cost lots of money and success depends on funding by the United States and Europe. Although the cost may seem extravagant, the cost of funding efforts to stop AIDS is only 5 percent of what these countries pay to subsidize large farmers in the their own countries, resulting in higher prices for food for consumers and rounds of retaliatory protectionism in world markets. A wiser use of money would be to protect rich farmers less and to prevent AIDS more.

Tough Love

Decades ago, conservatives such as William Buckley proposed mandatory testing for HIV and tattooing anyone who tested positive. Cuba initiated quarantine for anyone testing HIV+, which resulted in a very low rate of HIV infection there.

Cuba, of course, is a dictatorship, whereas quarantine could not legally be done in the United States because doing so would violate legal rights to liberty and freedom from incarceration without committing a crime of Americans who are HIV+. But it could be done in other parts of the world where AIDS threatens to wipe out entire generations, e.g., in South Africa where 1 in 10 adults is HIV+.

Such draconian measures would never work in America, where testing positive for HIV in North America gives one *presumptive disability* and benefits under a special branch of Social Security for those with disabilities. As such, HIV-infected people are protected under the Americans with Disabilities Act against being fired or evicted. As such, gay men who are HIV-infected ironically gain rights they otherwise would never have.

Mandatory testing followed by a tattoo somewhere on the body would identify someone as HIV+ and therefore as a risky sexual partner. Although invasive of privacy and personal bodily integrity, this practice might save some lives.

A major problem in stopping the spread of HIV is that the people prevented from acquiring HIV infection are statistical and anonymous, whereas the people who must be restricted or harmed to prevent spread of HIV are real and tangible. If a physician reveals to a patient's partner that the patient has infected him or her, over the patient's dissent, the physician injures the patient's interests. But if the partner may spread HIV further, either sexually, by using drugs, or by giving blood, then the physician's actions seem to be justified for the greater good.

Nevertheless, western medical ethics respect patient autonomy and the confidentiality of the physician–patient relationship. Notifying possibly infected partners of a patient violates confidentiality and values the good of others more than autonomy of patients.

Many people cringe at the idea of mandatory testing, contact tracing, tattoos, and quarantine, but stopping the spread of drastic epidemics requires drastic measures. If we merely do what we have done until now, in other words, try to educate potential victims about safe sex and drugs, then it seems likely that 30 to 40 million people will become HIV-infected in the next decades.

Are we really so weak that we must allow that to happen? Are autonomy and privacy really so important that this many people must be sacrificed for these values?

Besides, the expected increase in funding necessary for the preventive efforts of the Education View is unlikely to occur. So, where are we then? Back to watching the number of HIV-infected people soar to 60 million?

We need to triage countries such as South Africa where President Mubekki publicly resists the fact that HIV causes AIDS and where he not only does not lead the fight against spread of HIV but helps to spread it by his poor example. Similarly, in Zimbabwe, where the dictator Mugabe won't let starving people in his country eat genetically modified Starlink corn because he fears western science, the leadership is part of the problem of stopping the spread of AIDS.

Pouring money and time into these countries seems to be a waste. The point of triage is to leverage interventions to where they leverage at-risk life into life. So we ignore countries that don't need our help (North America, Europe) and also countries where nothing we do will make much difference. Then we focus on countries such as Thailand and Uganda, where leaders are ready for change and the people can be quickly educated.

The main problem with using Tough Love in stopping AIDS is that it hasn't been tough enough. In Cuba, NuShawn Williams would have been executed. What if the government of Ethiopia condemned to die any man who infected a woman with HIV and did a DNA matching test to prove which man infected her?

The Structuralist View

Some researchers, especially in anthropology, believe that colonialism, racism, class injustice, and imperialism spread AIDS and that AIDS will continue until these evils are stopped. Anthropologist Stephanie Kane believes that, "We have the scientific understanding and the technology to stop war, pollution, and AIDS." For her, conservative moralism cannot stop AIDS and actually spreads it:

> AIDS prevention can itself be used as an alibi for consolidating political and economic interests around archaic moral pretenses, such as perverted purveyors of abstinence-only sex education for sexually active youth or the closure of sex-related business to hasten the Disneyfication of New York City's Times Square.[17]

Early epidemiological studies that identified homosexuals, hemophiliacs, and intravenous drug users wrongly, in her opinion, "led to nearly universal overemphasis on individual behavioral change in AIDS prevention campaigns, campaigns that ignore underlying social forces that condition risk . . . in many people's lives.

In other words, education won't work unless people's lives improve to the point where they won't risk their life shooting drugs or having unprotected sex.

So how does she think we should stop the spread of AIDS? Her main idea is to legalize all drugs and use the money previously spent on fighting drugs to treat people with HIV and drug addiction. In addition, we need to "alleviate poverty as a cofactor in the epidemic." Finally, we need "to launch unflinching educational campaigns," by which she means be really tough and frank about sex, drugs, and HIV, teaching 6-year-olds how to use condoms and how not to get infected shooting up.

But poverty has been around a long time, and it may be easier to eliminate AIDS than to eliminate poverty, especially if some riches and some poverty result from people's free-willed decisions about their habits, choices, and lives.

Moreover, other social scientists have described the Exposure Problem: should drugs be legalized? When drugs are illegal, many fewer people are exposed to addictive drugs; if legalized, a much higher number of people will be exposed.

As with alcohol, about the same percentage will become addicted permanently whether addictive drugs are legal or illegal, but the numbers jump dramatically with legalization because millions more people sample previously banned drugs. So legalization of addictive drugs, even if done with clean needles, has a high human cost.

Finally, part of the culture of addictive drugs is the communal aspect, even the aspect of trust of sharing the same needle. Other social scientists such as Klerman emphasize the social construction of disease, and use of recreational drugs is paradigm of such a social construction. In other words, even with legalization, it is not clear how or why sharing of drugs would cease, and hence, how the spread of HIV would cease.

The Cynical View

Every American now knows he can be an organ donor or donate organs of a deceased relative, yet most people do not donate. Champions of the Education view say more education will get more people to donate, but if this were true, it would have worked by now.

Similarly, education and counseling will only go so far if people themselves don't care for their own safety. After 20 years, and regardless of whether you call it AIDS or "slim disease (a common name in Africa for AIDS), most adults on the planet know that having unprotected sex, getting a transfusion of blood, or sharing needles can get you infected with HIV. If your own motivation doesn't protect you from HIV, do-gooder education certainly won't.

Jeffrey Fisher, director of Center for HIV Prevention at the University of Connecticut at Storrs, criticizes most AIDS education as bland and generic, hence, of little value in teaching teenagers how to negotiate usage of condoms during sex or how to safely use hard drugs. "We lack the political will to implement these things," he says.[18]

Among large portions of the world, primal, recurring drives for sexual pleasure, fueled by poor judgment under the influence of alcohol and other drugs, lead people to practice unprotected sex. In Russia and China, despair over the conversion to capitalism has fueled widespread use of drugs.

All these forces will swamp any educational efforts. Wisdom lies in recognizing that we can't control the private actions of most people of the world. Here, wisdom lies in keeping a candle lit as the darkness grows.

Survivors will be fastidiously aware of what behaviors can kill them, and teach their children to be similarly aware. Sure, a billion people may die from AIDS, but humanity will go on. Plagues, flus, and floods have wiped out similar percentages of humanity before, but humanity has survived. It is all part of our Darwinian evolution.

Moralism, Resurrected

The Education view is way too permissive. It is time to rejuvenate old-fashioned moral condemnation. How can we prevent AIDS by countering unprotected sex and sharing of intravenous drugs when at the same time millions of teenagers are getting high on alcohol, ecstasy, and marijuana, as well as having premarital sex? Isn't it time that we call it like it is and say that current, permissive attitudes towards sex and drugs are not just part of the problem, but the real problem?

Of course, adopting this view would mean holding ourselves up for scrutiny. If we tell teenagers not to smoke or use drugs, then we must stop smoking cigarettes and drinking alcohol.

Maybe unfashionable, isn't old-fashioned moralism better than triaging 20 million people or worse, doing what cynics want, forgetting about them? At least, moralism directed at a person says that someone *cares* about the one condemned (versus the "belle indifference" of the lofty cynic looking down haughtily at the masses below).

Moralism can be implemented in small, faith-based communities, such as where a missionary wields power in an African village. Money, food, and supplies, combined with faith and good-will, can perhaps set a good example of abstinence and sex-within-marriage. Such an approach will also combat slavery and sexual exploitation of women and children, and be compatible with Islamic views popular in some African countries.

Secular public health proposals that emphasize education may be inappropriate for faith-based, poor communities, where many people are illiterate and ignorant of the most basic scientific facts. Because AIDS is lethal and because a person only has to get infected once to get a lethal disease, such populations cannot wait to be taught to read or to be taught basic science. They need a solution now, and moralism just might be the solution.

Public Health Responds

First, what's wrong with moralism in public health is that it really serves the emotions and ego of the moralizer, not the one condemned. Moralizing did nothing to stop gay men from having sex after AIDS was discovered, but fear of death did. Moralizing only made matters worse.

The key claim is that moralizing can change behavior. Is that true? One argument that it won't is that a lot of moralism has already been directed against using drugs, much less intravenous drugs. Similarly, a lot of moralism has been directed toward not having sex outside marriage, but has it worked?

Second, cynicism and triage are too pessimistic. Why not generalize that attitude and let everyone starve, too? Or go without penicillin? Why bother about the rest of the planet at all? Why not let the undeveloped world fight it out among themselves and let the rich nations keep them at a distance, away from their shores?

But is this a moral point of view? For us to have so many blessing and to refuse to share them with the rest of the planet? What would the Golden Rule say?

And to take it the other way, if we're not concerned about the rest of the planet, why should we be concerned with anyone farther than 5 miles away? Or anyone at all outside our friends and family?

Finally, the very essence of public health morality is to fight pragmatically for the good of the many, especially using governmental powers. If we give up on that assumption, we might as well give up on public health having any role at all in stopping the worldwide spread of AIDS.

The Cynic Replies

The Education View responds to our claim by sounding like a moralist, appealing to the Golden Rule and unselfishness. He has shifted his claim from a pragmatic claim about what *will* work, and what *can* be done to a claim about what we *should* still try, despite failures. But he begs the question against us by appealing to moral principles we may not share.

Indeed, we might reply, "You're right. If there are 6 billion people now on the planet and a billion of them die of AIDS, mostly on the other side of the planet and all unknown to me, I really don't care one way or the other. I change the channel when such stories come up on the news. I may be morally deficient, but I am at least honest in telling you that I have no moral feelings of compassion, shame, or outrage about such deaths from AIDS. It's going to happen: it's a fact of life; I don't think governments or missionaries can do anything about it, and that's just the way it is."

Conclusions

Stopping the spread of AIDS is not easy, and one reason is that people are divided ethically about how we should do it. One person's solution is another's problem.

If that conclusion is correct, there may be only two ways to stop AIDS. First, one implements his view on a small scale, perhaps in a province, where the view can be fully implemented, top to bottom of society. Whether that is moralism or education, given different religious backgrounds, provincial leaders, and scientific understanding, a particular view might work better in one region rather than another.

The most promising solution would be a workable vaccine. The Bill and Melinda Gates Foundation is funding work on such a vaccine, but so far, work over the last decades has failed to create one.

As we saw with the discovery of penicillin, even if we had a successful vaccine, we can anticipate resistance to implementing it from some of the views above. But just as penicillin was quickly accepted by the medical profession, it is likely that a vaccine for AIDS would be, too.

FURTHER READING

B. McCarthy et al., "Who Should Be Screened for HIV Infection?" *Archives of Internal Medicine*, vol. 153, May 10, 1993, pp.1107–1116.

Carol Pogash, *As Real As It Gets: The Life of a Hospital at the Center of the AIDS Epidemic*, Birch Lane, Carol Publishing Group, New York, 1992.

T. Quinn, "Screening for HIV Infection: Benefits and Costs," *New England Journal of Medicine*, vol. 327, no. 7, August 13, 1992, pp. 486–488.

Randy Shilts, *And the Band Played On*, St. Martin's, New York, 1987.

Abraham Verghese, *My Own Country*, Simon & Schuster, New York, 1994.

"Turning The Tide on the AIDS Epidemic," W. J. Clinton, and "Curbing the Global AIDS Epidemic." H. D. Gayle, New England Journal of Medicine, vol. 348, no. 18, May 1, 2003, pp. 1800–1805.

CHAPTER 18

Reforming the American Medical System

Expanding Medicare?

*S*hould you have to risk death because you work in a job that doesn't provide medical coverage? For over 40 million Americans, that is a question they wonder about every time they get sick and consider seeing a physician.

America has a strange system of medical finance that covers four groups of people through federal monies: seniors over age 65 (Medicare), very poor people through systems jointly funded by states (Medicaid), people with kidney disease (End Stage Renal Disease Act), and people declared disabled (covered under a special section of Social Security/Medicare). Every working person in America is taxed to pay for medical services for these four groups of people.

Yet many of the 40 million Americans without medical coverage also work. So they pay for medical coverage of others while getting nothing in return. Obviously this is unfair to them, but how should we change?

Some propose that we make small businesses purchase coverage for all their employees, but such businesses object that they should not be forced to bear the costs for an expansion of medical coverage. And such a proposal would not cover the self-employed or the unemployed under age 65.

This chapter explores how America got to this point, how countries such as Canada and Germany provide medical coverage in different ways, and arguments for and against a national, single-payer system like the one in Canada.

BACKGROUND: PROBLEMS OF MEDICAL CARE IN THE UNITED STATES

Problems of the System: Three Examples

Reformers of the American system of medical care want increased access to the system, or even *universal access*—that is, coverage for all Americans. The following cases illustrate problems of getting medical care in the United States.

William Hunter   When professional wrestler William Hunter lost his liver at age 27, possibly due to anti-seizure medication he had been taking, he entered the

444

Medical University of South Carolina at Charleston (MUSC) where liver transplants are done, without thinking about his medical insurance.[1] But MUSC did not have a contract for such transplants with Hunter's health plan, Physician's Health Plan (PHP), so Hunter was transferred to Duke Medical Center, which supposedly did have the PHP contract for liver transplants.

As Duke's surgeons searched for a liver for their sick patient, their financial coordinator realized that Hunter was "out of network" because Duke did not in fact have the liver contract with PHP. So Hunter might have an operation that could cost $1 million with no one to reimburse Duke.

When PHP was contacted, they wanted Hunter moved to a hospital where their capitation contract limited their financial exposure—in this case, to UAB, 600 miles away. Meanwhile, Hunter was deteriorating and Duke's surgeons were trying to do what was medically best for Hunter. Another call from PHP demanded that Hunter be moved to North Carolina Medical Center (UNC), 20 minutes away. The reason Hunter hadn't been moved there originally is that it was only a few days before that PHP had sold its liver business to United Resources Network (URN), which had cut a deal with UNC a few days before that.

While waiting for a liver at Duke, Hunter slipped into a coma, his skin turning yellow from jaundice, with PHP all the while demanding that he be transferred to UNC, the hospital that held the contract for liver transplants. A few days later, while he was still at Duke, a liver became available, and Hunter was transplanted there, with payment by PHP up in the air. To complicate matters, a general contract between PHP and Duke with a liver-transplant financial cap was under negotiation, and this case might sabotage it.

Hunter's transplant was successful, but he must take anti-rejection drugs for the rest of his life, at a monthly cost of $1,500. How much Duke will be reimbursed by PHP is unresolved; Hunter must stay in PHP because no other insurance company will insure him with his now preexisting condition.

Rosalyn Schwartz   Rosalyn Schwartz, age 47, white, lives in Ridgefield, New Jersey; she has one child, Andy. She lost her medical coverage when she and her husband divorced in 1987.[2] At that time, the gift-wrap company where she worked with five other employees (she was then making around $19,000 a year) provided no medical coverage, though it was considering doing so soon. When Rosalyn Schwartz tried to buy an individual policy, several insurance companies informed her that *if* they offered her a policy, the premiums would be about $4,000 a year, since she had a preexisting condition—an ulcer. Moreover, no policy would cover any treatment for the ulcer.

In 1988, Rosalyn Schwartz found a small lump in her breast. Her physician said it might be cancerous and recommended removing it; but she asked if that could wait until her employer provided medical coverage. The physician agreed to postpone the surgery.

In late 1989, while cooking, Rosalyn Schwartz turned abruptly, and pain suddenly tore through her hip. Unbeknownst to her, the breast cancer had metastazied and had eaten into her hip, making the hip bones as fragile as glass. When she fell to the floor, her hip socket shattered. In the ambulance, she sobbed and could think only of the costs. "Andy, you've just turned 18," she said. "I have no insurance. Tell them [at the hospital] I have no insurance. But don't sign anything or you'll be responsible."

Rosalyn Schwartz was hospitalized for 23 days, during which she had surgery three times. The total cost was over $40,000. Half of that was paid by a charity; the rest went onto her own bill, which she is now paying off—$10 a month to each of 12 physicians.

Her surgery has left her unable to work. She receives Medicare disability benefits, amounting to about $10,500 a year. When she tried again to buy medical coverage, she found that it would still cost her $4,000 a year, and that it would not cover any procedure for her cancer, since the cancer was now another preexisting condition.

Lacking insurance, she is not getting physical therapy to help her adjust to her hip replacement—nor can she afford a bone scan to make sure the cancer has not spread.

Denise and Randy Sadler   Many Americans have medical insurance but are afraid to use it. Women who are found to have a genetic marker for hereditary breast cancer are reluctant to tell their medical insurer why they want a radical mastectomy, since their premiums might then be raised or they might lose their coverage altogether.

Randy Sadler owns a tile business in Kernersville, North Carolina; his wife, Denise Sadler, is a part-time worker for the Census Bureau. Together, in 1992 they made about $35,000 a year—a figure that was close to the median in the United States. One of the Sadlers' sons has severe allergies and repeatedly develops pneumonia; Denise Sadler has migraine headaches and episodes of depression.

The Sadlers have two medical insurance policies: one for Denise and their sons, with a yearly deductible of $500; and another for Randy, with a $1,000 deductible. These policies cost them a total of $2,500 per year, and they are trying to get a 5 percent reduction in premiums by not filing a claim for 1 year. Because they do not feel that they can use their policies for anything short of a catastrophe they spend $100 to $200 each month on prescription drugs and physicians' bills. Denise says, "I still feel like we have no insurance."[3]

Problems of Costs: Richard Lamm's Critique

Richard Lamm, who was governor of Colorado from 1978 to 1987, set off a national debate about exorbitant medical costs in 1987 when he attacked the high costs of organ transplants and the amounts often spent on the last years of life. His remarks were published in 1987 in the journal *Dialysis and Transplantation*:

> Health care is clearly entering into a new era: Infinite health needs have run into finite resources. The miracles of medicine have outstripped our ability to pay, and some thoughtful and equitable thinking has to be done to ensure that America gets the most health care for its limited dollars.
>
> It is a very serious mistake to deny that a major change is in the wings. No sector of the economy, no matter how important, can continue to grow at two-and-a-half times the rate of inflation. We are heading rapidly toward an America that has

rusting plants, closed factories, staggering trade deficits. Health care cannot continue to operate under the illusion that it can continue business as usual.

Once we accept the fact that there are limits to what the nation can afford (and increasingly, people are recognizing this truth), then we will begin a process of asking how to get the most health benefits for the most Americans for our money. We should have asked this question years ago. It is outrageous that this country spends five to eight times what other countries spend, and yet has no better health outcome. America is going to demand more accountability for the more than one billion dollars a day it now spends on health care. Many countries give a high level of health care to all their citizens for a fraction of what we spend, and yet keep them healthier. We are no longer rich enough to give a blank check to an inefficient health care industry.

Once we start to apply even minimum management standards to the health care industry, we will see some substantial changes. If we ask how to get the most health benefits for the greatest number of Americans for our tax dollars, many of today's practices will not meet the test. If we zero-budget all that we now do in health care, we shall inevitably close unnecessary hospitals, close excess ICU units, and look much more closely at utilization factors and outcomes. We shall have to develop a concept of cost-effective medicine. Virtually every health care provider will agree that much of what we do today in medicine has "marginal utility." When a society faces fiscal reality and seeks to optimize its dollars, it not only starts on the road to financial sanity, but it also brings dramatic change to existing medical practices. Dialysis and transplantation will undoubtedly undergo major change. The "opportunity costs" in other areas of medicine are clearly greater than much of what is being done today. The bottom line is that we can save more lives and bring better health care to more Americans for many of the dollars we are spending today.

Economist Lester Thurow suggests that, to impress upon health providers what they are doing when they order marginal services, we should require them to imagine an American worker sentenced to a period of slavery long enough to pay the medical bill for that procedure. Dr. Thomas Starzl recently gave a liver transplant to a 76-year-old woman. It cost $240,000. Dr. Starzl should understand that with the average U.S. family making $24,000 a year, he has sentenced 10 U.S. families to work all year so that he could transplant a 76-year-old woman.

Such actions are cheating our children of resources they desperately need to build a better life and to revitalize the United States economically. If all of us, or even a significant percentage of us, take $240,000 in high-tech medicine as we are on our way out the door, we are stealing resources that our children and our grandchildren desperately need. Health care is important, but it cannot be the only value of our society. It cannot continue on its growth curve without bankrupting America.

Health providers are not used to thinking this way. Many of you will cry foul and think this heresy. But alas—it is true. A nation that runs $200 billion deficits and borrows 20 cents from its children out of every dollar it spends must one day demand more accountability from its politicians, from its industries, and from its health providers. That day is near at hand, and we should welcome it— for our children's sakes.[4]

When Governor Lamm's speech became widely quoted, the sharp knives of critics left Lamm bloody and politically wounded, but he addressed the common good of many Americans as no one else had done. His observations highlight many of the questions that arise when the cost of the American medical system is being evaluated. Specifically, should existing Americans borrow from future ones to pay their medical bills?

Problems of Allocation: Limiting Health Care

Rationing   During the 1980s, the American medical system operated increasingly by informal schemes of rationing. *Rationing* is a vague, ambiguous term, and in discussions of finances in American medicine, it refers to both social and individual decisions. That is, medical services can be limited by eliminating some category of service to everyone, by eliminating specific services to some category of people, or by limiting specific services to specific individuals.

The foremost example of medical rationing in the United States today is found in health maintenance organizations (HMOs), plans for group medical care. Physicians in HMOs are required to justify their decisions, and they must allocate care among the members of the plan—the patients—by rationing: HMOs try to provide only justifiable care and to deny unjustifiable care. Employers who offer medical insurance favor HMOs, because an HMO costs less than other kinds of coverage.

Here are examples of rationing by HMOs: Physicians are discouraged from prescribing antibiotics for common colds or giving cortisone injections for minor sprains. At the same time, physicians are encouraged to urge pregnant patients to come in for regular examinations. In theory, the money saved by denying unnecessary care, such as unneeded antibiotics and cortisone, makes it possible to spend more on preventive care, such as monitoring a pregnancy. Moreover, it is claimed (though perhaps on the basis more of ideology than of fact) that preventive care itself saves money by forestalling curative intervention.

It should be emphasized that members of HMOs do not always get what they want from their physicians. In an HMO, costs are reduced by denying some things which patients have traditionally received but which may not be financially or medically justified, such as immediate access to a physician for a minor complaint. A physician commonly must receive prior approval from an HMO official before starting an expensive treatment. Physicians in some HMOs receive yearly bonuses based on how much money has been saved by their rationing decisions, and this kind of financial incentive can pit physicians and administrators against patients.

Does the average independent American physician ration care? Yes and no.

In the past, physicians were not expected to ration care; today, new systems such as managed care plans are forcing physicians to consider costs at each step of treatment, and almost every physician has some patients whose coverage is managed or limited in some way. This creates conflicts for physicians: Their traditional self-concept as good Samaritans may contradict their new role as gatekeepers.[5] Their loyalties split between doing what is best for each patient and contributing to an efficient, prudent system.

Does American society ration? The answer is only indirectly. Priorities are established, but not in the conscious, nationally consistent way that has characterized medical systems in other western countries such as England and Canada. In the United States, to see where medical resources are flowing, we need to see which medical specialties are flourishing—and to discover that, we simply need to see which ones are reimbursed well. Because independent American physicians work on a fee-for-service system, and because they are increasingly allowed to own part of facilities providing medical care (to the consternation of some critics), they provide most medical services where the money is best. Thus Americans have the latest programs of angioplasty, oncology, and liver transplants because medical plans and their subscribers pay for these things. In other words, the American system rations, in effect, by deciding how well to reimburse each specialty.

Who makes social decisions about rationing? That is often very difficult to determine. Insurance companies make some decisions, of course: For instance, they pay "usual and customary" fees of surgeons, who steadily raise their fees and perform more and more surgery; then, insurers pass these increased costs along to policyholders in the form of higher premiums. This is a social system, of sorts, although Americans have never voted on it and have never agreed to be taxed to fund it. It just continues to career along—a strange situation.

To see how these levels of rationing—HMOs, independent physicians, and society—can operate, consider two medical situations: hemophilia and heart attacks.

Hemophiliacs need what is known as a *clotting factor.* The first clotting factor, which became available in the 1960s, was formed from the blood of 2,000 donors; some later donors were infected with human immunodeficiency virus (HIV), the causative agent in AIDS, and by 1985, over 70 percent of hemophiliac recipients in the United States had been infected[6]. Although today's natural clotting factors are much safer, they are not entirely risk-free for HIV. A new synthetic recombinant-DNA clotting factor is now available from a commercial producer, and this new factor would prevent the remaining 30 percent of hemophiliacs from being infected. However, it has been patented, and its pure form costs $45,000 to $50,000 a month—or more than $500,000 a year—per patient.[7]

With regard to heart attacks, there are two drugs that can reduce damage. The older drug, streptokinase, is made from bacteria and costs about $240 per dose. The new drug, tissue plasminogen activator (TPA), is a genetically engineered, patented substance costing $2,400 a dose. TPA appears to be slightly more effective than streptokinase,[8] but it costs 10 times as much. In other words, a slight improvement in outcome entails a disproportionate increase in costs, though if cost were not a consideration, most patients would prefer to receive TPA and most physicians would prefer to prescribe it.

In such situations, HMOs would typically opt for the cheaper treatment. An independent physician would typically opt for the more expensive treatment only if the patient's insurer would pay for it; however, in the specific case of the synthetic clotting factor probably no medical insurance plan could afford to pay that much, and in the specific case of TPA the general recommendation would probably be simply that a patient should get either streptokinase or TPA as opposed to nothing at all. On the social level, there is no real policy on the clotting factor or TPA.

These trends in rationing in the United States may not look very impressive. Rationing by HMOs often seems to be at odds with patients' interests; rationing by independent physicians seems to be based mainly on patients' coverage rather than on medical considerations; and rationing by society seems to be essentially unplanned (to take just one example, as discussed in Chapter 12, society continued to fund artificial hearts—despite very poor outcomes—until criticism became too intense). Nevertheless, as Lamm point outs, rationing is inevitable; without some kind of rationing, the American system of medical care will go bankrupt.

Organ replacement has come to symbolize unreasonable costs in the American medical system, a fact that is reflected in Lamm's commentary. As discussed in

Chapter 13, there has been no rationing at all for dialysis since Congress passed the End Stage Renal Disease Act (ESRDA) in 1972; and recent decisions about allocating organs for transplant have occurred largely behind closed doors within the medical profession. The issue with expensive treatments like dialysis and transplants is that enormous amounts of money are being spent on relatively few recipients while millions of Americans are not receiving basic medical care. Since almost no one can afford, say, a $250,000 liver transplant, such a transplant amounts to a transfer payment to one person from many others, enforced by public policy.

Expensive transplants therefore raise questions of justice, and these questions could become especially acute if there is a technical breakthrough—if, for instance, xenografts become feasible—or if the number of donor organs rises significantly, so that many more organ transplants are possible. So far, despite the high cost of each transplant, a persistent shortage of donor organs has constrained the total cost of transplants; but if the supply of donor organs rises, the total cost will skyrocket. Then, rationing will be essential.

The Oregon Plan   At least one state limited expensive, dramatic interventions for the few in order to extend basic medical care to more of the poor. In the late 1980s, Oregon established a bold plan, the Oregon Health Plan (OHP), for its state Medicaid fund. Medicaid is the system of medical care for the poor administered by each state, with matching funds from the federal government.

The Oregon legislature passed the first version of OHP in 1987. After much discussion, including debate in the legislature and town meetings for the public, certain conclusions had emerged about medical priorities; and under the original OHP, 709 medical conditions were listed in decreasing order of importance and outcomes. Funds saved by withholding low-priority care—interventions that were too expensive or promised only poor outcomes—would be used to provide basic care to people who were poor and uninsured, and also to help employers pay for private insurance. The goal was to require all employers, even small businesses, to offer basic coverage by 1995 or to pay a new payroll tax—hence the phrase "pay or play." Low-priority interventions which would not be funded by Oregon's Medicaid system included in vitro fertilization, experimental therapies for late-stage AIDS patients, heart transplants, liver transplants, bone-marrow transplants for leukemia (such a transplant costs $100,000), and care in neonatal intensive care units (NICUs) for premature babies weighing under 750 grams at birth. (With regard to the last item, it can be noted that the cost of care for these babies in NICUs is exorbitant, and as few as perhaps 12 percent will emerge unimpaired to lead a normal life; in one study of such babies, only about half lived, and 75 percent of those had neurological damage.[9])

Oregon democratically developed a public policy about medical financing and treatment. Not surprisingly, though, when the parents of a child with leukemia, 7-year-old Coby Howard, learned in 1988 that Medicaid would not pay for a bone-marrow transplant, they appealed to the news media, hoping the rule of rescue would work. The media were in a bind: Although journalists were well aware that they were being used, the case of Coby Howard was real news. Here was a patient who would be denied treatment under OHP and would therefore die. Would the public in Oregon simply accept his death? The Oregon legislature did hear a plea by Coby's mother, as well as pleas by relatives of two other patients who needed transplants, but it did not change OHP or grant exemptions. All three families also appealed for donations through the media, but the public did not respond. Coby Howard died a few months later.

The reaction outside Oregon was different. OHP was rejected by President Bush's Secretary of Health and Human Services (HHS), Louis Sullivan: He would not release federal matching funds for Oregon's Medicaid program. Sullivan was particularly concerned about OHP's exclusion of people with disabilities, especially since this exclusion also applied to premature babies whose birthweight was under 750 grams.

Oregon then modified OHP to comply with the Americans with Disabilities Act (ADA, 1992), providing coverage even for babies under 500 grams.[10] In March 1993, the Clinton administration accepted this new version of OHP; in fact, it was reportedly a model for Clinton's own Health Care Security bill.

However, OHP ran into trouble in 1993. The legislature had appropriated $34 million for Medicaid, but in that year the costs of the program rose to $84 million—at a time when the state budget was already facing a $1.2 billion shortfall.[11] In 2002, Oregonians voted 4 to 1 against creating a statewide system guaranteeing medical coverage to every Oregonian. The costs imposed on small businesses of doing so was the stumbling block. About 400,000 Oregonians were never covered by OHP.

A Comparative Perspective: Health Care in Germany and Canada

In discussing medical care in the United States, it is useful to have some points of comparison, so the German and Canadian systems will be discussed here.

Germany has a national health care system, financed by more than 1,100 insurance funds. Each person joins one fund early in life and remains in that fund thereafter. Germans see physicians of their choice, choose physicians who can order the treatments they want, and wait no longer for appointments or admission to hospitals than Americans do. In 1990, Germany spent 8.5 percent of its gross national product (GNP), or roughly $1,286 per person, on health care; that year the United States spent nearly 12 percent of its GNP on health care—roughly $3,500 per person. Germany, then, was succeeding in insuring all its citizens at a much lower cost.

There is an explanation for this difference. The German government plays a much greater role in health care than the American government; and in Germany, the government has put a ceiling on physicians' fees, that is, on how much a physician can charge a patient—a restraint which American physicians have vehemently resisted. (To earn more money, German physicians can only try to see more patients.) On the other hand, the decisions of German physicians are not second-guessed by third parties as they are in the United States, and this aspect of the German system appeals to many American physicians.[12]

In the 1990s, however, Germany's medical system came back to haunt it after the unification of East and West Germany, creating a situation where workers had lavish medical benefits, including two weeks at a spa, at a time when the economy could not create enough jobs for all the (formerly-employed) workers of East

Germany. Paying for medical benefits made hiring workers in Germany expensive and as a result, Daimler-Benz located new assembly plants for Mercedes cars in cheaper places such as Alabama. By the end of the decade, everyone agreed that the German system provided too many benefits and was too expensive, but no one knew quite how to reel it in.

•

Canada has a fund for national medical coverage, much like the American social security system. This fund covers the medical care of every Canadian; it is universal, portable (meaning you can carry it with you anywhere), and publicly administered through a single-payer system, and it covers all medically necessary services. The single-payer system is financed partly by high "sin" taxes on cigarettes and alcohol. Each of Canada's provinces sets its own policies and allocates medical care by regulating the supply of medical services. For example, each province funds only a small number of hospitals, CAT-scanners, and lithotripters (expensive machines that break up kidney stones with sound waves). So Canada rations the supply of expensive medical services.

Physicians in Canada do not work for the Canadian government; like independent American physicians, they work for themselves and bill on a fee-for-service basis. Canadian physicians cannot set their own fees, however, and this is what American physicians dislike about the Canadian system; but it should be noted that under the American system, costs are borne by the taxpayers and by people who insure themselves—and that Canadian physicians are far from poor. In American dollars, in 1991, cardiologists in Canada earned $290,500 on average; ophthalmologists, $240,500; dermatologists, $200,500; and general practitioners, $128,000.[13] There are fewer specialists in Canada than in the United States, though, because the Canadian system discourages specialization whereas the American system encourages it.

The Canadian system costs less than $2,000 (in American dollars) per capita and covers all Canadians; the American system costs $3,500 per capita and leaves over 40 million Americans uncovered.

Canadians are extremely proud of their medical system, especially when they contrast it with medical care in the United States. Here are some examples:

- In Canada, every pregnant woman gets free care. In the United States, 17 percent of women in childbirth experience not only the inevitable, natural fears and pain but also the anxiety of having no medical coverage to pay for their hospitalization or their physicians' bills.[14]
- In Canada, all citizens are eligible for long-term nursing home care. Although they must pay for a portion of such care (about $19 of the $67 which is the typical cost per day), this is an affordable option for most of them. In the United States, virtually no one has coverage for long-term care in a nursing home; to become eligible for Medicaid, which pays for bare-bones nursing home care, elderly Americans must "spend down" until their assets are virtually gone.[15]
- Canada generously covers people with extraordinary medical needs. In one Canadian family, for instance, the 8-year-old son was retarded and had a rare brain disease, tubular sclerosis, characterized by severe mood swings, tumors

on several organs, skin rashes, and seizures; he wore a diaper and had the mental age of a 4-year-old. The father earned the equivalent of $12,000 (American) a year. This boy had seen a physician 40 times within 2 years and had been hospitalized three times, but the family had never received a bill. In the United States, this family's income in many states would disqualify them from Medicaid.[16]

In one poll, only 3 percent of Canadians considered the American medical system superior to their own. (It must be admitted, though, that nearly 30 percent thought Elvis Presley might still be alive.)

American physicians often say that Canadians must wait for some kinds of care. Strictly speaking, that is true, but it may not be as significant as many Americans conclude. To take just one example, a lithotripter, a machine that breaks up kidney stones with sound waves, is available in the province of Nova Scotia only in one city, Halifax. Moreover, a patient in Nova Scotia may have to wait three months for an appointment to use it. However, most stone-busting is preventive; most kidney stones eventually drop and pass through the ureter; and surgery is available as an emergency alternative to lithotripsy. Furthermore, the only way to diminish the waiting list would be to buy more machines, at enormous expense—each one costs millions of dollars. The Canadian system rations and saves millions by purchasing fewer lithotripters, though there is some risk that some patients will need surgery before the appointment for lithotripsy comes around. Canadians are aware of this kind of decision and seem to accept it, although some wealthy Canadians go south to the States to purchase this service.

EXPANDING MEDICARE: A PROPOSAL
FOR A NEW SYSTEM

One system of American medical care organized by the federal government has won strong allegiance from the patients it covers. This is Medicare, the federal system of medical care for all American citizens over age 65.

Congress began to think about Medicare in the early 1960s, as part of the Great Society legislation, which also included Head Start, food stamps, VISTA, and Aid to Families with Dependent Children. Conceptualized by President John F. Kennedy, these programs were wrangled into law by President Lyndon Johnson in 1965. Medicare was intended to help elderly people during illness; originally, it was intended for the elderly poor, but almost immediately it was extended to everyone over 65.

Perhaps this was a mistake. Why should young tax payers pay for medical care for the wealthy elderly? For senior citizens who already had medical coverage?

For elderly people, Medicare alleviated the very great evil of uncertainty about medical treatment; it gave them security they had never known before. For many, the greatest worry had been whether they could afford physicians and hospitalization. Before Medicare, when workers retired—typically, in those days, at 65—many of them were on their own with regard to medical coverage. If they did not insure themselves, they would somehow have to pay for all their own medical expenses. Today, that is no longer true: The elderly now need to pay a maximum of 20 percent of their medical expenses, and most pay only 15 percent. Since Medicare is very comprehensive—and since medical expenses are so high, particularly for this age group—that is a great bargain.

Medicare covers 40 million Americans over age 65 and, in a supplemental system, 4 million disabled people under 65.[17] Together, Medicare and Medicaid, the system for the poor, cover about one in five Americans. Unlike Medicaid, which is run differently by each state with federal matching funds, Medicare is administered by the federal government and is financed from mandatory payroll taxes— indicated on paycheck stubs as FICA (that is, Federal Insurance Corporation of America). Medicare costs about $140 billion a year, 15 percent of the nation's health spending; Medicaid costs state taxpayers about $35 billion.[18]

Medicare is a *single-payer system*, and in this it contrasts sharply with private medical coverage in the United States. Since World War II, private insurance plans have multiplied; they now number over 1,500, each with its own rules, qualifications, reimbursement rates, and forms to be filled out by patients and physicians.[19] This private system is so complicated that special businesses have sprouted to help patients fill out all the different forms and to help physicians bill all the different plans.

Advocates of Medicare argue that, as a single-payer system, it has eliminated the overhead and waste of multiple private insurers. They point out that about 4 to 12 percent of health care costs represent fees and profits of private insurance plans[20]; by comparison, Medicare has maintained very reasonable administrative expenses, about 2.5 percent of its total expenditures.

Critics emphasize that Medicare covers no drugs at all, and costs for the elderly may run $1,000 a month. Getting Medicare to cover drugs has been a feature of several national political campaigns, but none has been successful.

Why not expand Medicare, therefore, to cover all Americans regardless of age? An expanded Medicare system could also absorb all other government systems of medical coverage, including Medicaid, insurance for federal employees, the CHAMPUS program for military personnel, and all government disability funds.

An expanded Medicare system would offer several significant advantages. To begin with, a single-payer system eliminates the wasteful duplication and conflicting rules that seem inevitable with multiple insurers. Second, such a system can control costs: It has enormous power in negotiating with physicians and hospitals; it can essentially say, "Take it or leave it." Third, a single-payer system eliminates cost-shifting to other payers.

The disadvantages of expanding Medicare are considerable. For one thing, the current system is financially unstable and, without changes, predicted to go broke in the early 2030s. What could also happen is that the age of eligibility will be raised, say to 70, and the payroll tax will increase, say from 2.9 percent to 5.5 percent.

More generally, what everyone pays for, nobody pays for, and there is a tendency for everyone to seek his or her own advantage to the detriment of the overall good. This is an age-old story, played out long ago in England in the *tragedy of the commons:* The owner of each flock increased the number of sheep he grazed on town land—the commons—until the commons were so overgrazed that the grass simply disappeared and the commons system was destroyed.[21]

A single-payer system might also create a bloated, unresponsive federal bureaucracy; the Veterans Administration hospitals are thought by some to be such a bureaucracy and are not an encouraging model. Third, many Americans feel that government, especially the federal government, simply cannot do certain things very well, and this feeling is particularly strong with regard to personal matters like medical care. Finally, as libertarian law professor Richard Epstein emphasizes, the cost of universalizing Medicare dramatically increases as the system moves to insure each smaller segment of the 40-plus million presently uninsured Americans.[22] Covering most of the half who are children is relatively cheap (except for NICU babies and kids with congenital diseases). Covering most of the adult, working poor is not exboritant. But covering the last 10 percent, 5 percent, or 1 percent is very, very expensive, because such percentages represent the real "outliers" and "cost-busters" that all private systems want to avoid. These are the patients needing heart-liver transplants, the untreatable schizophrenics with cancer, and the severely retarded babies born with maternal-fetal alcohol syndrome. Similarly, covering basic, generic drugs might be affordable but not so for the newest, designer drugs that are now advertised directly on television to potential customers. If a national system creates a sense that such people are entitled to the best care (given by people other than family members), it will be difficult for a national system to say when a just limit of care has been reached.

But these disadvantages might be offset by another important advantage: Medicare is a system which is *already in place.* Hospitals already get half their revenues from Medicare patients. Using Medicare for all age groups would entail simply broadening it, rather than creating some wholly new, untried system; thus its effects would probably be more predictable, and more manageable, than those of a new system. Medicare might even be expanded gradually, to each additional age group in turn; this would allow time for its effects to be assessed, and for corrections and modifications to be made.

ANOTHER PROPOSAL: THE HEALTH CARE SECURITY BILL AND MANAGED CARE PLANS

Soon after William Jefferson (Bill) Clinton became president in January 1993, he and his wife, Hillary Rodham Clinton, announced that reforming American medical care would be a top priority of their new administration; in fact, Clinton's promise to redress the inadequacies of the existing system had been a significant factor in his election. Clinton made two promises about medical care: to broaden access to it and to control its high costs—though whether both goals could be achieved simultaneously remained to be seen.

Originally, Clinton hoped to expand Medicare to include workers' compensation, the medical portion of automobile insurance, and Medicaid; and in May of 1993, it was expected that within 18 months Congress would pass "landmark legislation" to control medical costs and expand insurance coverage.[23] However, it was not until late 1993 that Bill and Hillary Clinton presented their actual plan to

Congress, and this plan—called the Health Care Security bill—was significantly different from their original idea.

The Health Care Security bill was based on two major concepts. The first of these was what came to be known as an *employer mandate:* All employers would be required to pay something toward medical insurance for their employees (the exact amount to be negotiated as the bill was debated).

The second major concept was the formation of large *managed care plans,* which were intended to reduce costs. Each of these managed care plans would sign up, on the supply side, a hospital or a large number of physicians and would offer to patients—the demand side—a broad range of medical services for a predetermined flat cost. This second concept had originated with an untested idea for lowering costs of supplies to the Pentagon from the defense industry.[24] It was based on the assumption that the various managed care plans would compete against each other, and that this competition would both provide adequate care and keep the costs of care low. The concept of managed care plans was also based on the profit motive: Any money left over after a plan had rendered all the services it advertised would be profit. Each plan would have an incentive to be efficient, since an efficient plan would lower its costs and would thus attract clients. Or so the theory went.

There were problems with both bases of the Health Care Security bill. The employer mandate came in for especially strong opposition. It appeared that the brunt of paying for medical insurance for people who are presently not covered might fall—unjustly—on small businesses, and it was estimated that the cost of mandated coverage for such businesses would be between $1,600 and $1,900 per employee. Many small businesses said they would simply not hire, or would fire, workers rather than provide mandated medical coverage. Even a surprising number of physicians in private corporations did not want to pay for medical insurance for their own employees.[25] A reaction like this creates a dilemma for public policy: How can we evaluate a tradeoff between medical insurance for some people and loss of jobs for others?

Another problem at that time was that American patients were simply not accustomed to any limitations at all on access to medical services. The idea that every American had to be in an HMO was not very popular.

It is interesting to note that the American College of Surgeons backed the Clinton plan, and that some physicians and surgeons felt that they would have been better off with it than they are under many new private plans. Their reasoning is that the federal government would have had to abide (as Medicare now must abide) by due process, ADA, and similar constraints. By contrast, a large company is free to deliver an ultimatum to, say, a group of ophthalmologists: "If you don't drop your fees by 50 percent, we have another group waiting in the wings who will provide services at the lower rate." In such a situation, there is very little room for physicians to maneuver.

In October 1994, after 2 years of intense public discussion and behind-the-scenes lobbying, the 103rd Congress went home without having passed, or even having voted on, a new medical plan for Americans. Clinton's Health Care Security bill had never gotten out of committee, and no alternative proposals had reached a vote. Medicare remained unchanged.

ETHICAL ISSUES: FROM COMMUNITY/ EXPERIENCE RATING TO RAWLSIAN JUSTICE

Facts and Misconceptions

In the debate over health care, there are a number of serious misconceptions. Let's examine these.

Who Pays for Medicare?   One widespread misconception, among the elderly and others, is that Medicare recipients have already paid for their benefits through FICA taxes. One popular book about Medicare benefits states, "The most fundamental point is that *Medicare is not a gift. You paid for it while you were working.* Medicare owes you services in just the same way that health insurer to whom you have paid premiums owes them to you."[26]

In fact, the Medicare benefits going to today's elderly people are being paid for almost entirely by the FICA taxes of today's workers.[27] It is true that retirees with yearly pensions over $25,000 are taxed on the amount over $25,000; this tax takes the form of reductions in social security payments, but it is modest and defrays only a very small fraction of the costs of Medicare. After the first few years on Medicare, most beneficiaries have received benefits amounting to what they paid in, plus all interest; thereafter, their benefits are paid for by taxes on current workers.

What Is Medical Insurance?   *Medical insurance* is a misleading phrase. Thirty years ago, medical insurance was really insurance—a hedge against a dreaded but rather remote possibility. At that time, people took out medical insurance policies in the hope that they would never need to receive any benefits, and policies covered mainly catastrophic situations such as hospital care after an automobile accident or a diagnosis of cancer.

Gradually, medical policies evolved into something quite different, though they have continued to be called *insurance:* They became plans for prepaid group medical care. Blue Cross Blue Shield (BCBS), for example, simply adds up all its medical costs (subtracting a small amount for administration), divides by the number of policyholders, and sends out the bills. Medical insurance next expanded to cover not just catastrophic care but all "major medical" expenses. This was a logical extension: If people were willing to pay small premiums to protect themselves against remote catastrophic risks, why not pay slightly larger premiums to protect against more common risks? Thus "insurance" grew and grew until it now includes almost any medical service; today, some people become indignant when their insurance doesn't cover absolutely everything and they have to pay for anything at all.

Another misconception about medical insurance has to do with who pays for private insurance. Couples on a family plan without children pay much higher rates than singles, and hence, subsidize parents with children. In commercial medical insurance plans, those who do not receive benefits subsidize those who do (this is also true, to some extent, of Medicare). Because premiums are raised when average use rises, many people believe that they have paid for their own care and are thus entitled to as much care as they want. This misconception virtually guarantees that costs and services will increase.

What Is Socialized Medicine?   *Socialized medicine* is another term that can be misleading. What does *socialized* mean? Why are so many Americans so afraid of it? If *socialized* means simply "publicly owned," then that is not necessarily a bad thing, or even an unusual thing: Americans are used to public ownership of highways and waterways, public schools, state colleges and universities, the armed forces, airwaves, the air, the skies, and national parks.

When Medicare was debated in Congress in 1965, the American Medical Association (AMA) opposed it as socialized medicine. American physicians feared that government-administered care financed by taxes would mean government-controlled care,[28] and that all physicians would end up as employees of the federal government. To placate physicians, a crucial decision was made: Under Medicare, physicians would be reimbursed on a fee-for-service basis. Eventually, this arrangement would make physicians rich and would give them the best of both worlds: freedom to work independently rather than as government employees, and freedom to order infinite services for their patients—services that would be taken care of by government-enforced payments in the form of higher and higher FICA taxes. Consider, moreover, that if *socialized medicine* does mean what AMA feared in 1965—working for a boss who decides how much to pay you—then many Americans today are in precisely that position.

One additional misconception about socialized medicine is that people pay for it in some way which involves more compulsion than Americans are used to. The truth here is that Americans are already paying FICA taxes to support Medicare, and federal taxes are about as compulsory as anything can be: For a typical taxpayer, it is equivalent to being forced to work an extra month to pay for the care of the elderly. What is more, under socialized medicine everyone is covered, which means—obviously enough—that everyone who pays taxes is covered; but today many Americans who pay FICA taxes are *not* covered themselves.

What Is a National Medical System?   There are also misconceptions about the terms *national health insurance* and *national health care system*. When we are considering reforms in the American medical system, it is important to be clear about how these terms are being used, since different people may have very different concepts in mind.

National health insurance and *national health care system* might mean any of the following:

1. An American medical service—a system in which all medical professionals would work for the federal government.
2. A single-payer system, such as a universalized Medicare, in which the federal government would tax all Americans and reimburse physicians on a fee-for-service basis.
3. A system based on a federal law requiring every employer to buy basic medical coverage for every employee and establishing a separate government-financed system for unemployed people.
4. A system in which all Americans would receive government-funded vouchers to buy medical care directly from providers (such as hospitals) or indirectly from companies selling medical coverage.

5. A mixed public-private system in which the government would run all hospitals and would fund all hospital care, but private insurers would cover outpatient costs.[29]

In this chapter, the present Canadian system and a universalized Medicare system are both examples of definition 2.

The "Market" Solution

It is sometimes argued that medical care could be provided and costs controlled by letting medicine operate as a *true market,* subject to the laws of supply and demand. Champions of a marketplace for medical care argue that many other goods and services are successfully provided by a market, and that a true marketplace for medical care would eliminate bloated bureaucracies and wasteful costs.

In a true market, people would buy medical care, such as the services of a physician or nurse, out of their own pockets; there would be no medical insurance and no reimbursement from insurers. Because people would have to pay for their service themselves, many prices would tumble drastically. For a routine eye examination, patients might be able to choose a nurse practitioner charging $10, a primary care physician charging $30, or an ophthalmologist charging $300. Given these alternatives, very few patients would choose the ophthalmologist, and so ophthalmologists would have to lower their fees to compete (unless they could somehow demonstrate that their services were really worth more). Another example is elective surgery to correct a cataract in an eye. This operation is now subsidized by other people's insurance premiums and is reimbursed at $6,000; but if patients had to pay for it themselves, the price might drop to $300.

A true market would certainly lower costs, but there are strong arguments against the market concept in the context of medical care.

The first counterargument is very basic: We do not have a true market for medical care, and we have not had such a market since World War II, half a century ago. In fact, since World War II medicine has operated as the opposite of a true market. In the area of Birmingham, Alabama, for example—where medical care has replaced the old steel factories as the chief employer—when more and more specialists were added, the cost of their services rose. In a true market, the cost would have dropped as a consequence of the law of supply and demand.

This development in Birmingham is typical, and there are two related explanations for it. First, insurance companies reimburse specialists on the basis of what is normal ("reasonable and customary"), and as more specialists enter a system, they can drive up costs by raising the "normal" level. Second, specialists are able to do this by creating demand for their services—a phenomenon known as *induced demand.* Each specialist tends to believe that people need his or her services (just as every instructor believes that students need more courses in his or her field). Thus more services are created, creating more costs. Without a gatekeeper, this effect cannot be controlled. Every patient wants the best care, and when a specialist says a certain procedure is "best" and an insurer will pay for it, the patient tends to go along.

There are additional arguments against the concept of a market solution: Even if we did have a true market for medical care, there are several reasons why it would probably not be a good thing.

One reason has to do with elderly patients. Applying a market solution to elderly patients might be dangerous; it is not at all clear how a market system could deliver minimal basic care to all elderly Americans fairly, efficiently, and inexpensively. On the twentieth anniversary of Medicare in 1985, the Harvard Medicare Project evaluated its successes and failures and concluded:

> The special nature of older persons and their health problems argues for caution in relying primarily on private solutions to providing health care for them.
>
> . . . In particular, the elderly are less equipped to deal with a marketplace of medical care than younger, working persons. Partly because elderly persons are more likely to suffer from physical and mental impairments (including eyesight, hearing, and memory), they have more trouble than younger persons in comprehending the increasingly complex insurance arrangements now available. The elderly also usually lack the counsel of the purchasing agents and benefits representatives who serve younger, employed populations. Although some retired persons may be able to navigate our health care system, many others will not fare well in the rough and tumble of a health care marketplace.
>
> Consequently, although we favor providing Medicare beneficiaries with more choices, we believe this can best be achieved by allowing them more options within the existing Medicare program and by encouraging a cooperative approach between the public and private sectors.[30]

Another argument against the market solution is that since the level of medical services would be significantly lower under a true market system (because consumers would have to pay for everything themselves), such a system might put millions of health professionals out of work. During the last few years, one-sixth of all new jobs created in the United States have been in health care, and one-seventh of the American economy has been concerned with providing health care.

One major argument against the market solution is that many people simply would not get the medical care they need because they could not afford it. In a true market, some people would remain untreated because they could not pay for their own care; and medical professionals would need to become very hardboiled, doing "wallet biopsies" before helping anyone, to avoid being "manipulated" into providing free care. A real market for medical care would be a harsh, cruel system where patients would have to bargain with professionals, and professionals no longer worked with patients to overcome illness and injury.

It is also true that if medical care were provided as other commercial commodities are—rather than being subsidized as it now is—many people who could afford care would not make wise decisions about what to buy and what to postpone or forgo. If we had to choose between a new car and a hip replacement, some of us would choose the car. Moreover, some people might be tempted, or pressured, to sacrifice medical care for the sake of their families: A parent might give up a hip replacement and put the money toward a house for the family.

In some more modest form, however, the market concept may still have something to offer. One intriguing idea is to make the present system more like a market by making medical coverage more like automobile insurance.[31] Because people pay for automobile insurance themselves, they usually shop around for the best or most appropriate policy. If this concept was applied to health care, people could increase or decrease their deductibles and coverage just as with automobile insurance: People who wanted to save money on premiums could opt for a higher deductible or less extensive coverage; people who wanted both prepaid group health care and catastrophe insurance could pay more.

This is called a *cafeteria plan,* where an employer gives an employee, say, $3,000 worth of coverage. The employee then selects whether he wants to be covered by IVF and transplants and with what deductible and co-pay. Dental and optical plans would be included. (Dental and optical might be more important for those under 40 than coverage for transplants.)

Costs of Increased Medical Care

A major issue about medical care is that increases in access and services seem to entail increases in costs. Fiscal conservatives say that our experience with Medicare has taught us an important lesson: The system cannot expand the number of patients covered or the range of services offered and simultaneously decrease costs.

The Clinton plan hoped to increase access by providing coverage for the 40 million Americans who are now uninsured or underinsured. Although some analysts have argued that this would cost only about 6 percent of current spending for medical care, still a sizable figure at $50 billion annually.[32] Moreover, Americans who now lack insurance may be generally unhealthier than those with insurance, and covering them would cost significantly more. Attempts to increase access do not bode well for controlling costs.

Reformers often have another goal—increased services. Each increase in service provided to all Americans will cost lots more money.

The increases in services that are most needed are:

- Coverage of prescription drugs.
- Long-term care in nursing homes (despite widespread belief that this is covered now).
- Auxiliary medical services such as home health care, hospice care, and transportation to medical facilities.
- Dental services, including preventive dental care.
- Services for mental illness—especially the most costly, inpatient care for substance abuse.

Each of these is extremely expensive. Long-term nursing home care can last 20 years or more. Costs of home health care rose even faster than other medical costs between 1988 and 1993.[33]

Experience with Medicare shows that reduction in costs is incompatible with expanding either access or services and certainly with an increase in both. Under Medicare the cost of health care has risen from 5.3 percent of the GNP in 1965 to 14 percent of the GNP in 1993.

Some argue that the cost of increases in access and services can be offset by reducing waste. Consumers Union estimated that $200 billion could be saved by eliminating waste and unnecessary procedures from the medical system.[34] This money saved could pay for medical care for the uninsured. However, this may be a fantasy, like reducing the federal deficit by eliminating waste.

Why? Well, defining *waste* in generally acceptable terms would be difficult. Some definitions of *waste* would be legally unacceptable: For example, if some services mandated by ADA were considered *waste,* they could not be eliminated without violating the law of the land. Other definitions of *waste* would be politically unacceptable: Each politician, for instance, would fight to preserve medical services and facilities in his or her own constituency, even if more objective evaluators considered them wasteful. One person's waste is another person's job, clinic, or hospital.

Also, even if waste could be significantly reduced, it would be a one-time saving. Reducing waste would have no effect on the cost escalation inherent in an aging population with greater medical needs, or on the escalation inherent in new, better devices and patented drugs.

In the end, then, Americans must choose between increasing medical care (in terms of access and services) and controlling costs; we may not be able to have both. And if we do increase access and services, an equally important choice may be whether to pay for expanded care ourselves or leave it to future generations.

Insurance Companies: Approaches to Coverage

Basically, there are two ways of conceptualizing medical insurance. First, there is the *moral* approach. With this concept, insurance is an enterprise of sharing risk among many people, and it is intended as a way of helping us protect ourselves against bad luck. One example of the moral approach is *community rating,* a system whereby the risk represented by an area (such as an entire state) is evaluated, and every policyholder in the area is charged the same rate. When insurance is sold on a communitywide rating system, it favors people who are less healthy, because they cannot be excluded and their benefits are subsidized by the premiums of healthier policyholders. Another example of the moral approach is rating an entire country, as in Canada's single-payer system: Healthier Canadians, who rarely use the medical system, subsidize those who are less healthy.

Second, there is the *profit* approach to medical insurance. With this concept, providing medical coverage is simply one way among many for a business to make profits; selling medical coverage is no different in nature from selling cars or encyclopedias. Profits are maximized by selling policies to healthy young people, who are unlikely to make claims; and by avoiding having to sell policies to people who are sick, old, disabled, or at high risk of accidents—that is, people who are likely to make claims. Thus insurers who operate on the profit concept often exclude many people from medical coverage. The profit approach is based on *experience rating:* a system of differential rates based on risks represented by individuals or groups.

Both approaches have been taken in the United States: Medical insurance here began with the moral concept, but most of it has evolved into the profit concept.

During the 1930s, when surgeons and physicians founded first Blue Cross and later Blue Shield, their highest priority was to make sure that patients would have enough money to pay the bills of surgeons and physicians after hospitalization for catastrophic conditions. By state law, the "Blues" were nonprofit organizations; as such, in many states they paid no federal taxes and no taxes on the premiums they collected. In return for their nonprofit status, Blue Cross Blue Shield (BCBS) companies were expected to insure as many people as possible, and to do this they adopted a community-rating scheme. Between the 1930s and the 1960s, because BCBS had a virtual monopoly on medical coverage, things worked out for everyone. BCBS insured everyone who wanted insurance, and rates remained reasonable.

In the early 1970s, changes in federal regulations allowed commercial insurance companies of a new kind to come into existence. These new commercial insurers were allowed to use experience rating, and they started "cherry picking" the healthiest customers of BCBS, leaving BCBS as an insurer of last resort for the unhealthiest and neediest customers.[35] Under these circumstances, what eventually happened to Empire BCBS, the organization serving New York State, was predictable. Empire BCBS suffered financial losses because commercial insurance companies took its best customers and left it with only the sickest customers, such as those with AIDS. As a result, Empire BCBS had to raise premiums for all its customers by nearly 100 percent. Another target of cherry picking, Kentucky BCBS, saw its share of policies statewide drop from 90 to 30 percent between the early 1960s and the late 1970s. Some states have now made cherry picking illegal.

Employment and Coverage

There is a widespread belief that most Americans without medical coverage are unemployed, but this is a myth: In fact, most of the 40 million Americans without good medical coverage are employed.[36] Most waiters and waitresses, for instance, have no employer-sponsored medical insurance. Only 1 of 10 businesses employing fewer than 10 people provides medical coverage.[37]

Most Americans—57 percent—get medical coverage though employment.[38] An employment-based medical system has both strengths and weaknesses.

The strengths of employment-based coverage show with large employers, who offer far better medical plans, than small employers. Large employers can spread risks over a pool of many employees. Also, large employers receive discounts from hospitals and, in effect, from insurance companies. Insurance companies now generally set different rates, based on how large an employer is (this is a type of experience rating), and employers with over 1,000 workers pay the lowest rates. Moreover, one factor keeping insurance affordable for many larger employers is demographics: workers tend to have fewer medical problems than other groups such as unemployed people, retired people, and people on disability.

The weaknesses of employment-based coverage appear, to begin with, when we consider small employers. Many small businesses—and most very small businesses—do not offer medical coverage at all, and this is not necessarily their fault.

Despite the demographics, insuring employees can be very expensive; under experience rating, employers with 50 to 100 workers pay higher rates for insurance than larger employers, and employers with fewer than 25 employees pay the highest rates of all. Thus small businesses trying to allocate capital for expansion—or struggling to make any profit at all—often cannot afford to offer insurance.

A second disadvantage of the American employment-based system is that when a worker leaves a job, medical coverage is likely to be cut off. For one thing, insurance is almost never transferable or *portable* to another company. Also, many young working people in the United States today do not realize that their employer pays most of the cost of medical coverage, and that if they quit or are fired they will have to bear this cost themselves, at least until they find another job. Essentially the same is often true of older workers who retire or lose their jobs before age 65 (when they will become eligible for Medicare); even if the employer agrees to continue coverage at the cheaper rates of the group plan, the former employee will have pay for it alone—the employer will no longer contribute.

A third disadvantage is *cost-shifting*. American hospitals are not reimbursed for providing care to the poor, but federal law forbids any hospital with an emergency room to turn patients away because of inability to pay. To make up for the cost of this care, hospitals shift costs: They charge more for services to insured patients. This effect, of course, falls on privately insured patients as well, but employers in particular resent it; cost-shifting forces them to act as charities by subsidizing medical care for the indigent. (For this reason, employers in Oregon supported OHP.) Large businesses also argue that they are subsidizing the care of uninsured employees of small businesses, who are likely to come to emergency rooms with very serious medical problems, or to enter the medical system at age 65, under Medicare, with serious conditions that would have been preventable earlier. It is estimated that cost-shifting rose from $1.6 billion in 1988 to $38.8 billion in 1992.[39]

A fourth disadvantage is that American employers say the cost of insuring their employees is much too high. In 1990, for instance, over $675 of the cost of each new Ford vehicle went to pay for medical coverage for employees of Ford and its suppliers.[40] Presumably in 2002, the costs are more like $1,500 per car.

This leads to a fifth disadvantage of employment-based insurance: In recent years, many employers have been trying to lower their costs in ways that can be harmful to workers. They replace one full-time worker with benefits with two part-time workers who have no benefits, or they contract "independent consultants" without benefits to replace managers and lower-level employees. Such a policy creates a two-class medical system in the United States: full-time employees with high salaries and benefits versus part-time employees and the unemployed with no benefits.

A sixth disadvantage of the employment-based system is that many workers are pushed into chronic unemployment because of an illness or injury. Many poor people are poor primarily because of medical conditions that make them unacceptable to employers who are seeking to reduce medical costs.

People who are unemployed or work for a small company that offers no medical insurance may, of course, try to buy individual policies. About 7 percent of Americans do; they include people who are self-employed, seasonal workers, adult students, and people who are between jobs. However, private individual policies are expensive because the policyholder is not part of a large pool of workers and because such policies are subject to experience rating.

Medical Care and the Federal Government

What is the proper role of the federal government with regard to medical care? This is a controversial question: Some Americans want more federal government, some want less, and many swing back and forth between these two positions.

Some of the critics who advocate a market approach to reforming medical care, for instance, are not really calling for a true market system but are simply expressing their distrust of big government. They say that federal funding for end-stage renal disease, artificial hearts, and AIDS is politicized and has been provided at the expense of other diseases. They also argue that American government is being asked to do too many things for too many different groups.

Some critics of a single-payer system are also dubious about a larger role for the federal government. With one-seventh of the American economy at stake, and perhaps one-sixth of new jobs, do we want to take the chance of a federally administered system? Suppose it flops?

The record of federal government is mixed, and how it is evaluated depends on who is being interviewed and when. For example, the armed forces—a prime example of a federally run institution—are notorious for cost overruns and inefficiency; on the other hand, of all American institutions which employ large numbers of people and have ever been racially segregated, the armed forces are now most nearly color-blind. Medicine was also once highly segregated and is now on the whole color-blind, and this has been brought about largely through federally enforced changes.

Medical Care and Political Philosophy

We cannot really discuss or evaluate systems of medical care without including some political philosophy. One way to consider political philosophy with regard to medical care is in terms of justice and the "right" to care.

The "Right" to Medical Care   Many people claim that Americans have a right to medical care. What does such a right mean?

A right to a medical care does *not* mean that everyone would receive the same kind of medical care. Nor does it mean equality of outcomes: Since health depends on so many factors—including genes, environment, and individual habits—no degree of equal medical treatment could possibly ensure equal results.

A right to medical care would, at most, probably mean a right to *basic care*, a decent minimum of care.[41] This would not preclude a system in which some people bought extra medical care above this minimum; a two-tiered system of this nature would not be unjust, and as a practical matter it could not be prevented in a democratic society.

Rawls: Medical Care in a Just Society   There are several bases for the claimed right to medical care.[42] One argument is provided by the theory of justice developed by the philosopher John Rawls.[43]

Rawls believes that the term *justice* best applies to the design of basic structures and institutions in a society, and a system of medical care is one such structure or institution. According to Rawls, principles of justice are part of a hypothetical social contract in which we all come together to make choices—but we must choose under a *veil of ignorance* about our own age, race, religion, sex, health, wealth, abilities, and talents. In other words, we cannot bias our choices by considering arbitrary personal characteristics.

Under these conditions, Rawls believes, rational people would not gamble with the structure of their most important institutions; they would choose those structures that gave people equal opportunities (such as the opportunity to get ahead in business by being free to make contracts and by receiving equal treatment under the law). To Rawls, inequality is justifiable only when it works to the advantage of those who are worst off, that is, when the worst-off group actually does better with the inequality than without it. This is Rawls's *difference principle.*

An essential part of Rawls's concept of justice is the recognition that the world is naturally unfair: Some people are born into rich families, some into poor ones; some people are born healthy, others with spina bifida. For Rawls, government can either exacerbate such inequalities or smooth them out. A government which sharpens inequality is unjust; only the government which mitigates inequality is just.

Rawls's veil of ignorance can be seen as a device for ensuring that the golden rule will become part of our decisions about the structure of society. Underlying this approach is the ability to imagine *ourselves* as worst off—to see ourselves as sick, hurt, poor, uninsured; to imagine how bad it would be to have a serious illness or accident, and how much worse it would be to have no way to pay for the care we need.

•

How might Rawls's approach be specifically applied to our own system?

The 1980s and 1990s were not good for the working poor or the lower middle class. By one measure, 70 percent of the increase in wealth between 1977 and 2000 went to the top 1 percent of Americans. The Center on Budget and Policy Priorities reported that, overall, the gap between the richest one-fifth of Americans and the lowest fifth widened greatly: The income of the highest fifth increased by 70 percent while the income of the lowest fifth decreased by 8 percent.[44] More and more workers had to work longer and longer just to keep what they had. More and more companies did not hire permanent full-time workers with full benefits such as medical coverage but rather used part-time workers and consultants. Some jobs that once paid $20 an hour now paid $7. If, as Rawls assumes, a just society is egalitarian, then American society became more unjust.

Our existing medical system, in which more than 44 million Americans are without insurance, may represent a structural inequality at a deep level, a level where life-and-death decisions are made. To make matters worse, those who suffer most from this structural inequality may be our children. As many as one-third of American children may spend part of their lives in poverty; far too many of their parents must choose between medical care for these children and basic necessities like food.

According to Rawls's difference principle, an unequal medical structure would be just only if the poor were better off under it than under an egalitarian system; and in the present, unequal American medical system, that is obviously not the case. Thus Rawls's theory of justice would call for reforming the American medical system, because almost any reform would improve the lot of the worst-off group.

Libertarian Critiques

Libertarians, such as University of Chicago law professor Richard Epstein, believe that it would be unwise, and perhaps immoral, to expand Medicare and that the Clinton Health Security Act (HSA) of 1993 shows exactly what would go wrong when the American government tried to mandate medical coverage for all Americans.[45]

The HSA first ran into trouble with Libertarians over its vague estimates of cost. Even advocates said it might entail an extra 10 percent "health insurance tax" to cover everybody (although hope remained that by exorcising the profits of private insurance companies, many savings could occur).

The plan anticipated worries about costs and thus tried to implement cost-containment strategies while also implementing universal access. It would have four levels of government (read "bureaucracy"): a national medical board, state boards under supervision of the national board, regional health-insurance purchasing cooperatives (HIPCs), and competing health plans.

One problem with a system where everyone gets the same care is what to do with people at the margins, specifically, illegal aliens working in the country. If they were entitled to the same benefits as working Americans, millions more would cross the borders, burdening working Americans with the costs of their medical care (and sick aliens might purposefully come to America to get free treatment).

Although it may be incorrect to call the present rationing system "immoral," libertarians call it unjust. People who are employed pay Federal Insurance Corporation of America (FICA) taxes, and we all pay sales taxes, to support Medicare and Medicaid—even if we ourselves have no medical coverage. As a result, many uninsured people are contributing to Medicare and Medicaid.[46] For example, waitresses with kids and no medical coverage pay for liver transplants for wealthy retirees.

Another problem was whether it was illegal to purchase extra medical care outside a nationally-approved plan. Whether or not it was the original intent to make such purchases illegal (this remains controversial even today), it was widely perceived by many people that it might be. It was one thing to guarantee everyone a basic minimum of medical care; it was quite another to force everyone into the same system and deny opportunities for paying for extra care. The latter seemed un-American.

Surprisingly, the American Association of Retired Persons opposed the HSA, perceiving that the cost-containment goals could only be obtained by limiting funds for Medicare. Put differently, the costs of giving care to the most expensive uninsured patients might conflict with the goal of giving the best care to the elderly.

Two other things doomed the plan: a provision to pay for abortions and a desire (from the Gores) to pay for mental health services. The first alienated conservative religious groups and the latter was a cost-buster.

Libertarians just do not believe that the American government can control costs and provide universal access the way the Canadian, German, and Australian governments did. They fear that governments will limit freedoms of physicians, businesses, and mandate expensive services requiring higher taxes. As the millennium was ending, governments in Canada, Germany, Australia, and elsewhere with single-payer systems were finding it very difficult to rein in costs and difficult not to provide extra services, for example, to the disabled.

UPDATE

As America's nonmedical system lurched into the next century, more people than ever are uninsured—as many as 40 million—and more people than ever fear that they may be hospitalized and have problems with their medical plan.

Two contrary movements rock proposals for national, single-payer systems. On the one hand, more and more companies use experience rating to exclude potentially costly employees and more and more insurance companies try to avoid issuing policies to small companies with expensive employees. The advent of presymptomatic genetic testing, which tests not just individuals but whole generations of families, is especially scary here because profit-seeking insurance companies could exclude costly, sick people with actuarial accuracy. The system seems to be moving toward one where those who are genetically healthy and young will be insured and those most likely to need insurance will not be able to get it. Such a reductio moves one to think that the only sensible, just system is a single-payer system with the nation as the "community."

On the other hand, such a single-payer system would be very costly, for reasons already explored, and hence, could only afford minimum treatment or basic care. Such notions have been notoriously difficult in the past to define and defend. Already, *Medicare is an income-redistribution system,* taking 159 percent of the lifelong salary of the self-employed richest to pay for the care of the poorest (who may have contributed little or nothing during their lives). Problems at the margins would also be difficult: Who is a citizen and entitled to national care? A baby born here? An immigrant? How long must one live here before becoming eligible? Already, no immigrant or foreigner can be denied treatment in an emergency room if he or she is in distress, even if such patients can never pay for treatment. In states with many illegal immigrants, such care is very costly. Would it be right to let someone move here and, after 7 years, for instance, have the same medical benefits as someone who had paid 30 years of her payroll taxes into the system?

The issue affecting most middle-class Americans in the 2000's was limitations on their choice of medical treatment imposed by a managed care plan. Stories abounded in the visual and print media of patients who were denied or delayed treatment for cancer, organ transplants, and especially, mental illness or substance-dependence because their managed care plan denied coverage for such treatment as inappropriate. Congress tried to override such denials with mandatory minimum stays in hospitals for pregnant women to avoid "drive-through deliveries." As our first case in this chapter shows, more and more Americans found their choice of physicians limited, especially when they became seriously ill and needed to see specialists. Philosophically, the dilemma remained that Americans could not have maximal choice of ever-expanding kinds of expensive medical treatment while simultaneously refusing to pay taxes or premiums to fund such treatment.

CHIP

One ray of hope occurred in 1997 when Congress passed CHIP, the Children's Health Insurance Plan, and President Clinton signed it. Under CHIP, children in a family of four making less than $25,000 can be seen by physicians or dentists and get prescriptions filled at no cost. Similar families making up to $33,000 can get the same care with small co-pays. The federal government pays for about 80 percent of CHIP's costs of covering uninsured children under age 18, with states picking up the rest.

At the start of 2003, over 8 million children are still uninsured despite the fact that the federal government allotted over 40 billion dollars of federal matching funds in 1997 towards the Children's Health Insurance Program (CHIP). Why is this so?

CHIP is designed for the working poor who earn too much money to qualify for Medicaid, yet are unable to insure their children through private insurance companies.

Under CHIP, little Timmy—whose parents have minimal wage jobs—can obtain regular checkups, prescriptions, dental and eye care, and hospital and physician services—which is just a small handful of the benefits provided through CHIP—for free.

So why are millions of kids still going uninsured? Why would any eligible family not pounce on the idea of insuring their kids for free? Answer: Many families do not know that they are eligible, and others are hesitant because of the stigma attached to public health insurance.

Many have the misconception that CHIP is a version of welfare. And like Free Lunch Programs, many families believe that they are ineligible if both parents are working.

Every state is given the option of using CHIP funds to expand Medicaid, create a new health insurance program, or do a combination of both. Every state is also responsible for spreading the word about these new benefits, and with numbers as large as 8 million, it seems that many states are failing.

Alabama, the first state to enact a CHIP program in 1998, has enrolled more than 52,000 children in the program, far more than their initial goal of 47,000. What is its secret of success?

First of all, Alabama has made application procedures easy for anyone. It uses joint application forms for Medicaid and CHIP, since many people who apply for CHIP end up being eligible for Medicaid. Paid advertisements get the word out in all major media areas in the state. An efficient staff, and social work consultants, leave only a 10-day turnaround time to process each application. And all application procedures are also accessible in Spanish. Last but not least, many volunteers help educate others on whether or not they are eligible.

FURTHER READING

Ezekiel Emanuel, *The Ends of Human Life: Medical Ethics in a Liberal Policy*, Harvard University Press, Cambridge, MA, 1992.

Richard Epstein, *Mortal Peril—Our Inalienable Right to Health*, Addison-Welsey, Reading, MA, 1997.

Frank Marsh and Mark Yarborough, *Medicine and Money: A Study of the Role of Beneficence in Health Care Cost Containment*, Greenwood, New York, 1990.

E. Haavi Morreim, ed., "Ethics and Alternative Health Systems," *Journal of Medicine and Philosophy*, vol.17, no. 1 (special issue), February 1992.

Notes

The following abbreviations (in addition to the customary bibliographic terms) are used in these notes:

AMN = American Medical News
AP = Associated Press
HCR = Hastings Center Report
JAMA = Journal of the American Medical Association
NEJM = New England Journal of Medicine
NYT = New York Times
UAB = University of Alabama at Birmingham
UPI = United Press International
WP = Washington Post
WSJ = Wall Street Journal

CHAPTER 2

1 The first NYT story on the Quinlan case is September 16, 1975, New Jersey sec., p. 32. The Quinlans' version is from Joseph Quinlan and Julia Quinlan with Phyllis Battelle, Karen Ann: The Quinlans Tell Their Story, Doubleday Anchor, New York, 1977.
2 Robert Morse, in In the Matter Of Karen Quinlan: The Complete Legal Briefs, Court Proceedings, and Decisions in the Superior Court of New Jersey, vols. 1 and 2, University Publications of America, Frederick, Md., 1982, p. 236 (hereafter, Proceedings 1, Proceedings 2).
3 Julius Korein, in Proceedings 1, pp. 34–35.
4 George Daggett, NYT, September 20, 1975, New Jersey sec.
5 Quinlan and Quinlan, op. cit., p. 22.
6 Ibid., p. 27.

7 Daniel Coburn, in Proceedings 1, p. 17.
8 Ibid., p. 29.
9 Thomas C. Oden, "Beyond an Ethic of Immediate Sympathy," HCR, February 1976, p. 12.
10 Daniel Coburn, in Proceedings 1, pp. 196–198.
11 Ralph Porzio, in Proceedings 1, pp. 202–206.
12 Julius Korein, in Proceedings 1, p. 329.
13 Fred Plum, in Quinlan and Quinlan, op. cit., p. 198.
14 Robert Morse, in Quinlan and Quinlan, op. cit., pp. 188–189.
15 Quinlan and Quinlan, op. cit., pp. 272–273 (the nun is not named).
16 Gino Concetti, quoted in Quinlan and Quinlan, op. cit., p. 284.
17 Quoted in Quinlan and Quinlan, op. cit.
18 Cruzan v. Director, Missouri Dept. of Health, 110 S. Ct. 2841, 1990.
19 George Annas, "Nancy Cruzan and the Right to Die," NEJM, vol. 323, no. 10, September 6, 1990, p. 670.
20 "Love and Let Die," Time, March 19, 1990, pp. 62ff.
21 Andrew M. Malcolm, "Nancy Cruzan: End to Long Goodbye," NYT, December 29, 1990, p. A3. See also, "A Conversation with Mr. and Mrs. Cruzan," Midwest Medical Ethics: The Nancy Cruzan Case, volume 5, Numbers 1 & 2, Winter/Spring 1989.
22 Linda Greenhouse, "Right to Reject Life," NYT, June 27, 1990, p. A1.
23 NYT, June 27, 1990, p. A14.
24 In 1991, an Indiana court (In re Lawrance, 579 N.E. 2d 32) ruled that a surrogate could judge the best interests of the person in a right-to-die case for a never competent patient in PVS. This standard is discussed further in Chapter 9.

25 Charles Baron, "On Taking Substituted Judgment Seriously," *HCR*, vol. 20, no. 5, September–October 1992, p. 7.

26 John Robertson, *"Cruzan:* No Rights Violated," *HCR*, vol. 20, no. 5, September–October 1992, p. 7.

27 Baron, op. cit., p. 8.

28 Ronald Cranford, lecture at UAB Medical School, January 19, 1991. See also Ellen Goodman, "Permanently Comatose Don't Live," *Boston Globe*, December 12, 1992.

29 Joanne Lynn and Jacqueline Glover, *"Cruzan* and Caring for Others," *HCR*, vol. 20, no. 5, September–October 1992, p. 11.

30 Carol Lewis in Judge Teel's office in Jasper County courthouse, Joplin, MO.

31 Annas, op. cit., p. 672.

32 President's Commission for the Study of Ethical Problems in Medicine and Biomedical and Behavioral Research, *Defining Death*, Superintendent of Documents, Washington, D.C., 1981, p. 14.

33 P. Mollaret and M. Goulon, "Le Coma Depasse," *Revue Neurologie*, vol. 101, no. 3, 1959.

34 Ad Hoc Committee of the Harvard Medical School to Examine the Definition of Brain Death," A Definition of Brain Death, "A Definition of Irreversible Coma," *JAMA*, vol. 205, no. 337, 1968.

35 The characteristics listed by the philosopher Mary Anne Warren in Chapter 5 (with regard to whether an aborted fetus is a person) might be used in a similar way to define the "higher person" standard: If *all* these characteristics are lacking, we do not have a "person."

36 National Conference of Commission on Uniform Laws, *Uniform Laws Annual*, vol. 15, supp., 1981.

37 Lance Stell, "Let's Abolish 'Brain-Death,'" *Community Ethics* (University of Pittsburg Center for Medical Ethics), vol. 4, no. 1, Winter 1997.

38 Multi-Society Task Force on PVS, "Medical Aspects of the Persistent Vegetative State," parts 1 and 2, *NEJM*, vol. 330, no. 22, pp. 1572–1579, May 26, 1994; June 2, 1994.

39 I. Durbroja, S. et al., "Outcome of Post-traumatic Unawareness Persisting for More Than a Month," *Journal of Neurological Neurosurgery Psychiatry*, vol. 58, no. 4, 1995, pp. 465–66.

40 R. Chen et al., "Prediction of Outcome in Patients with Anoxic Coma: a Clinical and Electrophysiologic Study," *Critical Care Medicine*, vol. 24, no. 4, April, 1996, pp. 672–78.

41 AP, "Policeman who Briefly Emerged from Coma-like State in '96 Dies," *Birmingham News*, April 16, 1997, p. 7A.

42. K. Payne et al., "Physicians' Attitudes about the Care of Patients in Persistent Vegetative State; A National Survey," *Annals of Internal Medicine 1996*; 125, pp. 104–110.

43 Quinlan and Quinlan, op. cit., p. 87.

44 American Academy of Neurology, amicus curiae brief in *Brophy v. New England Sinai Hospital, Inc.*, 1986; quoted in Ronald Cranford, "The Persistent Vegetative State: the Medical Reality (Getting the Facts Straight)," *HCR*, vol. 18, no. 1, 1988, p. 31.

45 Multi-Society Task Force on PVS, op. cit., pp. 1501–1502. The task force did not comment on the apparent contradiction between its claim that brain scans show no activity in PVS patients and the fact that seven patients made a "good recovery" after over 1 year in PVS.

46 Ibid.

47 "U.S.A.: Right to Live, or Right to Die?" *Lancet*, vol. 337, January 12, 1991.

48 Message posted on the Medical College of Wisconsin Discussion Forum on Medical Ethics by Hank Dunn, February 29, 1996. Hank Dunn, Chaplain, Fairfax Nursing Center, 10701 Main Street, Fairfax, VA 22030. A few weeks before Dunn's posting, a story updating Rita's condition appeared on the local CBS affiliate in Washington, D.C..

49 Daniel Callahan, "On Feeding the Dying," *HCR*, vol. 13, no. 5, October 1983, p. 22; Gilbert Meillander, "On Removing Food and Water: Against the Stream," *HCR*, vol. 14, no. 6, December 1984, pp. 11–13.

50 Ibid., app. B, p. 288.

51 W. May, R. Barry, O. Griese, et al., "Feeding and Hydrating the Permanently Unconscious and Other Vulnerable Persons," *Issues in Law and Medicine*, vol. 3, no. 3, Winter 1987, pp. 203–217; C. Sprung, "Changing Attitudes and Practices in Forgoing Life-Sustaining Treatments," *JAMA*, vol. 263, no. 16, April 25, 1990, pp. 2211–2221.

52 American Medical Association, *Opinions of the Judicial Council*, Chicago, IL., 1973.

53 Nat Hentoff, "The Deadly Slippery Slope," *Village Voice*, September 1, 1987.

54 Ibid.

55 Linda Greenhouse, "Right to Reject Life," *NYT*, June 27, 1990.

56 SUPPORT Principal Investigators, "A Controlled Trial to Improve Care for Seriously Ill Hospit alized Patients. The Study to Under-

stand Prognoses and Preferences for Outcomes and Risks of Treatment (SUPPORT)." *JAMA*, 1995, vol. 274, pp. 1591–1598.

57 Lisa Belkin, "As Family Protests, Hospital Seeks End to Woman's Life Support," *NYT*, January 10, 1991, pp. A1–2.

58 Steven Miles, "Interpersonal Issues in the Wanglie Case," *Kennedy Institute of Ethics Journal*, vol. 2, no. 1, March 1992, pp. 61–72.

59 For a review of these cases, see *Law, Medicine, and Health Care*, vol. 20, 1993, pp. 310–315.

60 R. Knox, "Americans' New Way of Dying: Don't Fight It," *Boston Globe*, June 5, 1994.

61 Irwin Molotsky, "Wife Wins Right-to-Die Case; Then a Governor Challenges It," *NYT*, October 2, 1998, p. A20.

CHAPTER 3

1 Quotations are from *Phaedo*, in E. Hamilton and H. Cairns, eds., *Plato: The Collected Dialogues*, Princeton University Press, Princeton, NJ, 1961.

2 Epictetus, *Dissertations*, 1.9, 16. Quoted in James Rachels, "Euthanasia," in T. Regan, ed., *Matters of Life and Death*, 3d ed., McGraw-Hill, New York, 1993, p. 35.

3 Seneca, *De Ira*, quoted in Rachels, op. cit.

4 Jean Paul Sartre, "The Humanism of Existentialism," in Wade Beck., ed., *The Philosophy of Existentialism*, Philosophical Library, New York, 1965.

5 Matthew 16:26–28; for similar predictions, see Mark 9:1, Matthew 10:23, Matthew 16:26–28; Luke 21:29–32; Matthew 24:32–33; Mark 13:28–30; and indirectly, Matthew 10:7.

6 Alasdair MacIntyre, *A Short History of Ethics*, Macmillan, New York, 1966, pp. 116–117.

7 Margaret Pabst Battin, *Ethical Issues in Suicide*, Prentice-Hall, Englewood Cliffs, NJ, 1982, p. 34.

8 Frederick Russell, *The Just War in the Middle Ages*, Cambridge University Press, Cambridge, England, 1975.

9 Battin, op. cit.

10 Paul Badham, "Christian Beliefs and the Ethics of In-Vitro Fertilization and Abortion," *Bioethics News*, vol. 6, no. 2, January 1987, p. 8.

11 Quoted in James Gutman, "Death and Dying in Western Culture," *Encyclopedia of Bioethics*, vol. 1, Free Press, New York, 1978, p. 240.

12 Baruch Spinoza, *Ethics*, William White and Amelia Stirling, trans., Hafner, New York, 1949.

13 Quoted in Derek Humphrey and Ann Wickett, *The Right to Die: Understanding Euthanasia*, Harper and Row, New York, 1986, pp. 8–9.

14 Immanuel Kant, "On Suicide" (1755–1780), *Lectures on Ethics*, L. Enfield, trans., Harper and Row, New York, 1963, pp. 148–154.

15 David Hume, "On Suicide" (1755), in Eugene Miller, ed., *Collected Essays of David Hume*, Liberty Classics, Indianapolis, IN, 1986.

16 Ibid.

17 John Stuart Mill, *On Liberty* (1859), Appleton-Century-Crofts, New York, 1974.

18 Quoted in Humphrey and Wickett, op. cit., p. 16.

19 AP, October 16, 1983.

20 Robert Steinbock and Bernard Lo, "The Case of Elizabeth Bouvia: Starvation, Suicide, or Problem Patient?" *Archives of Internal Medicine*, vol. 146, January 1986, p. 161.

21 Quoted in George Annas, "When Suicide Prevention Becomes Brutality: The Case of Elizabeth Bouvia," *HCR*, vol. 14, no. 2, April 1984, p. 20.

22 Steinbock and Lo, op. cit., p. 161.

23 *Bouvia v. County of Riverside*, California Superior Court, December 16, 1983.

24 Quoted in Arthur Hoppe, *San Francisco Examiner*, December 20, 1983.

25 Richard Scott, in "Patient's Suicide Wish Troubles Hospital MDs," *AMN*, January 20, 1984, p. 5.

26 AP, in *Birmingham Post-Herald*, December 14, 1984, p. A2.

27 Hoppe, op. cit.

28 Annas, op. cit., p. 46.

29 Quoted in Scott, op. cit.

30 Ibid., p. 16.

31 Annas, op. cit., p. 20.

32 The hospital's rationale in its brief to Judge Deering is quoted in Annas, "Elizabeth Bouvia: Whose Space Is This Anyway?" *HCR*, vol. 16, no. 2, April 1986, pp. 24–25.

33 *Bouvia v. Glenchur*, Los Angeles Superior Court, *California Reporter*, vol. 225, 1986, pp. 296–308.

34 *Bouvia v. Superior Court* (Glenchur), *California Reporter*, vol. 297, California Appellate 2 District, 1986.

35 Steinbock and Lo, op. cit., p. 162.

36 George Annas, "Elizabeth Bouvia: Whose Space Is This Anyway?"

37 Humphrey and Wickett, op. cit., p. 150.

38 Paul Longmore, "Elizabeth Bouvia, Assisted Suicide, and Social Prejudice," in *Issues in Law and Medicine*, vol. 2, no. 2, Fall 1987, p. 158.

39 Russ Fine, *UAB Report,* September 4, 1992, p. 4.

40 B. D. Colen, "His Life, to Take or Not," *Newsday,* September 25, 1989, pp. 5–19 (cover story). I am indebted to Doris Rippetoe for this reference.

41 Ibid., p. 19.

42 Ibid.

43 Susan Schindehette and Gail Wescott, "Deciding Not to Die," *People,* January 18, 1993, p. 86.

44 Ibid.

45 Fine, op. cit.

46 Ibid., p. 12.

47 Alan Meisel, *The Right to Die: Cumulative Supplement 1,* Wylie, New York, 1991, p. x.

48 Battin, op. cit., p. 22; James Rachels, *The End of Life,* Oxford University Press, Oxford, 1986, p. 182; Tom Beauchamp, "Suicide," in T. Regan, ed., *Matters of Life and Death,* 3d ed., McGraw-Hill, New York, 1993.

49 Meisel, op. cit., p. x.

50 Kevin D. O'Rourke, "Value Conflicts Raised by Physician-Assisted Suicide," *Linacre Quarterly,* vol. 57, no. 3, August 1990, pp. 38–49.

51 T. Woody, "Was His Act of Mercy Also Murder?" *NYT,* November 7, 1988.

52 H. Hendin, "Suicide in America," *Miami News,* August 30, 1982, p. B1.

53 Art Kleiner, "Life after Suicide," *High Wire,* Summer 1982, p. 30.

54 Quoted in Humphrey and Wickett, op. cit., p. 152.

55 Quoted ibid., p. 155.

56 Longmore, op. cit., p. 156.

57 Cowart's case became the topic of a famous videotape, *Please Let Me Die,* and a later film, *Dax's Case.* See also L. Kliever, *Dax's Case—Essays in Medical Ethics and Human Meaning,* SMU Press, Dallas, Texas, 1989.

58 John Shuster, talk at UAB Medical School, August 24, 2002.

59 Longmore, op. cit., p. 168.

60 Fine, op. cit., p. 12.

61 Ibid.

62 AP, "Thousands Retiring without Social Security," February 16, 1993.

63 "McAfee Tries to Cut Red Tape," *Birmingham Post-Herald,* June 18, 1990, p. C1.

64 J. Hogeland and L. Sellars, "McAfee Shouldn't Get Special Treatment," letter, *Birmingham Post-Herald,* July 9, 1990.

65 Jeff Wilson (AP), "Precedent-Setter Lives On after Plea to Die," *Indianapolis Star,* December 19, 1993, p. H7.

66 *UAB Report,* August 28, 1992, p. 12.

67 Fine, personal communication to author, May 16, 1994.

68 Griffith Thomas MD, JD, "Elizabeth Bouvia: 18 Years Later," *EOL Choices,* vol. 1, no. 1, Winter 2002.

69 Dax Cowart, personal communication to author at 6th Undergraduate Biothics Conference, College Station, TX, March 27, 2003.

70 Paul Longmore, Column in *Electric Edge,* January/February 1997. Also available at: www.ragged-edge-mag.com/

71 Douglas Martin, "Disability Culture: Eager to Bite the Hands That Would Feed Them," June 1, 1997; *NYT,* p. 1.

72 Douglas Martin, "Fearing for Gains Won by Disabled," *NYT,* 29 April 1997, A12.

CHAPTER 4

1 Ludwig Edelstein, *Ancient Medicine: Collected Essays of Ludwig Edelstein,* O. Temkin and L. Temkin, eds., Johns Hopkins University Press, Baltimore, MD, 1967.

2 G. E. R. Lloyd, "Introduction," *Hippocratic Writings,* J. Chadwick and W. N. Mann, trans., Penguin, New York, 1978 (trans. 1950), p. 13.

3 Leo Alexander, "Medical Science under Dictatorship," *NEJM,* vol. 42, July 14, 1949.

4 Robert Jay Lifton, *The Nazi Doctors,* Basic Books, New York, 1986.

5 J. C. Wilke, *Assisted Suicide and Euthanasia: Past and Present, Hayes Publications,* 1998, p. 9. I am indebted to Stephen W. Poff, M.D., for this reference and points made in this paragraph.

6 Quoted in Derek Humphrey and Ann Wickett, *The Right to Die: Understanding Euthanasia,* Harper and Row, New York, 1988, p. 172.

7 Johannes J. M. van Delden et al., "The Remmelink Study: Two Years later," *HCR,* vol. 23, no. 6, November–December 1993, p. 24.

8 H. Hendin et al., "Euthanasia and Physician-Assisted Suicide in the Netherlands," *NEJM,* vol. 336, no. 19, pp. 1385–1387, May 8, 1997. M. Angell, "Euthanasia in the Netherlands: Good News or Bad?" *NEJM,* vol. 336, no. 25, pp. 1795–1801. June 19, 1990.

9 Shana Alexander, at "Birth of Bioethics" conference, University of Washington Medical School, Seattle, October 22, 1992.

10 Lisa Belkin, "Doctor Tells of First Death Using His Suicide Device," *NYT,* June 8, 1990.

11 Jack Kevorkian, *Prescription: Medicide—The Goodness of Planned Death,* Prometheus, Buffalo, NY, 1991, p. 221. See also *Newsweek,* November 13, 1989.

12 Isabel Wilkerson, "Physician Fulfills a Goal: Aiding a Person in Suicide," *NYT,* June 7, 1990.

13 Jack Kevorkian, op. cit., p. 214.

14 Gloria Borger, "The Odd Odyssey of 'Dr. Death,'" *U.S. News and World Report,* August 27, 1990, p. 2.

15 Timothy Quill, "Death and Dignity: A Case of Individualized Decision Making," *NEJM,* vol. 324, no. 10, March 7, 1991, pp. 691–694.

16 Timothy Quill, ibid.

17 Timothy Egan, *NYT,* May 5, 1994, p. A1.

18 Clyde Farnsworth, "Canadian Who Lost Suicide Lawsuit Kills Herself," *NYT,* February 14, 1994, p. A8.

19 "Excerpts from Court's Decision," *NYT,* June 27, 1997, p. A18.

20 Timothy Egan, "In Oregon, Opening a New Front in the World of Medicine," *NYT,* November 6, 1997, p. A22.

21 Timothy Egan, ibid.

22 Timothy Egan, ibid.

23 M. A. Lee et al., "Legalizing Assisted Suicide—Views of Physicians in Oregon," *NEJM,* vol. 334, 1996, pp. 310–315.

24 Timothy Egan, "Assisted Suicide Comes Full Circle in Oregon," *NYT,* October 26, 1997.

25 Timothy Egan, "First Known Legal Suicide Reported in Oregon," *NYT,* March 26, 1998, p. A1.

26 Susan Tolle, "Care of the Dying: Clinical and Financial Lessons from the Oregon Experience," *Annals of Internal Medicine,* vol. 128, No. 7, April 1, 1998.

27 Timothy Egan, "Assisted Suicide Comes….", op. cit.

28 J. Groenewould, et. al, "Clinical Problems with the Performance of Euthanasia and Physician-Assisted Suicide in the Netherlands," *NEJM,* vol. 342:8 (February 24, 2000), p. 551.

29 Nat Hentoff, "The Coat Hanger of Assisted Suicide," *Washington Post,* December 12, 1997.

30 "What Are the Potential Cost Savings from Legalizing Physician-Assisted Suicide?" E. Emanuel and M. Batton, *NEJM,* vol. 339, no. 3, pp. 167–172.

31 I am thankful to Jarvis Ryals, M.D., for pointing this method out to me and showing me the article by F. Miller and D. Meier, "Voluntary Death: A Comparison of Terminal Dehydration and Physician-Assisted Suicide," *Annals of Internal Medicine,* vol. 128, no. 1, April 1, 1998, pp. 559–562.

32 Edith Hoover, "Oregon Assisted Suicide Legal; Roadblocks Remain," *The Oregonian,* March 1, 1998.

33 Susan Tolle et al., *A Guidebook for Health Care Providers: The Oregon Death with Dignity Act,* March, 1998, available from the Center for Ethics in Health Care, Oregon Health Services University, 3181 Southwest Sam Jackson Park Road, Portland, OR 97201.

34 Susan Tolle et al., ibid., p. 7.

35 Oregon's Death with Dignity Act, *Annual Report 2001,* Oregon Health Service, www.ohd.hr.state.or.us/chs/pas/ar-smmry.htm.

36 Susan Tolle et al., ibid., p. 23–25.

37 Christine Cassell, quoted in Michael Specter, "Suicide Device Fuels Debate," *Washington Post,* June 8, 1990.

38 James Rachels, "Active and Passive Euthanasia," *NEJM,* vol. 292, January 9, 1975, pp. 78–80.

39 Baruch Brody, "Ethical Questions Raised by the Persistent Vegetative Patient," *HCR,* vol. 18, no. 1, p. 35.

40 Ronald Cranford, lecture at UAB, January 11, 1991.

41 Jean Davies, "Raping and Making Love Are Different Concepts: So Are Killing and Voluntary Euthanasia," *Journal of Medical Ethics,* vol. 14, 1988, pp. 148–49.

42 Gina Kolata, "'Passive Euthanasia' in Hospitals is the Norm, Doctors Say," *NYT,* June 28, 1997, p. A1.

43 Gina Kolata, ibid.

44 Joan Teno and Joanne Lynn, "Voluntary Active Euthanasia: The Individual Case and Public Policy," *Journal of the American Geriatrics Society,* vol. 39, 1991, pp. 827–830.

45 Quoted in Barnard White Stack, "Doctors Divided Over the Very Ill," *Pittsburgh Post Gazette,* June 11, 1990.

46 Quoted in Alan Parachini, "A Dutch Doctor Carries Out a Death Wish," *Los Angeles Times,* July 5, 1987, sec. 6, p. 9.

47 Richard Brandt, quoted in Susan Ager, "When Suicide Is the Last Hope," *Detroit Free Press,* June 8, 1990.

48 Quoted in Barnard White Stack, op. cit.

49 Margaret Battin, "The Least Worst Death," *HCR,* vol. 13, no. 2, April 1983, pp. 13–16.

50 Douglas Walton, *Slippery Slope Arguments,* Oxford University Press, New York 1992.

51 Yale Kamisar, quoted in Earl Ubell, "Should Death Be a Patient's Choice?" *Parade Magazine,* February 9, 1992, p. 27.

52 Quoted in Mark Ward, "Experts Consider Legal and Ethical Aspects of Helping Amer-

icans Die," *Milwaukee Journal* (Wisconsin), June 7, 1990 (*NEWSBANK* microfiche).

53 Michael Specter, "Suicide Device Fuels Debate," *Washington Post*, June 8, 1990.

54 Quoted in Peter Steinfels, "Dutch Study Is Euthanasia Vote Issue," *NYT*, September 20, 1991.

55 Charlie LeDuff, "Prosecutors Say Ex-Doctor Killed Because it Thrilled Him," *NYT*, September 7, 2000, p. A29.

56 Leo Alexander, op. cit. p. 47.

57 For example, see Carlos Gomez, M.D., *Regulating Death: Euthanasia and the Case of the Netherlands*, Free Press/Macmillan, New York, 1991.

58 Nat Hentoff, "The Deadly Slippery Slope," *Village Voice*, September 1, 1987.

59 Nat Hentoff, "Decision on Euthanasia Will Create a Slippery Slope," nationally syndicated column, Newspaper Enterprise Association, October 6, 1992 (see also *Washington Post* of same date).

60 Norman Paradis, "Making a Living Off the Dying," *NYT*, April 25, 1992, p. 15.

61 Christiaan Barnard, *One Life*, Macmillan, New York, 1965.

62 Rufus E. Miles, "Quick and Painless Death Should Be a Right," letter, *NYT*, June 19, 1990.

63 Quoted in Linda Matchan, "Suicide Shocks Ethicists," *Boston Globe*, June 7, 1990.

64 Quoted in Earl Ubell, op. cit., p. 28.

65 Frank Bruni, "Theatrics Eclipse Ethics," *Detroit News and Free Press*, October 26, 1991.

66 Quoted in Brian T. Meehan, "Adkins Suicide Ignites Nationwide Debate," *The Oregonian*, June 8, 1990.

CHAPTER 5

1 Paul Badham, "Christian Belief and the Ethics of In Vitro Fertilization," *Bioethics News*, vol. 6, no. 2, January 1987, p. 10.

2 Paul Johnson, *A History of Christianity*, Atheneum, New York, 1983, chap. 3.

3 John R. Connery, "Abortion: Roman Catholic Perspectives," *Encyclopedia of Bioethics*, vol. I, Macmillan, New York, 1978.

4 Robert W. Mulligan, S. J., Jesuit Community at St. Louis University, personal communication.

5 Today, the official Catholic position on immediate animation is unclear, although the church does teach that the "greatest care" should be taken with the embryo from the moment of conception. See Connery, op. cit., p. 13.

6 *Roe* v. *Wade, Supreme Court Reporter*, 93, 410 US 151, pp. 709–762. Subsequent quotations from the decision are from this source.

7 Barbara Ehrenreich and Deirdre English, *For Her Own Good: 150 Years of the Experts' Advice to Women*, Doubleday, New York, 1987, pp. 319–320.

8 Alan Guttmacher Institute, *Abortion and Women's Health*, New York and Washington, D.C., 1990, p. 27.

9 Alan F. Guttmacher, *The Case for Legalized Abortion*, Diablo, Berkeley, CA, 1977, pp. 15–17.

10 In 1992 a movie called *A Private Affair* was made about this case; Sissy Spacek portrayed Sherri Finkbine.

11 Peter Steinfels, "Paper Birth-Control Letter Retains Its Grip," *NYT*, July 29, 1993, pp. A1, 13.

12 Among them can be counted Albert Jonsen, Paul Tong, and Warren Reich. Although Daniel Callahan was never a priest, his first book on abortion and his founding of the Hastings Center reflect the concerns of someone educated in the Catholic tradition and struggling to make sense of new ethical issues in medicine. (Personal communication from Warren Reich.)

13 Norma McCorvey, *I Am Roe—My Life: Roe v. Wade and Freedom of Choice*, Harper Collins, 1993.

14 CDC Fact Sheet: Abortion Surveillance, June 7, 2002.

15 Alan Guttmacher Institute, op. cit., p. 22.

16 Maggie Scarf, "The Fetus as Guinea Pig," October 19, 1975 *NYT Magazine*, 194–200.

17 Paul Ramsey, *The Ethics of Fetal Research*, Yale University Press, New Haven, Conn. 1975.

18 A. Philipson et al., "Transplacental Passage of Erythromycin and Clindamycin," *NEJM*, vol. 288, no. 23, June 7, 1973, pp. 1219–1221.

19 William Nolen, *The Baby in the Bottle*, Coward, McCann, and Geoghegan, New York, 1978.

20 Ibid., p. 203.

21 Ibid., p. 150.

22 "The Edelin Trial," transcript of trial for WBGH recreation for Bill Moyers documentary; Project of Legal-Medical Studies, Inc., Box 8219, John F. Kennedy Station, Government Station, Boston, MA 12134.

23 William F. Buckley, *National Review*, March 14, 1975; quoted in Nolen, op. cit., p. 221.

24 *Commonwealth* v. *Kenneth Edelin*, Mass. Supreme Court 359, N.E. 2d 4, 1976.

25 Kenneth Edelin, *Ob. Gyn. News*, January 1, 1977, p. 1.

26 Quoted in Paul Ramsey, *Ethics at the Edges of Life,* Yale University Press, New Haven, CT, 1978, p. 94.

27 Nolen, op. cit.

28 Ibid., p. 175.

29 Mary Anne Warren, "On the Moral and Legal Status of the Fetus," *Monist,* vol. 57, 1973, pp. 43–61.

30 Don Marquis, "Why Abortion Is Immoral," *Journal of Philosophy,* vol. 86, 1989, pp. 183–202; Warren Quinn, "Abortion: Identity and Loss," *Philosophy and Public Affairs,* vol. 13, 1984, pp. 24–54.

31 John T. Noonan, Jr. "An Almost Absolute Value in History," in John T. Noonan, Jr., ed., *The Morality of Abortion: Legal and Historical Perspectives,* Harvard University Press, Cambridge, MA, 1970, pp. 51–59.

32 Judith Jarvis Thomson, "A Defense of Abortion," *Philosophy and Public Affairs,* vol. 1, no. 1, Fall 1971, pp. 47–66.

33 Francis Kamm, *Creation and Abortion,* Oxford University Press, New York, 1992.

34 Connery, op. cit., pp. 9–13.

35 Ellen Willis, "Harper's Forum on Abortion," *Harper's Magazine,* July 1986, p. 38.

36 "Explosions over Abortion," *Time,* January 14, 1985, p. 17.

37 "New Skill For Future OB/GYN's: Abortion Training," Linda Villanova, 6/11/02, *NYT.*

38 Jeff Lyon, "The Doctor's Dilemma: When Abortion Gives Birth to Life, Physicians Become Troubled Saviors," *Chicago Tribune,* August 15, 1982, sec. 12, pp. 1, 3.

39 Consultants to the Advisory Committee to the Director, National Institutes of Health, *Report of the Human Fetal Tissue Transplantation Research Panel,* vol. I, National Institutes of Health (NIH), Bethesda, MD, 1988.

40 AP, "Easier Way Found for Abortion Pill," *NYT,* May 27, 1993, p. A13; "Scientists Push for Quick Approval of French Abortion Pill," *NYT,* September 9, 1993.

41 Gina Kolta, "Without Fanfare, Morning-After Pill Gets a Closer Look," *NYT,* 8 October 2000, A1.

42 For example, see the commentary by Phillip Stubblefield, "Self-Administered Emergency Contraception—A Second Chance," *NEJM,* vol. 339, no. 1, July 2, 1998, pp. 41–42.

43 James Trussel, "Emergency Contraceptives," *American Journal of Public Health,* vol. 87, no. 6, June 1997, pp. 909–910.

44 Anna Glasier and David Baird, "The Effects of Self-Administering Emergency Contraception," *NEJM,* vol. 339, no. 1, July 2, 1998, pp. 1–4.

45 Kenneth Jost, *American Bar Association Journal,* "Mother versus Child," April 1989, p. 86.

46 AP, "Mother Gets 6 Years for Drugs in Breast Milk," *NYT,* October 28, 1992, p. A11.

47 E. L. Abel and R. J. Sokol, "Fetal Alcohol Syndrome Is Now the Leading Cause of Mental Retardation," *Lancet,* vol. 8517, pp. 898–899 (letter).

48 Opinion in *Akron* v. *Akron Center for Reproductive Health* (1983), quoted in *Newsweek,* January 14, 1985, p. 28.

49 Harold Morowitz and James Trefil, *"Roe* v. *Wade* Passes a Lab Test," *NYT,* November 25, 1992, p. A13.

50 Excerpts from *Planned Parenthood* v. *Casey, NYT,* June 30, 1992, p. A8.

51 Tamar Lewin, "Parental Consent to Abortion: How Enforcement Can Vary," *NYT,* May 28, 1992, p. A9.

52 George Annas, "Partial-Birth Abortion, Congress, and the Constitution," *NEJM,* vol. 339, no. 4, July 23, 1998, pp. 279.

53 Hadley Arkes, "Courts Strike Down Laws Against Partial-Birth Abortion," *Wall Street Journal,* December 17, 1998, A31.

CHAPTER 9

1 Robert Weir, *Selected Nontreatment of Handicapped Newborns,* Oxford University Press, New York, 1984; John Boswell, *The Kindness of Strangers: The Abandonment of Children in Western Europe from Late Antiquity to the Renaissance,* Pantheon, New York, 1989.

2 William Lecky, *History of European Morals from Augustus to Charlemagne,* vol. II, Brazilier, New York, 1955, pp. 25–56 (originally published 1869).

3 W. L. Langer, "Europe's Initial Population Explosion," *American Historical Review,* vol. 69, 1963, pp. 1–17; quoted in G. Hardin, *Exploring New Ethics for Survival: The Voyage of the Spaceship Beagle,* Viking, New York, 1972, pp. 180–183.

4 James Gustafson, "Mongolism, Parental Desires, and the Right to Life," *Perspectives in Biology and Medicine,* vol. 16, Summer 1973, p. 529.

5 Some important details of these cases come from conversations with Norman Fost, a well-known ethicist and pediatrician at the University of Wisconsin medical school.

6 *Who Should Survive?* produced by the Joseph P. Kennedy Jr. Foundation; available from Film Service, 999 Asylum Avenue, Hartford, CT, 06105. Norman Fost, who was

then a resident at Hopkins, appears briefly in the film (in the background).

7 Quoted in *Who Should Survive?*

8 Gustafson, op. cit.

9 Ibid.

10 R. Duff and A. Campbell, "Moral and Ethical Dilemmas in the Special-Care Nursery," *NEJM*, vol. 289, no. 17, October 25, 1973, pp. 890–894.

11 John Lorber, "Results of Treatment of Myelomeningocele: An Analysis of 524 Unselected Cases, with Special Reference to Possible Selection for Treatment," *Developmental Medicine and Child Neurology*, vol. 13, no. 3, 1971, pp. 279–303.

12 *Dorland's Illustrated Medical Dictionary*, Saunders, Philadephia, PA, 1987.

13 Mary Tedeschi, "Infanticide and Its Apologists," *Commentary*, November 1984, p. 34.

14 Shari Staaver, "Siamese Twins' Case 'Devastates' MDs," *AMN*, October 9, 1981, p. 15–16.

15 Bonnie Steinbock, "Whatever Happened to the Danville Siamese Twins?" *HCR*, vol. 17, no. 4, August–September 1987, pp. 3–4.

16 John Robertson, "Dilemma in Danville," *HCR*, vol. 11, no. 5, October 1981, p. 7.

17 U.S. Commission on Civil Rights, "Medical Discrimination against Children with Disabilities," September 1989, p. 391.

18 Ibid., pp. 36, 323.

19 Adrian Peracchio, "Government in the Nursery: New Era for Baby Doe Cases," *Newsday*, November 13, 1983. (This story and Kathleen Kerr's story, cited in note 21, are available from *Newsday* as a reprint, "The Baby Jane Doe Story: Winner of the 1984 Pulitzer Prize for Local Reporting.")

20 This result is according to *Newsday*'s investigation.

21 Kathleen Kerr, "An Issue of Law and Ethics," *Newsday*, October 26, 1983.

22 Kathleen Kerr, "Legal, Medical Legacy of Case," *Newsday*, December 7, 1987.

23 Ibid.

24 Bonnie Steinbock, "Baby Jane Doe in the Courts," *HCR*, vol. 14, no. 1, February 1984, p. 15.

25 Kerr, "Legal, Medical Legacy of Case"; see also Kathleen Kerr, "Reporting the Case of Baby Jane Doe," *HCR*, vol. 14, no. 4, August 1984.

26 "Baby Jane Doe Has Surgery to Remove Water from Brain," *NYT*, April 7, 1984, p. 28.

27 Kerr, "Legal, Medical Legacy of Case."

28 *HCR*, vol. 24., no. 3, May–June 1994, p. 2.

29 Rhoda Amon, "A Long-Running Morality Play," www.lihistory.com/9/hs9moral.htm

30 Gustafson, op. cit.; C. Everett Koop, "The Slide to Auschwitz," *Whatever Happened to the Human Race?* Revell, Old Tappan, NJ, 1979.

31 John Paris, "Right to Life Doesn't Demand Heroic Sacrifice," *WSJ*, November 28, 1983, p. 30.

32 *Who Should Survive?*

33 Fred Bruning, "The Politics of Life," *Newsday*, December 12, 1983, p. 17.

34 C. Everett Koop, "The Seriously Ill or Dying Child: Supporting the Patient and the Family," in D. Horan and D. Mall, eds., *Death, Dying and Euthanasia*, University Publications of America, Frederick, MD, 1977, pp. 537–539.

35 Koop, "The Slide to Auschwitz."

36 R. McCormick, "To Save or Let Die: The Dilemma of Modern Medicine," *JAMA*, vol. 229, no. 8, July 1974, pp. 172–176.

37 Peter Singer, *Practical Ethics*, Cambridge University Press, New York, 1979, p. 137; Tristam Engelhardt, "Ethical Issues in Aiding the Death of Young Children," in Marvin Kohl, ed., *Beneficent Euthanasia*, Prometheus, Buffalo, NY, 1975; Michael Tooley, "Abortion and Infanticide," *Philosophy and Public Affairs*, vol. 2, no. 1, Fall 1972, pp. 37–65.

38 Kerr, "Legal, Medical Legacy of Case."

39 Weir, op. cit.

40 R. B. Zachary, "Life with Spina Bifida," *British Medical Journal*, vol. 2, 1977, p. 1461.

41 David Gibson, "Dimensions of Intelligence," in *Down Syndrome: The Psychology of Mongolism*, Cambridge University Press, New York, 1978, pp. 35–77; Janet Carr, "The Development of Intelligence," in David Lane and Brian Stafford, eds., *Current Approaches to Down Syndrome*, Praeger, New York, 1985, pp. 167–186.

42 J. Freeman, "To Treat or Not to Treat: Ethical Dilemmas of Treating the Infant with Myelomeningocele," *Clinical Neurosurgery*, vol. 20, 1973, p. 137.

43 Peter Singer, "Sanctity of Life or Quality of Life?" *Pediatrics*, vol. 72, no. 1, July 1983, pp. 128–129.

44 Letters reacting to Singer's article appeared in *Pediatrics*, vol. 73, no. 2, February 1984.

45 B. D. Colen, "A Life of Love—and Endless Pain," *Newsday*, October 26, 1983. (Available from *Newsday* in the reprint "The Baby Jane Doe Story: Winner of the 1984 Pulitzer Prize for Local Reporting.")

46 Steven Baer, "The Half-Told Story of Baby Jane Doe," *Columbia Journalism Review*, November–December 1984, pp. 35–38.

47 Tedeschi, op. cit., pp. 31–35.

48 *Gleitman* v. *Cosgrove,* quoted in M. Coppenger, ed., *Bioethics: A Casebook,* Prentice-Hall, Englewood Cliffs, NJ, 1985, pp. 8–12.

49 Brenda Coleman, "Moral Floodgates Opened by Father Pulling Plug on Son," AP, May 1, 1989.

50 E. M. Maragakis, "EMTALA Rears its Ugly Head: The Case of Baby K," *Utah Law Review,* 1996, pp. 109–130.

51 A. Gallo, "Spina Bifida: The State of the Art of Medical Management," *HCR,* vol. 14, no. 1, February 1984, pp. 10–13.

52 Ibid.

53 Spina Bifida Association, Brief Amicus Curiae of the Spina Bifida Association of America, *Weber* v. *Stony Brook Hospital,* New York State Supreme Court, Appellate Division, 2d Department, *New York Law Journal,* October 28, 1983; quoted in Steinbock, "Baby Jane Doe in the Courts," p. 19.

54 Loretta Kopelman, "Do the 'Baby Doe' Rules Ignore Suffering?" *Second Opinion,* vol. 18., no. 4, April 1983, pp. 101–113.

55 Gina Kolata, "Parents of Tiny Infants Find Care Choices Are Not Theirs," *NYT,* September 30, 1991, p. A1.

56 Norman Fost, comment made on the email listserv of the Medical College of Wisconsin. Quoted with permission.

57 Norman Fost, personal communication, August 1, 1998, quoted with permission.

58 Bill Bartholomene, personal communication, whom I also thank for reading the chapter.

59 Marc Kaufman, "Ruling Upheld on Baby with Brain Damage," *Washington Times,* August 6, 1999, p. A1.

60 Mathew Rarey, "Wrongful-birth Lawsuits Put Doctors in Ethical Dilemma," *Washington Times,* August 5, 1999, p. A20.

61 "High Court Rules 'Wrongful Birth' Suits Invalid," *Atlanta Journal-Constitution,* July 7, 1999, p. E1.

62 Suzanne Daley, "France Bans Damages for 'Wrongful Births'," *NYT,* January 1, 2002, A8.

63 Norman Fost, "Decisions Regarding Treatment of Seriously Ill Newborns," *JAMA* 281, June 2, 1999, pp. 2041–2043.

CHAPTER 10

1 Nicholas Fontaine, *Memoires pour servir l'histoire de Port-Royal,* vol. 2 (originally published in Cologne in 1738); quoted in L. Rosenfield, *From Beast-Machine to Man-Machine: The Theme of Animal Soul in French Letters from Descartes to La Mettrie,* Oxford University Press, New York, 1940, pp. 52–53; also quoted in Peter Singer, *Animal Liberation, New York Review of Books,* 1975.

2 C. S. Lewis, *How Human Suffering Raises Almost Intolerable Intellectual Problems,* Macmillan, New York, 1940, pp. 131–133.

3 David Hume, *A Treatise of Human Nature,* 1789.

4 Office of Technology Assessment, *Animal Usage in the United States,* Superintendent of Documents, Washington, D.C., 1986, p. 12; Andrew Rowan, *Of Mice, Models, and Men: A Critical Evaluation of Animal Research,* State University of New York Press, Albany, 1984, pp. 67–70; *Newsweek,* December 26, 1988, p. 51.

5 Bernard Rollins, *Animal Rights and Human Morality,* Prometheus, Buffalo, NY, 1981, pp. 97–99.

6 W. Robbins, "Animal Rights: A Growing Movement in the U.S.," *NYT,* June 15, 1984, p. A16.

7 "The Use of Animals in Research," *NEJM,* vol. 313, no. 6, pp. 395–400.

8 *Evaluation of Experimental Procedures Conducted at the University of Pennsylvania Experimental Head-Injury Laboratory 1981– 1984 in Light of the Public Health Science Animal Welfare Policy,* Office for Protection of Research Risks, National Institutes of Health, 1985, p. 37.

9 Quoted in "Animals in the Middle," in the television series *Innovation,* sponsored by Johnson and Johnson on A & E Network, September 5, 1987.

10 James Kilpatrick, "Animal-Rights Suporters Claim Well-Won Victory," nationally syndicated column, July 23, 1985.

11 Robbins, op. cit.

12 Robert Marshak, quoted in *NYT,* July 29, 1984, p. A12.

13 Donald Abt, quoted in *NYT,* August 12, 1984, p. B1.

14 *NYT,* December 10, 1984, p. A10.

15 Ibid.

16 Edward Taub, "The Silver Spring Monkey Incident: The Untold Story," *Coalition for Animals and Animal Research Newsletter,* vol. 4, no. 1, Winter–Spring 1991, pp. 1–8.

17 Tony Dajer, "Monkeying with the Brain," *Discover,* January 1992, p. 70–71. See also Warren E. Leary, "Sharp Brain Healing Found in Disputed Monkey Tests, *NYT,* June 28, 1991, p. A9.

18 Edward Taub, *Topics in Stroke Rehabilitation,* vol. 3, pp. 38–61.

19 Sandra Blakeslee, "Pushing Injured Brains and Spinal Cords to New Paths," *NYT*, August 28, 2001, p. D6.

20 Singer, op. cit.

21 Quoted in Marsha Mercer, "Animal Rights Group Willing to Use Violence for Cause," Scripps Howard/Media General Newspapers, May 1, 1989.

22 Susan Wolf, "Moral Saints," *Journal of Philosophy*, vol. 79, no. 8, August 1982.

23 Quoted in S. Isen, "Laying the Foundation for Animal Rights: Interview with Tom Regan," *Animals Agenda*, July–August, 1984, pp. 4–5.

24 Tom Regan, *The Case for Animal Rights*, University of California Press, Berkeley, 1983.

25 Quoted in "Animals in the Middle."

26 Ibid.

27 Carl Cohen, "The Case for Animal Rights," *NEJM*, vol. 315, no. 14, October 4, 1986, pp. 865–870.

28 R. G. Frey, *Rights, Killing, and Suffering*, Basil Blackwell, Oxford, England, 1983, p. 65.

29 Quoted in Katie McCabe, "Who Will Live, Who Will Die?" *Washingtonian Magazine*, April 1986, p. 115.

30 Rebecca Dresser, "Measuring Merit in Scientific Research," *Theoretical Medicine*, vol. 10, no. 1, 1989, pp. 21–34. It is relevant to note that the discovery of the gene for colon cancer apparently resulted from "hard-core, undirected research" (Natalie Angier, "Scientists Isolate Novel Gene Linked to Colon Cancer," *NYT*, December 3, 1993, p. A10).

31 *NYT*, August 12, 1984.

32 Quoted in J. Duschek, "Protestors Prompt Halt in Animal Research," *Science News*, July 27, 1985, p. 53.

33 Quoted by O. Cusak, "Direct Action for Animals: Interview with England's Marley Jones," *Animals Agenda*, vol. 7, no. 3, April 1987, pp. 32–34.

34 Bernard Levin, "The Animals Lovers Lusting for Blood," *The Times*, July 3, 1985, p. 15.

35 "Of Pain and Progress," *Newsweek*, December 26, 1988, p. 53.

36 Donald Barnes, "Debating the Values of Animal Research," *Animals Agenda*, vol. 7, no. 3, April 1987, pp. 32–34.

37 Another example of a person who has changed sides on a moral issue is the former abortionist Barnard Nathanson.

38 D. Moss and P. Greanville, "The Emerging Face of the Movement," *Animals Agenda*, March–April 1985, p. 11.

39 L. Jewell and D. Frazier, "Annual Questionaire Results," *Physiologist*, vol. 29, no. 2, 1986, p. 23.

40 F. Feretti, "Forsaken Vacation Animals," *NYT*, September 5, 1984, p. C1.

41 Deborah Blum, *The Monkey Wars*, Oxford University Press, New York, 1994, p. 118.

42 Phil McCombs, "Activist Battles Animal-Rights Movement," *Los Angeles Times-Washington Post*, April 27, 1992.

43 John Durant, quoted in John Hargrove, "Bush Signs Heflin Bill to Protect Researchers," *Birmingham Post-Herald*, August 28, 1992.

44 Stephen Labaton, "Judge Orders Rules Tightened to Protect Animals in Research," *NYT*, February 26, 1993.

45 Madhusree Mukerjee, "Trends in Animal Research," *Scientific American*, February, 1997, p. 89. See also M. S. Russell and Rex L. Burch, *The Principles of Humane Experimental Technique*, Methuen, London, 1959, p. 594; F. Barbara Orlans and Tom Beauchamp, eds., *The Human Use of Animals: Case Studies in Ethical Choice*, Oxford University Press, New York, 1998.

46 Bo Emerson, "Dying for Space," *Atlanta Journal-Constitution*, p. C7-8, September 24, 2000.

CHAPTER 11

1 S. Gomer, H. Powell, and G. Rolino, "Japan's Biological Weapons"; H. Powell, "A Hidden Chapter in History," *Bulletin of Atomic Scientists*, October 1981, pp. 43, 44.

2 Eugene Kogon, *The Theory and Practice of Hell*, Farrar, Straus, and Cudahy, New York, 1950; Berkeley reprint, 1980, p. 166.

3 Ibid., pp. 164ff.

4 Gerald Posner and Jerome Ware, *Mengele: The Complete Story*, McGraw-Hill, New York, 1986, p. 11.

5 Vera Alexander, *The Search for Mengele*, Home Box Office, October 1985; interviewed by Central Television (London) and quoted in Posner and Ware, op. cit., p. 37.

6 Miklos Nyiszli, quoted in R. Lifton, "What Made This Man Mengele?" *NYT Magazine*, July 21, 1985, p. 22; see also Posner and Ware, op. cit., p. 39.

7 William Curran, "The Forensic Investigation of the Death of Joseph Mengele," *NEJM*, vol. 315, no. 17, Ocober 23, 1985, pp. 1071–1073.

8 Hannah Arendt, *Eichman at Jerusalem*, Penguin, New York, 1977.

9 Stanley Milgram, *Obedience to Authority*, Harper Collins, New York, 1980.

10 Leo Alexander, "Medical Science under Dictatorship," *NEJM*, vol. 42, July 14, 1949.

11 David Rothman, "Ethics and Human Experimentation," *NEJM*, vol. 317, no. 19, November 5, 1987, p. 1198.

12 Robert Bazell, "Growth Industry," *New Republic*, March 15, 1993, p. 14.

13 Constance Pechura, "From the Institute of Medicine," *JAMA*, vol. 269, no. 4, January 27, 1993, p. 453.

14 Rothman, op. cit., p. 1198.

15 Ibid., p. 1199.

16 H. Beecher, "Ethics and Clinical Research," *NEJM*, vol. 274, 1966, pp. 1354–1360.

17 H. Pappworth, *Human Guinea Pigs*, Beacon, Boston, MA, 1968.

18 Molly Selvin, "Changing Medical and Societal Attitudes toward Sexually Transmitted Diseases: A Historical Overview," in King K. Holmes et al., eds., *Sexually Transmitted Diseases*, McGraw-Hill, New York, 1984, p. 3–19.

19 Alan Brandt, "Racism and Research: The Case of the Tuskegee Syphilis Study," *HCR*, vol. 8, no. 6, December 1978, pp. 21–29.

20 Paul de Kruif, *Microbe Hunters*, Harcourt Brace, New York, 1926, p. 323.

21 R. H. Kampmeier, "The Tuskegee Study of Untreated Syphilis" (editorial), *Southern Medical Journal*, vol. 65, no. 10, October 1972, pp. 1247–1251.

22 J. E. Bruusgaard, "Über das Schicksal der nicht spezifisch behandelten Luetiker" ("Fate of Syphilitics Who Are Not Given Specific Treatment"), *Archives of Dermatology of Syphilis*, vol. 157, April 1929, pp. 309–332.

23 Todd Savitt, *Medicine and Slavery: The Disease and Health of Blacks in Antebellum Virginia*, University of Illinois Press, Champaign, 1978.

24 James Jones, *Bad Blood*, Free Press, New York, 1981.

25 H. H. Hazen, "Syphilis in the American Negro," *JAMA*, vol. 63, August 8, 1914, p. 463.

26 Jones, op. cit., p. 74.

27 Ibid.

28 Ibid.

29 Brandt, op. cit.

30 Quoted in E. Ramont, "Syphillis in the AIDS Era," *NEJM*, vol. 316, no. 25, June 18, 1987, pp. 600–601.

31 R. A. Vonderlehr, T. Clark, and J. R. Heller, "Untreated Syphilis in the Male Negro," *JAMA*, p. 107, no. 11, September 12, 1936, pp. 856–860.

32 *Archives of National Library of Medicine*; quoted in Jones, op. cit., p. 127.

33 Jones, op. cit., pp. 190–193.

34 Quoted ibid., p. 196.

35 W. J. Brown et al., *Syphilis and Other Venereal Diseases*, Harvard University Press, Cambridge, MA, 1970, p. 34.

36 Jean Heller, "Syphilis Victims in U.S. Study Went Untreated for 40 Years," *NYT*, July 26, 1972, pp. 1, 8.

37 Ibid., p. 8.

38 Jones, op. cit., insert following p. 48.

39 Tuskegee Syphilis Study Ad Hoc Panel to Department of Health, Education, and Welfare, *Final Report*, Superintendent of Documents, Washington, D.C., 1973.

40 David Tase, "Tuskegee Syphilis Victims, Kin May Get \$1.7 Million in Fiscal 1989," AP, September 11, 1988.

41 Heller, op. cit., p. 8.

42 Kampmeier, op. cit. It is not clear whether Kampmeier himself was involved in the Tuskegee study, or if so in what capacity.

43 Thomas Benedek, "The 'Tuskegee Study' of Untreated Syphilis: Analysis of Moral Aspects versus Methodological Aspects," *Journal of Chronic Diseases*, vol. 31, 1978, p. 35–50. I have drawn considerably on this excellent article.

44 Heller, op. cit., p. 1.

45 Kampmeier, op. cit.

46 "The Tuskegee Study of Untreated Syphilis: The Thirtieth Year of Observation," *Archives of Internal Medicine*, vol. 114, 1961, pp. 792–798.

47 "Malpractice Suit Settled for \$2.7 Million," *Burlington Free Press* (Alabama), December 21, 1988.

48 Benedek, op. cit., p. 44.

49 Personal correspondence, April 25, 1985. Benjamin Friedman is Professor Emeritus of Medicine, UAB.

50 Benedek, op. cit.

51 G. W. Hayes et al., "The Golden Anniversary of the Silver Bullet," *JAMA*, vol. 270, no. 13, October 6, 1993, p. 1610.

52 R. H. Kampmeier, "Final Report of the 'Tuskegee Study' of Syphilis," *Southern Medical Journal*, vol. 67, no. 11, 1974, pp. 1349–1353. Kampmeier advances a fourth argument which is somewhat more technical. Penicillin achieves seroreversal in latent syphilis, but Kampmeier insists that such seroreversal has never been proved to be associated with decreased morbidity or mortality. A related point is possible uncertainty over diagnosis and thus over therapeutic effects. (S. Edberg and S. Berger, *Antibiotics and Infection*, Churchill Livingstone, New York, 1983, pp. 141–142; K. Holmes et al., *Sexually Transmitted Diseases*, McGraw-Hill, New York,

1984, p. 1352; John Hotson, "Modern Neuro-syphilis: A Partially Treated Chronic Meningitis, *Western Journal of Medicine,* vol. 135, September 1981, pp. 191–200; Sarah Polt, Professor of Pathology, UAB, personal correspondence.)

53 Kampmeier, "Final Report of the 'Tuskegee Study' of Syphilis."

54 Quoted in Jim Auchemutey, "Ghosts of Tuskegee," *Atlanta Journal-Constitution,* September 6, 1992, pp. M1, M6.

55 It is only fair to add that when people like Sidney Olansky (and Kampmeier) took up syphilology in the 1930s, the field was avoided by physicians who wanted to have upper-class, paying patients. Only idealists—physicians who wanted to help people on the margins of society—went into syphilology.

56 "The Deadly Deception" (with George Strait), *Nova,* January 28, 1992.

57 Allison Mitchell, "Survivors of Tuskegee Study Get Apology from Clinton," *NYT,* May 17, 1997, p. A1.

58 Carol Yoon, "Families Emerge as Silent Victims of Tuskegee Syphilis Experiments," *NYT,* May 9, 1998, p. A1.

59 Carol Yoon, Ibid.

60 Robert Burns, "Radiation Experiments Were Far-Reaching," AP, August 18, 1995, *Birmingham Post-Herald,* p. E6.

61 Philip J. Hilts, "Healthy People Secretly Poisoned in 40s Test," *NYT,* January 19, 1995, p. A13.

62 Keith Schneider, "Scientists Are Sharing the Anguish over Nuclear Experiements on People," *NYT,* March 2, 1994, p. A9.

63 Philip J. Hilts, "U.S. Is Urged to Repay Some Radiation Tests," *NYT,* July 17, 1995, p. A9. See also *Final Report,* Advisory Committee on Human Radiation Experiments, Washington, DC: US Government Printing Office.

64 Arthur Caplan, "Rethinking the Cost of War," *Due Consideration,* John Wiley & Sons, New York, 1998, pp. 123–124.

65 Marcia Angell, "The Ethics of Clinical Research in the Third World," *NEJM,* vol. 337, no. 12, September 18, 1997, pp. 847–849.

66 Marcia Angell, "Tuskegee Revisited," *WSJ,* October 28, 1997.

67 Public Citizen News Release, April 22, 1997.

68 Ruth Macklin, "Ethics and International Collaborative Research, Part I," *American Society for Bioethics and Humanities Exchange,* vol. 1, no. 2, p. 1.

69 Ellen Goodman, "Is Tuskegee Study OK Abroad?," *The Boston Globe.*

70 D. Bagenda and P. Musoke-Mudido, "We're Trying to Help Our Sickest People, Not Exploit Them," *Washington Post,* September 28, 1997, p. C3.

71 Ruth Macklin, op. cit.

72 Ellen Goodman, op. cit.

73 Marcia Angell, "Tuskegee Revisited," *WSJ,* October 28, 1997.

74 Sheryl Gay Stolberg, "U.S. Ends Overseas H.I.V. Studies Involving Placebos," *NYT,* February 19, 1998

75 Ellen Goodman, op. cit.

CHAPTER 12

1 This account in places draws heavily on the excellent account of the history of transplantation of Calvin Stiller in the 2nd edition of the *Encyclopedia of Bioethics,* pp. 1871–1872.

2 Thomas Starzl, *The Puzzle People: Memoirs of a Transplant Surgeon,* Pittsburgh University Press, PA, 1992, p. 151.

3 Donald R. Kahn, personal communication to author, April 14, 1993; Norman Shumway, personal communication to author, January 10, 1994. One reason why Shumway may have given implicit permission was that he himself was being held back by the problem of declaring a donor "brain-dead"; in 1967, criteria for brain death had not yet been established in the United States.

4 Christiaan Barnard and Curtiss Bill Pepper, *One Life,* Macmillan, New York, 1969, p. 310.

5 Ibid., p. 332.

6 Ibid., p. 343.

7 Ibid., p. 372.

8 "The Ultimate Operation," *Time,* December 15, 1967, p. 65.

9 "Heart Transplant Keeps Man Alive in South Africa," *NYT,* December 4, 1967, p. A1.

10 Barnard and Pepper, op. cit., p. 378.

11 Ibid., p. 406.

12 "The Ultimate Operation," p. 66.

13 Barnard and Pepper, op. cit., p. 444.

14 Christiaan Barnard, *The Second Life,* Vlaeberg Publishers, South Africa, 1993.

15 The events of this story are described in Renée Fox and Judith Swazey, *The Courage to Fail,* 2nd ed., University of Chicago Press, IL, 1978, Chapter 6.

16 Thomas Preston, "Who Benefits from the Artificial Heart?" *HCR,* vol. 15, no. 1, February 1985, p. 5; see also *NYT,* December 5, 1988, p. A2.

17 Denise Grady, "Summary of Discussion of Ethical Perspectives," in Margery Shaw, ed.,

After Barney Clark, University of Texas Press, Austin, p. 52.

18 *NYT,* December 5, 1982, p. 48.

19 *Time,* December 9, 1982, p. 43.

20 *NYT,* December 3, 1982, p. A1.

21 *NYT,* March 25, 1983, p. A1.

22 *NYT,* December 5, 1982, p. 48.

23 *Time,* March 14, 1983, p. 74.

24 Preston, op. cit., p. 6.

25 *WP,* May 1, 1983, p. A2.

26 William A. Check, "Lessons from Barney Clark's Artificial Heart," *Health,* April 1984, pp. 22, 26.

27 *NYT,* April 17, 1983, p. 44.

28 *NYT,* editorial, December 16, 1982, p. A26.

29 "Knife to the Heart," with Connie Chung, January 27, 1997; television series on history of surgery.

30 *NYT,* December 6, 1967.

31 Peter Hawthorne, *The Transplanted Heart,* Keartland, Johannesburg, South Africa, 1968, pp. 188.

32 Gideon Gil, "Burcham Dies after Blood Accumulates in Chest," *Louisville Courier-Journal* (Kentucky), April 26, 1985.

33 Ibid., p. 117.

34 Eric Cassell, "How Is the Death of Barney Clark to Be Understood?" in Shaw, op. cit., p. 48.

35 P. M. Park, "The Transplant Odyssey," *Second Opinion,* vol. 12, November 1989, pp. 27–32; quoted in Fox and Swazey, *Spare Parts,* p. 200.

36 William Pierce, "Permanent Heart Substitution: Better Solutions Ahead," editorial, *JAMA,* vol. 259, no. 6, February 12, 1988, p. 891.

37 Quoted from *Newsweek* in Fox and Swazey, *Spare Parts.* Renée Fox and Judith Swazey, *Spare Parts: Organ Replacement in American Society,* Oxford University Press, New York, 1992, p. 141.

38 *Progressive,* February 1983, pp. 12–13.

39 Renée Fox and Judith Swazey, *The Courage to Fail: A Social View of Organ Transplants and Dialysis,* 2d ed., rev., University of Chicago Press, IL., 1974, 1978

40 Barnard and Pepper, op. cit., p. 361.

41 Starzl, op. cit., p. 148.

42 Werner Forssmann, quoted in Barnard and Pepper, op. cit., p. 360.

43 Institute of Medicine, *Non-Heart-Beating Organ Transplantation: Medical and Ethical Issues in Procurement,* Washington, D.C., National Academy Press, 1997, p. 24.

44 Charles Junkerman and David Schiedermayer, *Practical Ethics for Students, Interns, and Residents: A Short Reference Manual,* Uni-versity Publishing Group, Frederick, MD, 1994, p. 3.

45 Robert Arnold and Stuart Younger, "Back to the Future: Obtaining Organs from Non-Heart-Beating Cadavers," *Kennedy Institute of Ethics,* vol. 3, no. 2, p. 106.

46 Alan Weisbard, "A Polemic on Principles: Reflections on the Pittsburgh Protocol," *Kennedy Institute of Ethics,* vol. 3, no. 2, pp. 217–230.

47 Renée Fox, "An Ignoble Form of Cannibalism": Reflections on the Pittsburgh Protocol for Procuring Organs from Non-Heart-Beating Cadavers," *Kennedy Institute of Ethics,* vol. 3, no. 2, pp. 207–216.

48 Institute of Medicine, p. 4.

49 Ibid., p. 5.

CHAPTER 13

1 Renée Fox and Judith Swazey, *The Courage to Fail: A Social View of Organ Transplants and Dialysis,* 2d ed. rev., University of Chicago Press, IL, 1974, 1978; *Spare Parts: Organ Replacement in American Society,* Oxford University Press, New York, 1992.

2 Fox and Swazey, *Spare Parts,* p. 45.

3 Dale H. Cowan, ed., *Human Organ Transplantation: Social, Medical-Legal, Regulatory, and Reimbursement Issues,* Health Administration Press, Ann Arbor, MI. 1987, p. 60.

4 Ibid., p. 45; and data from United Organ Sharing Network, Research Department, Richmond, VA.

5 K. Isserson, "Voluntary Organ Donation: Autonomy . . . Tragedy," letter, *JAMA,* vol. 270, no. 16, October 27, 1993, p. 1930.

6 W. Kearney and A. Caplan, "Parity for the Donation of Bone Marrow: Ethical and Policy Considerations," in A. Bonnicksen and R. Blank, eds., *Emerging Issues in Biomedical Policy,* Columbia University Press, New York, 1991.

7 Fox and Swazey, *Courage,* p. 206.

8 James Childress, "Who Shall Live When Not All Can Live?" *Soundings: An Interdisciplinary Journal,* vol. 53, no. 4, Winter 1970.

9 Fox and Swazey, *Courage,* p. 235.

10 One of the first organized interdisciplinary discussions took place in 1967, at a conference funded by a company, CIBA.

11 Belding Scribner, unpublished manuscript, 1972; quoted in Fox and Swazey, *Courage,* p. 227.

12 Shana Alexander at "The Birth of Bioethics," conference at University of Washington Medical School, Seattle, September 23, 1992.

13 H. M. Schmeck, Jr., "Panel Holds Life-or-Death Vote in Allotting of Artificial Kidney," *NYT,* May 6, 1962, pp. 1, 83.

14 Shana Alexander, "They Decide Who Lives, Who Dies: Medical Miracle Puts a Burden on a Small Committee," *Life,* vol. 53, no. 102, November 9, 1962.

15 Fox and Swazey, *Courage,* p. 234.

16 Ibid., p. 209.

17 Belding Scribner, Presidential Address to American Society for Artificial Internal Organs, 1964.

18 *Who Shall Live?* NBC documentary narrated by Edwin Newman, 1965. (This was re-shown on September 23, 1992, at "The Birth of Bioethics" conference, University of Washington Medical School, Seattle.)

19 Judith Swazey at "The Birth of Bioethics" conference, University of Washington Medical School, Seattle, September 24, 1992.

20 David Sanders and Jesse Dukeminier, "Medical Advance and Legal Lag: Hemodialysis and Kidney Transplantation," *UCLA Law Review,* vol. 15, 1968, pp. 357–412.

21 Belding Scribner at "The Birth of Bioethics" conference, University of Washington Medical School, Seattle, September 23, 1992.

22 Alexander followed Scribner at the conference cited above and made this denial immediately after Scribner finished.

23 C. E. Norton, "Chronic Hemodialysis as a Medical and Social Experiment," *Annals of Internal Medicine,* vol. 66, June 1967, pp. 1267–1277.

24 Of course, there were hundreds of moral issues in medicine before this one, and some scholars had tried, though unsuccessfully, to bring them to the public. An example of a pioneering work is Joseph Fletcher, *Morals and Medicine,* Anchor, New York, 1955.

25 *Spare Parts* and *Courage,* cited above.

26 Fox and Swazey, *Courage,* p. 232.

27 Sanders and Dukeminier, op. cit.

28 George Annas, "The Prostitute, the Playboy, and the Poet: Rationing Schemes for Organ Transplantation," *American Journal of Public Health,* vol. 75, no. 2, 1985, pp. 187–189.

29 Nicholas Rescher, "The Allocation of Exotic Medical Lifesaving Therapy," *Ethics,* vol. 79, April 1969.

30 Fox and Swazey, *Courage,* chap. 9.

31 Robert Veatch, "Voluntary Risks to Health: The Ethical Issues," *JAMA,* vol. 243, January 4, 1980, pp. 50–55.

32 Herbert Fingarette, *Heavy Drinking,* University of California Press, Berkeley, 1988.

33 Alvin Moss and Mark Seigler, "Should Alcoholics Compete Equally for Liver Transplantation?" *JAMA,* vol. 265, no. 10, March 13, 1992, p. 1295.

34 C. Cohen and M. Benjamin, "Alcoholics and Liver Transplantation," *JAMA,* vol. 265, no. 10, March 13, 1992, pp. 1295–1301.

35 Tracy E. Miller, "Multiple Listing for Organ Transplantation: Autonomy Unbounded," *Kennedy Institute of Ethics Journal,* vol. 2, no. 1, March 1992, pp. 43–57.

36 Ibid., p. 49.

37 M. Michaels et al., "Ethical Considerations in Listing Fetuses as Candidates for Neonatal Heart Transplantation," *JAMA,* vol. 269, no. 3, January 20, 1993, pp. 401–402.

38 P. Ubell, R. Arnold, and A. Caplan, "Rationing Failure: The Ethical Lessons of the Retransplantation of Scarce Vital Organs," *JAMA,* November 24, 1993, vol. 270, no. 20, pp. 2469–2474.

39 Ibid., p. 2471.

40 Albert R. Jonsen, "(Bentham in a Box)," *Law, Medicine and Health Care,* vol. 14, 1986, pp. 172–174.

41 Gina Kolata, "Doctors Are Questioning the Use of Waiting Lists for Receiving Organs," *NYT,* January 20, 1993, p. B7.

42 Quoted in Michael Kroman, "Dialyzing for Dollars," *Reason,* August 1984, pp. 21–30.

43 N. G. Levinsky and R. A. Rettig, eds., *Kidney Failure and the Federal Government,* National Academy Press, Washington, D.C., 1991.

44 Michael Stoll, "A New Waiting Game for Hearts," *Philadelphia Inquirer,* February 7, 2000.

CHAPTER 14

1 Renée Fox and Judith Swazey, *The Courage to Fail: A Social View of Organ Transplants and Dialysis,* 2d ed., rev., University of Chicago Press, IL., 1974, 1978; Harmon Smith, "Heart Transplantation," *Encyclopedia of Bioethics,* vol. 2, Free Press, New York, 1978, pp. 654–660; Richard Howard and J. Najarian, "Organ Transplantation—Medical Perspective," *Encyclopedia of Bioethics,* vol. 3, Free Press, New York, 1978, pp. 1160–1165.

2 Smith, op. cit.; Howard and Najarian, op. cit.

3 Denise Breo, "Interview with 'Baby Fae's' Surgeon," *AMN,* November 16, 1984, p. 13.

4 "Baby Fae Stuns the World," *Time,* November 12, 1984, p. 70.

5 Tom Regan, "The Other Victim," *HCR,* vol. 15, no. 1, February 1985, pp. 9–10.

6 "Pro and Con: Use Animal Organs for Human Transplants?—Interview with Tom Regan," *U.S. News and World Report*, November 12, 1984, p. 58.

7 Thomasine Kushner and Raymond Belotti, "Baby Fae: A Beastly Business," *Journal of Medical Ethics*, vol. 11, 1985, pp. 178–183.

8 Breo, op. cit. p. 18.

9 "Interview with Dr. Jack Provonsha," *U.S. News and World Report*, November 12, 1984, p. 59.

10 Dan Chu and Eleanor Hoover, "Helped by a Baboon Heart, An Imperiled Infant, 'Baby Fae,' Beat the Medical Odds," *People Weekly*, November 18, 1984.

11 Charles Krauthammer, "The Using of Baby Fae," *Time*, December 3, 1984, pp. 87–88.

12 Breo, op. cit. p. 18.

13 Ibid., p. 13.

14 Ibid., p. 14.

15 Thomas Starzl, *The Puzzle People: Memoirs of a Transplant Surgeon*, University of Pittsburgh Press, Pa., 1992, p. 123.

16 "Baby Fae Stuns the World," p. 70.

17 *Animals Voice*, vol. 2, no. 3, December 1984.

18 Jacques Loman, *Journal of Heart Transplantation*, vol. 4, no. 1, November 1984, pp. 10–11.

19 George Annas, "The Anything Goes School of Human Experimentation," *HCR*, vol. 15, no. 1, February 1985, pp. 15–17.

20 *Nature*, vol. 88, no. 312, November 8, 1984, p. 5990.

21 Krauthammer, op. cit.

22 "Judicial Council Offers New Guidelines," *AMN*, vol. 27, December 14, 1984, p. 46.

23 Breo, op. cit., p. 18.

24 Chu and Hoover, op. cit., p. 74.

25 Quoted ibid.

26 Starzl, op. cit.

27 Breo, op. cit., p. 18.

28 Annas, op. cit.

29 Paul Ramsey, "The Enforcement of Morals: Nontherapeutic Research on Children," *HCR*, vol. 6, no. 4, August 1976, pp. 21–30.

30 Richard McCormick, "Proxy Consent in the Experimentation Situation," *Perspectives in Biology and Medicine*, vol. 18, no. 1, Autumn 1974, pp. 2–20.

31 Alexander Capron, "When Well-Meaning Science Goes Too Far," *HCR*, vol. 15, no. 1, February 1985, pp. 8–9.

32 Annas, op. cit.

33 "Celebrity surgery" was a term coined in *New Republic*, editorial, December 17, 1984.

34 Keith Reemtsma, *HCR*, February 1985, p. 10.

35 Alex Capron, *HCR*, February 1985, p. 8.

36 S. Twedl, "Second Recipient of Baboon Liver Dies," *Pittsburgh Post-Gazette*, February 6, 1993.

37 Philip Hilts, "Gene Transfers Offer New Hope for Interspecies Organ Transplants," *NYT*, October 19, 1993, p. B6.

38 Debra Berger, "The Infant with Anencephaly: Moral and Legal Dilemmas," *Issues in Law and Medicine*, vol. 5, no. 1989, p. 68.

39 Medical Task Force on Anencephaly, "The Infant with Anencephaly," *NEJM*, vol. 332, no. 10, March 8, 1990, p. 669.

40 Robert D. Trough and John D. Fletcher, "Can Organs Be Transplanted before Brain Death? *NEJM*, vol. 321, no. 6, 1989, p. 388.

41 A. Kantrowitz et al., "Transplantation of the Heart in an Infant and an Adult," *American Journal of Cardiology*, vol. 22, no. 782, 1968.

42 AP, "Hospital Sets Policy on Organ Donor Use," February 23, 1988.

43 Joan Heilman, "Tiny Gabriel's Gift of Life," *Redbook*, December 1988, p. 162. (I am indebted to Lynn Bondurant for bringing this article to my attention.)

44 J. Peabody et al., "Experience with Anencephalic Infants as Prospective Organ Donors," *NEJM*, vol. 321, no. 6, August 10, 1989, pp. 344–350.

45 AP, "Ethicists Debate Death and Baby's Lacking Brain," March 31, 1992; in *Birmingham News*, p. A1.

46 Brian Udell, quoted in *USA Today*, March 30, 1992, p. 3A.

47 "In Re T.A.C.P.," *Southern (Law) Reporter*, 2d Series, Supreme Court of Florida, November 12, 1992, p. 588–595.

48 D. Shewmon, "Anencephaly: Selected Medical Aspects," *HCR*, vol. 18, no. 5, 1988, pp. 1–9.

49 Laurie Abrahman, "The Use of Anencephalic Infants as Organ Sources," *AMN*, vol. 261, no. 12, March 24–31, 1989, pp. 1773–1781.

50 Debra H. Berger, *Issues in Law and Medicine*, vol. 67, 1989, pp. 84–85; quoted by Estella Moriarty in "In Re T.A.C.P.," p. 595.

51 D. Medearis and L. Holmes, "On the Use of Anencephalic Infants as Organ Donors," *NEJM*, vol. 321, no. 6, August 10, 1989, p. 392.

52 Beth Brandon, "Anencephalic Infants as Organ Donors: A Question of Life and Death," *Case Western Law Review*, vol. 40, 1989–1990, p. 781; quoted by Estella Moriarty in "In Re T.A.C.P."

53 "In Re T.A.C.P.," p. 590.

54 A. Capron, "Anencephalic Donors: Separate the Dead from the Dying," *HCR*, vol. 17,

no. 1, February 1987, pp. 5–8; John Arras, "Anencephalic Newborns as Organ Donors: A Critique," *JAMA*, vol. 259, no. 15, April 15, 1986, pp. 2284–2285.

55 Shewmon, op. cit.

56 John Antczak, "Oldest Living Survivor of Infant Heart Transplant Reaches 10-Year Mark," *LA Times*, November 21, 1995, p. 63.

57 David Wasserman, "Killing Mary to Save Jodie: Conjoined Twins and Individual Rights," *Philosophy and Public Quarterly*, vol. 21, No. 1 (Winter, 2001), pp. 9–14.

CHAPTER 15

1 Julian Jaynes, *The Origin of Consciousness and the Breakdown of the Bicameral Mind*, Houghton Mifflin, Boston, MA, 1976.

2 Plato, *The Republic*, in E. Hamilton and H. Cairns, eds., *Collected Works of Plato*, Princeton University Press, Princeton, NJ, 1961.

3 Thomas Szasz, "Involuntary Mental Hospitalization: A Crime against Humanity," in *Ideology and Insanity*, Doubleday, New York, 1970.

4 Ibid.

5 D. Rosenhan, "On Being Sane in Insane Places," *Science*, vol. 179, 1973, pp. 250–258.

6 *O'Conner v. Donaldson*, 422 U.S. 563. 95 S. Ct. 2486, June 26, 1975.

7 John Petrilia, "Mental Health Therapies," *Biolaw*, University Publications of America, Frederick, MD, 1986, pp. 177–215.

8 Quoted in Charles Krauthammer, "How to Save the Homeless Mentally Ill, *New Republic*, February 8, 1988, p. 24.

9 Saul Feldman, "Out of the Hospitals, into the Streets: The Overselling of Benevolence," *HCR*, vol. 13, no. 3, June 1983, pp. 5–7.

10 Paul Chodoff, "The Case for Involuntary Hospitalization of the Mentally Ill, " *American Journal of Psychiatry*, vol. 133, no. 5, May 1976.

11 *NYT*, November 7, 1987, p. B1.

12 *NYT*, November 6, 1987, p. B1.

13 Ibid.

14 *NYT*, November 13, 1987, p. B21.

15 *NYT*, November 14, 1987, p. B1.

16 *NYT*, November 13, 1987, p. A1.

17 Ibid.

18 "Brown versus Koch," *60 Minutes*, 1988.

19 "Court Backs Treatment of Woman Held under Koch Plan," *NYT*, December 19, 1987, p. A1. (Why the Appellate Court referred to Joyce Brown as "Ms. Boggs" was unclear.)

20 The previous hospitalizations mentioned in the dissent had been undisclosed; presumably the justices had seen Joyce Brown's medical records.

21 *60 Minutes*, interview with Ed Bradley, 1988.

22 Harold Evans, "Joyce Brown's Freedom," editorial, *U.S. News and World Report*, May 23, 1988, p. 78.

23 *NYT*, January 20, 1988, p. A16.

24 Charles Krauthammer, "Billie Boggs Revisited," *New York Daily News*, December 27, 1988, p. 21.

25 Krauthammer, "How to Save the Homeless Mentally Ill," pp. 22–25.

26 J. Livermore, C. Malmquist, and P. Meehl, "On the Justification of Civil Commitment, *University of Pennsylvania Law Review*, vol. 117, November 1968, pp. 75–96.

27 A. M. Rosenthal, "Questions to a Judge," *NYT*, November 27, 1987.

28 Virginia Abernethy, "Compassion, Control, and Decisions about Competence," *American Journal of Psychiatry*, vol. 141, no. 1, 1984, pp. 53–58.

29 *NYT*, November 13, 1987, p. A1.

30 *The Donahue Show*, Transcript #0128788.

31 *NYT*, November 14, 1987, p. 30.

32 Robert Levy and Robert Gould, "Psychiatrists as Puppets of Koch's Round-Up," *NYT*, November 27, 1987.

33 Chodoff, op. cit.

34 John Doe, personal communication to author, 1987.

35 Harold Evans, "Joyce Brown's Freedom," *U.S. News and World Report*, May 23, 1988, p. 78.

36 Ellen Goodman, "Before They Die with Their Rights On," *WP*, November 21, 1987.

37 Livermore, Malmquist, and Meehl, op. cit., p. 95.

38 Alice Baum and Donald Burnes, *A Nation in Denial: The Truth about Homelessness*, Westview, Boulder, CO, 1993.

39 C. Dugger, "Judge Orders Homeless Man Hospitalized," *NYT*, December 23, 1992, p. B1.

40 E. Rosenthal, "Who Will Turn Violent? Hospitals Have to Guess," *NYT*, April 7, 1993, p. A1.

41 C. Dugger, "Ruling Draws Debate to Mentally Ill Homeless," *NYT*, February 2, 1993, p. A13.

42 http://www.psychlaws.org/PressRoom/stmt%20-%20subwayperez.htm

43 http://www.omh.state.ny.us/omhweb/Kendra_web/KHome.htm

CHAPTER 16

1 J. Watson and F. Crick, "Molecular Structure of Nucleic Acids: A Structure for Deoxyribose Nucleic Acid," *Nature*, vol. 171, 1953, pp. 737–738.

2 "Interview with Nancy Wexler," *U.S. News and World Report*, 1985, p. 75.

3 See: www.hcbi.nim.nih.gov/omin/stats/mimstats/html

4 Dennis Breo, "Altered Fates: An Interview with Francis Collins," *JAMA*, vol. 209, no. 15, August 21, 1993, p. 2021.

5 Daniel Kevles, *In the Name of Eugenics: Genetics and the Uses of Human Heredity*, Knopf, New York, 1985, pp. 3–19.

6 Kenneth Ludmerer, "History of Eugenics," *Encyclopedia of Bioethics*, vol. 1, Free Press, New York, 1978, p. 460.

7 Kevles, op. cit., pp. 93–94.

8 Robert Lacey, *Ford: The Man and the Machine*, Little, Brown, New York, 1987.

9 Kevles, op. cit., p. 117.

10 Ibid., p. 116.

11 Ibid., p. 97.

12 Ibid., p. 110.

13 *Buck* v. *Bell*, Superintendent, *United States Supreme Court Reporter*, 1927.

14 Ibid.

15 Kevles, op. cit., p. 53.

16 Richard Herrnstein, "I.Q.," *Atlantic*, September 1971, pp. 63–64.

17 Herman J. Muller, *Out of the Night: A Biologist's View of the Future*, Vanguard, New York, 1935; quoted in Kevles, op. cit., p. 164.

18 Ronald W. Clark, *The Life and Work of J. B. S. Haldane*, Coward-McCann, New York, 1968, p. 70; quoted in Kevles, op. cit., p. 127.

19 J. B. S. Haldane, "Toward a Perfected Posterity," *World Today*, vol. 45, December 1924; quoted in Kevles, op. cit.

20 J. Huxley and A. C. Haddon, *We Europeans: A Survey of "Racial" Problems*, Cape, London, 1935, p. 184; quoted in Kevles, op. cit., p. 133.

21 Jim Heintz, Associated Press, "Sweden Forced to Face a Painful Past," August 26, 1997.

22 Tabitha Powledge, "Genetic Screening," *Encyclopedia of Bioethics*, Free Press, New York, 1978, pp. 567–572.

23 Gina Kolata, "Nightmare or the Dream: Of a New Era in Genetics," *NYT*, December 6, 1993, p. A1.

24 John Rennie, "Grading the Gene Tests," *Scientific American*, June 1994, p. 91.

25 Ibid.

26 Maya Pines, "In the Shadow of Huntington's," *Science* 84, May 1984, p. 33.

27 Quoted in *Boston Globe*, March 24, 1993; and in *Current Biography*, Wilson, New York, August 1994, p. 53.

28 M. R. Hayden, *Huntington's Chorea*, Springer-Verlag, New York, 1981.

29 Pines, op. cit., p. 33.

30 Ibid., p. 34.

31 One of Mendel's laws is that genes without alternative forms (i.e., without alleles) mix independently of each other in reproduction. However, small bits of genetic material close together on the same chromosome may be inherited together in 50 percent of cases and are then said to be linked. Genetic linkage is a major exception to Mendel's law of independent assortment.

32 *Current Biography*, Wilson, New York, August 1994, p. 53.

33 Pines, op. cit., p. 39.

34 J. F. Gusella, N. S. Wexler, P. M. Connealy, et al., "A Polymorphic DNA Marker Genetically Linked to Huntington Disease," *Nature*, vol. 306, 1983, pp. 234–238.

35 Denise Grady, "The Ticking of a Time Bomb in the Genes," *Discover*, June 1987, p. 30.

36 *60 Minutes*, May 1987.

37 "Confronting the Killer Gene," NOVA, March 28, 1989.

38 Ibid.

39 Natalie Angier, "Team Reports Genetic Cause of Huntington's," *NYT*, March 24, 1993, p. A1.

40 Ibid.

41 Alice Wexler, *Mapping Fate* (New York, Random House, 1995), p. 235.

42 Alice Wexler, *Mapping Fate*, p. 236.

43 D. Schrag et al., "Decision Analysis—Effects of Prophylactic Mastectomy and Oophorectomy on Life Expectancy among Women with BRCA1 and BRCA2 mutations," *NEJM*, 1997, vol. 36, no. 3, pp. 1465–1471.

44 Gina Kolata, "Breaking Ranks, Lab Offers Test to Assess Risk of Breast Cancer," Gina Kolata, *NYT*, April 1, 1996, p. A1.

45 S. Wiggins et al., "The Psychological Consequences of Predictive Testing for Huntington's Disease," *NEJM*, 1992, vol. 327, no. 20, pp. 1401–1405.

46 M. Hayden, AP, November 12, 1993.

47 Catherine Hayes, "Genetic Testing for HD—A Family Issue," *NEJM*, vol. 327, no. 20, November 11, 1992, pp. 1449–1451.

48 I am indebted to Michael Connealy for this case study.

49 *American Journal of Law and Medicine,* special issue on Human Genome Project, 1991.

50 Ibid.

51 *Current Biography,* p. 54.

52 C. Norton, "Absolutely Not Confidential," *Hippocrates,* March–April 1989, pp. 53–59; see also *Medical Records: Getting Yours,* Public Citizen, Washington, D.C., 1986.

53 Marc Lappe, "The Limits of Genetic Inquiry," *HCR,* vol. 17, no. 4, August 1987, pp. 5–10.

54 Rennie, op. cit., p. 96.

55 Grady, op. cit., p. 34.

56 Quoted in M. Waldoz, "Probing the Cell: The Diagnostic Power of Genetics Is Posing Hard Medical Choices," *WSJ,* April 1986, p. A1.

57 D. Craufurd and R. Harris, "Ethics of Predictive Testing for Huntington's Disease: The Need for More Information," *British Medical Journal,* vol. 293, July 26, 1986, pp. 249–251.

58 Grady, op. cit., p. 34.

59 Ibid., p. 30.

60 Grady, op. cit., p. 30.

61 G. Meissen et al., "Predictive Testing for Huntington's Disease with Use of a Linked DNA Marker," *NEJM,* vol. 318, no. 9, March 3, 1988, pp. 538ff.

62 Ibid., p. 538.

63 Catherine Hayes, op. cit (note 47).

64 Ibid, pp. 1459–1461.

65 President's Commission for the Study of Ethical Problems in Medicine and Biomedical and Behavioral Research, *Screening and Counseling for Genetic Conditions: The Ethical, Social, and Legal Implications for Genetic Screening, Counseling, and Educational Problems,* U.S. Government Printing Office, Washington, D.C., 1983.

66 Arthur Beaudet of Baylor College of Medicine, quoted in Waldoz, op. cit.

67 Case study presented by Nancy Wexler at talk at UAB, May 14, 1995.

68 Waldoz, op. cit., p. A1.

69 Rennie, op. cit., p. 91.

70 Waldoz, op. cit., p. 91.

71 Quoted in Rennie, op. cit., p. 97.

72 Ibid., p. 79.

73 Both quoted in Rennie, op. cit., p. 97.

74 My discussion of the history of biology's understanding of human genetics is indebted to Kelly Cox Smith (Duke) doctoral dissertation, *The Emperor's New Genes: The Role of the Genome in Development and Evolution* (Ann Arbor, MI: UMI Dissertation Services, 1994).

75 Cited in Kelly Smith, "The Emperor's New Genes . . ." 50. [Dalenpatius (de Plantage's pseudonym) (1699) "Extrait d'une lettre de M. Dalenpatius a l'auteur de ces nouvelles contenant une de'couverte curieuse, faite par le moyen du microscope," abstracted in Leeuwoenhoek, *Philosophical Transactions of the Royal Society,* 21.]

76 "The Science and Application of Cloning," National Bioethics Advisory Commission, *Cloning Human Beings,* 32–33.

77 Richard Jerome, "Death by Research," *People Magazine,* February 21, 2000, 123.

78 Deborah Nelson and Rick Weiss, "Hasty Decisions in the Race to a Cure? Gene Therapy Proceeded Despite Safety, Ethics Concerns," *Washington Post,* November 21, 1999, A1.

79 Complaint for Civil Action filed by John Gelsinger for estate of Jesse Gelsinger against Trustees of University of Pennsylvania et al., posted on web at: www.sskrplaw.com/links/healthcare2.html

80 Deborah Nelson and Rick Weiss, "Hasty Decisions."

81 Satya Shreenivas, "Who Killed Jesse Gelsinger: Ethical Issues in Human Gene Therapy," *Monash Bioethics Review* 19, No. 3, July 2002, pp. 37–38.

82 I am indebted to Matt Malone for research writing this case.

CHAPTER 17

1 A. Zuger and S. Miles, "Physicians, AIDS, and Occupational Risk," *JAMA* 258, no. 14, October 9, 1987, pp. 1924–1928.

2 Daniel Defoe, *Journal of the Plague Year (1723),* New American Library, New York, 1960, p. 86.

3 Barbara Tuchman, *A Distant Mirror,* Knopf, New York, 1978, p. 119.

4 Hahn, B., Shaw, G., Gao, F., *Nature* 397: pp. 436–441 (February 4, 1999). The authors also offered proof that the three major phylogenetic groups of HIV-1 (M, N, and O) arose from three independent transmissions to man of simian immunodeficiency virus, SIVcpz, which they hypothesized had existed in chimps for hundreds of thousands of years.

5 Centers for Disease Control, "Overview of HIV/AIDS" and "Human Immunodeficiency Virus Type 2," www.cdc.gov/hiv/hivinfo.

6 www.cdc.gov/hiv/hivinfo.

7 Margaret Heckler, quoted in Randy Shilts, *And the Band Played On,* St. Martin's, New York, 1987, p. 345.

8 Joseph Bove, quoted in Randy Shilts, op. cit., p. 345.

9 Joseph Bove, quoted from Randy Shilts, op. cit., p. 345.

10 Greg Dixon "Stop Homosexuals before They Infect Us All," *USA Today,* January 16, 1983.

11 "Television evangelists Jerry Falwell and Pat Robertson, two of the most prominent voices of the religious right, said 'liberal civil liberties groups, feminists, homosexuals and abortion rights supporters bear partial responsibility for Tuesday's terrorist attacks because their actions have turned God's anger against America.'" "'God Gave U.S. What We Deserve,' Falwell Says," John F. Harris, *Washington Post,* September 14, 2001, p. C3.

12 Charles Stanley, quoted in Scripps-Howard News Service, *Birmingham Post-Herald,* January 21, 1986.

13 Interviewed on Cross Fire, CNN, November 16, 1987.

14 Quoted in Randy Shilts, op. cit., p. 311.

15 Jonathan Lieberson, "The Reality of AIDS," *New York Review of Books,* January 16, 1986.

16 Larry Kramer, "Who Says AIDS Is Hard to Get?" *Newsweek,* 19 June 1992.

17 Stephanie Kane, *AIDS Alibis: Sex, Drugs, and Crime in the Americas,* Philadelphia, PA: Temple University Press, 1998, p. 4.

18 Jeffrey Fisher, quoted in L. A. McKeown, "Preventing AIDS in the Next Generation," *WebMD Medical News,* December 1, 1999.

CHAPTER 18

1 From "A Week in the Life of a Hospital," *Time,* October 12, 1998, pp. 93–99.

2 Lisa Belkin, "Victim of Both Cancer and Care System," *NYT,* March 26, 1992, p. B12.

3 Consumers Union, "Does Canada Have the Answer?" *Consumer Reports,* September 1992, p. 580.

4 Richard D. Lamm, "Health Care as Economic Cancer," *Dialysis and Transplantation,* vol. 16, 1987, pp. 432–433.

5 Albert Jonsen, *The New Medicine and the Old Ethics,* Harvard University Press, Cambridge, MA, 1992.

6 Mireya Navarro, "Hemophiliacs Demand Answers as AIDS Toll Rises," *NYT,* May 10, 1993, pp. A1, A12.

7 *60 Minutes,* September 28, 1992.

8 Lawrence K. Altman, "A Surprise in War between Heart Drugs," *NYT,* May 1, 1993, p. A13.

9 Gina Kolata, "Parents of Tiny Infants Find Care Choices Are Not Theirs," *NYT,* September 30, 1991, p. A1.

10 Robert Pear, "U.S. Backs Oregon's Health Plan for Covering All Poor People," *NYT,* March 20, 1993, p. A1.

11 Courtney S. Campbell, "Gridlock on the Oregon Trail," *Hastings Center Report,* vol. 23, no. 4, July–August 1993, p. 6.

12 Interview with James Todd on *Good Morning America,* May 10, 1993.

13 Consumers Union, op. cit., p. 580.

14 Alan Guttmacher Institute, quoted in AP, December 15, 1987.

15 Consumers Union, op. cit., p. 586.

16 Ibid.

17 Robert Pear, "Health Aides Plan to Place Medicare under New System," *NYT,* May 11, 1993, p. A1.

18 "Health Care Costs," *USA Today,* May 12, 1993, p. A2.

19 This has been repeatedly claimed by members of Physicians for a National Health Program; see, e.g., John V. Walsh, *Providence Journal* (Scripps-Howard), column, July 14, 1993.

20 Consumers Union, "Medicare for All Americans," *Consumer Reports,* September 1992, p. 592.

21 Garrett Hardin, "The Tragedy of the Commons," *Science,* vol. 162, 1968, pp. 1243–1248.

22 Richard Epstein, remarks made at UAB, Conference on the Ethics of Managed Care, April 12, 1997. See also his *Mortal Peril,* Addison-Wesley, Reading, MA, 1997, especially Chs. 7 and 8.

23 Pear, op. cit.

24 A. C. Enthoven, "Consumer Choice Health Plan," parts I and II, *NEJM,* vol. 298, March 23 and 30, 1978, pp. 650, 709–720; A. C. Enthoven and R. Kronick, "A Consumer-Choice Health Plan for the 1990s: Universal Health Insurance in a System Designed to Promote Quality and Economy," parts I and II, *NEJM,* vol. 320, January 5 and 12, 1989, pp. 29–37, 94–101.

25 John Inglehart, "National Health Reform and the American Medical Association," *NEJM,* March, 1994.

26 Charles B. Inlander and Charles K. MacKay, *Medicare Made Easy,* Addison-Wesley, Reading, MA, 1992, p. 14.

27 Some accountants, such as Peter Peterson, predict that the Medicare Hospital and Insurance fund will be broke when present "baby boomers" retire; instead of the present ratio of 2 workers supporting 1 retiree, Peterson says, the ratio will then be 1 worker supporting 2 retirees. (Peter Peterson, *Facing Up*, Simon and Shuster, New York, 1994.)

28 Paul Starr, *The Social Transformation of American Medicine*, Basic Books, New York, 1982.

29 Paul Menzel, "Equality, Autonomy, and Efficiency: What Health Care System Should We Have?" *Journal of Medicine and Philosophy*, vol. 17, no. 1, February 1992, p. 34.

30 David Blumenthal et al., "The Future of Medical Care," *NEJM*, vol. 314, no. 11, March 13, 1986, p. 723.

31 Michele Davis, "Make Health Insurance More Like Auto Insurance," *Birmingham News*, July 6, 1992.

32 Henry J. Aaron, "The Oregon Experiment," in Martin Strasberg, ed., *Rationing America's Medical Care: The Oregon Plan and Beyond*, Brookings Institute, Washington, D.C., 1991.

33 Lisa Hoffman and Andrew Schneider, "When the House Doubles as a Hospital," *Birmingham Post-Herald* and Scripps-Howard Newspapers, May 18, 1993, p. A1.

34 Consumers Union, "Wasted Health Care Dollars," *Consumer Reports*, July 1992, p. 436.

35 Consumers Union, "The Crisis in Health Insurance," *Consumer Reports*, August 1990, p. 543.

36 Robert Wood Johnson Foundation, quoted in AP, May 16, 1993.

37 Consumers Union, "Wasted Health Care Dollars."

38 Employee Benefit Research Institute, quoted in Marcy Mullins, *USA Today*, May 13, 1993, p. 2A.

39 George Strait, reporting on *ABC World News*, May 11, 1993.

40 Jack K. Shelton and Julia Mann Janosi, "Unhealthy Health Care Costs," *Journal of Medicine and Philosophy*, vol. 17, no. 1, February 1992, p. 8.

41 David Ozar, "Justice and a Universal Right to Basic Care," *Social Science and Medicine*, vol. 15F, 1981, pp. 135–141; Alan E. Buchanan, "The Right to a Decent Minimum of Health Care," in President's Commission for the Study of Ethical Problems in Medicine and Behavioral Research, *Securing Access to Health Care: The Ethical Implications of Differences in the Availability of Health Services 2*, apps., *Social and Philosophical Studies*, Superintendent of Documents, Washington, D.C., 1983, pp. 208–238.

42 Pat Milmoe McCarrick, "Scope Note 20: A Right to Health Care," biblio., *Kennedy Institute of Ethics Journal*, December 1992, pp. 388–405.

43 John Rawls, *A Theory of Justice*, Harvard University Press, Cambridge, Mass., 1971.

44 Sylvia Nasar, "However You Slice the Data, the Richest Did Get Richer," *NYT*, May 11, 1992.

45 The following critique of the HSA of 1993 is taken from Chapter 8, "Clintoncare; The Shipwreck," of Richard Epstein's *Mortal Peril: Our Inalienable Right to Health Care?*, Addison-Wesley, Reading, MA, 1997.

46 Martha Angle, "Social Security Is Much More Than a Personal Bank," *Congressional Quarterly*, May 18, 1993; reprinted in Scripps-Howard Newspapers, May 19, 1993.

Indexes

Name Index

For additional names, *see* "Further Reading" in each chapter, and "Notes."

Subject Index